Handbook of Thyroid Hormone

Handbook of Thyroid Hormone

Edited by **Benjamin Copes**

FOSTER ACADEMICS

New Jersey

Published by Foster Academics,
61 Van Reypen Street,
Jersey City, NJ 07306, USA
www.fosteracademics.com

Handbook of Thyroid Hormone
Edited by Benjamin Copes

International Standard Book Number: 978-1-63242-218-7 (Hardback)

Printed in China.

Contents

Preface

This book provides extensive information regarding the thyroid hormone. Thyroid hormone is necessary for controlling metabolism and several other body functions. Alterations in thyroid hormone physiology, its regulation and diseases pose a significant challenge for the humankind. Comprehension of thyroid hormones has continuously undergone updates and revisions. Authors from distinct specialties have contributed in this book. Its aim is to serve as a useful reference for furthering the knowledge on thyroid and help in establishing novel vistas of research.

The researches compiled throughout the book are authentic and of high quality, combining several disciplines and from very diverse regions from around the world. Drawing on the contributions of many researchers from diverse countries, the book's objective is to provide the readers with the latest achievements in the area of research. This book will surely be a source of knowledge to all interested and researching the field.

In the end, I would like to express my deep sense of gratitude to all the authors for meeting the set deadlines in completing and submitting their research chapters. I would also like to thank the publisher for the support offered to us throughout the course of the book. Finally, I extend my sincere thanks to my family for being a constant source of inspiration and encouragement.

Editor

Section 1

Thyroid Hormone Physiology

Chapter 1

Paracrine Regulation of Thyroid-Hormone Synthesis by C Cells

José María Fernández-Santos, Jesús Morillo-Bernal,
Rocío García-Marín, José Carmelo Utrilla and Inés Martín-Lacave

Additional information is available at the end of the chapter

1. Introduction

Thyroid hormone secretion by follicular cells is mainly regulated by thyroid-stimulating hormone (TSH) from the pituitary gland, which in turn is controlled by thyrotropin releasing hormone (TRH) of hypothalamic origin. However, there are a number of additional endocrine mediators, such as estrogens and corticosteroids, which are also involved in the regulation of the biosynthesis of T_3 and T_4. Besides this extrathyroidal main regulation, thyroid function and growth are under the influence of intrathyroidal peptides. Thus, there is evidence of the role played by some local factors released by nerve endings, such as vasointestinal peptide (VIP) or neuropeptide Y [1], by follicular cells themselves, such as insulin-like growth factors (IGFs) [2], and, specifically, by C cells through a paracrine mechanism, acting locally upon neighboring follicular cells [1]. This last intrathyroidal mechanism of regulation of follicular-cell activity by C cells is the main subject of the present review.

2. Histological organization of the thyroid gland

The thyroid gland consists of two lobes connected by a narrow band of thyroid tissue called the isthmus, located in the midportion of the neck, immediately in front of the larynx and trachea. Each lobe of the thyroid gland consists of numerous follicles, the **thyroid follicles,** which constitute the structural and functional unit of the gland. Each follicle consists of a simple layer of cuboidal epithelial cells, the **follicular epithelium,** enclosing a central lumen containing a **colloid** substance rich in **thyroglobulin,** an iodinated glycoprotein, yielding a periodic-Schiff (PAS)-positive reaction. The shape of the normal follicles varies from round to oval and they show a considerable size variation depending on the degree of gland activity (Figure 1).

The thyroid follicles are composed of two different endocrine cell populations: (1) the **follicular cells**, the most abundant endocrine cells in the gland and responsible for secreting T_3 and T_4, hormones that control the basal metabolism; (2) **C cells** or **parafollicular cells**, which are very scarce and mainly known for producing calcitonin (CT), a hypocalcemic and hypophosphatemic hormone (Figure 1).

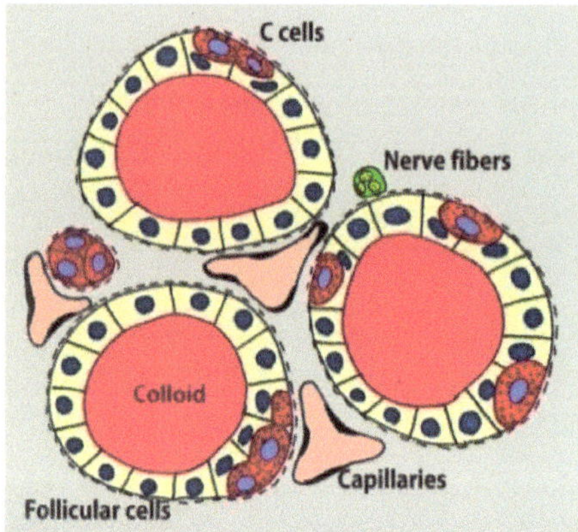

Figure 1. Schematic diagram of the histological components of the normal thyroid gland.

2.1. Embryological development of the thyroid gland and origin of C cells

The thyroid gland has a dual embryonic origin. Most of the thyroid gland derives from the medial anlage, a ventral outpocketing of the foregut endoderm at the level of the first pair of pharyngeal pouches. The medial anlage appears as a bilobulate vesicular structure at the foramen caecum of the tongue. It then descends as a component of the thyroglosal duct to reach its definitive position in the neck. After involution of the thyroglosal duct, the thyroid anlage begins to expand laterally to form two lateral lobes and a medial isthmus between them. Consequently, the medial anlage gives rise to most, if not all, of the follicular epithelium [3].

On the other hand, C cells derive from the ultimobranchial bodies (UBB), two outpocketings of the forth-fifth pharyngeal pouch complexes that lose their connection and migrate centrally to fuse with the medial thyroid anlage. Fusion typically occurs slightly above to the middle of the lateral lobes. After incorporation into the larger medial anlage, cells of the UBB disperse into the surrounding thyroid tissue and give rise to C cells. UBB may also contribute to the formation of a minimal part of thyroid follicular cells [4]. Finally, portions of the UBB persist in the postnatal thyroid glands as small cystic structures -the "**ultimobranchial follicles**"- in rodents [5], or as "**solid cell nests**" in humans [6]. Estimates of the relative contributions to thyroid weight from the lateral anlage range from less than 1 to 30% in humans [7]. In non-mammal vertebrates, the embryonic thyroid and UBB develop as separate structures, thus, C cells are confined to the ultimobranchial glands derived from the UBB, where they secrete calcitonin [8].

Since Le Douarin and Le Lievre study [9] confirmed, using chick-quail chimeras, that avian ultimobranchial C cells originate from the neural crests, it was assumed, without much supporting evidence, that mammalian thyroid C cells also originate from the neural crest via the UBB. Nevertheless, the neuroectodermical origin of C cells in mammals is currently a controversial subject. In fact, Kameda et al. [10] have recently presented evidence that murine C cells are derived from the endodermal epithelial cells of the last pharyngeal pouch -UBB- and do not originate from neural crest cells.

2.2. C cells as a member of the Diffuse Neuroendocrine System

Classically, C cells formed part of the APUD system (term created by Pearse in 1966 [11] from the initial letters of *Amine Precursor Uptake and Decarboxylation*), a collection of cells of neuroectodermal origin, characterized by having as their primary function the production of endocrine peptides which are stored in secretory granules, and the common possession of a number of cytochemical and ultrastructural properties, in whatever situation they occur. Subsequently, further evidence indicated that only very few of the original series of APUD cells were definitively derived from the neural crests.

Nevertheless, according to Pearse [12], whenever APUD cells occur they could properly be regarded as "neuroendocrine cells" for synthesizing peptides (neuropeptides) common to both the nervous and endocrine systems. Additionally, as not all of these cells accumulate amine precursors, the designation APUD was finally replaced by Pearse in 1977 [12] with a new concept, the *Diffuse Neuroendocrine System* (DNES). The DNES includes, besides C cells, gastroenteroendocrine cells, pancreatic islet cells, bronchopulmonary and urogenital endocrine cells, adenohypophyseal cells, parathyroid cells and chromaffin cells of the adrenal medulla, carotid body, and sympathetic ganglia [13].

2.3. Normal morphology and distribution of C cells

C cells represent the neuroendocrine cells that produce calcitonin in the thyroid gland. Since their discovering by Baber in 1876, these cells have been given many different terms. However, the two most common denominations employed are *C cells* and *parafollicular cells*. The name "C cell" was coined by Pearse in 1966 and it is reflective of calcitonin production; this term is preferred to that of "parafollicular cell" as these cells are not always related to follicles in parafollicular position and may, furthermore, be found outside the thyroid gland, unrelated to follicles, as occurs in the ultimobranchial glands in non-mammal vertebrates [11].

C cells are difficult to identify in formalin-fixed, paraffin-embedded sections stained with H&E. Generally, their nuclei are somewhat larger and paler than those of follicular cells. Therefore, the most reliable procedure for the identification of C cells involves the use of immunohistochemical procedures with antibodies for calcitonin (Figure 2).

C cells have variable shapes ranging from polygonal to spindled. The location of C cells relative to follicular cells also varies. They may be found between follicular cells or completely peripheral to the follicular epithelium. C cells are typically separated from the colloid by the cytoplasm of follicular cells and the basal aspects of C cells are usually in contact with follicular basal lamina. Occasionally, C cells emit cytoplasmic processes that surround adjacent follicular cells (see Figure 3). At ultrastructural level, many dense secretory granules are observed in the cytoplasm of C cells [13, 14].

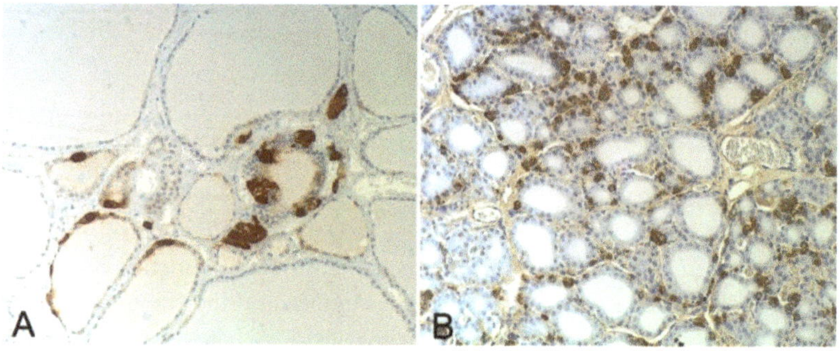

Figure 2. Visualization of C cells using an immunohistochemical method for calcitonin. (A) Human thyroid gland; (B) Rat thyroid gland. C cells are more abundant in rat in comparison with the human thyroid gland. 200x.

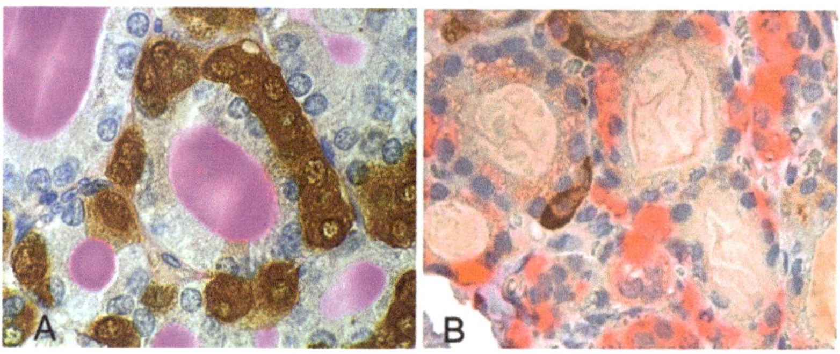

Figure 3. Immunohistochemical demonstration of C cells in the normal rat thyroid gland. (A) Immunostaining for calcitonin followed by the PAS method for carbohydrates. (B) Double immunostaining for calcitonin (red) and somatostatin (brown). In Fig.A, the "parafollicular" ubication of C cells can be observed. In Fig. B, all C cells are immunostained for calcitonin but only very few of them are also immunopositive for somatostatin. This somatostatin-positive C cell exhibits a cytoplasmatic process surrounding neighbouring follicular cells. (x500).

The distribution of C cells within the thyroid lobes has also been reported to vary among species. In most species, C cells are located primarily in the centre of thyroid lobes, including humans [15, 16], mice [17], rats [18] and rabbits [17]. The area where C cells predominate has been termed as 'C-cell region' [19], which is also the place where the most-active follicles of the gland predominate [20]. In general, portions of the thyroid containing the highest concentration of C cells correspond to the typical fusion sites of between the UBB and the medial thyroid anlage. As another reminder of their embryonic origin, C cells could also be located within the parathyroid gland and thymus in some species, such as rabbits and cats [17].

The ratio of C cells to follicular cells in the thyroid gland differs markedly among species. In humans, C cells comprise less than 1% of the total endocrine-cell population [21], while the proportion of C cells to follicular cells is at least 5% in rats [18]. Furthermore, C cell concentration may vary according to age. In humans, however, data are very contradictory: Wolfe et al. in 1974 found that the number of C cells per unit area appeared to decrease with age [15], while Gibson et al. in 1982 found an age-dependant increase in C cells [16]. In contrast, thyroid glands of adult rodents have clearly more numerous C cells than those of neonates [14, 18].

2.4. Substances synthesized by C cells

The C cells share with other neuroendocrine cells the expression of different characteristic neuroendocrine markers, such as chromogranin, synaptophysin and NSE, with chromogranin A as the most reliable marker generally used to characterize cells of DNES (see Figure 4). Most of those neuroendocrine markers are shared with different populations of nervous cells (Table 1).

Neuroendocrine markers	Species	Authors
NSE (*Neuron-Specific Enolase*)	Human	Lloyd et al. 1983 [22]
PGP 9.5 (*Protein Gene Product 9.5*)	Human	Thompson et al., 1983 [23]
Chromogranins (A, B)	Human	O'Connor et al., 1983 [24, 25]); Weiler at al., 1989 [24, 25]
7B2 protein	Human, rat, pig	Marcinkiewicz et al., 1988 [26]
Synaptophysin	Human	Weiler at al., 1989 [25]
Secretogranin-II/chromogranin C	Human	Weiler at al., 1989 [25]
Secretoneurin	Human	Schmid et al., 1995 [27]
MMP-2 and MMP-9	Human	Tomita, 1997 [28]
SV2 (*Synaptic Vesicle Protein 2*)	Human	Weiler at al., 1989 [25]
PC1 and PC2 (*Prohormone Convertases*)	Mouse	Kurabuchi et al., 2002 [29]

Table 1. Characteristic substances identified in different neuroendocrine cells, including C cells, according to a chronological order.

In addition to calcitonin, C cells may also contain many other regulatory peptides (Table 2), such as calcitonin gene-related peptide (CGRP) [30], katacalcin [31] or GRP [32]. Somatostatin has also been identified within C cells of most species. In the adult rabbits, bats and guinea pigs, most calcitonin-positive cells also contain somatostatin; however, in adult human and rat thyroid glands, only a small proportion of the calcitonin-positive cells are also somatostatin positive [33]. Similarly, peptides including neuromedin U [34] and helodermin-like peptide [35], have been demonstrated to colocalize with CT in normal C cells. Lately, a new generation of regulatory peptides, similar to those characteristically found in some hypothalamic nuclei, such as TRH [36], CART [37] or ghrelin [38], has increased the long list of substances synthesized by C cells.

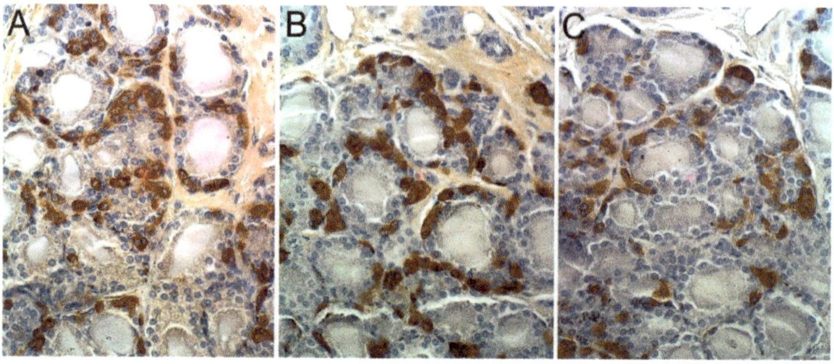

Figure 4. Immunohistochemical demonstration of chromogranin A (A), calcitonin (B) and CGRP (C) in consecutive sections of the rat thyroid gland. All C cells express the different markers, being slightly less intense CGRP-positive C cells. (x400).

Regulatory factors	Species	Authors
Calcitonin (CT)	Pig, dog	Bussolati and Pearse, 1967 [39]
Somatostatin	Mammals	Kameda et al., 1982 ([33]
Katacalcin-I/CCP-I/PDN-21	Human	Ali-Rachedi et al., 1983 [31]
CGRP (*Calcitonin Gene-Related Peptide*)	Mammals	Sabate et al., 1985 [30, 40]; Kameda, 1987 [30, 40]
Serotonin	Sheep	Barasch et al., 1987 [41]
GRP (*Gastrin-Releasing Peptide*)	Human	Sunday et al., 1988 [32]
Helodermin-like peptide	Human, rat, pig, dog, etc.	Grunditz et al., 1989 [35]
CCK/ C-terminal gastrin	Rat	Arias et al., 1989 [42]
TRH (*Thyroid Releasing Hormone*)	Rat	Gkonos et al., 1989 [36]
Neuromedin U	Rat	Domin et al., 1990 [34]
CCP-II (*CT Carboxyl terminal Peptide*)	Human	Cohen et al., 1992 [43]
PTHrP (*Parathyroid Hormone-related Protein*)	Sheep	Okada et al., 1995 [44]
Melatonin	Rat	Kvetnoy, 1999 [45]
Neuropéptide Y	Human	Scopsi et al., 1990 [46]
Ghrelin	Rat, human	Raghay et al., 2006 [38]
Pneumadin	Rat	Kosowicz et al., 2003 [47]
CART (*Cocaine- and Amphetamine-Regulated Transcript*)	Pig	Wierup et al., 2004 [37]
Motilin	Human	Xu et al., 2008 [48]
NERP (*NeuroEndocrine Regulatory Peptide*)	Human	Matsuo et al., 2010 [49]

Table 2. Regulatory factors identified in the cytoplasm of C cells, according to a chronological order.

In addition to the regulatory peptide products, C cells also contain a variety of biologically active amines including serotonin [41] and melatonin [45] (see Table 2). Additionally, C cells are also implicated in the synthesis of many other different substances, such as tetranectin [50] or CEA [51] (see Table 3).

Other substances	Species	Authors
CEA (*Carcinoembryonic Antigen*)	Human	Kodama et al., 1980 [51]
Tetranectin	Human	Christensen et al., 1987 [50]
PAM (*Peptidylglycine Alpha-amidating Monooxygenase*)	Rat	Braas et al., 1992 [52]
E-cadherin	Rat	Nishiyama et al., 1996 [10, 53]; Kameda et al., 2007 [10, 53]
NCAM (*Neural Cell Adhesion Molecule*)	Rat	Nishiyama et al., 1996 [53]
RESP18 (*Regulated Endocrine-Specific Protein 18*)	Rat	Darlington et al., 1997 [54]
c-erbB-2-like product	Human, guinea pig	Martín-Lacave and Utrilla, 2000 [55]

Table 3. Other substances synthesized by C cells, according to a chronological order.

2.5. Paracrine role played by C cells

Apart from their role in calcium homeostasis, C cells are also probably involved in the intrathyroidal regulation of follicular cells. This hypothesis is supported by different features, such as their characteristic 'parafollicular' position, their predominance in the central region of the thyroid lobe – the so-called "C-cell region" [19]– where the most-active follicles of the gland predominate [20], and their implication in the secretion of many different regulatory factors [1, 46, 56]. Some of these regulatory peptides display an inhibiting action on thyroid hormone secretion, such as calcitonin, calcitonin gene-related peptide (CGRP) and somatostatin [1], whereas others act as local stimulators of thyroid hormone synthesis, such as gastrin-releasing peptide (GRP), helodermin, and serotonin [35, 57, 58]. For any of those peptides, a requirement to exert an effective paracrine regulation of follicular cells is the presence of their specific receptors in this endocrine cell population. At this point, the existence of some of those receptors on follicular cells, such as somatostatin or serotonin receptors, has already been described [58, 59]. Furthermore, we have recently demonstrated the expression of TRH-receptor on follicular cells [60].

There is additional evidence that C cells and follicular cells somehow interact functionally. Thus, C cells, in the normal-appearing thyroid tissue adjacent to follicular tumours, have been reported to display reactive changes. These changes may include the development of a C cell hyperplasia [61] or the presence of an increased percentage of immunopositive C cells for GRP [32] or somatostatin [62], being the latter a potent inhibitor of TSH-enhanced mitotic activity and T_3 and T_4 synthesis by follicular cells. Moreover, we have found hyperplastic changes in the C-cell population of rat thyroid glands in a model of non-hypercalcemic hypothyroidism induced by propylthiouracil administration [63]. As we have recently demonstrated the presence of TSH receptors on C cells [64], we can infer that those hyperplastic changes may be due to the corresponding increased TSH-serum levels. Nevertheless, the influence of local secretion of growth factors by follicular cells themselves, or by the surrounding tissue could not be discarded.

The main secretagogue of C cells is calcium, which is concordant with the classical role of calcitonin as a plasma calcium- and bone metabolism-related hormone. Nevertheless, C-cell activity appears to be subjected to a more complex regulation, for which different regulatory peptides, either with inhibitory (somatostatin) or stimulatory effect (glucagon, pentagastrin), have being reported [65]. Furthermore, Suzuki et al. in 1998 [66] reported that C cells expressed the thyroid transcription factor 1 (TTF-1), which is typically expressed by follicular cells and known for its critical role in thyroid-specific gene expression. According to these authors, TTF-1 is calcium-modulated and coordinately regulates genes involved in calcium homeostasis in C cells. All these data constitute new evidence of interdependence between the two endocrine cell populations of the thyroid gland.

3. Description of the different regulatory factors synthesized by C cells and their potential effects on thyroid hormone synthesis

The most important objective of the current review is to present new evidence of the paracrine regulation exerted by C cells upon follicular cells, through the secretion of numerous factors synthesized by C cells in the immediate vecinity of the follicular epithelium, which could act in a synergistic or antagonist manner. To accomplish that objective, we will expose the functional role played by the most studied C-cell secreted factors on the activity of follicular cells mediated through their specific receptors.

3.1. Calcitonin and calcitonin family of peptides

In 1961, Copp et al. were the first in postulating the existence of a hypocalcemic hormone secreted by the thyro-parathyroid complex which was named calcitonin (CT) [67]. Subsequently, in 1963, Kumar et al. [68] confirmed the secretion of this hypocalcemic hormone by the thyroid gland. The evidence that parafollicular cells contained calcitonin was provided by immunofluorescent techniques in dog and pig thyroids [39], and these findings led to the name of 'C' cells for parafollicular cells. In more recent years, however, accumulating evidence supports the existence of nonthyroidal calcitonin or CT-like peptides in brain, prostate and uterus, although their biological role is unknown [69].

Calcitonin is expressed in many species including fish, amphibians, reptiles, birds and mammals, and it is normally a 32 amino acid peptide with a carboxy terminal proline amide and a disulfide bridge between cysteine residues at positions 1 and 7 [70, 71]. The CT amino acid sequence in the amino terminal loop region is highly conserved within species, but displays less homologies in the rest of the sequence [69].

The hypocalcemic action of calcitonin is due to inhibition of bone resorption and to effects on other tissues indirectly related to bone remodeling such as kidneys. Additional cellular actions of calcitonin include its effect on the growth of breast cancer cells [72].

Calcitonin is synthesized as a 136 amino acid precursor which is processed by proteolytic cleavage and by amidation of the carboxy terminal proline residue before being secreted. The gene transcript encoding CT also encodes calcitonin gene related peptide (CGRP), another peptide in the CT family of peptides. The CT/CGRP gene was one of the first described examples of tissue-specific alternative RNA processing, it has six exons, of which the first four are spliced together to generate calcitonin mRNA in C cells, which encodes calcitonin and katacalcin (CCP), while the transcripts from CT/CGRP gene in neurons are processed into CGRP mRNA containing exons 1-3, 5 and 6 [30, 73] (see figure 5). In thyroid C cells 95% of the transcripts encode calcitonin, while more than 98% of the transcripts encode CGRP in the nervous system [69].

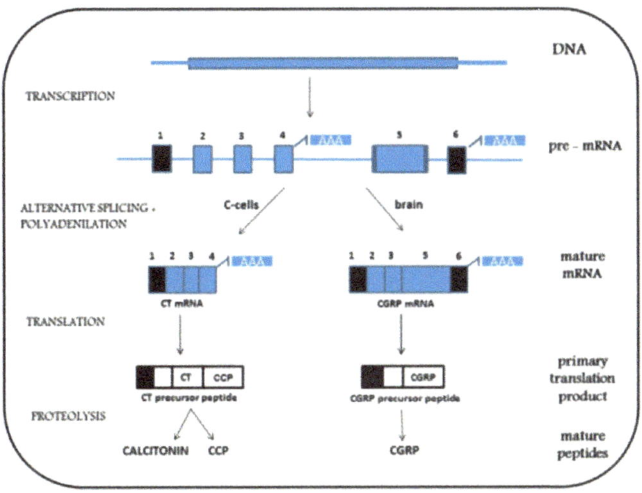

Figure 5. Schematic representation of alternative RNA processing of CT/CGRP gene. Transcription of the CT/CGRP gene produces a pre-mRNA, which has two polyadenylation sites. From the primary transcript two different mRNAs are produced, one coding for the calcitonin (CT)/katacalcin (CCP) precursor and the other coding for the CGRP precursor. The blue boxes indicate sequences complementary to exons, the lines between them are the sequences complementary to introns and the black boxes indicate the noncoding sequences of RNA.

The alternative product of the CT/CGRP gene, a neuropeptide referred to as CGRP, is a 37 amino acid peptide widely expressed in nerves in both the central and peripheral nervous systems and in several neuroendocrine tissues [74]. CT and CGRP have some homologies in the amino terminal region, but are almost entirely different in the rest of the molecule [74]. CGRP is a potent vasodilator, relaxant of mesangial cells and has functional roles in response to painful stimuli [75].

CT interacts with a member of seven-transmembrane-domain G-protein-coupled receptor superfamily cloned in 1991 [76]. High-affinity CT receptors (CTRs) were characterized on isolated osteoclasts, the physiological CT target cells. Moreover, calcitonin receptors have been identified in a variety of tissues, such as brain, testis, spermatozoa, kidney, skeletal muscle, breast cancer cell lines and human primary breast cancer cells [77]. Numerous studies have demonstrated that multiple CTR mRNA isoforms are present in a number of species. In humans, two isoforms (h-CTR1 and h-CTR2) differing by a 16 amino-acid insert in the first intracellular loop have been reported [78]. Finally, studies have revealed h-CTR2 expression in normal thyroid glands, in medullary thyroid carcinoma (MTC), and in a model of human MTC cell line (TT), suggesting an autocrine regulation of CTR in C cells [79]. Nevertheless, there is still no evidence of the CTR expression in follicular cells.

A family of receptors for CGRP and CT has been demonstrated throughout the nervous systems of both man and rat. CGRP-specific binding sites have been found in the cerebellum, spinal cord and other brain regions including vessels and pia mater. In contrast to calcitonin receptors found in bone, these receptors are not linked to adenylate cyclase, however, CGRP stimulates adenylate cyclase activity by acting at the calcitonin receptor in more than one tissue. Furthermore, specific cAMP linked CGRP receptors have been identified both in the intima and media of vessels as well as the atria and ventricles of the heart [80]. Seifert et al. [81] demonstrated the presence of a novel specific receptor for CGRP in the acinar cells of the pancreas. Finally, specific CGRP binding has also been demonstrated on cloned lung and bone cancer cells [82].

CGRP has a double location in the thyroid, one in nerve fibers around blood vessels and follicles and the other in C cells. This may suggest a functional role on the follicular cells; however, it seems not to affect basal or TSH-stimulated thyroid hormone secretion [83]. In contrast, CT, CGRP and katacalcin, which have been demonstrated to have no effect on basal and TSH-stimulated thyroid hormone secretion when separately administered alone, inhibited TSH-stimulated thyroid hormone secretion when the three peptides were applied together [83]. Despite this, further studies about the CTRs or calcitonin like receptors (CLRs) expression in follicular cells are necessary to dilucidate the role of CT/CGRP family peptides in the thyroid gland function.

3.2. Somatostatin

Somatostatin (SS) was first identified in 1973 in ovine hypothalamus as a tetradecapeptide (SS-14) with a disulfure bond between 3 and 14 cysteines. Its main function was to inhibit the release of growth hormone [84]. Subsequently, a big family of functional and structural peptides related to somatostatin was discovered. Over the years several forms of somatostatin depending on the tissue and species have been described.

SS-like immunoreactivity has been found in all vertebrates as well as in some invertebrate species and in the plant kingdom. SS-producing cells occur at high densities throughout the central and peripheral nervous systems, such as the hypothalamus, pituitary, cerebellum, limbic lobe, retina, sympathetic ganglia and the vagus and sciatic nerves. SS-producing cells have also been reported in the endocrine pancreas, the gut and in small numbers in the thyroid, adrenals, submandibular glands, kidneys, prostate, and placenta [85-87].

SS has many physiological actions, it functions as a neurotransmitter in the brain with effects on cognitive, locomotor, sensory, and autonomic functions [88]. Moreover, it has inhibitory effects on the endocrine system, gut exocrine secretion, adrenal glands, kidneys, and on proliferation of lymphocytes, cartilage and bone precursor cells [86, 87, 89, 90]. Other effects consist on the inhibition of the release of growth factors (IGF1, EGF, PDGF) and cytokines (IL6, IFN-g) [91]. All of these diverse effects of SS can be explained by the inhibitory actions of the peptide on two key cellular processes: secretion and cell proliferation.

The above-listed functions of SS are mediated by a family of receptors that recognizes these ligands with different affinities [92]. Originally, five different somatostatin receptor types (SSR1-5) were identified, cloned and found able to bind not only native SS forms (SS-14 and SS-28), but also their synthetic analogues [93]. SS receptors belong to the family of G protein-coupled receptors, typically consisting of extracellular domains forming the ligand binding site, a single polypeptide chain with seven transmembrane domains and intracellular domains mediating signal transduction. Each SS receptor subtype mediates different biological actions of SS, via the activation of different intracellular systems such as inhibition of adenylate cyclase (with decrease of intracellular cyclic AMP levels), reduction of intracellular calcium levels, and stimulation of phosphotyrosine phosphatase or MAP kinase activity [94].

Within the thyroid, SS coexists with CT in a subpopulation of C cells, with a variable extension. Thus, while the frequency for somatostatin-immunoreactive (SS-IR) CC varies in rats throughout their lives, as they are scarce in the foetus, abundant at the time of birth and scarce again in adults (see Figure 6) [33, 95-97], the majority of calcitonin immunoreactive (CT-IR) CC in guinea pigs and rabbits are also SS-IR, besides positivity is seen in the parathyroid gland [33]. On the contrary, SS-IR CC are observed very occasionally in normal pig and human thyroid glands [98].

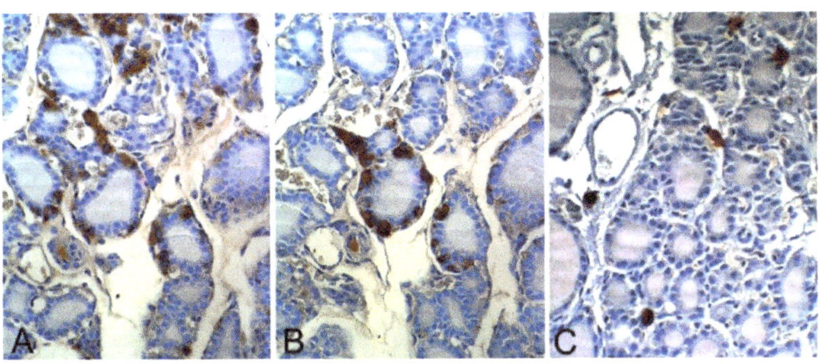

Figure 6. Immunohistochemical demonstration of calcitonin (A), somatostatin (B) and serotonin (C) in consecutive sections of the rat thyroid gland. Only a subpopulation of calcitonin-positive C cells is also immunopositive for somatostatin. Serotonin is exclusively located in mast cells, being C cells negative in the rat. (x400).

The effects of SS on the thyroid include the inhibition of the TSH-stimulated release of T_4 and T_3 [99], as well as the inhibition of TSH-stimulated radioiodine turnover accumulation in thyroid glands of euthyroid volunteers [100]. SS inhibition of basal as well as TSH-stimulated adenyl cyclase activity has been demonstrated in normal and neoplastic human thyroid tissues [101] as well as in cultures of human thyrocites [102]. Besides its effects on thyroid function, suppression of thyroid follicular cell growth has been demonstrated by the inhibition of both TSH and IGF-1 proliferative stimulation [103].

These evidences of the expression of SS in thyroid, more precisely limited to the C cells, and the actions in the follicular cells have led us to the speculation that this peptide could elicit local effects on thyroid hormone release acting locally in a paracrine fashion.

3.3. TRH

Thyrotropin-releasing hormone (TRH) is a tripeptide (pGlu-His-ProNH2) that was originally described to be synthesized in the mammalian hypothalamus, released into the hypothalamic–pituitary portal system and has the capability of inducing the release of thyroid-stimulating hormone (TSH) from the anterior pituitary [104, 105]. TRH binds to specific seven transmembrane domain, Gq/11-protein-coupled receptors of which, two subtypes have been cloned and characterized so far: TRHR1 and TRH-R2 [106, 107]. The two receptor subtypes exhibit similar affinities to TRH but different tissue distribution [108] and basal activities [109].

Besides stimulation of TSH secretion at the pituitary, main role of TRH as key factor in the hypothalamic-pituitary-thyroid axis, numerous morphological and pharmacological studies have described TRH as neurotransmitter or neuromodulator in the CNS affecting behaviour, temperature regulation, food intake, and nociception [110, 111]. Furthermore, as suggested by the wide tissue-distribution of TRH and TRH receptors, TRH is implicated in many physiological and pathological processes of prostate, pancreas, testis, adrenal gland, heart, skin and thyroid tissues [112-119].

In the case of thyroid, it has been well established that C cells express TRH at both mRNA and protein levels (see Figure 7) [36]. Furthermore, our research group have described that C-cell cultures express TRH-R1 and TRH-R2, whereas only TRH-R2 subtype is expressed by PC-Cl3 rat thyrocytes [60]. It has also been reported that TRH inhibits the TSH-induced increase of cAMP and subsequent release of thyroid hormones by the dog thyroid gland [120, 121], suggesting that TRH could participate in the regulation of thyroid hormone secretion as an antagonist to TSH [122].

In accordance to this point, Rausell et al. in 1999 [122] found that the levels of TRH and TRH-like peptides in the thyroid were strongly influenced by thyroid status. Furthermore, Rausell et al. demonstrated that TRH exerted a direct effect on thyroid hormone release in vitro [123] and administration of TRH to hyperthyroid patients with very low levels of TSH resulted in decreased levels of circulating thyroid hormones [124].

Although the effects of TRH on thyroid hormone secretion could, at least in part, be due to hypothalamic TRH, the results so far published in the literature and reviewed above would open the possibility of a paracrine regulation of follicular cell activity through C-cell released TRH as a putative additional mechanism for thyroid function.

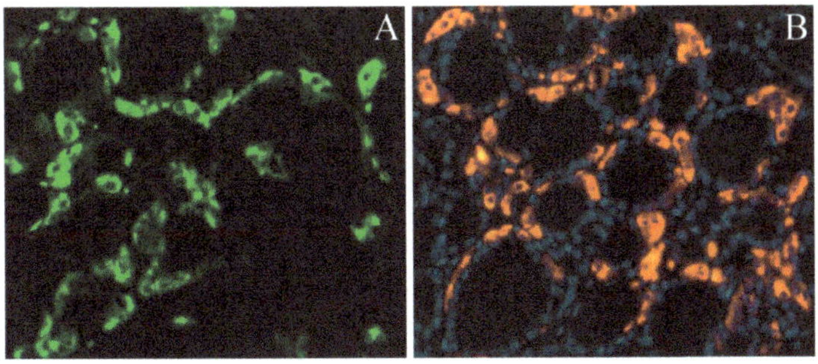

Figure 7. Immunofluorescent staining for calcitonin (A) and TRH (B) in rat thyroid tissue. All calcitonin-immunopositive C cells are also immunopositive for TRH. (x400).

3.4. Ghrelin

Ghrelin, is a 28 amino-acid acylated-peptide with powerful GH-releasing, orexigenic and adipogenic functions that, at hypothalamic level, regulates appetite, food-intake and energy metabolism in mammals [125, 126]. Since its initial description in 1999 [125], a variety of new functions for ghrelin have been characterized in the literature. Thus, apart from its GH-releasing and orexigenic effects, ghrelin has been reported to influence sleep and behaviour [127, 128], and the pituitary-gonadal axis at both peripheral [129] and central levels [130, 131].

The enteroendocrine cells of the stomach mucosa are the main source of circulating ghrelin [132]. Ghrelin synthesis and plasma levels rise and fall in relation to food intake, increasing with fasting and decreasing after eating [133, 134].Besides its gastric secretion, ghrelin is also expressed in many other tissues and organs [38, 135, 136] and despite the fact that molecular mechanisms have not yet been characterized, recent investigations have implicated ghrelin in many pathological conditions of heart, bone, liver, kidney and, specifically thyroid tissues [137].

The first observation regarding the presence of ghrelin in thyroid tissue was that by Kanamoto et al. in 2001 [138], describing the production of ghrelin in human medullary thyroid carcinoma tissue. Also, Gnanapavan et al. in 2002 [139] showed a very low expression of ghrelin at mRNA level and suggested to be carried-out by a very minor thyroid cell-population in normal human thyroid tissue. Those findings were concordant to those from Volante et al. [140] who failed to detect ghrelin-immunopositive cells in normal human adult thyroid gland. This last fact, being probably due to the very scarce presence of C cells in the human adult thyroid gland as compared to rats, where their percentage, in relation to follicular cells, ranges from 4.5 to 10.4% [18]. These observations were supported by the study by Raghay et al. in 2006 [38] in which ghrelin was described in the thyroid gland to be synthesized only by C cells.

Moreover, the ghrelin functional receptor has been demonstrated to be expressed in the neighbouring follicular cells [141], supporting, one more time the idea, increasingly found in the literature, that C cells would modulate thyroid function [38, 60, 63, 64], in this case, in a paracrine fashion, via ghrelin. Addressing this last point, up to date there are evidences that would help to elucidate some aspects of this putative new mechanism. Thus, Volante et al. showed differences in ghrelin content in foetal and pathologic thyroid as compared to normal adult glands, [140]. Moreover, Park et al. [141] demonstrated that ghrelin, via GHS-receptor and calcium signalling, enhanced the TSH-induced proliferation of FRLT5 rat follicular cells, suggesting the thyroid function as a target for ghrelin, via GHS-receptor and protein kinase C, one of the key signal-pathways for thyroid follicular-cell function and thyroid hormone synthesis [142].

In regard to the implication of ghrelin in thyroid hormone synthesis, after the demonstration of the ghrelin receptor in human thyroid tissue [143], Kluge et al. [144] described a ghrelin-mediated decrease in TSH levels and an increase of serum T_4, probably due to a ghrelin direct stimulatory action on the thyroid gland. These results has been supported by a study from our research group which have demonstrated that, effectively, ghrelin has a direct effect on the three tissue-specific genes involved in thyroid hormone synthesis: thryroperoxidase (TPO), Na^+/I^- symporter (NIS) and thyroglobulin [144, 145]. This direct effect on follicular-cell activity could be responsible for the effects observed at the hypothalamus-pituitary-thyroid axis [144, 145].

3.5. CART

Cocaine and amphetamine related transcript (CART) is an abundantly expressed and widely distributed neuropeptide that has been implicated in a number of physiologic processes. The existence of a CART peptide fragment was first reported by Spiess et al. in 1981 in extracts of ovine hypothalamus as a somatostatine-like polypeptide [146], but its functional significance was not explored further. Almost fifteen years later, Douglass et al. found the first evidence of the existence of mRNA encoding neuropeptide CART in the rat brain after psychostimulant drugs were administered [147].

CART gene is composed of 3 exons and 2 introns, with rats and mice having alternatively spliced variants resulting in the production of two peptides, the longest of which has 129 amino acids (lCART) while the shortest is composed by 116 amino acids (sCART) [148]. The C-terminal end of CART, consisting of 48 amino acid residues and three disulfide bonds, it is thought to constitute the biologically active part of the molecule, and several fragments, notably, rlCART 55-102 and rlCART 62-102, have been shown to be active *in vivo*. In humans, only the short form is expressed (116 amino acids).

Distribution of CART mRNA and peptides has been demonstrated by several techniques showing a wide distribution throughout the nervous system, including sensory processing areas, central autonomic control areas, pathways involved in drug reward and reinforcement (*nucleus accumbeus*, lateral hypothalamus and projections to dopaminergic ventral tegmental area neurons), areas controlling feeding and body weight (hypothalamic nuclei), and stress related brain regions [149-152]. Furthermore, CART expressing cells have been found in the anterior pituitary, adrenal gland, islets of Langerhans, myenteric plexus of small intestine and in the ovary [153, 154]. Wierup et al. [155] reported for the first time the existence of CART IR in C cells in the porcine thyroid, in addition to porcine pancreas, gastrointestinal tract and adrenal gland, thus suggesting that the widespread expression of CART reveals a role for CART as modulator of neurohormonal functions.

Besides as nervous system neurotransmitters , CART peptides have been implicated in the regulation of feeding and body weight, drug reward and reinforcement and other processes [156]. They also have neuroprotective properties and promote the survival and differentiation of neurons in vitro [157]. Moreover, there is some evidence of its role as a modulator of anxiety and stress response [158].

While the importance of CART peptides is clear, little is known about the cellular mechanisms by which CART exert their effects. No receptor for CART peptides has yet been identified, but some cellular effects have been observed, such as the induction of c-Fos activity in brain areas that are related to feeding and energy expenditure [159] or the induction of phosphorylation of ERK in AtT20 cells [160] which activates the MAP kinase pathways.

Due to important CART roles in the regulation of food intake and energy balance, where the thyroid plays a relevant function, several studies have been focused in the effects of CART in the regulation of Hypothalamus-Pituitary-Thyroid axis (HPT) and whether the thyroid status could regulate the expression of CART in the hypothalamus. CART-IR neurons in the paraventricular hypothalamic nucleus are reported to co-express thyrotropin releasing hormone (TRH) in rats, this neuronal populations co-containing TRH and CART project their axons to the median eminence, suggesting that CART peptides may have an important role in the regulation of thyroid-stimulating hormone (TSH) in the anterior pituitary [161]. In 2002, López et al. [162] demonstrated the existence of functional interrelations of the HPT axis with CART peptides. In other studies, the importance of the CART signaling system in the regulation of the HPT axis is suggested by the potent stimulatory effect of CART on the TRH gene expression of hypophysiotropic neurons [163]. Intracerebroventricular administration of CART increases TRH mRNA in hypophysiotropic neurons of fasting animals, and CART increases TRH content and release of hypothalamic cells in vitro [163]. These results together with those from Wierup et al. [155] described above provide the basis for future studies of the role played by C-cell secreted CART on thyroid function.

3.6. Serotonin

Serotonin or 5-hydroxytryptamine (5-HT) is a biogenic amine synthesized by serotonergic neurons of the CNS, pineal gland and enterochromaffin cells of the gastrointestinal tract of humans and other mammals. Serotonin was isolated for the first time by Rapport et al. in 1948 [164] as a vasoconstrictor plasma agent. In fact, platelet serotonin is released to blood clots contributing to the haemostasis regulation. Serotonin synthesized by enterochromaffin cells is mainly involved in intestinal motility, whereas that synthesized in CNS acts as a neurotransmitter implicated in the regulation of mood, appetite, sleep, memory and learning. Besides, serotonin has antidepressant actions and regulates behaviour, cardiovascular function, muscle contraction, endocrine activity and body temperature [165].

Serotonin is derived from the essential amino acid L-tryptophan. The biosynthetic pathway of serotonin has two enzymatic steps: the first is catalyzed by the enzyme tryptophan-hydroxylase (TPH), which converts the tryptophan in 5-hydroxytryptophan (5-HTP), while the second is catalyzed by an amino-acid decarboxylase which removes a carboxyl group from 5-hydroxytryptophan, forming 5-hydroxytryptamine or serotonin. TPH has been shown to exist in two forms: TPH1, found in several tissues, and TPH2, which is a brain-specific isoform [58].

In 1960, Giarman and Freedman confirmed that the pineal gland was the richest site of serotonin in the brain [166]. This discovery suggested the pineal gland as an important site of serotonergic activity. In the pineal gland, much of this serotonin is acetylated and then methylated to yield melatonin during the night. In fact, there are day-night variations in pineal serotonin-content which is low at night, as opposite to plasmatic melatonin, which is low during the day and increases to a peak during the night [167].

Many regulatory factors that control thyroid activity at hypothalamic level have been described. Specifically, serotonin stimulates hypothalamic TRH production, leading to an increase in TSH production from the pituitary. Adequate serotonin production is necessary to maintain thyroid hormone levels. In fact, in depressed patients with low levels of serotonin, treatment with thyroid hormones has increasing effects on *selective serotonin re-uptake inhibitors* (SSRI) [168].

In normal mouse and rat thyroid glands, serotonin is stored as a component of mast-cell granules (see Figure 6C) [169, 170]. Variations on mast-cell exocytosis and serotonin-content seem to be chronobiologically-linked to circadian variations of thyroid activity [169]. In rats, thyrotropin induces a gradual amine release from mast cells within the thyroid gland, where 5-HT stimulates thyroid blood flow and/or vascular permeability [170, 171]. In addition, a 5-HT-inactivating transporter (SERT), identical to that of serotonergic neurons has been found in follicular cells of several mammals [172]. Furthermore, follicular cells express specific 5-HT_2 receptors through which serotonin modulates TSH response and stimulates thyroid hormone synthesis [58].

Besides mast-cell synthesis, serotonin is also expressed by thyroid C cells of different mammal species, however, as far as we know only sheep, goats, cows, bats and marmosets apparently convert endogenous 5-HTP into 5-HT [173-175]. Mice and rats belong to these many species in which endogenous 5-HT has not yet been found in adult C cells, unless the thyroid gland is pretreated with 5-HTP. C cells store serotonin in the same secretory granules as calcitonin [41, 176], where 5-HT is linked to a specific protein called serotonin-binding-protein (SBP) [41, 177-179]. Furthermore, C cells have been proposed as a serotonergic neuron study model since they exhibit some properties of serotonergic neurons, including biosynthesis and storing of serotonin and regulated release and expression of both the 5-HT autoreceptor and the 5-HT transporter [180]. Finally, C cells have been demonstrated to be stimulated by both: extracellular calcium and, in the same way to that described for mast cells, by TSH; these results support the putative regulatory role of the C-cell secreted serotonin [181].

The effects observed on thyroid function could be partly due to extrathyroidal serotonin and, on the other hand, serotonin-synthesis is not a general feature of C cells of every animal model. Nevertheless, in accordance to the literature published so far, C-cell secreted serotonin could be, at least for some animal models, considered as a local factor involved in the control of the follicular-cell activity through the hypothalamic-pituitary-thyroid axis.

3.7. Melatonin

Melatonin, chemically known as *N*-acetyl-5-methoxytryptamine, is an indoleamine rhythmically secreted by the pineal gland and involved in the regulation of circadian and, sometimes, seasonal rhythms [182]. Although it was originally discovered as a skin-lightening molecule acting on frog and fish melanocytes [183], melatonin is present in all vertebrates and is also produced by bacteria, protozoa, plants, fungi and invertebrates [184, 185].

Pineal melatonin biosynthesis, that takes place during the night, it is activated by norepinephrine through its specific receptor located in the membranes of pinealocytes and consists of four enzymatic reactions. The first two are common to the synthesis of serotonin. Then, serotonin is converted to N-acetylserotonin (NAS) by the enzyme arylalkylamine N-acetyltransferase (AANAT) [186]. NAS is subsequently methylated by hydroxyindole-O-methyltransferase (HIOMT) to form melatonin [187] (see Figure 8).

Melatonin has a wide spectrum of biological activities and it is considered as a pleiotropic compound with important chronobiotic properties. This indoleamine has the capacity to resynchronize circadian rhythms [188-190] and regulate sleep-wake-cycles [191]. Besides playing an important role as a transmitter of photoperiodic information, melatonin has well-characterized antioxidant capacities, either, directly as a free-radical neutralizer or, indirectly by enhancing the activity or the expression of antioxidant enzymes [192, 193]. In certain aspects, related to these last activities, there is evidence in the literature that describes potential anti-aging and anticarcinogenic effects for melatonin [194].

Action mechanisms of melatonin are very varied. In this respect, this hormone can bind to specific G-protein coupled membrane receptors, of which there are two subtypes in mammals: melatonin-receptor 1a (MT_1) and melatonin-receptor 1b (MT_2) [195]. MT_1 and MT_2 possess high-affinity binding sites for melatonin and are widely distributed in CNS and in a wide-spectrum of peripheral tissues [196, 197]. Furthermore, and in addition to its abilities as a free-radical scavenger described above, melatonin has been described to interact with nuclear receptors [198, 199] as well as cytoplasmic proteins such as calmodulin and protein kinase C.

Since its discovery, melatonin had been considered an exclusive hormone of the pineal gland. However, numerous published studies have changed this view, describing many extrapineal tissues, such as retina [200], Harderian gland [201], gut [202], ovary [203, 204], immune system [205, 206], skin [207], and testes [208], as melatonin synthesizers.

Moreover, melatonin has also been found in the rat thyroid-gland, specifically, immunopositive C cells for melatonin have been detected [45]. Furthermore, our research group has recently demonstrated endogenous melatonin biosynthesis by rat thyroid C cells through the expression of the two key melatonin biosynthetic enzymes, AANAT and

HIOMT and, moreover, melatonin membrane receptors have also been found in the rat thyroid gland, specifically, on follicular-cell and C-cell membranes [209] (see Figure 8).

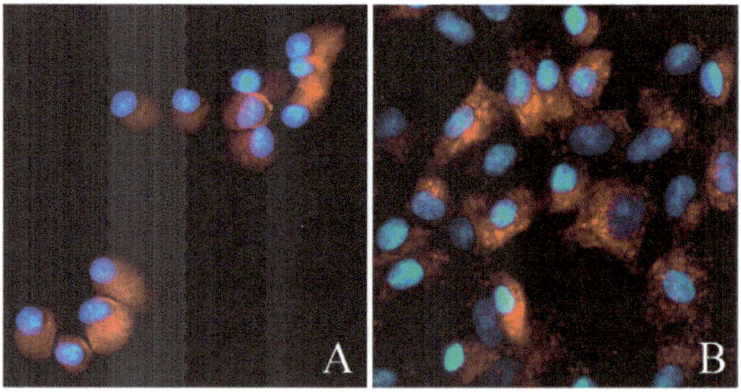

Figure 8. Immunolocalization of AANAT in a rat C-cell line (CA77) (A), and melatonin receptor (MT1) in a follicular-cell line (PC-Cl3) (B) by immunofluorescence.

Many effects of melatonin on the thyroid gland have been described so far in the literature. In rodents, high doses of melatonin inhibit basal and TSH-stimulated mitotic activity of thyroid follicular cells *in vivo* and in primary culture [210]. Besides, melatonin has a direct inhibitory effect on T_4 secretion and, also, depresses the response of the thyroid to TSH [211]. Furthermore, melatonin plays a protective role against oxidative stress in the rat thyroid gland [212-214].

As regard to the latter, reactive oxygen species (ROS) are deeply involved in cellular processes of the thyroid gland. Follicular cells are subjected to high oxidative stress since they require hydrogen peroxide (H_2O_2) for thyroid hormones biosynthesis and moreover, a large number of diseases associated with H_2O_2 accumulation in the thyroid gland have been described. For example, H_2O_2 participates in the Wolff-Chaikoff's effect and in hypothyroidism caused by iodine excess in the thyroid [213]. Melatonin has been suggested to be able to directly scavenge H_2O_2 [215]; in accordance to this last point melatonin synthesized by C cells might play a role in thyroid antioxidant defense against oxidative stress. Endogenous synthesized intrathyroidal melatonin could, thus, be a kind of local regulator that could regulate redox homeostasis and modulate thyroid function [216].

3.8. Other C-cell secreted peptides

The data presented here describe, according to our criteria, the most significant regulatory factors produced by C cells and their effects and pathways involved on follicular-cell activity according to the literature. Nevertheless, as illustrated in the present review, the list of C-cell secreted peptides and their putative paracrine functions on follicular cells is constantly being enlarged.

In addition to those described along the present chapter, and despite the fact that there is still limited evidence in the literature, there is a small group of regulatory factors such as bombesin/GRP, CCK (cholecystokinin) and helodermin, that should be observed as potential new candidates for thyroid local-modulators.

Bombesin/GRP (gastrin-releasing peptide) was first described as being expressed by neoplastic C cells from MTCs by the group of Kameya et al. In 1983 [217]. Moreover, Ahren in 1989 [57] confirmed that GRP had the capacity to stimulate both basal and TSH-stimulated thyroid hormone secretion in mice. Furthermore, differences in GRP synthesis among developing thyroid C cells, normal adult C cells, and neoplastic C cells led Sunday et al [32] to hypothesize that C-cell GRP gene-expression might play a role in both normal and neoplastic growth processes.

In the case of CCK, its expression in C cells was described by Arias et al. in rat thyroid gland [42]. Recently, its receptor CCK2R, which is shared with gastrin, has been described to be expressed at different intensities in normal and malignant C cells by Blakër et al. [218]. No additional data has been published with regard to the putative functional role of CCK signalling in thyroid, however, there are initial encouraging therapeutic results with the use of CCK/Gastrin R2-binding peptides in patients with MTC [219, 220].

The last factor from this "other" group is the amidated peptide helodermin. Originally isolated from *Heloderma suspectum* [221, 222], helodermin was described to be expressed by rat C cells by Grunditz et al. in 1999 [35]. Furthermore, these authors reported dose and time course experiments which showed a consistent stimulatory effect of helodermin on thyroid hormone synthesis.

Although some of these data seemed to have well-characterized new pathways for C-cell and thyrocytes interrelationships, surprisingly no further studies that illustrated new insights for this evidence have been reported so far. Therefore, to our knowledge, future studies are still necessary to finally clarify their involvement in thyroid function and homeostasis.

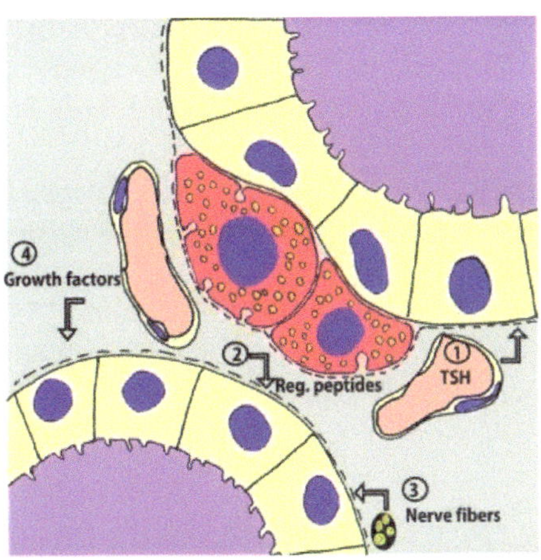

Figure 9. Schematic diagram of the different mechanisms of regulation of the synthesis of thyroid hormones by follicular cells.

4. Conclusion

In conclusion, according to the data published so far in the literature and revised through this chapter, a number of regulatory factors are produced at thyroid level by C cells and have direct effects on follicular-cell activity at both proliferative and thyroid hormone synthesis levels (Figure 9). These new paracrine regulatory mechanisms would justify, from a phylogenetic point of view, the parafollicular localization of C cells in mammals and might open new molecular approaches for the treatment of human thyroid disease.

Author details

José María Fernández-Santos, Jesús Morillo-Bernal, Rocío García-Marín,
José Carmelo Utrilla and Inés Martín-Lacave*
Department of Cytology and Histology. School of Medicine, University of Seville, Spain

Acknowledgement

This work was supported by grants from the Consejería de Innovación, Ciencia y Empresa, Junta de Andalucía, Spain (refs. CTS-439/2009 and P08-CVI-03598).The authors thank Mr. John Brown for the corrections of the English language.

5. References

[1] Ahren B (1991) Regulatory peptides in the thyroid gland -a review on their localization and function. Acta Endocrinol (Copenh). 124: 225-32.
[2] Eggo MC, Quiney VM, Campbell S (2003) Local factors regulating growth and function of human thyroid cells in vitro and in vivo. Mol Cell Endocrinol. 213: 47-58.
[3] Biddinger PW, Ray M (1993) Distribution of C cells in the normal and diseased thyroid gland. Pathol Annu. 28 Pt 1: 205-29.
[4] Conde E, Moreno AM, Martin-Lacave I, Fernandez A, Galera H (1992) Immunocytochemical study of the ultimobranchial tubule in Wistar rats. Anat Histol Embryol. 21: 94-100.
[5] Martin-Lacave I, Conde E, Moreno A, Utrilla JC, Galera H (1992) Evidence of the occurrence of calcitonin cells in the ultimobranchial follicle of the rat postnatal thyroid. Acta Anat (Basel). 144: 93-6.
[6] Harach HR (1988) Solid cell nests of the thyroid. J Pathol. 155: 191-200.
[7] Sugiyama S (1971) The embryology of the human thyroid gland including ultimobranchial body and others related. Ergeb Anat Entwicklungsgesch. 44: 3-111.
[8] Copp DH, Cockcroft DW, Kueh Y (1967) Calcitonin from ultimobranchial glands of dogfish and chickens. Science. 158: 924-5.

* Corresponding Authors

[9] Le Douarin N, Le Lièvre C (1970). [Demonstration of neural origin of calcitonin cells of ultimobranchial body of chick embryo C R Acad Sci Hebd Seances Acad Sci D. 270:2857-60.

[10] Kameda Y, Nishimaki T, Chisaka O, Iseki S, Sucov HM (2007) Expression of the epithelial marker E-cadherin by thyroid C cells and their precursors during murine development. J Histochem Cytochem. 55: 1075-88.

[11] Pearse AG (1966) Common cytochemical properties of cells producing polypeptide hormones, with particular reference to calcitonin and the thyroid C cells. Vet Rec. 79: 587-90.

[12] Pearse AG (1977) The diffuse neuroendocrine system and the APUD concept: related "endocrine" peptides in brain, intestine, pituitary, placenta, and anuran cutaneous glands. Med Biol. 55: 115-25.

[13] DeLellis RA, Dayal Y (1992) Neuroendocrine System. In: Sterberg SS, Editor. Histology for Pathologists. New York: Reven Press. p. 347-62.

[14] Conde E, Martin-Lacave I, Utrilla JC, Gonzalez-Campora R, Galera-Davidson H (1995) Postnatal variations in the number and size of C-cells in the rat thyroid gland. Cell Tissue Res. 280: 659-63.

[15] Wolfe HJ, Voelkel EF, Tashjian AH, Jr. (1974) Distribution of calcitonin-containing cells in the normal adult human thyroid gland: a correlation of morphology with peptide content. J Clin Endocrinol Metab. 38: 688-94.

[16] Gibson WG, Peng TC, Croker BP (1982) Age-associated C-cell hyperplasia in the human thyroid. Am J Pathol. 106: 388-93.

[17] Kameda Y (1971) The occurrence and distribution of the parafollicular cells in the thyroid, parathyroid IV and thymus IV in some mammals. Arch Histol Jpn. 33: 283-99.

[18] Martin-Lacave I, Conde E, Montero C, Galera-Davidson H (1992) Quantitative changes in the frequency and distribution of the C-cell population in the rat thyroid gland with age. Cell Tissue Res. 270: 73-7.

[19] McMillan PJ, Heidbuchel U, Vollrath L (1985) Number and size of rat thyroid C cells: no effect of pinealectomy. Anat Rec. 212: 167-71.

[20] Kalisnik M, Vraspir-Porenta O, Kham-Lindtner T, Logonder-Mlinsek M, Pajer Z, Stiblar-Martincic D, et al. (1988) The interdependence of the follicular, parafollicular, and mast cells in the mammalian thyroid gland: a review and a synthesis. Am J Anat. 183: 148-57.

[21] Roediger WE (1975) The oxyphil and C cells of the human thyroid gland. A cytochemical and histopathologic review. Cancer. 36: 1758-70.

[22] Lloyd RV, Sisson JC, Marangos PJ (1983) Calcitonin, carcinoembryonic antigen and neuron-specific enolase in medullary thyroid carcinoma. Cancer. 51: 2234-9.

[23] Thompson RJ, Doran JF, Jackson P, Dhillon AP, Rode J (1983) PGP 9.5--a new marker for vertebrate neurons and neuroendocrine cells. Brain Res. 278: 224-8.

[24] O'Connor DT, Burton D, Deftos LJ (1983) Chromogranin A: immunohistology reveals its universal occurrence in normal polypeptide hormone producing endocrine glands. Life Sci. 33: 1657-63.

[25] Weiler R, Cidon S, Gershon MD, Tamir H, Hogue-Angeletti R, Winkler H (1989) Adrenal chromaffin granules and secretory granules from thyroid parafollicular cells have several common antigens. FEBS Lett. 257: 457-9.
[26] Marcinkiewicz M, Benjannet S, Falgueyret JP, Seidah NG, Schurch W, Verdy M, et al. (1988) Identification and localization of 7B2 protein in human, porcine, and rat thyroid gland and in human medullary carcinoma. Endocrinology. 123: 866-73.
[27] Schmid KW, Kunk B, Kirchmair R, Totsch M, Bocker W, Fischer-Colbrie R (1995) Immunohistochemical detection of secretoneurin, a novel neuropeptide endoproteolytically processed from secretogranin II, in normal human endocrine and neuronal tissues. Histochem J. 27: 473-81.
[28] Tomita T (1997) Matrix metalloproteinases and tissue inhibitors of metalloproteinases in thyroid C-cells and medullary thyroid carcinomas. Histopathology. 31: 150-6.
[29] Kurabuchi S, Tanaka S (2002) Immunocytochemical localization of prohormone convertases PC1 and PC2 in the mouse thyroid gland and respiratory tract. J Histochem Cytochem. 50: 903-9.
[30] Sabate MI, Stolarsky LS, Polak JM, Bloom SR, Varndell IM, Ghatei MA, et al. (1985) Regulation of neuroendocrine gene expression by alternative RNA processing. Colocalization of calcitonin and calcitonin gene-related peptide in thyroid C-cells. J Biol Chem. 260: 2589-92.
[31] Ali-Rachedi A, Varndell IM, Facer P, Hillyard CJ, Craig RK, MacIntyre I, et al. (1983) Immunocytochemical localisation of katacalcin, a calcium-lowering hormone cleaved from the human calcitonin precursor. J Clin Endocrinol Metab. 57: 680-2.
[32] Sunday ME, Wolfe HJ, Roos BA, Chin WW, Spindel ER (1988) Gastrin-releasing peptide gene expression in developing, hyperplastic, and neoplastic human thyroid C-cells. Endocrinology. 122: 1551-8.
[33] Kameda Y, Oyama H, Endoh M, Horino M (1982) Somatostatin immunoreactive C cells in thyroid glands from various mammalian species. Anat Rec. 204: 161-70.
[34] Domin J, Al-Madani AM, Desperbasques M, Bishop AE, Polak JM, Bloom SR (1990) Neuromedin U-like immunoreactivity in the thyroid gland of the rat. Cell Tissue Res. 260: 131-5.
[35] Grunditz T, Persson P, Hakanson R, Absood A, Bottcher G, Rerup C, et al. (1989) Helodermin-like peptides in thyroid C cells: stimulation of thyroid hormone secretion and suppression of calcium incorporation into bone. Proc Natl Acad Sci U S A. 86: 1357-61.
[36] Gkonos PJ, Tavianini MA, Liu CC, Roos BA (1989) Thyrotropin-releasing hormone gene expression in normal thyroid parafollicular cells. Mol Endocrinol. 3: 2101-9.
[37] Wierup N, Kuhar M, Nilsson BO, Mulder H, Ekblad E, Sundler F (2004) Cocaine- and amphetamine-regulated transcript (CART) is expressed in several islet cell types during rat development. J Histochem Cytochem. 52: 169-77.
[38] Raghay K, Garcia-Caballero T, Nogueiras R, Morel G, Beiras A, Dieguez C, et al. (2006) Ghrelin localization in rat and human thyroid and parathyroid glands and tumours. Histochem Cell Biol. 125: 239-46.

[39] Bussolati G, Pearse AG (1967) Immunofluorescent localization of calcitonin in the 'C' cells of pig and dog thyroid. The Journal of endocrinology. 37: 205-9.

[40] Kameda Y (1987) Localization of immunoreactive calcitonin gene-related peptide in thyroid C cells from various mammalian species. Anat Rec. 219: 204-12.

[41] Barasch JM, Tamir H, Nunez EA, Gershon MD (1987) Serotonin-storing secretory granules from thyroid parafollicular cells. J Neurosci. 7: 4017-33.

[42] Arias J, Scopsi L, Fischer JA, Larsson LI (1989) Light- and electron-microscopical localization of calcitonin, calcitonin gene-related peptide, somatostatin and C-terminal gastrin/cholecystokinin immunoreactivities in rat thyroid. Histochemistry. 91: 265-72.

[43] Cohen R, Delehaye MC, Minvielle S, Segond N, Taboulet J, Noel M, et al. (1992) CCP II: a novel calcitonin carboxy terminal peptide is expressed in normal thyroid tissue. Biochem Biophys Res Commun. 185: 330-4.

[44] Okada H, Capen CC, Rosol TJ (1995) Immunohistochemical demonstration of parathyroid hormone-related protein in thyroid gland of sheep. Vet Pathol. 32: 315-7.

[45] Kvetnoy IM (1999) Extrapineal melatonin: location and role within diffuse neuroendocrine system. Histochem J. 31: 1-12.

[46] Scopsi L, Pilotti S, Rilke F (1990) Immunocytochemical localization and identification of members of the pancreatic polypeptide (PP)-fold family in human thyroid C cells and medullary carcinomas. Regul Pept.30: 89-104.

[47] Kosowicz J, Miskowiak B, Konwerska A, Tortorella C, Nussdorfer GG, Malendowicz LK (2003) Tissue distribution of pneumadin immunoreactivity in the rat. Peptides. 24: 215-20.

[48] Xu L, Zhong F, Guo FF, Zhao WJ, Sun XR, Wei XF (2008) [Expression of motilin and its precursor mRNA in normal parenchyma, benign and malignant tumors of human thyroid]. Zhonghua Bing Li Xue Za Zhi. 37: 243-9.

[49] Matsuo T, Yamaguchi H, Kageyama H, Sasaki K, Shioda S, Minamino N, et al. (2010) Localization of neuroendocrine regulatory peptide-1 and-2 in human tissues. Regul Pept. 163: 43-8.

[50] Christensen L, Johansen N, Jensen BA, Clemmensen I (1987) Immunohistochemical localization of a novel, human plasma protein, tetranectin, in human endocrine tissues. Histochemistry. 87: 195-9.

[51] Kodama T, Fujino M, Endo Y, Obara T, Fujimoto Y, Oda T, et al. (1980) Identification of carcinoembryonic antigen in the C-cell of the normal thyroid. Cancer. 45: 98-101.

[52] Braas KM, Harakall SA, Ouafik L, Eipper BA, May V (1992) Expression of peptidylglycine alpha-amidating monooxygenase: an in situ hybridization and immunocytochemical study. Endocrinology. 130: 2778-88.

[53] Nishiyama I, Ogiso M, Oota T, Kimura T, Seki T (1996) Developmental change in expression of highly polysialylated neural cell adhesion molecule in C-cells in rat thyroid gland. Anat Embryol (Berl). 194: 419-26.

[54] Darlington DN, Schiller MR, Mains RE, Eipper BA (1997) The expression of regulated endocrine-specific protein of 18 kDa in peptidergic cells of rat peripheral endocrine tissues and in blood. J Endocrinol. 155: 329-41.

[55] Martin-Lacave I, Utrilla JC (2000) Expression of a neu/c-erbB-2-like product in neuroendocrine cells of mammals. Histol Histopathol. 15: 1027-33.
[56] Sawicki B (1995) Evaluation of the role of mammalian thyroid parafollicular cells. Acta Histochem. 97: 389-99.
[57] Ahren B (1989) Effects of gastrin-releasing peptide on basal and stimulated thyroid hormone secretion in the mouse. Acta Endocrinol (Copenh). 120: 245-9.
[58] Tamir H, Hsiung SC, Yu PY, Liu KP, Adlersberg M, Nunez EA, et al. (1992) Serotonergic signalling between thyroid cells: protein kinase C and 5-HT2 receptors in the secretion and action of serotonin. Synapse. 12: 155-68.
[59] Forssell-Aronsson EB, Nilsson O, Bejegard SA, Kolby L, Bernhardt P, Molne J, et al. (2000) 111In-DTPA-D-Phe1-octreotide binding and somatostatin receptor subtypes in thyroid tumors. J Nucl Med. 41: 636-42.
[60] De Miguel M, Fernandez-Santos JM, Utrilla JC, Carrillo-Vico A, Borrero J, Conde E, et al. (2005) Thyrotropin-releasing hormone receptor expression in thyroid follicular cells: a new paracrine role of C-cells? Histol Histopathol. 20: 713-8.
[61] Albores-Saavedra J, Monforte H, Nadji M, Morales AR (1988) C-cell hyperplasia in thyroid tissue adjacent to follicular cell tumors. Hum Pathol. 19: 795-9.
[62] Scopsi L, Di Palma S, Ferrari C, Holst JJ, Rehfeld JF, Rilke F (1991) C-cell hyperplasia accompanying thyroid diseases other than medullary carcinoma: an immunocytochemical study by means of antibodies to calcitonin and somatostatin. Mod Pathol. 4: 297-304.
[63] Martin-Lacave I, Borrero MJ, Utrilla JC, Fernandez-Santos JM, de Miguel M, Morillo J, et al. (2009) C cells evolve at the same rhythm as follicular cells when thyroidal status changes in rats. J Anat. 214: 301-9.
[64] Morillo-Bernal J, Fernandez-Santos JM, Utrilla JC, de Miguel M, Garcia-Marin R, Martin-Lacave I (2009) Functional expression of the thyrotropin receptor in C cells: new insights into their involvement in the hypothalamic-pituitary-thyroid axis. J Anat. 215: 150-8.
[65] Raue F, Zink A, Scherubl H (1993) Regulation of calcitonin secretion in vitro. Horm Metab Res. 25: 473-6.
[66] Suzuki K, Lavaroni S, Mori A, Okajima F, Kimura S, Katoh R, et al. (1998) Thyroid transcription factor 1 is calcium modulated and coordinately regulates genes involved in calcium homeostasis in C cells. Mol Cell Biol. 18: 7410-22.
[67] Copp DH, Cameron EC (1961) Demonstration of a hypocalcemic factor (calcitonin) in commercial parathyroid extract. Science. 134: 2038.
[68] Kumar MA, Foster GV, MacIntyre I (1963) Further Evidence for Calcitonin. A Rapid-Acting Hormone Which Lowers Plasma-Calcium. Lancet. 2: 480-2.
[69] Pondel M (2000) Calcitonin and calcitonin receptors: bone and beyond. Int J Exp Pathol. 81: 405-22.
[70] Perez Cano R, Girgis SI, Galan Galan F, MacIntyre I (1982) Identification of both human and salmon calcitonin-like molecules in birds suggesting the existence of two calcitonin genes. J Endocrinol. 92: 351-5.

[71] Perez Cano R, Girgis SI, MacIntyre I (1982) Further evidence for calcitonin gene duplication: the identification of two different calcitonins in a fish, a reptile and two mammals. Acta Endocrinol (Copenh). 100: 256-61.
[72] Inzerillo AM, Zaidi M, Huang CL (2002) Calcitonin: the other thyroid hormone. Thyroid. 12: 791-8.
[73] Amara SG, Jonas V, Rosenfeld MG, Ong ES, Evans RM (1982) Alternative RNA processing in calcitonin gene expression generates mRNAs encoding different polypeptide products. Nature. 298: 240-4.
[74] Rosenfeld MG, Mermod JJ, Amara SG, Swanson LW, Sawchenko PE, Rivier J, et al. (1983) Production of a novel neuropeptide encoded by the calcitonin gene via tissue-specific RNA processing. Nature. 304: 129-35.
[75] Fischer JA, Tobler PH, Henke H, Tschopp FA (1983) Salmon and human calcitonin-like peptides coexist in the human thyroid and brain. J Clin Endocrinol Metab. 57: 1314-6.
[76] Lin HY, Harris TL, Flannery MS, Aruffo A, Kaji EH, Gorn A, et al. (1991) Expression cloning of an adenylate cyclase-coupled calcitonin receptor. Science. 254: 1022-4.
[77] Pondel MD, Jagger C, Hebden C, Partington G, Mould R (2002) Transcriptional regulation of the calcitonin receptor gene. Biochem Soc Trans. 30: 423-7.
[78] Gorn AH, Rudolph SM, Flannery MR, Morton CC, Weremowicz S, Wang TZ, et al. (1995) Expression of two human skeletal calcitonin receptor isoforms cloned from a giant cell tumor of bone. The first intracellular domain modulates ligand binding and signal transduction. J Clin Invest. 95: 2680-91.
[79] Frendo JL, Delage-Mourroux R, Cohen R, Pichaud F, Pidoux E, Guliana JM, et al. (1998) Calcitonin receptor mRNA is expressed in human medullary thyroid carcinoma. Thyroid. 8: 141-7.
[80] Breimer LH, MacIntyre I, Zaidi M (1988) Peptides from the calcitonin genes: molecular genetics, structure and function. Biochem J. 255: 377-90.
[81] Seifert H, Sawchenko P, Chesnut J, Rivier J, Vale W, Pandol SJ (1985) Receptor for calcitonin gene-related peptide: binding to exocrine pancreas mediates biological actions. Am J Physiol. 249: G147-51.
[82] Zaidi M, Chambers TJ, Bevis PJ, Beacham JL, Gaines Das RE, MacIntyre I (1988) Effects of peptides from the calcitonin genes on bone and bone cells. Q J Exp Physiol. 73: 471-85.
[83] Ahren B (1989) Effects of calcitonin, katacalcin, and calcitonin gene-related peptide on basal and TSH-stimulated thyroid hormone secretion in the mouse. Acta Physiol Scand. 135: 133-7.
[84] Brazeau P, Vale W, Burgus R, Ling N, Butcher M, Rivier J, et al. (1973) Hypothalamic polypeptide that inhibits the secretion of immunoreactive pituitary growth hormone. Science. 179: 77-9.
[85] Patel YC (1999) Somatostatin and its receptor family. Front Neuroendocrinol. 20: 157-98.
[86] Reichlin S (1983) Somatostatin. N Engl J Med. 309: 1495-501.
[87] Reichlin S (1983) Somatostatin (second of two parts). N Engl J Med. 309: 1556-63.
[88] Epelbaum J, Dournaud P, Fodor M, Viollet C (1994) The neurobiology of somatostatin. Crit Rev Neurobiol. 8: 25-44.

[89] Aguila MC, Rodriguez AM, Aguila-Mansilla HN, Lee WT (1996) Somatostatin antisense oligodeoxynucleotide-mediated stimulation of lymphocyte proliferation in culture. Endocrinology. 137: 1585-90.
[90] Karalis K, Mastorakos G, Chrousos GP, Tolis G (1994) Somatostatin analogues suppress the inflammatory reaction in vivo. J Clin Invest. 93: 2000-6.
[91] Elliott DE, Blum AM, Li J, Metwali A, Weinstock JV (1998) Preprosomatostatin messenger RNA is expressed by inflammatory cells and induced by inflammatory mediators and cytokines. J Immunol. 160: 3997-4003.
[92] Patel YC, Srikant CB (1997) Somatostatin receptors. Trends Endocrinol Metab. 8: 398-405.
[93] Raynor K, Coy DC, Reisine T (1992) Analogues of somatostatin bind selectively to brain somatostatin receptor subtypes. J Neurochem. 59: 1241-50.
[94] Reisine T, Woulfe D, Raynor K, Kong H, Heerding J, Hines J, et al. (1995) Interaction of somatostatin receptors with G proteins and cellular effector systems. Ciba Foundation symposium. 190: 160-7; discussion 7-70.
[95] Van Noorden S, Polak JM, Pearse AG (1977) Single cellular origin of somatostatin and calcitonin in the rat thyroid gland. Histochemistry. 53: 243-7.
[96] Alumets J, Hakanson R, Lundqvist G, Sundler F, Thorell J (1980) Ontogeny and ultrastructure of somatostatin and calcitonin cells in the thyroid gland of the rat. Cell Tissue Res. 206: 193-201.
[97] Zabel M, Surdyk J, Biela-Jacek I (1987) Immunocytochemical studies on thyroid parafollicular cells in postnatal development of the rat. Acta Anat (Basel). 130: 251-6.
[98] Fierabracci A, Castagna M, Baschieri L (1993) Calcitonin and somatostatin containing C cells in rat and human thyroid. Immunohistochemical study by a double-staining method. Pathologica. 85: 467-74.
[99] Ahren B, Hedner P, Melander A, Westgren U (1977) Inhibition by somatostatin of mouse thyroid activity following stimulation by thyrotrophin, isoprenaline and dibutyryl cyclic-AMP Acta Endocrinol (Copenh). 86: 323-9.
[100] Loos U, Raptis S, Birk J, Escobar-Jimenez F, Meyer G, Rothenbuchner G, et al. (1978) Inhibition of TSH-stimulated radioiodine turnover and release of T4 and T3 in vivo by somatostatin. Metabolism. 27: 1269-73.
[101] Siperstein AE, Levin KE, Gum ET, Clark OH (1992) Effect of somatostatin on adenylate cyclase activity in normal and neoplastic thyroid tissue. World J Surg. 16: 555-60.
[102] Brandi ML, Toccafondi R (1985) Neuropeptidergic control of cyclic AMP accumulation in human thyroid cell. Peptides. 6: 641-4.
[103] degli Uberti EC, Hanau S, Rossi R, Piva R, Margutti A, Trasforini G, et al. (1991) Somatostatin reduces 3H-thymidine incorporation and c-myc, but not thyroglobulin ribonucleic acid levels in human thyroid follicular cells in vitro. J Clin Endocrinol Metab. 72: 1364-71.
[104] Lechan RM, Wu P, Jackson IM (1986) Immunolocalization of the thyrotropin-releasing hormone prohormone in the rat central nervous system. Endocrinology. 119: 1210-6.
[105] Lechan RM, Wu P, Jackson IM, Wolf H, Cooperman S, Mandel G, et al. (1986) Thyrotropin-releasing hormone precursor: characterization in rat brain. Science. 231: 159-61.

[106] de la Pena P, Delgado LM, del Camino D, Barros F (1992) Two isoforms of the thyrotropin-releasing hormone receptor generated by alternative splicing have indistinguishable functional properties. J Biol Chem. 267: 25703-8.
[107] O'Dowd BF, Lee DK, Huang W, Nguyen T, Cheng R, Liu Y, et al. (2000) TRH-R2 exhibits similar binding and acute signaling but distinct regulation and anatomic distribution compared with TRH-R1. Mol Endocrinol. 14: 183-93.
[108] Cao J, O'Donnell D, Vu H, Payza K, Pou C, Godbout C, et al. (1998) Cloning and characterization of a cDNA encoding a novel subtype of rat thyrotropin-releasing hormone receptor. J Biol Chem. 273: 32281-7.
[109] Deflorian F, Engel S, Colson AO, Raaka BM, Gershengorn MC, Costanzi S (2008) Understanding the structural and functional differences between mouse thyrotropin-releasing hormone receptors 1 and 2. Proteins. 71: 783-94.
[110] Griffiths EC (1985) Thyrotrophin releasing hormone: endocrine and central effects. Psychoneuroendocrinology. 10: 225-35.
[111] Sun Y, Zupan B, Raaka BM, Toth M, Gershengorn MC (2009) TRH-receptor-type-2-deficient mice are euthyroid and exhibit increased depression and reduced anxiety phenotypes. Neuropsychopharmacology. 34: 1601-8.
[112] Satoh T, Feng P, Kim UJ, Wilber JF (1994) Identification of thyrotropin-releasing hormone receptor in the rat testis. Neuropeptides. 27: 195-202.
[113] Mellado M, Fernandez-Agullo T, Rodriguez-Frade JM, San Frutos MG, de la Pena P, Martinez AC, et al. (1999) Expression analysis of the thyrotropin-releasing hormone receptor (TRHR) in the immune system using agonist anti-TRHR monoclonal antibodies. FEBS Lett. 451: 308-14.
[114] Morley JE (1979) Extrahypothalamic thyrotropin releasing hormone (TRH) -- its distribution and its functions. Life Sci. 25: 1539-50.
[115] Pekary AE, Reeve JR, Jr., Smith VP (1986) Evidence for thyrotropin-releasing hormone (TRH) biosynthesis in rat prostate. Life Sci. 39: 2565-70.
[116] Iversen E, Weeke J, Laurberg P (1984) TRH immunoreactivity in the thyroid gland. Scand J Clin Lab Invest. 44: 703-9.
[117] Montagne JJ, Ladram A, Grouselle D, Nicolas P, Bulant M (1997) Thyrotropin-releasing hormone immunoreactivity in rat adrenal tissue is localized in mast cells. J Histochem Cytochem. 45: 1623-7.
[118] Bacova Z, Baqi L, Benacka O, Payer J, Krizanova O, Zeman M, et al. (2006) Thyrotropin-releasing hormone in rat heart: effect of swelling, angiotensin II and renin gene. Acta Physiol (Oxf). 187: 313-9.
[119] Yamada M, Shibusawa N, Ishii S, Horiguchi K, Umezawa R, Hashimoto K, et al. (2006) Prolactin secretion in mice with thyrotropin-releasing hormone deficiency. Endocrinology. 147: 2591-6.
[120] Delbeke D, Van Sande J, Cochaux P, Decoster C, Dumont JE (1983) Effect of thyrotropin-releasing hormone on dog thyroid in vitro. Biochim Biophys Acta. 761: 262-8.
[121] Iversen E, Laurberg P (1985) Thyrotrophin-releasing hormone (TRH) and hormone secretion from the follicular and C-cells of perfused dog thyroid lobes. Acta Endocrinol (Copenh). 109: 499-504.

[122] Rausell V, Fraser HM, Tobaruela M, del Rio-Garcia J, Smyth DG (1999) Identification of the TRH-like peptides pGlu-Glu-Pro amide and pGlu-Phe-Pro amide in rat thyroid: regulation by thyroid status. Reg Pept. 81: 55-60.
[123] Raspe E, Laurent E, Andry G, Dumont JE (1991) ATP, bradykinin, TRH and TSH activate the Ca(2+)-phosphatidylinositol cascade of human thyrocytes in primary culture. Mol Cell Endocrinol. 81: 175-83.
[124] Sato A, Yamada T, Aizawa T, Ichikawa K, Komiya I, Takasu N, et al. (1995) Effect of thyrotropin-releasing hormone on serum thyroid hormones: a study in the patients with untreated and treated Graves' disease and subacute thyroiditis. J Clin Endocrinol Metab. 80: 2173-7.
[125] Kojima M, Hosoda H, Date Y, Nakazato M, Matsuo H, Kangawa K (1999) Ghrelin is a growth-hormone-releasing acylated peptide from stomach. Nature. 402: 656-60.
[126] Arvat E, Maccario M, Di Vito L, Broglio F, Benso A, Gottero C, et al. (2001) Endocrine activities of ghrelin, a natural growth hormone secretagogue (GHS), in humans: comparison and interactions with hexarelin, a nonnatural peptidyl GHS, and GH-releasing hormone. J Clin Endocrinol Metab. 86: 1169-74.
[127] Korbonits M, Goldstone AP, Gueorguiev M, Grossman AB (2004) Ghrelin--a hormone with multiple functions. Front Neuroendocrinol. 25: 27-68.
[128] Van der Lely AJ, Tschop M, Heiman ML, Ghigo E (2004) Biological, physiological, pathophysiological, and pharmacological aspects of ghrelin. Endocr Rev. 25: 426-57.
[129] Caminos JE, Tena-Sempere M, Gaytan F, Sanchez-Criado JE, Barreiro ML, Nogueiras R, et al. (2003) Expression of ghrelin in the cyclic and pregnant rat ovary. Endocrinology. 144: 1594-602.
[130] Fernandez-Fernandez R, Tena-Sempere M, Aguilar E, Pinilla L (2004) Ghrelin effects on gonadotropin secretion in male and female rats. Neurosci Lett. 362: 103-7.
[131] Kluge M, Schussler P, Uhr M, Yassouridis A, Steiger A (2007) Ghrelin suppresses secretion of luteinizing hormone in humans. J Clin Endocrinol Metab. 92: 3202-5.
[132] Date Y, Kojima M, Hosoda H, Sawaguchi A, Mondal MS, Suganuma T, et al. (2000) Ghrelin, a novel growth hormone-releasing acylated peptide, is synthesized in a distinct endocrine cell type in the gastrointestinal tracts of rats and humans. Endocrinology. 141: 4255-61.
[133] Cummings DE, Purnell JQ, Frayo RS, Schmidova K, Wisse BE, Weigle DS (2001) A preprandial rise in plasma ghrelin levels suggests a role in meal initiation in humans. Diabetes. 50: 1714-9.
[134] Bagnasco M, Kalra PS, Kalra SP (2002) Ghrelin and leptin pulse discharge in fed and fasted rats. Endocrinology. 143: 726-9.
[135] Raghay K, Garcia-Caballero T, Bravo S, Alvarez CV, Gonzalez R, Dieguez C, et al. (2008) Ghrelin localization in the medulla of rat and human adrenal gland and in pheochromocytomas. Histol Histopathol. 23: 57-65.
[136] Morillo-Bernal J, Fernandez-Santos JM, De Miguel M, Garcia-Marin R, Gordillo-Martinez F, Diaz-Parrado E, et al. (2011) Ghrelin potentiates TSH-induced expression of the thyroid tissue-specific genes thyroglobulin, thyroperoxidase and sodium-iodine symporter, in rat PC-Cl3 Cells. Peptides. 32:2333-9

[137] Katergari SA, Milousis A, Pagonopoulou O, Asimakopoulos B, Nikolettos NK (2008) Ghrelin in pathological conditions. Endocr J. 55: 439-53.
[138] Kanamoto N, Akamizu T, Hosoda H, Hataya Y, Ariyasu H, Takaya K, et al. (2001) Substantial production of ghrelin by a human medullary thyroid carcinoma cell line. J Clin Endocrinol Metab. 86: 4984-90.
[139] Gnanapavan S, Kola B, Bustin SA, Morris DG, McGee P, Fairclough P, et al. (2002) The tissue distribution of the mRNA of ghrelin and subtypes of its receptor, GHS-R, in humans. J Clin Endocrinol Metab. 87: 2988.
[140] Volante M, Allia E, Fulcheri E, Cassoni P, Ghigo E, Muccioli G, et al. (2003) Ghrelin in fetal thyroid and follicular tumors and cell lines: expression and effects on tumor growth. Am J Pathol. 162: 645-54.
[141] Park YJ, Lee YJ, Kim SH, Joung DS, Kim BJ, So I, et al. (2008) Ghrelin enhances the proliferating effect of thyroid stimulating hormone in FRTL-5 thyroid cells. Mol Cell Endocrinol. 285: 19-25.
[142] Riesco-Eizaguirre G, Santisteban P (2006) A perspective view of sodium iodide symporter research and its clinical implications. Eur J Endocrinol. 155: 495-512.
[143] Ueberberg B, Unger N, Saeger W, Mann K, Petersenn S (2009) Expression of ghrelin and its receptor in human tissues. Horm Metab Res. 41: 814-21.
[144] Kluge M, Riedl S, Uhr M, Schmidt D, Zhang X, Yassouridis A, et al. (2010) Ghrelin affects the hypothalamus-pituitary-thyroid axis in humans by increasing free thyroxine and decreasing TSH in plasma. Eur J Endocrinol. 162: 1059-65.
[145] Sosic-Jurjevic B, Stevanovic D, Milosevic V, Sekulic M, Starcevic V (2009) Central ghrelin affects pituitary-thyroid axis: histomorphological and hormonal study in rats. Neuroendocrinology. 89: 327-36.
[146] Spiess J, Villarreal J, Vale W (1981) Isolation and sequence analysis of a somatostatin-like polypeptide from ovine hypothalamus. Biochemistry. 20: 1982-8.
[147] Douglass J, McKinzie AA, Couceyro P (1995) PCR differential display identifies a rat brain mRNA that is transcriptionally regulated by cocaine and amphetamine. J Neurosci. 15: 2471-81.
[148] Kuhar MJ, Adams LD, Hunter RG, Vechia SD, Smith Y (2000) CART peptides. Reg Pept. 89: 1-6.
[149] Broberger C (1999) Hypothalamic cocaine- and amphetamine-regulated transcript (CART) neurons: histochemical relationship to thyrotropin-releasing hormone, melanin-concentrating hormone, orexin/hypocretin and neuropeptide Y. Brain Res. 848: 101-13.
[150] Couceyro P, Paquet M, Koylu E, Kuhar MJ, Smith Y (1998) Cocaine- and amphetamine-regulated transcript (CART) peptide immunoreactivity in myenteric plexus neurons of the rat ileum and co-localization with choline acetyltransferase. Synapse. 30: 1-8.
[151] Koylu EO, Couceyro PR, Lambert PD, Kuhar MJ (1998) Cocaine- and amphetamine-regulated transcript peptide immunohistochemical localization in the rat brain. J Comp Neurol. 391: 115-32.
[152] Smith Y, Kieval J, Couceyro PR, Kuhar MJ (1999) CART peptide-immunoreactive neurones in the nucleus accumbens in monkeys: ultrastructural analysis, colocalization

studies, and synaptic interactions with dopaminergic afferents. J Comp Neurol. 407: 491-511.
[153] Koylu EO, Couceyro PR, Lambert PD, Ling NC, DeSouza EB, Kuhar MJ (1997) Immunohistochemical localization of novel CART peptides in rat hypothalamus, pituitary and adrenal gland. J Neuroendocrinol. 9: 823-33.
[154] Kobayashi Y, Jimenez-Krassel F, Ireland JJ, Smith GW (2006) Evidence of a local negative role for cocaine and amphetamine regulated transcript (CART), inhibins and low molecular weight insulin like growth factor binding proteins in regulation of granulosa cell estradiol production during follicular waves in cattle. Reprod Biol Endocrinol. 4: 22.
[155] Wierup N, Gunnarsdottir A, Ekblad E, Sundler F (2007) Characterisation of CART-containing neurons and cells in the porcine pancreas, gastro-intestinal tract, adrenal and thyroid glands. BMC Neurosci. 8: 51.
[156] Hunter RG, Philpot K, Vicentic A, Dominguez G, Hubert GW, Kuhar MJ (2004) CART in feeding and obesity. Trends in endocrinology and metabolism: TEM. 15: 454-9.
[157] Leshan RL, Opland DM, Louis GW, Leinninger GM, Patterson CM, Rhodes CJ, et al. (2010) Ventral tegmental area leptin receptor neurons specifically project to and regulate cocaine- and amphetamine-regulated transcript neurons of the extended central amygdale. J Neurosci. 30: 5713-23.
[158] Koylu EO, Balkan B, Kuhar MJ, Pogun S (2006) Cocaine and amphetamine regulated transcript (CART) and the stress response. Peptides. 27: 1956-69.
[159] Vrang N, Tang-Christensen M, Larsen PJ, Kristensen P (1999) Recombinant CART peptide induces c-Fos expression in central areas involved in control of feeding behaviour. Brain research. 818: 499-509.
[160] Lakatos A, Prinster S, Vicentic A, Hall RA, Kuhar MJ (2005) Cocaine- and amphetamine-regulated transcript (CART) peptide activates the extracellular signal-regulated kinase (ERK) pathway in AtT20 cells via putative G-protein coupled receptors. Neuroscience letters. 384: 198-202.
[161] Fekete C, Lechan RM (2006) Neuroendocrine implications for the association between cocaine- and amphetamine regulated transcript (CART) and hypophysiotropic thyrotropin-releasing hormone (TRH). Peptides. 27: 2012-8.
[162] Lopez M, Seoane L, Tovar S, Senaris RM, Dieguez C (2002) Thyroid status regulates CART but not AgRP mRNA levels in the rat hypothalamus. Neuroreport. 13: 1775-9.
[163] Fekete C, Mihaly E, Luo LG, Kelly J, Clausen JT, Mao Q, et al. (2000) Association of cocaine- and amphetamine-regulated transcript-immunoreactive elements with thyrotropin-releasing hormone-synthesizing neurons in the hypothalamic paraventricular nucleus and its role in the regulation of the hypothalamic-pituitary-thyroid axis during fasting J Neurosci. 20: 9224-34.
[164] Rapport MM, Green AA, Page IH (1948) Serum vasoconstrictor, serotonin; isolation and characterization. J Biol Chem. 176: 1243-51.
[165] Berger M, Gray JA, Roth BL (2009) The expanded biology of serotonin. Annu Rev Med. 60: 355-66.
[166] Giarman NJ, Freedman DX (1960) Serotonin content of the pineal glands of man and monkey. Nature. 186: 480-1.

[167] Ganguly S, Coon SL, Klein DC (2002) Control of melatonin synthesis in the mammalian pineal gland: the critical role of serotonin acetylation. Cell Tissue Res. 309: 127-37.
[168] Cooper R, Lerer B (2010) [The use of thyroid hormones in the treatment of depression]. Harefuah. 149: 529-34, 50, 49.
[169] Catini C, Legnaioli M (1992) Role of mast cells in health: daily rhythmic variations in their number, exocytotic activity, histamine and serotonin content in the rat thyroid gland. Eur J Histochem. 36: 501-16.
[170] Melander A, Sundler F (1972) Significance of thyroid mast cells in thyroid hormone secretion. Endocrinology. 90: 802-7.
[171] Melander A, Westgren U, Sundler F, Ericson LE (1975) Influence of histamine- and 5-hydroxytryptamine-containing thyroid mast cells on thyroid blood flow and permeability in the rat. Endocrinology. 97: 1130-7.
[172] Tamir H, Hsiung SC, Liu KP, Blakely RD, Russo AF, Clark MS, et al. (1996) Expression and development of a functional plasmalemmal 5-hydroxytryptamine transporter by thyroid follicular cells. Endocrinology. 137: 4475-86.
[173] Falck B, Owman C (1968) 5-hydroxytryptamine and related amines in endocrine cell systems. Adv Pharmacol. 6: 211-31.
[174] Machado CR (1976) Monoamines in the C cells of the thyroid gland of callithricid primates. Histochemistry. 48: 187-90.
[175] Nunez EA, Gershon MD (1972) Synthesis and storage of serotonin by parafollicular (C) cells of the thyroid gland of active, prehibernating and hibernating bats. Endocrinology. 90: 1008-24.
[176] Zabel M (1984) Ultrastructural localization of calcitonin, somatostatin and serotonin in parafollicular cells of rat thyroid. Histochem J. 16: 1265-72.
[177] Bernd P, Gershon MD, Nunez EA, Tamir H (1981) Separation of dissociated thyroid follicular and parafollicular cells: association of serotonin binding protein with parafollicular cells. J Cell Biol. 88: 499-508.
[178] Tamir H, Liu KP, Hsiung SC, Adlersberg M, Nunez EA, Gershon MD (1990) Multiple signal transduction mechanisms leading to the secretion of 5-hydroxytryptamine by MTC cells, a neurectodermally derived cell line. J Neurosci. 10: 3743-53.
[179] Tamir H, Liu KP, Payette RF, Hsiung SC, Adlersberg M, Nunez EA, et al. (1989) Human medullary thyroid carcinoma: characterization of the serotonergic and neuronal properties of a neurectodermally derived cell line. J Neurosci. 9: 1199-212.
[180] Solcia E, Sampietro R (1968) New methods for staining secretory granules and 5-hydroxytryptamine in the thyroid C-cells. In: Taylor S, Editor. Calcitonin: Proceedings of the symposium on thyrocalcitonin and the C cells. New York: Springer-Verlag. p. 127-32.
[181] Liu KP, Russo AF, Hsiung SC, Adlersberg M, Franke TF, Gershon MD, et al. (2003) Calcium receptor-induced serotonin secretion by parafollicular cells: role of phosphatidylinositol 3-kinase-dependent signal transduction pathways. J Neurosci. 23: 2049-57.
[182] Reiter RJ (1993) The melatonin rhythm: both a clock and a calendar. Experientia. 49: 654-64.

[183] Lerner AB, Case JD, Takahashi Y (1958) Isolation of melatonin, pineal factor that lightens melanocytes. J Am Chem Soc. *80*: 2057-8.
[184] Hardeland R, Fuhrberg B, Uria H, Behrmann G, Meyer TJ, Burkhardt S, et al. (1996) Chronobiology of indoleamines in the dinoflagellate Gonyaulax polyedra: metabolism and effects related to circadian rhythmicity and photoperiodism. Braz J Med Biol Res. 29: 119-23.
[185] Hardeland R, Poeggeler B (2003) Non-vertebrate melatonin. J Pineal Res. 34: 233-41.
[186] Voisin P, Namboodiri MA, Klein DC (1984) Arylamine N-acetyltransferase and arylalkylamine N-acetyltransferase in the mammalian pineal gland. J Biol Chem. 259: 10913-8.
[187] Axelrod J, Weissbach H (1960) Enzymatic O-methylation of N-acetylserotonin to melatonin. Science. 131: 1312.
[188] Redman J, Armstrong S, Ng KT (1983) Free-running activity rhythms in the rat: entrainment by melatonin. Science. 219: 1089-91.
[189] Lewy AJ, Emens JS, Sack RL, Hasler BP, Bernert RA (2002) Low, but not high, doses of melatonin entrained a free-running blind person with a long circadian period. Chronobiol Int. 19: 649-58.
[190] Hack LM, Lockley SW, Arendt J, Skene DJ (2003) The effects of low-dose 0.5-mg melatonin on the free-running circadian rhythms of blind subjects. J Biol Rhythms. 18: 420-9.
[191] Sharkey KM, Fogg LF, Eastman CL (2002) Effects of melatonin administration on daytime sleep after simulated night shift work. J Sleep Res 10: 181-92.
[192] Reiter RJ, Tan DX, Maldonado MD (2005) Melatonin as an antioxidant: physiology versus pharmacology. J Pineal Res. 39: 215-6.
[193] Mogulkoc R, Baltaci AK, Oztekin E, Aydin L, Sivrikaya A (2006) Melatonin prevents oxidant damage in various tissues of rats with hyperthyroidism. Life Sci. 79: 311-5.
[194] Lewinski A, Karbownik M (2002) Review. Melatonin and the thyroid gland. Neuro Endocrinol Lett. 23 Suppl 1: 73-8.
[195] Witt-Enderby PA, Bennett J, Jarzynka MJ, Firestine S, Melan MA (2003) Melatonin receptors and their regulation: biochemical and structural mechanisms. Life Sci. 72: 2183-98.
[196] Pang SF, Dubocovich ML, Brown GM (1993) Melatonin receptors in peripheral tissues: a new area of melatonin research. Biol Signals. 2: 177-80.
[197] Ishii H, Tanaka N, Kobayashi M, Kato M, Sakuma Y (2009) Gene structures, biochemical characterization and distribution of rat melatonin receptors. J Physiol Sci. 59: 37-47.
[198] Rafii-El-Idrissi M CJ, Harmouch A, García-Mauriño S, Guerrero JM. (1998) Specific binding of melatonin by purified cell nuclei from spleen and thymus of the rat. J Neuroimmunol. 86: 190-7.
[199] Smirnov AN (2001) Nuclear melatonin receptors. Biochemistry (Mosc). 66: 19-26.
[200] Iuvone PM, Brown AD, Haque R, Weller J, Zawilska JB, Chaurasia SS, et al. (2002) Retinal melatonin production: role of proteasomal proteolysis in circadian and photic control of arylalkylamine N-acetyltransferase. Invest Ophthalmol Vis Sci. 43: 564-72.

[201] Djeridane Y, Vivien-Roels B, Simonneaux V, Miguez JM, Pevet P (1998) Evidence for melatonin synthesis in rodent Harderian gland: a dynamic in vitro study. J Pineal Res. 25: 54-64.
[202] Konturek SJ, Konturek PC, Brzozowska I, Pawlik M, Sliwowski Z, Czesnikiewicz-Guzik M, et al. (2007) Localization and biological activities of melatonin in intact and diseased gastrointestinal tract (GIT). J Physiol Pharmacol. 58: 381-405.
[203] Itoh MT, Ishizuka B, Kudo Y, Fusama S, Amemiya A, Sumi Y (1997) Detection of melatonin and serotonin N-acetyltransferase and hydroxyindole-O-methyltransferase activities in rat ovary. Mol Cell Endocrinol. 136: 7-13.
[204] Itoh MT, Ishizuka B, Kuribayashi Y, Amemiya A, Sumi Y (1999) Melatonin, its precursors, and synthesizing enzyme activities in the human ovary. Mol Hum Reprod. 5: 402-8.
[205] Carrillo-Vico A CJ, Abreu P, Lardone PJ, García-Mauriño S, Reiter RJ, Guerrero JM. (2004) Evidence of melatonin synthesis by human lymphocytes and its physiological significance: possible role as intracrine, autocrine, and/or paracrine substance. FASEB J. 18: 537-9.
[206] Naranjo MC, Guerrero JM, Rubio A, Lardone PJ, Carrillo-Vico A, Carrascosa-Salmoral MP, et al. (2007) Melatonin biosynthesis in the thymus of humans and rats. Cell Mol Life Sci. 64: 781-90.
[207] Fischer T.W. SA, Zmijewski M.A., Reiter R.J. and Paus R (2008) Melatonin as a major skin protectant: from free radical scavenging to DNA damage repair. Exp Dermatol. 9: 713-30.
[208] Tijmes M, Pedraza R, Valladares L (1996) Melatonin in the rat testis: evidence for local synthesis. Steroids. 61: 65-8.
[209] Garcia-Marin R, De Miguel M, Fernandez-Santos JM, A. C-V, Utrilla JC, Morillo-Bernal J, et al. (2012) Melatonin-Synthesizing Enzimes and Melatonin Receptors in rat Thyroid Cells. Histol Histopathol. Paper in press.
[210] Lewinski A, Sewerynek E (1986) Melatonin inhibits the basal and TSH-stimulated mitotic activity of thyroid follicular cells in vivo and in organ culture. J Pineal Res. 3: 291-9.
[211] Wright ML, Pikula A, Babski AM, Labieniec KE, Molan RB (1996) Effect of Melatonin on the Response of the Thyroid to Thyrotropin Stimulation in Vitro. Gen Comp Endocrinol. 108: 298-305.
[212] Makay B, Makay O, Yenisey C, Icoz G, Ozgen G, Unsal E, et al. (2009) The interaction of oxidative stress response with cytokines in the thyrotoxic rat: is there a link? Mediators Inflamm. 2009: 391682.
[213] Karbownik M, Lewinski A (2003) Melatonin reduces Fenton reaction-induced lipid peroxidation in porcine thyroid tissue. J Cell Biochem 90: 806-11.
[214] Rao MV, Chhunchha B (2010) Protective role of melatonin against the mercury induced oxidative stress in the rat thyroid. Food Chem Toxicol. 48: 7-10.
[215] Tan DX, Manchester LC, Reiter RJ, Plummer BF, Limson J, Weintraub ST, et al. (2000) Melatonin directly scavenges hydrogen peroxide: a potentially new metabolic pathway of melatonin biotransformation. Free Radic Biol Med. 29: 1177-85.
[216] Sainz RM, Mayo JC, Reiter RJ, Tan DX, Rodriguez C (2003) Apoptosis in primary lymphoid organs with aging. Microsc Res Tech. 62: 524-39.

[217] Kameya T, Bessho T, Tsumuraya M, Yamaguchi K, Abe K, Shimosato Y, et al. (1983) Production of gastrin releasing peptide by medullary carcinoma of the thyroid. An immunohistochemical study. Virchows Arch A Pathol Anat Histopathol. 401: 99-107.
[218] Blaker M, de Weerth A, Tometten M, Schulz M, Hoppner W, Arlt D, et al. (2002) Expression of the cholecystokinin 2-receptor in normal human thyroid gland and medullary thyroid carcinoma. Eur J Endocrinol. 146: 89-96.
[219] Behr TM, Behe M, Angerstein C, Gratz S, Mach R, Hagemann L, et al. (1999) Cholecystokinin-B/gastrin receptor binding peptides: preclinical development and evaluation of their diagnostic and therapeutic potential. Clin Cancer Res. 5: 3124s-38s.
[220] Aloj L, Aurilio M, Rinaldi V, D'Ambrosio L, Tesauro D, Peitl PK, et al. (2011) Comparison of the binding and internalization properties of 12 DOTA-coupled and (1)(1)(1)In-labelled CCK2/gastrin receptor binding peptides: a collaborative project under COST Action BM0607. Eur J Nucl Med Mol Imaging. 38: 1417-25.
[221] Hoshino M, Yanaihara C, Hong YM, Kishida S, Katsumaru Y, Vandermeers A, et al. (1984) Primary structure of helodermin, a VIP-secretin-like peptide isolated from Gila monster venom. FEBS Lett. 178: 233-9.
[222] Parker DS, Raufman JP, O'Donohue TL, Bledsoe M, Yoshida H, Pisano JJ (1984) Amino acid sequences of helospectins, new members of the glucagon superfamily, found in Gila monster venom. J Biol Chem. 259: 11751-5.

Chapter 2

Thyroid Hormone Effects on Sensory Perception, Mental Speed, Neuronal Excitability and Ion Channel Regulation

Irmgard D. Dietzel, Sivaraj Mohanasundaram, Vanessa Niederkinkhaus, Gerd Hoffmann, Jens W. Meyer, Christoph Reiners, Christiana Blasl and Katharina Bohr

Additional information is available at the end of the chapter

1. Introduction

Although thyroid hormone effects on the brain are most prominent in development, also in adult-acquired hypothyroidism symptoms such as sensory impairments, disagreeable smells and taste, slowness of thought and action, changes of speech, irritability, headaches, sleep disturbances, confusion up to delusions and hallucinations, impairments of memory, of vision as well as of hearing frequently occur. This involvement of the nervous system was already discussed in the first reports on myxoedema (1–3) and a systematic description included in the first extensive investigation by the Committee of the Clinical Society of London (4). Many of these symptoms have since been studied in considerable detail. The conspicuous slowing of movements of hypothyroid subjects has been shown to correlate with peripheral sensory and motor nerve dysfunctions and abnormal neuromuscular transmission (5–10). The slowing of thoughts and mental function occurs concomitant with a decrease in the frequency of the alpha rhythm of the EEG (11–15). In addition to the slowing of the alpha-rhythm increased latencies of visual, auditory and somatosensory evoked potentials in adult-onset hypothyroidism indicate a slowed conduction of information in the central nervous system (16–24). In addition to a slowing of neuronal conduction velocity, changes in the threshold of hearing (25–29) and of the sensation of smell have been reported (30, 31). Cognitive and memory tests revealed impaired performances, which could at least partially be reversed by hormone substitution (24, 32–34). The extent of the reversibility of these symptoms is still a matter of debate (35).

Since many of the neurological symptoms observed in hypothyroidism point to a conspicuous mental slowing as leading symptom of hypothyroidism, we here were interested to test in a small sample of 6 patients, whether already a transient hypothyroid state, induced by 4 weeks of total thyroid hormone withdrawal, would result in detectable changes in the speed of sensory perception and cognitive functions. For this aim we combined different psychophysical tests shown to be sensitive in previous studies of hypothyroidism with some new examinations. While cognitive tests, such as the trail making test as well a calculation task showed a non-significant tendency toward slowing, a more complex visual- spatial performance test revealed a significant slowing of mental function after four weeks of hypothyroidism. The speed of speech was significantly reduced and a fast Fourier analysis showed a shift to lower frequencies in the hypothyroid test persons. A significant decrease in red-green colour fusion frequency was found, indicating an impaired temporal resolution of visual stimuli. Smelling of two odorants tested, odorant discrimination (Sniffin`sticks) and the hearing thresholds were slightly, but insignificantly impaired in the hypothyroid test persons. The results of these tests indicate that the most prominent and first significant clinical symptom to develop in hypothyroidism is a slowing of speech and of visual perception.

Slowing of conduction velocity can be explained by a reduced myelination. A second mechanisms is a decrease in voltage-gated sodium current density, leading to a slowed charging of the membrane capacitor thus resulting in a decreased slope of the action potential upstroke velocity which in turn decreases conduction velocity. Although several investigations support the concept that thyroid hormone affects myelination, recently evidence has accumulated, that thyroid hormone also increases sodium current density in neurons from several species. We will thus discuss reports on the regulation of voltage gated ion currents in neurons and muscle cells later in the chapter, which could offer an explanation for the observed slowing of thoughts and movements at the cellular and molecular level.

Furthermore, it has been known for a long time, that thyroid hormone regulates energy expenditure (see also Yehuda-Shnaidman et al. in this issue). Pumping of Na^+ out of the cells has been accounted for the expense of 40% of energy consumed at rest (36, 37). Thus an increased influx of Na^+ due to enhanced voltage-gated Na^+-influx will most likely also stimulate Na^+/K^+-ATPase activity, and could also account at least to some extent for the stimulation of an enhanced expression of Na^+/K^+-ATPase subunits in the membranes. We thus conclude the chapter by reviewing data on the regulation of Na^+/K^+-ATPase by thyroid hormone in the brain and its potential link to Na^+ current regulation.

2. Clinical symptoms during transient severe hypothyroidism quantified by psychophysical investigations in adult human test persons

To illustrate some conspicuous effects of thyroid hormone on brain function we studied 6 patients after total thyroidectomy for thyroid carcinoma who had discontinued taking thyroid hormone prior to routine diagnostic ^{131}I- scanning and who thus showed a reproducible degree and duration of hypothyroidism. Symptoms described to occur a few weeks after discontinuation of thyroid hormone therapy are changes in peripheral conduction velocity and in the EEG (15). Furthermore, subjective impairments of the quality of life (38–40) as well as changes in mood (41, 42) and decreases in working memory (43) have been reported.

3. Methods

Test persons. A test battery was developed to allow a relatively fast examination of several aspects of sensory and cognitive function. To integrate the investigation into the normal clinical examination procedures the whole testing protocol was designed to be completed within 1.5 hours. All tests were carried out on 6 patients after thyroid hormone withdrawal for 26 to 28 days and on 6 healthy volunteers which were age (maximal difference: 3 years) and sex matched (with the exception of one female control person for a male patient). Patients were retested after at least 6 weeks of hormone substitution, after obtaining low TSH values. To elaborate the optimal test parameters some of the tests had been performed in more detail on an additional hypothyroid test person, the data of which are included in the appropriate results sections. In the 7 test persons (age 42-64, 4 female, 3 male) TSH-suppressive thyroid hormone substitution after total thyroidectomy and radioiodine therapy for thyroid carcinoma had been discontinued for 26-28 days for routine diagnostic application of ^{131}I. Thyroid hormone levels measured in hypothyroidism were FT3: < 2.0 pmol/l, FT4: <2.6 pmol/l in 6 patients and FT3: 2.6 pmol/l, FT4: 4.8 pmol/l in the remaining patient, TSH was > 80 mU/l in three patients and 48.7 ± 10.4 mU/l (mean ± SE) in the remaining four patients. After 6 - 10 weeks of hormone substitution these values were: FT3: 6.2 ± 0.5 pmol/l, FT4: 26.0 ± 3.0 pmol/l and TSH: 0.09 ± 0.04 mU/l, n=7 (normal ranges: FT3: 3.4 - 7.6 pmol/l (SPART, Amerlex MAB, Johnson & Johnson); FT4: 11 - 23 pmol/l (SPART, Amerlex MAB, Johnson & Johnson), TSH: 0.3 - 4.0 mU/l (IRMA, Dynotest, Brahms). Results are given as means ± standard error. Statistical analysis was performed using paired Student`s t-test. Informed consent was obtained from all individuals before performing the tests.

Speed of speech. To investigate possible changes in the speed of speech we asked the test persons to repeat four times the same word as fast as possible (in this case the word „Apfelmus"). They were asked the repeat the series of four words four times and were encouraged to accelerate their speech as much as possible. The four series of words were stored on magnetic tape with a SONY WTC-D6C stereo cassette recorder and analysed off-line using a Digidata 1200A analog-digital converter with "Axoscope" software (Axon Instruments). The time needed to pronounce the four words was then read from a digital storage oscilloscope. In addition a fast Fourier analysis was performed on the record of the second syllable ("mus") selected from the two fastest traces obtained from each test person in the hypothyroid and the euthyroid condition. The section of the record to be analysed was selected with "Axoscope" and then analysed with "Origin 5" software.

Tests of cognitive performance:

a. *Calculation and Correlation.* To test more complex mental performances patients were first handed a sheet of paper and asked to complete a set of 24 simple calculation tasks of third grade difficulty (like: 23+11=?). Each result of a calculus task was assigned one of five colours (yellow, red, green, dark and light blue). After completing the calculation task the test persons were asked to fill a second form, consisting of an outline drawing containing 54 numbered areas, where each number equalled one of the results of the preceding calculus task (some numbers were used several times). The patients were handed coloured pencils and asked to assign the appropriate colour from the result of the calculus task to each of the numbers given in the drawing. This procedure finally resulted in the appearance of a meaningful picture (in this case a boat). The time taken by the patients to complete the calculus task and to assign the colours to the figures in the drawing was monitored.

b. *Trail making*. The test consisted of a piece of DIN A4 paper, containing randomly distributed numbers (24 pt size, black, surrounded by a black circle). The paper was placed on a table in front of the test persons who were asked to connect the numbers from one to 25 (version A). In version B numbers from 1 to 13 and letters from A to L were distributed randomly and the test persons asked to connect them alternating between the numbers and the succession of the alphabet, e.g., 1-A 2-B- 3-C etc. The time needed for completion of the test was recorded (44).

Tests to determine time resolution of visual perception and colour contrast perception:

a. *Flicker fusion frequency*. Light flashes delivered with a sufficiently high frequency fuse to give the impression of a continuous light source. The lowest frequency at which an intermittent light source is perceived as a continuous one is termed the „flicker fusion frequency". A light source containing red (660nm), green (565 nm) or blue (470nm) diodes of 1 cm^2 diameter with an intensity of 14 Cd m^2 (determined with a Minolta luminance meter) was displayed to the test persons at a distance of 52 cm (to excite a 1° area of the visual field). The screen was positioned at the back of a 50 x 50 cm wide and 52 cm deep box with black walls. The flicker frequency was generated with a square wave pulse generator with a 50% duty cycle. The frequency could be changed with a dial. Test persons were asked to focus on the light with both eyes while the frequency was increased and to give a sign when they perceived the flashes to fuse to a continuous light source. Since it turned out to be too time-consuming to test the right or the left eyes, foveal and peripheral illumination separately and to use lights of different colours and since preliminary experiments showed no qualitative differences in the results, most patients were only retested with the red colour fixed by two eyes. The average value of three determinations of flicker fusion frequency always starting from low frequencies was determined.

b. *Red-Green fusion*. Changes in the perception of chromatic flicker were tested in addition to the critical flicker fusion frequency of luminance flicker. In this test a rotating disk of 12 cm diameter was shown to the test persons. The disk was diagonally partitioned into four sections which were painted alternatively in light red (Plaka Nr. 82) and light green (Plaka No. 90; 16 – 20 Cd/m^2, determined with a Minolta LS 100 luminance meter). The speed of rotation was increased continuously and the number of rotations per minute was electronically counted. Increasing the speed of rotation first gave the impression of a luminance flicker. A further increase in the speed of rotation resulted in the impression of a homogenous dark yellow colour. The patients were asked to give a sign at the frequency were they saw the first signs of a luminance flicker and as soon as they perceived the impression of a homogenous yellow colour. Each test was repeated three times starting with low frequencies and the average value of the three determinations was noted.

Sense of Smell. Two tests were used to detect possible changes in the sense of smell: First a test for the recognition and discrimination of 16 different odorants, including familial smells like cinnamon and rather unusual flavours, like leather, was used. Then the threshold of perception was tested using two different odours, one that tests the excitation of the olfactory nerve (phenylethyl alcohol (Phe)), smelling like rose, and one, exciting both, trigeminal and olfactory nerves (eugenol (Eu)), Sniffing´sticks, (45)). In brief, for the odorant tests, caps were removed from plastic sticks containing odorants of different concentrations filled into the sticks ending in felt tips extruding about 5 mm from the tip of the stick. A stick was gently moved at a distance of about 1 cm below the nostril of the test person. Sticks containing the test solution in ascending concentration (descending numbers on the stick) were presented to the test person in series of three sticks, two of which contained distilled water. The threshold was defined as the concentration at which the patient correctly recognised the odour in two out of three presentations.

Hearing threshold. Hearing thresholds were determined for 8 different frequencies using an Ascom Audiosys Maico ST20 audiometer. Changes in threshold for sinusoidal tones of 1 and 8 kHz were evaluated.

3.1. Experimental results

Speed of speech. Figures 1A and B show digitized traces of speech records of a female test person in hypothyroidism (upper trace, a) and after hormone substitution (lower trace, b). After hormone substitution this test person pronounced the four words faster. As shown in Fig. 1C, on average the test persons needed a significantly longer time to pronounce the same words in the hypothyroid condition as compared to the euthyroid control persons or after thyroid hormone substitution. Figure 1D gives a more elaborate example of the development of the slowing of speech during hormone withdrawal and resubstitution. Here an additional test person was asked to repeat a short poem in regular intervals at maximal speed and the time taken to complete this poem was recorded. During hormone withdrawal the time needed to finish the poem became increasing longer. During resubstitution with thyroid hormone the time to finish the poem gradually decreased during the following month. To find out whether the increase in speed of speech during hormone resubstitution was accompanied by an increase in pitch a fast Fourier analysis was performed on the syllable "mus" (encircled by the rectangles in Fig. 1A). The analysis of the pronounciation of this syllable, consisting with predominant amplitude of the noun "u" showed several clear frequency peaks (Fig. 1B). The records from four of the five male subjects included in the study showed a peak between 100 and 200 Hz which was not seen in the records from any of the female test persons. Since the most prominent peak in all test persons was found between 200 and 300 Hz this peak was evaluated in hypothyroidism and after hormone substitution. As shown in Table 2 and illustrated in Fig. 1B the peak frequency was shifted by an average of about 30 Hz to higher frequencies by the hormone substitution. This shift was found in all subjects with the exception of one test person, aged 61, who suffered from paresis of the *n. recurrens*.

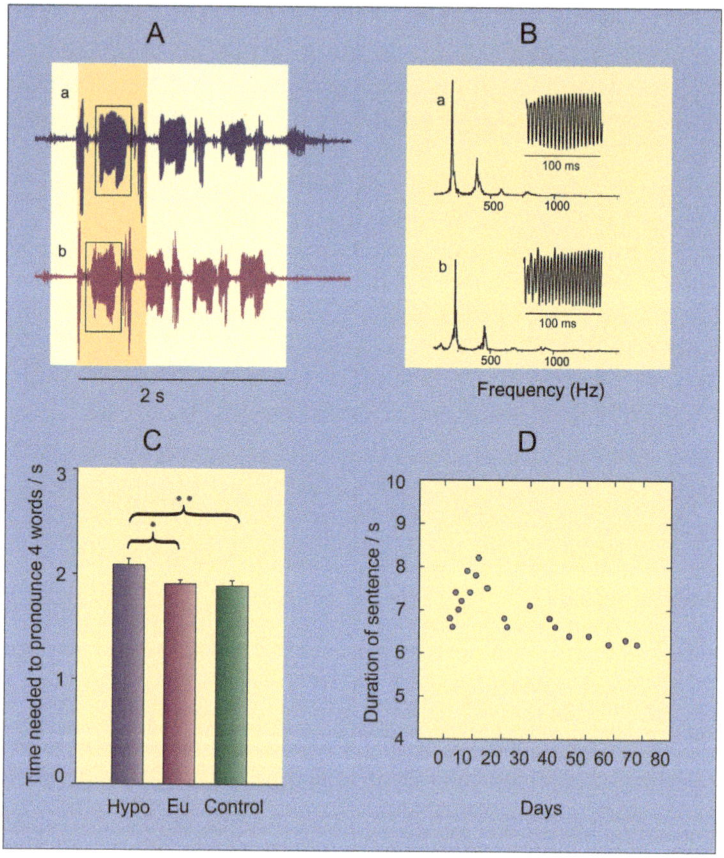

Figure 1. *Changes of speech during thyroid hormone withdrawal.* Original voltage traces of a record from a female test person (A) repeating four times the word "Apfelmus" as fast as possible after four weeks of thyroxine withdrawal (a) and after 10 weeks of hormone resubstitution (b). The darker yellow shadow indicates the time needed to pronounce the first word in the hypothyroid condition. B: Fast Fourier analysis of sections of the speech record shown within the squares in A. Inset: 100 ms long sections from the analysed traces. C: average time needed to pronounce the four words after hormone withdrawal (Hypo), resubstitution (Eu) and by control subjects (mean ± SE, n=6) asterisk: $p<0.05$, 2 asterisks: $p<0.01$. D: time needed to complete a short poem of an additional test person recorded daily during last 20 days of thyroxine withdrawal and during the following 60 days of resubstitution. Note the gradual decline in speed of speech with increasing time of thyroid hormone withdrawal.

Speed of visual perception. In hypothyroidism, the frequency, at which patients first reported to perceive a flickering light source as a continuous one was slightly but insignificantly smaller than the frequency determined in the control group. The hypothyroid group showed no significant improvement after 6 weeks of hormone therapy (Figure 2Ab). In a single test person, where the flicker fusion frequency was recorded daily for blue, green and red light and both eyes tested separately, however, a significant decrease in flicker fusion frequency was shown in the third week after the arrest of hormone substitution. After six weeks of hormone resubstitution the flicker fusion frequency had significantly recovered with respect to the last week without the hormone (Table 1 and Figure 2 Aa).

	6 days during first week of thyroid hormone withdrawal			Days 17-22 of hormone withdrawal			P (1st week versus 3rd week)	40-46 days after beginning of thyroid hormone resubstitution			P (6 weeks after resubstitution versus 3 weeks after hormone withdrawal)
	n	mean	SEM	n	mean	SEM		n	mean	SEM	
CFF (Hz), green 2600 Cd/m²	12	37.4	0.4	12	36.6	0.6	0.27	12	40.6	0.3	0.000006
CCF (Hz), red 100 Cd/m²	12	35.8	0.6	12	32.8	0.4	0.0003	12	36.3	0.3	0.0000002
CCF (Hz), blue 30 Cd/m²	12	35.3	0.6	12	29.9	0.5	0.0000004	12	37.2	0.3	<0.0000000001

Table 1. Critical flicker fusion frequency for three different colours (12 measurements on 2 eyes determined on 6 successive days were pooled from one test person, SEM: standard error of the mean, unpaired t-test), the original data for red light are displayed in Figure 2Aa.

The critical colour fusion frequency (CCFF), determined with a rotating wheel of alternating green and red sectors was significantly reduced in the hypothyroid test persons compared with the control subjects. The frequencies at which the rotating, red-green disk was perceived as starting to show a luminance flicker (Fig. 2 Ba) as well as the frequency at which a uniform yellow colour was reported (Fig. 2Bb) were both significantly smaller in the hypothyroid test persons as compared to the control group.

Cognitive performance. Since several cognitive tests have been shown to be sensitive for thyroid hormone we here tested whether hypothyroidism for 4 weeks has an effect on calculation and visual-spatial orientation. A slight but insignificant slowing of the speed with which the hypothyroid persons completed the calculation task compared with the euthyroid control group was observed (Table 2, Figure 3A). A stronger effect was seen, however, if a more complex performance task, like the correlation of numbers with colours and finding and colouring the appropriate numbered area, had to be accomplished (visual-spatial orientation). Here the hypothyroid patients performed somewhat slower than the control subjects. After 6 weeks of hormone substitution the formerly hypothyroid persons showed a significantly improved performance (Figure 3B). Hypothyroid persons completed the trail making test insignificantly slower than the euthyroid controls or after hormone substitution, (Figure 3C, D).

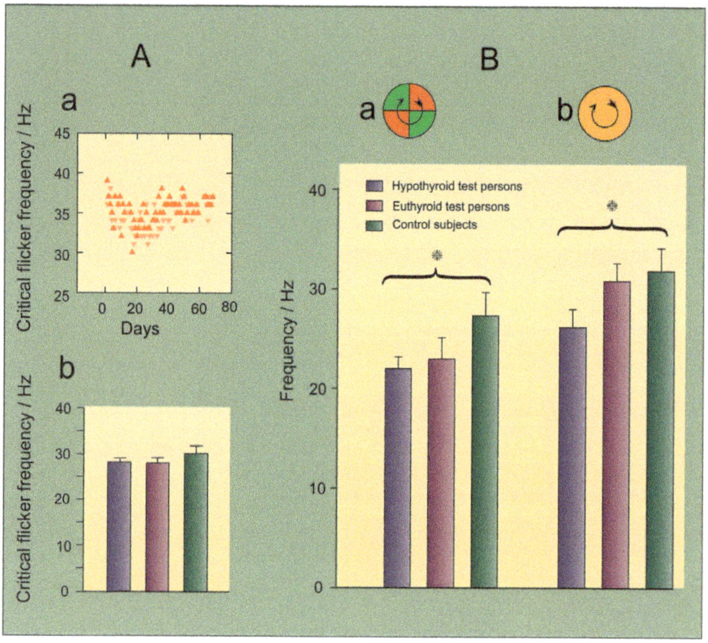

Figure 2. *Speed of visual perception.* Aa: critical flicker fusion frequency for a luminance flicker of red light, 100 Cd/m² measured once daily at the same time in the morning in a test person during the last 20 days of thyroxine withdrawal and during resubstitution. Note the gradual continuous decrease in CFF with increased time of thyroxine withdrawal and the gradual increase after hormone resubstitution. Dark red symbols: right eye, light red symbols: left eye. Ab: average critical flicker fusion frequency determined in six separate test persons after four weeks of hormone withdrawal (green bars), resubstitution (violet bars) and in control subjects (pink bars). B: critical colour fusion frequency in same test persons for luminance flicker of red and green sectors of a rotating disk (a) and fusion of the red-green sectors to homogenous yellow (b) (mean ± SE, n=6) asterisk: $p<0.05$.

Hearing threshold. Since thyroid hormone has been reported to also affect the auditory system here we tested whether thyroid hormone withdrawal for several weeks has a measurable effect on hearing thresholds. No changes in hearing threshold were obvious for frequencies below 8 kHz. Hence only the measurements at 1 kHz and 8 kHz were evaluated (Table 2). If data from both ears were pooled, the improvement of 8 dB seen after hormone substitution at the test frequency of 8 kHz just reached significance.

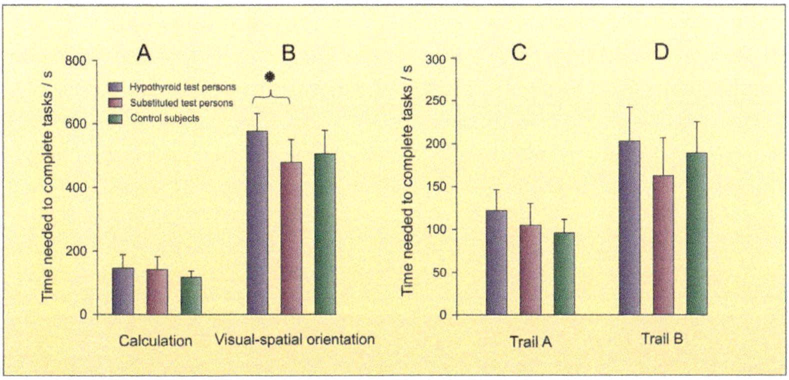

Figure 3. *Performance in cognitive tests.* A: Average time needed by test persons after four weeks of hormone withdrawal (light bars), thyroid hormone resubstitution for at least nine weeks (grey bars) and by control subjects (black bars) to complete a set of simple calculations. B: Average time needed by the same subjects to combine numbers in an outline drawing with corresponding colours. C: Average time needed by the same subjects to complete the Trail A test and D: the Trail B test (mean ± SE, n=6). Asterisk: $p<0.05$

Sense of smell. Finally, thyroid hormone might also affect the sense of smell. Of the six test persons tested one had been anosmic since childhood and a second subject did not want to repeat the smelling threshold test. Hence only 4 persons could be retested in the euthyroid state (Table 2). Using the odorant discrimination task, the hypothyroid test persons rated 66% of the presented flavours correctly. After hormone substitution they showed a slightly increased performance rating 72% of the presented flavours correctly, while the controls gave 70% correct answers. After four weeks of hypothyroidism, small but insignificant decreases in the threshold of odorant detection were found for both odorants which were still below the thresholds determined for the control subjects (Table 2).

Age-dependence of thyroid hormone effects

Although hypothyroid subjects performed on average slower in several tests it could have been possible that some test persons showed only a slowing of speech while others showed a slower resolution of visual signals. To find out whether some subjects were on average, slower or faster than others for each of seven tests, the speed of speech, calculation time, picture filling, Trail A, Trail B, critical flicker fusion frequency for red luminance flicker and fusion frequency for chromatic flicker, all twelve test persons were assigned numbers of 1 to 12 for each test, were the fasted was scored with 1 and the slowest with 12. If two persons showed the same speed of performance they were assigned an equal score, such that the highest value was less than 12 for several tests. For each test person the average score in the seven tests was calculated (Fig. 4). If differences in performance in the different tests were random, then the scores would scatter around a value of somewhere below 6.5 (assuming that in some tests several test persons showed the same speed). As Fig. 4 shows, this was not the case. As expected, the hypothyroid test persons were on average slower than the control subjects (Fig. 4A). As also somewhat expected the speed of performance showed a tendency to decline with age, such that the older test persons, displayed at the right side of the series of columns in Fig 4A, scored on average higher than the younger subjects. In comparison of the performance of the test persons during hormone substitution with the control subjects an increase in overall speed of performance of the formerly hypothyroid subjects was seen, such that the average speed of the substituted test persons became indistinguishable from that of the controls (Fig. C). Interestingly, the relative increase in speed seemed to be larger in the younger than the older test persons (compare Fig. 4A with Fig. 4B).

	Hypothyroid Test Persons (HypoTP)			Substituted Test Persons (SubTP)			P (HypoTP versus SubTP)	Controls			P (HypoTP versus Controls)
	n	mean	SEM	n	mean	SEM		n	mean	SEM	
Speed of speech / s	12	2.09	0.05	12	1.91	0.04	0.03	12	1.88	0.05	0.003
Pitch of „u" /Hz	12	236	13	12	263	10	0.008	12	264	10	0.16 NS
CFF /Hz	6	28.3	1.0	6	28.2	1.1	0.90 NS	6	30.3	1.6	0.38 NS
CCFF I /Hz	6	22.0	1.2	6	23.0	2.1	0.73 NS	6	27.3	2.4	0.03
CCFF II /Hz	6	26.2	1.8	6	30.8	1.8	0.21 NS	6	31.8	2.3	0.02
Calculation time /s	6	146	42	6	142	40	0.75 NS	6	118	19	0.51 NS
Visual-spatial orientation/s	6	576	56	6	478	71	0.02	6	504	74	0.44 NS
Trail A /s	6	122	25	6	105	26	0.16 NS	6	96	16	0.40 NS
Trail B /s	6	203	40	6	163	44	0.13 NS	6	189	36	0.79 NS
Odour recognition (%)	5	66	6	5	72	6	0.32 NS	5	70	6	0.48 NS
Smell threshold (eugenol)	5	6.7	0.6	4	6.9	1.2	0.91 NS	5	7.8	0.5	0.19 NS
Smell threshold (Phe)	5	5.9	1.1	4	6.7	0.5	0.54 NS	5	7.8	0.5	0.23 NS
Smell threshold (Pyr)	5	5.1	0.5	4	5.4	0.8	0.37 NS	5	5.9	1.1	0.50 NS
Hearing threshold for 8 kHz /-dB	12	32	5	12	24	6	0.05	12	25	4	0.24 NS
Hearing threshold for 1 kHz /-dB	12	22	3	12	21	4	0.43 NS	12	23	2	0.83 NS

Speed and pitch of speech: the two fastest measurements of each test and control persons were included. CFF: critical flicker fusion frequency, CCFF: critical colour fusion frequency, Smell thresholds: a lower threshold of smell corresponds to a higher test score: Phe: Phenylethylalcohole, Eu: Eugenol: Pyr: pyridine, hearing thresholds: data from right and left ears were pooled, SEM: standard error of the mean, paired t-Test

Table 2. Summary of the effects of hypothyroidism on performance in the different psychophysical tests in hypothyroid test persons, hormone substituted hypothyroid test persons and euthyroid control subjects.

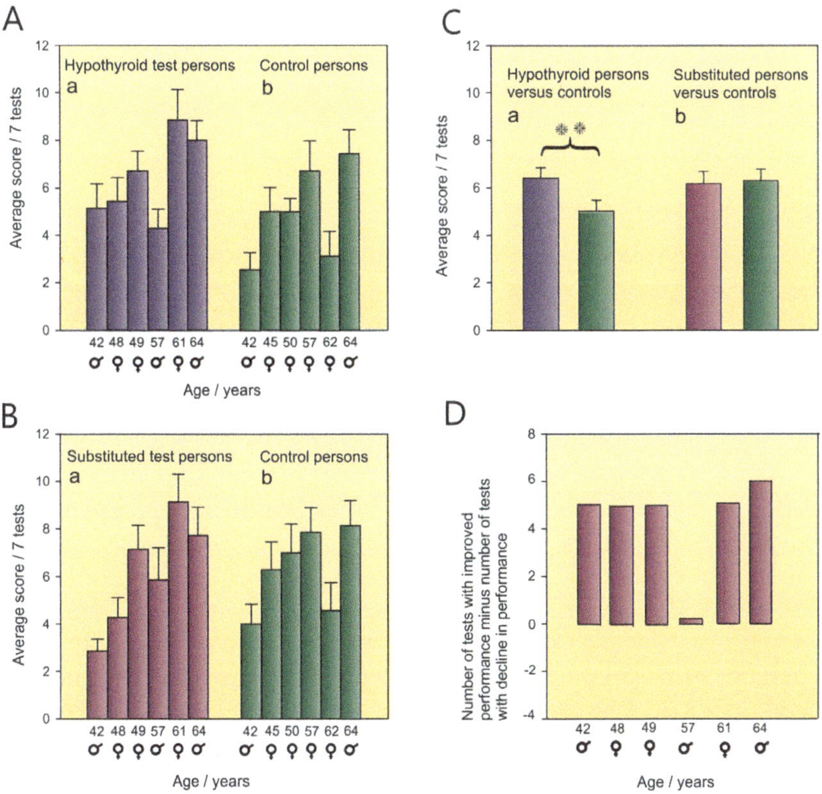

Figure 4. *Effects of age and thyroid status on speed of performance of individual test persons.* Mean scores obtained by the 12 test and control subjects in 7 tests. A: Comparison of speed of performance in the sum of 7 tests in hypothyroid subjects with control subjects. Smallest score: fastest person, largest score: slowest person. B: Comparison of former hypothyroid subjects after at least 6 weeks of hormone substitution (a) with controls (b). C: Mean values of scores of all six persons after thyroid hormone withdrawal compared with control subjects (a) and of test persons after hormone replacement with controls (b). Light bars: test persons after hormone withdrawal, grey bars: test persons after hormone resubstitution, black bars: control subjects.**: $p<0.01$.D: Overall improvement in speed of performance after hormone substitution. For each of the 6 test persons the number of tests in which performance was speeded minus the number of tests in which performance was slowed was determined (maximal value of improvement: 8, maximal value of slowing: -8). While 5 persons considerably increased their speed of performance (e.g. an increase in speed in 6 tests and a decrease in performance in 1 test) only 1 test person showed no average increase in speed.

To investigate whether only the younger test persons responded with an increase in the speed of neuronal information processing to thyroid hormone we evaluated the individual change in performance of each test person. For each of the 6 test persons and eight tests (the speed of speech, pitch of speech, calculation time, picture filling, Trail A, Trail B, critical flicker fusion frequency for red luminance flicker and fusion frequency for chromatic flicker) we rated an increase in the speed of performance in a test assigning a 1 to an increase in speed, a 0 for an unchanged performance and a –1 for a slowing of performance at retesting during hormone resubstitution. If a person showed no overall change in speed of performance, a score scattering around 0 should result, if the subject slowed considerably the score should be in the negative range and if a subject speeded in all tasks, the maximal score would reach 8. As depicted in Fig. 4D out of the 6 persons tested with all 8 identical tests 5 showed a considerable speeding which corresponded to an increased performance in at least 6 out of 8 tests. Only one of the test persons, aged 57, showed an increased performance in only 4 tests and a decreased performance in 4 tests. This person was the only one who showed no increase in the speed of speech with thyroid hormone substitution. Nevertheless Fourier- analysis revealed an increase in pitch by 11% after prolonged hormone resubstitution in this test person.

Our findings, that younger persons are more impaired than older subjects after thyroid hormone withdrawal is in accordance with recent findings by Heinzel et al., who reported a stronger subjective impairment in younger patients after thyroid hormone withdrawal than in older patients (46). This is in accordance with observations of age-dependent effects on heart action potential parameters observed to parallel age-related thyroid states (47, 48). This observation might relate to a down-regulation of thyroid hormone receptors with aging (49).

4. Evaluation of the experimental data in the context of previous observations of the action of thyroid hormone on mental speed

Taken together, this short survey of measurable changes in sensory perception and reaction after a period of a few weeks of severe hypothyroidism indicates that the first effects of hypothyroidism to become significantly evident concern changes in the speed of speech and visual perception.

Speed of speech

Although slowing of speech and thinking had already been noticed in the first description of myxedema (2) and by the Committee of the Clinical Society in 1888 (4) to be one of the most prominent symptoms of hypothyroidism we are aware of only one published attempt to quantify changes in speech due to different thyroid states. This study reported a negative correlation between the basal frequency of speech and the duration of the achilles tendon reflex (50). These authors performed investigations before and after treatment of hypo- and hyperthyroidism with reported time intervals from 7 days to 17 weeks, but did not further comment on the severity of thyroid dysfunction and the time course of development of recovery of the changes in pitch. A further study observed a decrease of the fundamental frequency of speaking 4 days after thyroid ablation (51). Although the cause for the slowing of speech is difficult to interpret, increased intervals between the different words (see Fig. 1A) suggest, that in addition to a possible slowing of muscle contraction and a potential decrease in tension of the vocal cords a central slowing of neuronal information processing is likely to occur.

Speed of processing of visual signals

The second most prominent effect of hypothyroidism revealed by our tests is a slowing of the speed of perception of visual information. These results confirm several previous studies, one of which reported critical flicker fusion frequencies (CFF) up to 41 - 48 Hz in 23 hyperthyroid patients and a decrease in flicker fusion frequency to the normal value of 37 Hz within one month after treatment of the hyperthyroidism (52). Decreased values of the critical flicker fusion frequency as well as of the maximal speed of finger movements were shown in hypothyroid patients (53). A third study revealed an increase in CFF in hypothyroid subjects with a delay of 2-3 weeks after an increase in dose of thyroid hormone substitution (54). We could find no previous reports on influences of thyroid hormone on the critical colour-fusion frequency (CCFF) which tests the speed of processing of chromatic pathways in addition to the CFF, which tests the speed of luminance processing. CCFF occurs at a lower frequency as CFF (55). The lower frequency of colour processing compared to luminance flicker already starts to arise at the level of the retina (56).

Since thyroid hormone affects the renewal rate of the photoreceptor outer segments in the rat (57, 58) one locus of action of thyroid hormone could be the retina. This is confirmed by the finding of increased amplitudes of chiefly the b-waves of the electroretinogram in hyperthyroidism and a decrease in hypothyroidism (59, 60), suggesting that thyroid hormone influences retinal sensitivity to light. Since there is evidence that thyroid releasing hormone (TRH) in the circulation decreases the critical flicker fusion frequency (61) the effect could also be due to the enhanced TRH level in the investigated test persons. Since, however, no effects of hypothyroidism on peripheral circulating TRH values have been found (62) it seems presently more likely that the decrease in flicker fusion frequency is due to a direct effect of thyroid hormone.

Increased voltages of EEG records and a decreased duration of arousal responses to photic stimulation after administration of thyroid hormone (63) could be explained by an increased light-sensitivity of the retina, but additionally also by an increased transmission of sensory signals to the visual cortex. Substantial experimental evidence has been obtained to show that the upper frequency limit with which signals are transmitted in the visual pathways decreases with the number of synaptic stations traversed (for review see (64)). Hence a modulation of synaptic transmission at the thalamic level seems to be responsible for the increase of CFF by psychotropic stimulants and the decrease by sedatives (for reviews see (65, 66)). Furthermore, investigations of the relation between CFF and intelligence revealed only non-significant relations between different scores for intelligence and CFF (67, 68), however a decrease of 4 Hz of was found in mentally retarded persons (69) suggesting that a larger decline of cognitive function may be accompanied by decreases in CFF. In addition a correlation was found between the decline of CFF and the decline in performance on cognitive tests in old age (70).

Complementary to a reduction in CFF, flash evoked potentials showed increased latencies and reduced amplitudes in hypothyroid patients 6 weeks after thyroidectomy which were reversed after 8 weeks of treatment (16). Consistently, visual evoked potentials using chequerboard reversal patterns showed reversible increases in latencies and reductions in amplitudes in hypothyroidism (17, 19–21, 23, 24, 71–73). However, this increase in latency is not consistently observed in all cases of hypothyroidism and thus it is still controversial after which duration and or severity of hypothyroidism significant increases in latency can be observed (74). Nevertheless, blink reflex prolongation could be consistently observed in hypothyroid patients confirming a slowing in visual pathways in adult onset hypothyroidism (75). From the available studies no definitive conclusion concerning the targets for thyroid hormone action in the visual pathways can be drawn. Thyroid hormone could already effect photoreceptor sensitivity as well as increase the speed of impulse propagation and synaptic transmission in any of the following relay stations.

Cognitive performance

Several reports have described mental changes in hypothyroidism, ranging from difficulties to perform simple calculations to memory impairments and finally to hallucinations (76–79). Although these impairments are probably the most troublesome symptoms for the patients, it has been difficult to quantify cognitive problems in adult-onset hypothyroidism. Daytime sleepiness as well as mental and physical fatigue are complaints in 70 - 80% of the hypothyroids (80, 81). Disturbances of sleep during thyroid dysfunction might account for some of the problems delineated above, as the different sleep stages are necessary for memory consolidation (82, 83). Sleep fragmentation in hypothyroids is not necessarily caused by nocturnal breathing disorders (sleep apnea) (84, 85).

The trail making test, which tests skills including vigilance, concentration, visual scanning and visuomotor tracking speed was shown by Reitan (44, 86) to respond to different types of organic brain damage. Later on slowed performance on the trail making test (part B) was shown in hypothyroid patients (78, 87). Subsequently Osterweil et al. (24) observed that the performance for Trail A was significantly slowed in old and very old hypothyroid patients as compared to age-matched controls and Wahlin et al. (88) reported that TSH was predictive for Trail-B in very old persons. Our finding of a non-significant slowing in the trail making tests confirms the observation of Osterweil et al., that carcinoma patients off thyroid hormone replacement show no statistically significant differences in test performance compared to euthyroid controls. However, 5 of the six persons tested showed an increase in performance when retested after hormone replacement, which escaped statistical significance because of the large scatter between the different individuals. This suggests that thyroid hormone withdrawal of longer duration is necessary before changes in this test become statistically significant.

Apart from this relatively simple test effects of thyroid hormone on more complex cognitive tasks have been investigated. The first measurement of an increase in the intelligence level by a mean of 20 I. Q. points of three adult myxedematous patients after three months of treatment with thyroid hormone has been reported by Crown (32). Especially in older hypothyroid persons, reversible decreases in the Folstein mini mental state score were found (24, 89, 90). In a double-blind study on adult persons with subclinical hypothyroidism out of 17 patients 4 showed improved performance on at least two and 7 test persons improved in one of a reaction time, an object memory and a figure identification test after a six month period of thyroxine supplementation (33). Likewise, in subclinically hypothyroid adults the Wechsler Memory Scale indicated a significant decrease in logical memory (91, 92) as well as verbal and visual memory (93) (for a recent review see (94)) and severe hypothyroidism for a short time decreased working memory (43). Using fMRI changes in hypothyroid subjects during working memory tasks could be visualized (95). Finally also changes in the estimation of time spans have been observed in hypothyroid subjects (96). All these experiments were performed after a longer period of hypothyroidism or latent thyroid dysfunction. To be able to complete our test battery in a reasonably short time we designed a short tests for calculation and visual-spatial performance. Our present results indicate that a severe hypothyroidism of a short duration already causes significantly slowed performance in a visuo-spatial orientation task. This is in line with findings of increased latencies of event-related evoked potentials in hypothyroidism (97, 98).

Perception of smells

Although perversions of taste and smell during myxoedema have already been noticed in the first descriptions of this disease (99, 100) there have only been a few investigations on this subject, which provided no clear answers concerning the prevalence of olfactory disorders during hypothyroidism. Reversible increases in the threshold of smell and taste have previously been found in hypothyroid subjects (30, 31, 101). In addition to the reduced threshold, hypothyroid persons rated bitter and salty tastes as more agreeable than euthyroid control persons in the latter study. Interestingly, a more general study concerned with smell and taste disorders reported a more than average complaint of patients taking levothyroxine about a loss of the sense of taste. The investigation of these patients revealed, in contrast to their subjective impressions, higher scores on a taste-identification test. Additionally, the patients taking thyroxine perceived a test concentration of coffeine as having a greater intensity as the other patients, without showing significantly different taste thresholds (102). The discrepancy between subjective impression and test results could have resulted from increases in thresholds of taste preceding hormone substitution resulting in an increased awareness of the sense of smell. A study of taste thresholds, measured in 11 hypothyroid subjects after total thyroid ablation, which had stopped taking replacement for 4-8 weeks prior to a ^{131}I scan showed no increases in recognition thresholds to NaCl and urea (103). These patients showed, however, a decrease in intensity rating for the two tastants and less dislike to both substances at higher concentrations as compared to control subjects. Although the authors conclude that hypothyroidism probably has to persist for a longer time in order to develop more pronounced changes in taste, the preference and intensity rating tests could indicate the beginning of changes in taste after this period. Our present findings of an insignificant tendency towards a higher threshold of smell for both odours in the hypothyroid compared with the euthyroid subjects are in line with the assumption of a beginning loss of taste and smell after 4 weeks of hypothyroidism. In contrast, however, a study by Lewitt et al. (104) found no significant changes in the thresholds for taste and smell even in longer standing hypothyroidism. Since this study, in addition, reported no increase in the latencies of visual evoked potentials, in contrast to seven other available reports, it could be possible, that the discordant findings of this report were due to the high median age of the investigated subjects (61 ± 16 years) which could already have displayed age-dependent declines in sensory function. In addition, the possibility exists, that only a fraction of the hypothyroid subjects shows changes in taste thresholds (105).

Possible causes of a loss in smell during hypothyroidism have also been investigated in rats. Here prolonged hypothyroidism has been shown to result in deficits in migration of olfactory receptor neurones while the mitotic rates of basal cells remained unaltered in postnatal (106) as well as in adult rats (107). The effects of propylthiouracil (PTU) – induced hypothyroidism were reversed by thyroxine therapy. Further experiments could, however, not confirm increases in the threshold to olfactory and taste stimuli in adult rats rendered hypothyroid with PTU for 5 weeks (108, 109) in which only changes in taste preferences for sour, bitter and salty, not of detection threshold were found. Additional confusion arose from several case reports describing thyreostatic drugs to also induce decreases in the sense of taste and smell in patients (methylthiouracil, - (110); methimazole - (111); thiamazol and carbimazol, (112–114). Sometimes, only the sensation of taste, sometimes also olfaction was impaired. Some patients could have actually become hypothyroid, but in some patients no other symptoms of hypothyroidism were noted and the symptoms did not reappear during thyroidectomy-induced hypothyroidism (110). A histological examination showing destruction of the olfactory epithelium, sparing the basal cells already after 32 hours of methimazol administration to rats further substantiates the possibility of toxic effects of antithyroid medication (115), which lead to apoptosis of rat olfactory receptor neurons (116). However, in studies of methimazol toxicology effects of hypothyroidism should be carefully excluded. Likewise, we cannot presently exclude, that changes in taste, which have been reported to occur frequently in patients as side effects of a high dose ^{131}I therapy (117) could also have resulted to some extent from the accompanying hypothyroidism, which also has been reported as a potential cause of a "bourning mouth symptom" (118).

Hearing

Impairments of hearing have long been reported to occur in hypothyroidism (for reviews see (27, 119)). The incidence of decreases in hearing threshold observed in hypothyroid patients varies from study to study, ranging from 85% (28), 80% (29), 62% (120), 55% (121) 43% (122), 31% (80) to as low as 12% [98].

The only study showing no evidence of reversible hearing losses in hypothyroid patients (123) was performed on old patients between 61-92 years, in which the effects of presbyacusis may have a stronger effect on hearing threshold than those of thyroid hormone. The most dramatic hearing impairments arise if the thyroid hormone supply is insufficient during development, where irreversible structural impairments in the cochlea, presumably a disruption of the smooth fit of the tectorial membrane to the hair cells occurs (see e.g. (124–126). While a thyroid-hormone induced selective expression of neurotrophin-receptors could underly the morphogenetic changes shaping the inner ear (127) the acceleration of the expression of a fast potassium conductance (128) and the development of rapidly activating Ca^{2+}- and voltage-activated K+ (BK) conductances in inner hair cells (129) could be necessary for the proper development of cochlear sensory transduction. Furthermore, hypothyroidism causes delays in the development of synaptic inhibition in the auditory brainstem (130). In line with a larger susceptibility of the immature auditory system to thyroid hormone deficiency Heinemann (131) reported no case of hearing impairment in 23 patients with primary hypothyroidism if treated in time but in 4 out of 7 cases if hormone substitution had been delayed. Besides the irreversible effects of thyroid hormone on the development of inner ear function, reversible changes of hearing acuity have already been described in early reports on the symptoms of adult-onset hypothyroidism (132, 133). Improvements of hearing threshold with treatment in some patients with hypothyroidism have since been shown with pure tone audiometric testing (25, 28, 29, 134, 135). Especially noteworthy in this context is the finding, that in 7- 11 year old, normal, but latently hypothyroid schoolchildren living in endemic areas of severe iodine deficiency iodine prophylaxis led to an average improvement of hearing (30 children tested in each village) by 15 db over the course of three years (136). Smaller changes in hearing threshold were reported after a total thyroid hormone withdrawal for a few weeks: 6 - 12 weeks after hormone withdrawal Post (137) reported 26 normal audiograms, decreased hearing thresholds which did not reverse after 3- 12 months of treatment in 5 patients and small, partially subjective improvements with hormone substitution in 4 patients from a total of 35 patients. No acute changes in hearing were also found by Mra and Wax (138) in 10 patients 2-6 weeks after total thyroidectomy. In contrast, Rubenstein et al. (120) described a case of a reversible hearing loss of 20 dB in a 5 year old child, that had been induced by stopping thyroid hormone therapy for four weeks. Another case report, where audiometric investigations were available 2 months before thyroidectomy a high frequency hearing loss started on the 40th day of hormone withdrawal, which was partially reversible after hormone substitution (139). These inconsistent findings correspond to our results of borderline significant increases in hearing thresholds of about 8 dB for high frequencies after 4 weeks of thyroid hormone withdrawal.

Animal experiments showed that in guinea pigs thyroid ablation caused decreased amplitudes of cochlear microphonic potentials (140) and cochlear action potentials of decreased amplitudes and increased delay when recorded four to eight months after administration of an ablative dose of radioactive iodine (124). Likewise, increased hearing thresholds have been observed in adult guinea pigs (125) at high frequencies of 8kHz (141) after 120 days of hypothyroidism. In contrast, Ritter (26) measured only deafness in five out of 166 experimental rats rendered hypothyroid on the 21st day of life. Interestingly, changes in the number of spines/per shaft of pyramidal neurones (indicating synaptic densities) could be shown in the auditory cortex of adult rats thyroidectomized at 120 days of age and investigated 120 days later (142). The authors note that in auditory pyramidal cells these changes develop much more slowly than in pyramidal cells of the visual cortex, which could indicate that the adult auditory system may respond to hypothyroidism on a slower time scale than the visual system. Perhaps these considerations could also explain why, in contrast to visual evoked potentials which consistently show slowing in hypothyroidism, some authors found no changes in auditory evoked potentials (24, 143) while other studies (18, 21, 22) found reversible increases in latencies of auditory evoked potentials in hypothyroidism.

Taken together, the auditory system may lose its sensitivity to thyroid hormone with increasing age and this may also depend on an individual susceptibility. In addition, effects on hearing may develop only after a thyroid hormone withdrawal for more than five weeks in the adult.

Effects of thyroid hormone on sensory perception and brain function

The present tests performed on a small number of patients indicate that the most prominent symptom after 4 weeks of thyroid hormone withdrawal is a beginning decline in the speed of central neuronal information processing, which was reflected in decreases in the speed of visual perception, speed of speech as well as of visual-spatial orientation. Hearing and smelling thresholds were only slightly changed, and in the context with the publications discussed above this indicates that auditory and olfactory perception may change only with thyroid dysfunctions of longer duration or are more sensitive to thyroid hormone in development. The experiments illustrated here complement previous findings, that hypothyroidism slows peripheral conduction velocity (144), reduces EEG frequencies and increases latencies of evoked potentials (73). The conception that thyroid hormone deficiency causes a general decrease in neuronal excitability was recently supported by the observation of a decreased cortical excitability and increased motor thresholds using transcranial magnetic stimulation in adult patients (145). Accordingly, in a small percentage of epileptic seizures in humans (146) thyrotoxicosis was identified as sole cause of the seizures and the seizures were found to fully subside after restoration of euthyroidism, again indicating an effect of thyroid hormone on cortical excitability. An increased susceptibility to seizures was also noticed in hyperthyroid animals such as cats (147) and mice (148).

5. Explanations of thyroid hormone effects on the brain at the molecular and cellular level

Owing to the complex actions of thyroid hormone there is currently no concluding explanation concerning the molecular mechanisms underlying the effects of thyroid hormone on cortical excitability. At the morphological level, in the mature brain thyroid hormone excess (149) as well as deficiency (150) have been reported to decrease the number of dendritic spines, assumed to represent postsynaptic endings, already after 5 days in adult rats. Even more dramatically, hypothyroidism leads to a reduction of the neuropile in CA1 and CA3 hippocampal areas and in addition to a loss of pyramidal cells in the CA1 area (151). Thus it seems possible that adult-onset hypothyroidism may actually cause neuronal degeneration, as already occasionally observed in autopsies of early cases of patients who had died with myxedema (152, 153). A reversible shrinkage of neuropile could also explain the findings of reversibly widened ventricular spaces in the brains of hypothyroid subjects (154, 155).

The development of cholinergic terminals in rat forebrain, hippocampus and amygdala is regulated to a considerable extent by thyroid hormone (see e.g. (156)). Although smaller and more localized effects are reported in adults, several lines of evidence suggest that acetylcholine -release may be enhanced by thyroid hormone and decreased in hypothyroidism in the adult nervous system as well (157, 158). A decrease of cholinergic activity could perhaps also explain the occurrence of slow EEG waves (159) as well as the cognitive impairments frequently seen in hypothyroid subjects. A regulation of cholinergic function also fits to the observation of a regulation of nerve growth factor which has been suggested to be involved in maintaining the function of cholinergic hippocampal projections by thyroid hormone in adult rat brain (160). Thyroid hormone, however, does not seem to interfere exclusively with cholinergic forebrain neurons but to regulate the balance of a variety of other neurotransmitters in a region-specific manner. Hence dopamine levels were found to be increased in the midbrain of hyperthyroid rats (161) and decreased in hypothyroid rats (162). Also the dopaminergic input into striatal neurons could be upregulated by thyroid hormone (163). Furthermore, a differential regulation of serotonin levels (162, 164) as well as 5-HT_2 receptors have been found (165). Regulations of various adrenoceptors as well as GABA-receptors have been described see e.g. (166–168). In addition T3 could act as a cotransmitter to modulate noradrenergic action (169) or as a modulator of endogenous benzodiazepine action (170). While it is believed that thyroid hormone exerts its effects predominantly via nuclear receptors possible direct effects on membrane receptors further complicate the picture (157, 171, 172). In addition to a membrane action via $\alpha V\beta 3$intergins, high doses of 20 μM T3 or T4 have been shown to directly act on GABA receptors to down-regulate GABAergic postsynaptic currents in cultured hippocampal neurons (173, 174), which could explain acute increases in neuronal excitability induced by iontophoretecally injected T4 and T3 (171). Although the regulatory influences exerted by thyroid hormone are complex it seems that T3 regulates to some extent the release of neurotransmitters such as acetylcholine, dopamine, 5-HT and noradrenalin in specific pathways as well as the density of the corresponding receptors (166).

A stimulating effect of thyroid hormone on transmitter synthetic enzymes or precursor-uptake systems as well as the protein synthesis of the receptors could in principle explain the decrease in cerebral responsiveness in hypothyroid subjects. Furthermore, a down-regulation of postsynaptic inhibitory currents in hyperthyroidism, as suggested by Puia and Losi (174), could account for the increased irritability seen in hyperthyroid subjects. A diminished postsynaptic current density due to a decrease in transmitter release or receptor density or activation could also explain some of the increased latencies since a smaller current density would lead to a delay in the charging of the membrane capacitance. However, investigations using transcranial magnetic stimulation provided evidence that in hypothyroid patients the cortical excitability as such is decreased (145). Furthermore, experiments on peripheral nerves of hyperthyroid rats indicated enhanced afferent spikes and a drop in the chronaxia for direct activation of action potentials in rat peripheral nerves (175). Hence thyroid hormone could also influence neuronal excitability directly, which could secondarily result in a decrease in transmitter release.

Changes in conduction velocity, action potential waveform and the regulation of voltage-gated ion currents by thyroid hormone

Changes in Achilles tendon reflexes and the slowing of peripheral conduction velocity in hypothyroidism have so far mostly been explained by a reduction in myelination, and the gene for myelin basic protein is, in fact, regarded as one of the few genes known to be directly regulated by thyroid hormone (for review see (176)). However, a decrease in sodium current density could as well explain the decreases in peripheral conduction velocities and increases in latencies of evoked potentials found in hypothyroidism (16–24) and reversely the increased amplitudes in hyperthyroidism (177, 178). Since there seems to be an optimal density of sodium channels that ensures maximal neuronal conduction velocity (179), beyond which no further increase or even a slowing of conduction velocity occurs, an upregulation of sodium currents by thyroid hormone could also explain the inconsistent findings concerning latencies of evoked visual potentials in hyperthyroidism, where some authors found decreases in latencies (180) or even increases with increases in thyroid hormone (21, 71, 177, 178). Because of the temperature sensitivity of the activation of sodium and calcium currents the fall in core temperature during hypothyroidism and its increase in hyperthyroidism could further exacerbate the symptoms (19).

Influences of thyroid hormone on action potentials and underlying ion currents in the heart

Evidence that thyroid hormone could indeed change action potential waveforms became available from electrical recordings performed in ventricular cells from guinea pig hearts, that showed decreases in action potential length in the course of hours after application of thyroxine, which then gradually recovered over the course of days (181). In line with these observations, prolongations of action potential durations were observed in hypothyroid rat heart cells (182) and guinea pig ventricular myocytes (183). That thyroid hormone directly effects the electrical properties of heart cells, and not just alters sympathetic receptors was shown by Valcavi et al. (184), who demonstated an increase in the intrinsic activity of the sinus node in hyperthyroid patients that persisted after chemical blockage of autonomous innervation. Patch clamp recordings revealed that in heart cells from neonatal rats (185, 186) and in cat atrial myocytes (187), acute applications of 5-20 nM T3 increased voltage activated sodium currents. Single channel recordings revealed that the application of 5-50 nM T3 induced bursting of Na^+-channels in rabbit ventricular myocytes (188). Later studies showed, that T3 increases the sodium channel open probability by binding directly inside the membrane and that the interaction with a pertussis toxin sensitive G-protein greatly enhances this effect (189). More recent experiments by Schmidt et al. (190), confirmed rapid effects of T3 on human hearts, however, suggesting a contribution of the sympathetic nervous system. After a period of prolonged hyperthyroidism in rats, in contrast to acute effects, no changes in Na^+current density as well as of inward potassium currents were found. At that time increased rates of rise of the action potentials could be rather explained by an increase in Ca^{2+}-currents and a shortened action potential duration by an increase in a delayed rectifier current (191). Although it is presently not completely understood, which channel regulations exactly determine short and long term effects of thyroid hormone, it is safe to conclude, that an upregulation of voltage activated Na^+-, Ca^{2+} and K^+-currents plays a pivotal role in decreases in action potential duration, the acceleration of the heart beat and modulation of contraction amplitude by thyroid hormone.

Influences of thyroid hormone on action potentials and underlying ion currents in the central nervous system

The influence of thyroid hormone on the electrical properties of neurons has been studied in less detail. The first experiments using whole cell patch clamp recordings were carried out on cultured postnatal rat hippocampal neurons and showed an upregulation of voltage-gated Na^+-currents (I_{Nav}) by T3 (192). An upregulation of the density of voltage-gated Na^+ currents was also found in acutely isolated neurons from the occipital cortex of hyperthyroid rats and a down regulation observed in cells from hypothyroid rats. The changes in Na^+current density led to increased action potential upstroke velocities as well as to enhanced discharge rates in thyroid hormone treated cells in response to identical stimulus strengths (193). Similarly, increases in voltage-gated Na^+ currents were observed in human neuroepithelial cells as well as mesenchymal stem cells after incubation with 1 nM T3 for 72h to 6 days in culture. Neuroepithelial cells additionally responded with increases in Ca^{2+} currents to prolonged T3-treatment (194). In the in *vivo* situation thyroid hormone effects seem to be more complex: Thus in CA1 neurons of the rat hippocampus changes in the bursting pattern have been observed, which could be explained by an upregulation of a low-threshold Ca^{2+} current (195). Furthermore, consistent with Hoffmann and Dietzel, 2004, decreases in action potential depolarization rate and decreases in discharge rate were observed by thyroid hormone withdrawal. In contrast to the action of thyroid hormone in the heart these authors additionally observed a shortening of action potential duration upon thyroid hormone withdrawal, that could be explained by the upregulation of an A-type potassium current (196). Finally in a somewhat distant animal, in Rohon-Beard neurons from the embryonic zebrafish rapid increases of voltage-gated Na^+currents by thyroxine were found (197). This Na^+current regulation was shown to be essential for the further development of the embryo and depended on $\alpha V\beta 3$ integrin activation and the MAPK (p38) pathway (198). An increase in voltage-gated Na^+current density by thyroid hormone would cause a general speeding of mental functions as illustrated in figure 5:

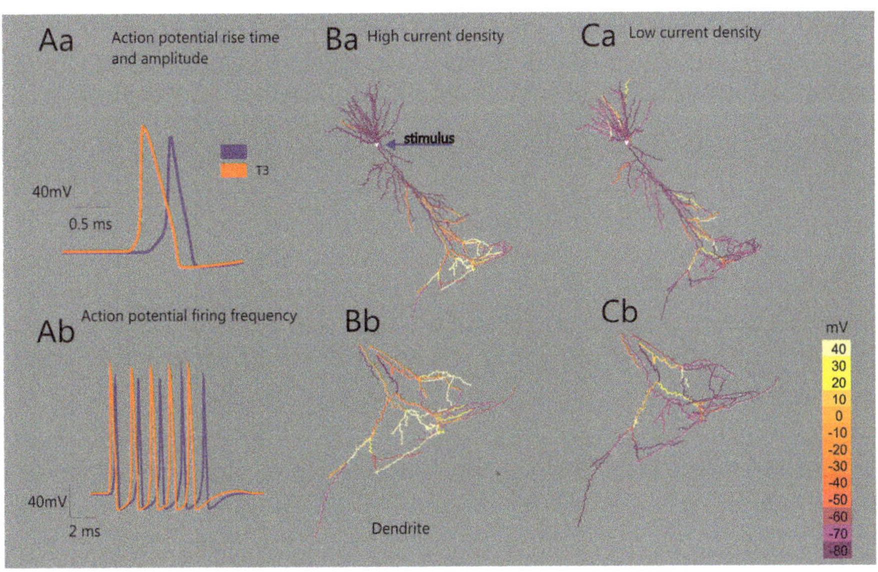

Figure 5. Simulation of action potential spread in a hippocampal model neuron, for action potential with high (A-red) and low (A-blue) Na^+-current density. A an increase in Na^+current density increases action potential depolarization (Aa), amplitude and discharge frequency (Ab). B. Simulation of action potential spread in a ramified neuron 1 ms after application of a stimulus at t=1ms.

B shows the spread for the neuron with high current density and B' for the neuron with low current density. The magnified inserts (Ba and Cb) clearly show, that the overshoot of the action potential (light colours) reaches the synapses much earlier in the cell with high current density than in the cell with lower current density (Cb). Simulations performed using the Hodgkin-Huxley equations and the program Neuron version 3.2.3 (199).

Hypothyreosis also affects a prominent EEG pattern, namely the alpha rhythm (11–15). This may be also related to altered Na^+ channel function, since TTX-insensitive Na^+ currents of cortical bursting neurones have been implicated in the generation of the alpha rhythm (200). Subsequently, the presence of SCN5A mRNA, encoding the TTX-resistant Na^+ channel had been demonstrated in the mammalian brain (201, 202).

It is noteworthy that the mental symptoms observed with the psychophysical tests used in the present study developed gradually, as most prominently demonstrated in the continuous observations on a single person and only recovered with a similar slow time course in the first weeks of hormone resubstitution (see Fig. 1D and 2A). Prolonged recovery phases for the reversal of several of the symptoms accompanying hypothyroidism have been described (20, 84, 203–205) and subjective improvements of well-being, quantified with a "Quality of life-Thyroid scale" were found only after four weeks compared to one week of thyroid hormone replacement (38).

This corresponds to the observation of a lack of acute effects of T3 in hippocampal slices (206) and the observation of a slow upregulation of Na^+current density in hippocampal cultures (207). In the later study the Na^+current regulation was shown to depend on the presence of glial cells in the culture medium. Thyroid hormone has been shown to induce protein secretion from glial cells (208), including *basic fibroblast growth factor* (FGF-2) (209) and *epidermal growth factor* (210). Furthermore, thyroid hormone has been shown to elevate *nerve growth factor, neurotrophin-3* and *brain derived neurotrophic factor* (BDNF) in the brain (see e.g.(211)). A first indication that intermediate steps, including growth factors could be involved in the regulation of Na^+currents by thyroid hormone were experiments, that showed, that the effect of T3 on Na^+ currents could be reduced by a simultaneous incubation of cultures with antibodies against FGF-2, leading to the hypothesis depicted in Figure 6.

Concerning the action of thyroid hormone on neuronal excitability there seems to be a common finding that the density of voltage-gated Na^+currents is up-regulated by thyroid hormone rendering the cells more excitable. This mechanism would explain many of the symptoms observed in thyroid disease, such as slowed peripheral conduction velocity and decreased excitability of the hypothyroid brain. In other tissues, such as various epithelial cells, thyroid hormone could, likewise, play an essential role in the regulation of the expression of amiloride sensitive, epithelial Na^+channels (see e.g. (212)). The molecular mechanisms, leading to Na^+current upregulation, may however, differ in different species and tissues and warrant further elucidation.

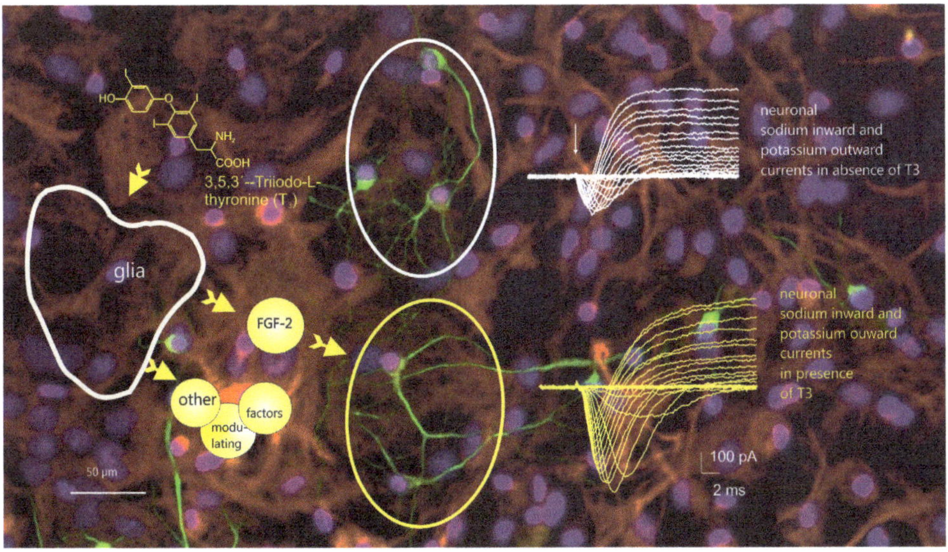

Figure 6. Illustration of a potential mechanism leading to Na^+-current regulation in the hippocampus of rats: T3 stimulates glial cells (stained red by antibodies against GFAP) to secrete growth factors (such as FGF-2) which in turn up-regulate Na^+currents in neurons. (stained green by antibodies against βIII tubulin). Thus in addition to regulating the neuronal environment and stimulating synapse formation glial cells could also be involved in modulating neuronal excitability.

Regulation of Na^+/K^+-ATPase expression by thyroid hormone

Since thyroid hormone has long been known to increase energy expenditure, and about 40% of energy at rest is consumed by activity of the Na^+/K^+-ATPase (36, 37, 213) many researchers focused on studying effects of thyroid hormone on Na^+/K^+-ATPase activity and expression. The Na^+/K^+-ATPase is a heterodimeric membrane spanning protein complex composed of three catalytic alpha subunits ($\alpha 1$, $\alpha 2$ and $\alpha 3$) with molecular weights of ~97-116kDa and two glycosylated β subunits (β1 and β2 of ~35-55kDa). While the α subunits contain the Na^+, K^+ and the intracellular ATP binding site, the β subunits are required to insert the catalytic α subunits into the appropriate locations of the cell membrane (214). An intracellular Na^+ load of the cell leads to binding of three Na-ions to their intracellular binding sites, thus triggering phosphorylation of the α subunit and inducing a conformational change of the pump to expose the Na-ions to the extracellular surface at the expense of ATP (see e.g. (37)). Thus an increased intracellular Na^+-load, as induced by a larger or longer Na^+ influx will increase energy consumption by stimulating the demand for ATP. Interestingly, the Na^+/K^+-ATPase shows a 10-12 fold increase in expression during postnatal development of the brain (215) which parallels the postnatal increase in Na^+ current density (216).

The different isoforms of the Na^+/K^+-ATPase were reported to be distributed in a cell and tissue dependent manner. Thus in brain tissue the $\alpha 3$ isoform transcript is expressed abundantly in comparison with the mRNA for the $\alpha 1$ and α 2 subunits. The $\alpha 3$ expression increases 10 fold within the first 7 days after birth and remains at this elevated level until the 55th day of age in the rat. In contrast, the mRNA for the $\alpha1$, $\alpha2$ and β isoforms reach their maximal expression levels only after the rats are at 25 days old (215).

In general, thyroid hormone was found to up-regulate Na^+/K^+-ATPase activity and expression in many tissues: For instance, in rat cardiomyocytes, T3 was observed to increase the mRNA pattern of Na^+/K^+-ATPase $\alpha1$ and $\beta1$ subunits 4fold after 48hrs and the $\alpha2$ mRNA expression even 7fold after 72hrs of treatment (217). A similar effect of T3 was found in a rat liver cell line. Here, a non transformed continuous cell line derived from adult rat liver treated with T3 showed a 1.3 fold increased activity of Na^+/K^+-ATPase. More specifically, the mRNA expression of the $\alpha1$ and $\beta1$ isoforms of the Na^+/K^+-ATPase increased 1.5 and 2.9 fold respectively compared with controls maintained in T3 free (hypothyroid) media (218).

In rat brains thyroid hormone has been shown to up-regulate Na^+/K^+-ATPase activity and protein expression in synaptosomes only in the first two postnatal weeks (219). In addition Schmitt *et al.*, in 1988 showed that the hypothyroid condition reduces the expression of the mRNA for Na^+/K^+-ATPase α isoforms in rat brain (220). However, observing thyroid hormone effects in identified brain regions in the adult rat indicated, that hypothyroidism could down-regulate Na^+/K^+-ATPase activity in specific brain regions, such as the adult hippocampus (221, 222). Further experiments showed that the predominant brain cell specific $\alpha3$ isoform of the Na^+/K^+-ATPase decreased in hypothyroid rat brain as well and that the relative sensitivity of the different Na^+/K^+-ATPase α subunits in brain cells for thyroid hormone is $\alpha3>\alpha1>\alpha2$ (223). The expression of all Na^+/K^+-ATPase isoforms and their regulation by T3 was also observed in primary neuronal cell cultures of rat brain at the mRNA and protein level using northern and western blot techniques (224). In contrast to neurons, glia cells express $\alpha1$, α 2 and $\beta1$, 2 not $\alpha3$. The mRNAs as well as the proteins of the four subunits expressed in glia cells showed an upregulation when the cells were grown with the supplement of T3 for 5 and 10 days respectively (225).

Although a T3-responsive element has been found in the promotor region of the $\alpha3$ subunit (226) two reports on muscle cells indicate, that the regulation of the Na^+/K^+-ATPase by thyroid hormone might be at least to some extent secondary to an enhanced sodium influx. Thus Brodie and Sampsom (227) observed that a blockage of Na^+-influx by tetrodotoxin to block the voltage-gated Na^+currents or by amiloride to block further Na^+transport routes both reduced the T3-induced increase of ^{3}[H]-ouabain binding sites, which represent membrane inserted Na^+/K^+-ATPase in cultured myotubes. These results were confirmed by Harrison and Clausen (228) in skeletal muscle, who showed that an increase in saxitoxin binding (reflecting Na^+channel density) preceded an increase in ^{3}[H]-ouabain binding (reflecting membrane inserted Na^+/K^+-ATPases). These experiments indicate a link between Na^+ current regulation and the regulation of the Na^+/K^+-ATPase by thyroid hormone. This is in agreement with other experiments in chick skeletal muscle that suggested that the activation of voltage-gated Na^+channels by veratridine leads to an increased biosynthesis of Na^+/K^+-ATPase in chick myogenic cultures (229). Whether these findings also apply to neurons, or whether some subunits are regulated directly by thyroid hormone receptors and others are regulated by the sodium load of the cells remains, however, to be clarified.

6. Conclusions

Thyroid hormone deficiency leads to a general slowing of many body functions, including a slowing of heart rate, a slowing of intestinal movements as well as of thoughts and movements. As demonstrated here in an exemplary fashion on a small sample of patients the most conspicuous symptom to develop during a short period of severe hypothyroidism is a gradual, quantifiable slowing of speech and of critical flicker fusion frequency. Although several explanations at the cellular and molecular level are feasible an intriguing hypothesis is, that a central aspect of the origin of many of these symptoms might be a regulation of the sodium current density that is a key player of neuronal and cellular excitability. In fact, some effects of thyroid hormone can to some extent be blocked by the sodium channel blocker TTX: Thus the upregulation of the membrane Na^+/K^+ATPase expression in myotubes (227) and skeletal muscle (228) as well as of soma growth in L-GABAergic neurons (230) by thyroid hormone were all to some extent blockable by TTX, suggesting that some effects of thyroid hormone occur downstream of sodium channel regulation. In future it will be exciting to elucidate the full signal cascade involved in the regulation of the different sodium channel subunits as well as to conclusively sort out the primary and the secondary targets of thyroid hormone action. It will be interesting to study whether some of these thyroid hormone actions decline in the aging brain.

Author details

Irmgard D. Dietzel
Department of Molecular Neurobiochemistry, Ruhr-University Bochum, Bochum, Germany

Sivaraj Mohanasundaram
Department of Molecular Neurobiochemistry, Ruhr-University Bochum, Bochum, Germany

International Graduate School of Neuroscience (IGSN), Ruhr-University Bochum, Germany

Vanessa Niederkinkhaus
Department of Molecular Neurobiochemistry, Ruhr-University Bochum, Bochum, Germany

International Graduate School of Neuroscience (IGSN), Ruhr-University Bochum, Germany

Gerd Hoffmann
Department of Molecular Neurobiochemistry, Ruhr-University Bochum, Bochum, Germany

PFM Medical AG, Köln, Germany

The late Jens W. Meyer
JM Technische Entwicklungen, Bochum, Germany

Christoph Reiners
Department of Nuclear Medicine, University Hospital, Würzburg, Germany

Christiana Blasl
Department of Nuclear Medicine, University Hospital, Würzburg, Germany

Diagnostische Gemainschaftspraxis Karlstrasse, Karlsruhe, Germany

Katharina Bohr
Neuro Reha Zentrum Plau, Plau am See, Germany

7. Acknowledgement

V. Niederkinkhaus and S. Mohanasundaram were supported by fellowships from the International Graduate School of Neuroscience (IGSN) at the Ruhr University. We want to thank U. Eysel, the Physiological Institutes of the Universities of Bochum and Würzburg for lending us a luminance meter and audiometers, N.E. Meyer for help with the design of the visual-spatial orientation test, and H. Schatz, R.A. Deisz, M. Kreissl and B. Igelhorst for many helpful discussions.

8. References

[1] Gull WW. On a cretinoid state supervening in adult life in women. Trans.Clin.Soc.Lond 1874; 7:180–5.
[2] Ord WM. On myxoedema, a term proposed to be applied to an essential condition in the "cretinoid" affection occasionally observed in middle-aged women. Med.Chir.Trans 1878; 61:57–78.
[3] Blaise H. De la cachexie pachydermique: Observation nouvelle avec aliénation mental transitoire. Arch.Neurol.(Paris) 1882; 3: 60-79 and 141-159.
[4] Clinical Society of London. Report of a Commitee of the Clinical Society of London to Investigate the Subject of Myxoedema. London: Longmans, Green & Co; 1888. (Suppl. vol. 21).
[5] Goldblatt S. Pallhypesthesia. Depression of the appreciation of vibration in trauma and in disease; a preliminary report. Arch.Neurol.Psychiat 1948; 59:292–301.
[6] Fincham RW, Cape CA. Neuropathy in Myxedema. Arch.Neurol 1968; 19:464–6.
[7] Scarpalezos S, Lygidakis C, Papageorgiou C, Maliara S, Koukoulommati AS, Koutras DA. Neural and muscular manifestations of hypothyroidism. Arch.Neurol 1973; 29:140–4.
[8] Rao SN, Katiyar BC, Nair KRP, Misra S. Neuromuscular status in hypothyroidism. Acta Neurol.Scand 1980; 61:167–77.
[9] Beghi E, Delodovici ML, Bogliun G, Crespi V, Paleari F, Gamba P et al. Hypothyroidism and polyneuropathy. J.Neurol.Neurosurg.Psychiatr 1989; 52:1420–3.
[10] Torres CF, Moxley RT. Hypothyroid neuropathy and myopathy: clinical and electrodiagnostic longitudinal findings. J.Neurol 1990; 237:271–4.
[11] Bertrand I, Delay J, Guillain J. L'électro-encéphalogramme dans le myxoedème. Comp.Rend.Soc.Biol 1938; 129:395–8.
[12] Ross DA, Schwab RS. The cortical alpha rhythm in thyroid disorders. Endocrinol 1939; 25:75–9.
[13] Browning TB, Atkins RW, Weiner H. Cerebral metabolic disturbances in hypothyroidism. Clinical and electroencephalographic studies on the psychosis of myxedema and hypothyroidism. AMA Arch.Int.Med 1954; 93:938–50.
[14] Lansing RW, Trunnell JB. Electroencephalographic changes accompanying thyroid deficiency in man. J.clin.Endocrinol.Metab 1963; 23:470–80.

[15] Pohunková D, Šulc J, Vána S. Influence of thyroid hormone supply on EEG frequency spectrum. Endocrinol.Exp 1989; 23:251–8.
[16] Nishitani H, Kooi KA. Cerebral evoked responses in hypothyroidism. EEG clin.Neurophysiol 1968; 24:554–60.
[17] Mastaglia FL, Black JL, Collins DWK, Gutteridge DH, Yuen RWM. Slowing of conduction in visual pathway in hypothyroidism. Lancet 1979; 1, Feb.18:387–8.
[18] Himelfarb MZ, Lakretz T, Gold S, Shanon E. Auditory brain stem responses in thyroid dysfunction. J.Laryngol.Otol 1981; 95:679–86.
[19] Abbott RJ, O'Malley BP, Barnett DB, Timson L, Rosenthal FD. Central and peripheral nerve conduction in thyroid dysfunction: the influence of L-thyroxine therapy compared with warming upon the conduction abnormalities of primary hypothyroidism. Clin.Sci 1983; 64:617–22.
[20] Ladenson PW, Stakes JW, Ridgway EC. Reversible alteration of the visual evoked potential in hypothyroidism. The American Journal of Medicine 1984; 77:1010–4.
[21] Huang T, Chang Y, Lee S, Chen F, Chopra IJ. Visual, brainstem auditory and somatosensory evoked potential abnormalities in thyroid disease. Thyroidol 1989; 3:137–42.
[22] Höhmann D, Kahaly G, Warzelhan J. Einfluß von Hyperlipidämien und Hypothyreosen auf die akustisch evozierten Hirnstammreizantworten. HNO 1990; 38:446–50.
[23] Avramides A, Papamargaritis K, Mavromatis I, Saddic G, Vyzantiadis A, Milonas I. Visual evoked potentials in hypothyroid and hyperthyroid patients before and after achievement of euthyroidism. J.Endocrinol.Invest 1992; 15:749–53.
[24] Osterweil D, Syndulko K, Cohen SN, Pettler-Jennings PD, Hershman JM, Cummings JL et al. Cognitive function in non-demented older adults with hypothyroidism. J.Am.Geriatr.Soc 1992; 40:325–35.
[25] Howarth AE, Lloyd HED. Perceptive Deafness in Hypothyroidism. Br.Med.J 1956; Feb. 25:431–3.
[26] Ritter FN. The effects of hypothyroidism upon the ear, nose and throat. A clinical and experimental study. Laryngoscope 1967; 67:1427–79.
[27] Meyerhoff WL. The thyroid and audition. Laryngoscope 1976; 86:483–9.
[28] van't Hoff W, Stuart DW. Deafness in myxoedema. Q.J.Med 1979; 48:361–7.
[29] Anand VT, Mann SBS, Dash RJ, Mehra YN. Auditory investigations in hypothyroidism. Acta Otolaryngol.(Stockh.) 1989; 108:83–7.
[30] McConnell RJ, Menendez CE, Smith FR, Henkin RI, Rivlin RS. Defects of taste and smell in patients with hypothyroidism. The American Journal of Medicine 1975; 59:354–64.
[31] Bhatia S, Sircar SS, Ghorai BK. Taste disorder in hypo and hyperthyroidism. Indian J.Physiol.Pharmacol 1991; 35:152–8.
[32] Crown S. Notes on an experimental study of intellectual deterioration. Br.Med.J 1949; Sept.24:684–5.
[33] Nyström E, Caidahl K, Fager G, Wikkels C, Lundberg P, Lindstedt G. A double-blind cross-over 12-month study of L-thyroxine treatment of women with "subclinical" hypothyroidism. Clin.Endocrinol 1988; 29:63–76.
[34] Monzani F, Pruneti CA, Negri F de, Simoncini M, Neri S, Di Bello V et al. Ipotiroidismo preclinico: precoce interessamento delle funzioni mnestiche, della reattività comportamentale e della contrattilità cardiaca. Minerva Endocrinol 1991; 16:113–8.

[35] Davis JD, Tremont G. Neuropsychiatric aspects of hypothyroidism and treatment reversibility. Minerva Endocrinol 2007; 32(1):49–65.
[36] Gill M, France J, Summers M, McBride BW, Milligan LP. Simulation of the energy costs associated with protein turnover and Na+,K+-transport in growing lambs. J. Nutr 1989; 119(9):1287–99.
[37] Kelly JM, McBride BW. The sodium pump and other mechanisms of thermogenesis in selected tissues. Proc Nutr Soc 1990; 49(2):185–202.
[38] Dow KH, Ferrell BR, Anello C. Quality-of-life changes in patients with thyroid cancer after withdrawal of thyroid hormone therapy. Thyroid 1997; 7:613–9.
[39] Taïeb D, Sebag F, Cherenko M, Baumstarck-Barrau K, Fortanier C, Farman-Ara B et al. Quality of life changes and clinical outcomes in thyroid cancer patients undergoing radioiodine remnant ablation (RRA) with recombinant human TSH (rhTSH): a randomized controlled study. Clin. Endocrinol. (Oxf) 2009; 71(1):115–23.
[40] Lee J, Yun MJ, Nam KH, Chung WY, Soh E, Park CS. Quality of life and effectiveness comparisons of thyroxine withdrawal, triiodothyronine withdrawal, and recombinant thyroid-stimulating hormone administration for low-dose radioiodine remnant ablation of differentiated thyroid carcinoma. Thyroid 2010; 20(2):173–9.
[41] Denicoff KD, Joffe RT, Lakshmanan MC, Robbins J, Rubinow DR. Neuropsychiatric manifestations of altered thyroid state. Am.J.Psychiatry 1990; 147:94–9.
[42] Constant EL, Adam S, Seron X, Bruyer R, Seghers A, Daumerie C. Anxiety and depression, attention, and executive functions in hypothyroidism. J Int Neuropsychol Soc 2005; 11(5):535–44.
[43] Schraml FV, Goslar PW, Baxter L, Beason-Held LL. Thyroid stimulating hormone and cognition during severe, transient hypothyroidism. Neuro Endocrinol. Lett 2011; 32(3):279–85.
[44] Reitan RM. The relation of the trail making test to organic brain damage. J.consult.Psychol 1955; 19:393–4.
[45] Kobal G, Hummel T, Sekinger B, Barz S, Roscher S, Wolf SR. "Sniffin' Sticks": Screening of olfactory performance. Rhinology 1996; 34:222–6.
[46] Heinzel A, Kley K, Mueller H, Hautzel H. A comparison of rh-TSH and thyroid hormone withdrawal in patients with differentiated thyroid cancer: preliminary evidence for an influence of age on the subjective well-being in hypothyroidism. Horm. Metab. Res 2012; 44(1):54–9.
[47] Felzen B, Rubinstein I, Lotan R, Binah O. Developmental changes in ventricular action potential properties in guinea-pigs are modulated by age-related changes in the thyroid state. J Mol.Cell Cardiol 1991; 23:787–94.
[48] Di Meo S, Martino Rosaroll P de, Piro MC, Leo T de. Modification of electrophysiological properties of rat heart with age. Arch Int.Physiol.Biochim.Biophys 1992; 100:7–11.
[49] Enderlin V, Alfos S, Pallet V, Garcin H, Azaïs-Braesco V, Jaffard R et al. Aging decreases the abundance of retinoic acid (RAR) and triiodothyronine (TR) nuclear receptor mRNA in rat brain: effect of the administration of retinoids. FEBS Lett 1997; 412(3):629–32.
[50] Pohunková D, Šulc J, Zamrazil V, Němec J, Veränderungen der menschlichen Stimme und Sprechweise in bezug zu Schilddrüsenfunktionsstörungen. Radiobiol.Radiother 1985; 26:192–4.

[51] Debruyne F, Ostyn F, Delaere P, Wellens W. Acoustic analysis of the speaking voice after thyroidectomy. J Voice 1997; 11(4):479–82.
[52] Beck K. Optische Messung der Verschmelzungsfrequenz zur Prüfung stoffwechselgebundener oder rein nervöser Funktionszustände. Klin.Wochenschr 1949; 27:210.
[53] Enzer N, Simonson E, Blankenstein SS. The state of sensory and motor centers in patients with circulatory insufficiency and in patients with hypothyroidism. Am.J.Physiol 1941; 133:269.
[54] Levander S, Rosenqvist U. Cerebral function in hypothyroid patients. A study of the vigilance level in patients with hypothyroidism before and during substitution therapy. Neuropsychobiol 1979; 5:274–81.
[55] Wisowaty JJ. Estimates for the temporal response characteristics of chromatic pathways. J Opt Soc Am 1981; 71:970–7.
[56] Gouras P, Zrenner E. Enchancement of luminance flicker by color-opponent mechanisms. Science 1979; 205:587–9.
[57] Takeda M, Onoda N, Suzuki M. Characterization of thyroid hormone effect on the visual system of the adult rat. Thyroid 1994; 4:467–74.
[58] Takeda M, Kakegawa T, Suzuki M. Effect of thyroidectomy on photoreceptor cells in adult rat retina. Life Sci 1996; 58:631–7.
[59] Torrents E, Cervino J, Maggiolo J, Navarro A, Zaldua Delfino E de, Mussio Fournier J. Modifications de l'électrorétinogramme (E.R.G.) dans le myxoedème. Presse Medicale 1954; 62:1716–7.
[60] Pearlman JT, Burian HM. Electroretinographic findings in thyroid dysfunction. Am.J.Ophthalmol 1964; 58:216–26.
[61] Miliczek K. Der Einfluß des Thyreotropin-Releasing-Hormons (TRH) auf retinale Adaptationsvorgänge. MD Thesis, University of Tübingen; 1993.
[62] Mallik TK, Wilber JF, Pegues J. Measurements of thyrotropin-releasing hormone-like material in human peripheral blood by affinity chromatography and radioimmunoassay. J. Clin. Endocrinol.Metab 1982; 54:1194–8.
[63] Wilson WP, Johnson JE, Feist FW. Thyroid hormone and brain function. II. Changes in photically elicited EEG responses following the administration of triiodothyronine to normal subjects. EEG Clin. Neurophysiol 1964; 16:329–31.
[64] van de Grind WA, Grüsser O, Lunkenheimer H. Temporal transfer properties of the afferent visual system. Psychophysical, neurophysiological and theoretical investigations. In: Autrum H, Jung R, Loewenstein W, MacKay D, Teuber H, editors. Handbook of Sensory Physiology, Vol VII/3 Central processing of visual information A. Heidelberg, New York: Springer; 1973. p. 433–573 .
[65] Simonson E, Brožek J, Flicker fusion frequency. Background and applications. Physiol.Rev 1952; 32:349–78.
[66] Smith JM, Misiak H. Critical flicker frequency (CFF) and psychotropic drugs in normal human subjects-a review. Psychopharmacol 1976; 47:175–82.
[67] Zlody RL. The relationship between critical flicker frequency (CFF) and several intellectual measures. Am.J.Psychol 1965; 78:596–602.
[68] Jensen AR. Critical flicker frequency and intelligence. Intelligence 1983; 7:217–25.

[69] Ali MR, Al-Shatti A, Khaleque A, Khanam M, Ahmed RU. Critical flicker frequency of mentally retarded and normal persons. Percept.Mot.Skills 1994; 79:1235–8.
[70] Misiak H, Loranger AW. Cerebral dysfunction and intellectual impairment in old age. Science 1961; 134:1518–9.
[71] Dhamija RM, Verma A, Maheshwari MC, Kochupillai N. Visual evoked response in thyroid disorders. J.Assoc.Physicians India 1990; 38:246–7.
[72] Jalonen T, Akerman KEO. Single Transient Potassium Channels in Human Neuro-Blastoma Cells Induced to Differentiate Invitro. Neurosci.Lett 1988; 86(1):99–104.
[73] Khedr EM, El Toony LF, Tarkhan MN, Abdella G. Peripheral and central nervous system alterations in hypothyroidism: electrophysiological findings. Neuropsychobiology 2000; 41(2):88–94.
[74] Nazliel B, Akbay E, Irkeç C, Yetkin I, Ersoy R, Törüner F. Pattern visual evoked potential (PVEP) evaluation in hypothyroidism. J. Endocrinol. Invest 2002; 25(11):955–8.
[75] Nazliel B, Ylmaz M, Gökce M, Yetkin I, Baysal AI. Blink Reflex in Hypothyroidism. The Endocrinologist 2007; 17(3):144–7.
[76] Sanders V. Neurologic manifestations of myxedema. New England J.Med 1962; 266:547–52.
[77] Tonks CM. Mental illnesses in hypothyroid patients. Brit.J.Psychiat 1964; 110:706–10.
[78] Whybrow PC, Prange AJ, Treadway CR. Mental changes accompanying thyroid gland dysfunction. Arch.Gen.Psychiat 1969; 20:48–63.
[79] Haggerty JJ, JR, Evans DL, Prange AJ, JR. Organic brain syndrome associated with marginal hypothyroidism. Am.J.Psychiatry 1986; 143:785–6.
[80] Nickel SN, Frame B. Neurologic manifestations of myxedema. Neurology 1958; 8:511–7.
[81] Kudrjavcev T. Neurologic complications of thyroid dysfunction. Adv.Neurol 1978; 19:619–36.
[82] Goodenough DR, Sapan J, Cohen H, Portnoff G, Shapiro A. Some experiments concerning the effects of sleep on memory. Psychophysiology 1971; 8(6):749–62.
[83] Maquet P, Peigneux P, Laureys S, Boly M, Dang-Vu T, Desseilles M et al. Memory processing during human sleep as assessed by functional neuroimaging. Rev. Neurol. (Paris) 2003; 159(11 Suppl):6S27-9.
[84] Kales A, Heuser G, Jacobson A, Kales JD, Hanley J, Zweizig JR et al. All night sleep studies in hypothyroid patients, before and after treatment. J.Clin.Endocrinol.Metab 1967; 27:1593–9.
[85] Blasl C, Bohr KC, Dietzel ID, Reiners C. Tagesmüdigkeit bei Hypothyreose:Schlaf gestört, aber nicht durch Apnoe. Nuclear Med 1997; 36:A84.
[86] Reitan RM. Validity of the trail making test as an indicator of organic brain damage. Percept.Mot.Skills 1958; 8:271–6.
[87] Treadway CR, Prange AJ, JR, Doehne EF, Edens CJ, Whybrow PC. Myxedema Psychosis: Clinical and biochemical changes during recovery. J.Psychiat.Res 1967; 5:289–96.
[88] Wahlin TR, Bäckman L, Wahlin A, Winblad B. Trail Making Test performance in a community-based sample of healthy very old adults: effects of age on completion time, but not on accuracy. Arch.Gerontol.Geriatr 1996; 22:87–102.
[89] Smith CL, Granger CV. Hypothyroidism producing reversible dementia. Am.J.Phys.Med.Rehabil 1992; 71:28–30.

[90] Monzón Monguilod MJ, Pérez López-Fraile I. Hipotiroidismo subclínico como causa de deterioro cognitivo reversible. Neurología 1996; 11:353–6.

[91] Monzani F, Del Guerra P, Caraccio N, Pruneti CA, Pucci E, Luisi M et al. Subclinical hypothyroidism: neurobehavioral features and beneficial effect of L-thyroxine treatment. Clin.Investig 1993; 71:367–71.

[92] Baldini M, Vita A, Mauri MC, Amodei V, Carrisi M, Bravin S et al. Psychopathological and cognitive features in subclinical hypothyroidism. Prog.Neuro-Psychopharmacol.& Biol.Psychiat 1997; 21:925–35.

[93] Jensovsky J, Ruzicka E, Spackova N, Hejdukova B. Changes of event related potential and cognitive processes in patients with subclinical hypothyroidism after thyroxine treatment. Endocr Regul 2002; 36(3):115–22.

[94] Samuels MH. Cognitive function in untreated hypothyroidism and hyperthyroidism. Current Opinion in Endocrinology, Diabetes and Obesity 2008; 15(5):429–33.

[95] He X, Ma N, Pan Z, Wang Z, Li N, Zhang X et al. Functional magnetic resource imaging assessment of altered brain function in hypothyroidism during working memory processing. Eur. J. Endocrinol 2011; 164(6):951–9.

[96] Stern MH. Thyroid function and activity, speed, and timing aspects of behaviour. Canad.J.Psychol 1959; 13:43–8.

[97] Nazliel B, Yilmaz M, Kocer B, Yetkin I, Yesilbudak Z. Event related potentials in hypothyroidism. Electromyogr Clin Neurophysiol 2008; 48(5):203–8.

[98] Anjana Y, Tandon OP, Vaney N, Madhu SV. Cognitive status in hypothyroid female patients: event-related evoked potential study. Neuroendocrinology 2008; 88(1):59–66.

[99] Savage GH. Myxodema and its nervous symptoms. J.Mental Science 1880; 25:517–9.

[100] White EW. Myxoedema associated with insanity. The Lancet 1884; May 31:974–6.

[101] Schaupp H, Seilz J. Geruch und Geschmack bei endokrinen Erkrankungen. Arch.klin.exp.Ohr.-,Nas.-u.Kehlk.Heilk 1969; 195:179–91.

[102] Deems DA, Doty RL, Settle RG, Moore-Gillon V, Shaman P, Mester AF et al. Smell and taste disorders, a study of 750 patients from the university of Pennsylvania smell and taste center. Arch.Otolaryngol.Head Neck Surg 1991; 117:519–28.

[103] Mattes RD, Heller AD, Rivlin RS. Abnormalities in suprathreshold taste function in early hypothyroidism in humans. In: Meiselman H, Rivlin R, editors. Clinical Measurement of Taste and Smell. New York, Toronto, London: Macmillan; 1986. p. 467–86

[104] Lewitt MS, Laing DG, Panhuber H, Corbett A, Carter JN. Sensory perception and hypothyroidism. Chemical Senses 1989; 14:537–46.

[105] Pittman JA, Beschi RJ. Taste thresholds in hyper- and hypothyroidism. Clin.Endocrinol.Metabolism 1967; 27:895–6.

[106] Paternostro MA, Meisami E. Developmental plasticity of the rat olfactory receptor sheet as shown by complete recovery of surface area and cell number from extensive early hypothyroid growth retardation. Dev.Brain Res 1993; 76:151–61.

[107] Mackay-Sim A, Beard MD. Hypothyroidism disrupts neural development in the olfactory epithelium of adult mice. Dev.Brain Res 1987; 36:190–8.

[108] Brosvic GM, Doty RL, Rowe MM, Harron A, Kolodiy N. Influences of hypothyroidism on the taste detection performance of rats: a signal detection analysis. Behav.Neurosci 1992; 106:992–8.

[109] Brosvic GM, Risser JM, Mackay-Sim A, Doty RL. Odor detection performance in hypothyroid and euthyroid rats. Physiology & Behavior 1996; 59:117–21.
[110] Schneeberg NG. Loss of sense of taste due to methylthiouracil therapy. JAMA 1952; 149:1091–3.
[111] Hallmann BL, Hurst JW. Loss of taste as toxic effect of methimazole (tapazole) therapy. JAMA 1953; 152:322.
[112] Erikssen J, Seegaard E, Naess K. Side-effect of thiocarbamides. The Lancet 1975; January 25:231–2.
[113] Kolenda K. Geschmacksstörungen und Leberparenchymschäden bei der Behandlung mit Thiamazol. Dtsch.med.Wschr 1976; 101:84–6.
[114] Neundörfer B. Geruchs- und Geschmacksstörungen unter der Behandlung mit Thiamazol und Carbimazol. Nervenarzt 1987; 58:61–2.
[115] Genter MB, Deamer NJ, Blake BL, Wesley DS, Levi PE. Olfactory toxicity of methimazole: dose-response and structure- activity studies and characterization of flavin-containing monooxygenase activity in the long-evans rat olfactory mucosa. Toxicol.Pathol 1995; 23:477–86.
[116] Sakamoto T, Kondo K, Kashio A, Suzukawa K, Yamasoba T. Methimazole-induced cell death in rat olfactory receptor neurons occurs via apoptosis triggered through mitochondrial cytochromec-mediated caspase-3 activation pathway. J. Neurosci. Res. 2007; 85(3):548–57.
[117] Alexander C, Bader JB, Schaefer A, Finke C, Kirsch C. Intermediate and long-term side effects of high-dose radioiodine therapy for thyroid carcinoma. J.Nuclear Med 1998; 39:1551–4.
[118] Femiano F, Lanza A, Buonaiuto C, Gombos F, Nunziata M, Cuccurullo L et al. Burning mouth syndrome and burning mouth in hypothyroidism: proposal for a diagnostic and therapeutic protocol. Oral Surgery, Oral Medicine, Oral Pathology, Oral Radiology, and Endodontology 2008; 105(1):e22.
[119] Haubrich J. Tierexperimentelle histologisch-histochemische Untersuchungen zur Formalgenese der hypothyreotisch bedingten Schwerhörigkeit. Acta Otolaryngol. (Stockh.) 1975; Suppl. 332:1-56.
[120] Rubenstein M, Rubenstein C, Theodor R. Hearing dysfunction associated with congenital sporadic hypothyroidism. Ann.Otol 1974; 83:815–9.
[121] Vos JA de. Deafness in hypothyroidism. J.Laryngol.Otol 1963; 77:390–414.
[122] Bhatia PL, Gupta OP, Agrawal MK, Mishr SK. Audiological and vestibular function tests in hypothyroidism. Laryngoscope 1977; 87:2082–9.
[123] Parving A, Ostri B, Bretlau P, Hansen JM, Parving H. Audiological and temporal bone findings in myxedema. Ann.Otol.Rhinol.Laryngol 1986; 95:278–83.
[124] Rubinstein M, Perlstein TP, Hildesheimer M. Cochlear action potentials in experimentally induced hypothyroidism in guinea pigs. Acta Otolaryngol.(Stockh.) 1975; Suppl.331:1-10.
[125] Meyerhoff WL. Hypothyroidism and the ear: electrophysiological, morphological, and chemical considerations. Laryngoscope 1979; 89, Suppl. 19:1–25.
[126] Legrand C, Bréhier A, Clavel MC, Thomasset M, Rabié A. Cholecalcin (28-kDa CaBP) in the rat cochlea. Development in normal and hypothyroid animals. An immunocytochemical study. Dev.Brain Res 1988; 38:121–9.

[127] Knipper M, Gestwa L, Cate W ten, Lautermann J, Brugger H, Maier H et al. Distinct thyroid hormone-dependent expression of TrkB and p75 NGFR in nonneuronal cells during the critical TH-dependent period of the cochlea. J.Neurobiol 1999; 38:338–56.

[128] Rüsch A, Erway LC, Oliver D, Vennström B, Forrest D. Thyroid hormone beta-dependent expression of a potassium conductance in inner hair cells at the onset of hearing. Proc.Natl.Acad.Sci 1998; 95:15758–62.

[129] Brandt N, Kuhn S, Munkner S, Braig C, Winter H, Blin N et al. Thyroid hormone deficiency affects postnatal spiking activity and expression of Ca2+ and K+ channels in rodent inner hair cells. J Neurosci 2007; 27(12):3174–86.

[130] Friauf E, Wenz M, Oberhofer M, Nothwang HG, Balakrishnan V, Knipper M et al. Hypothyroidism impairs chloride homeostasis and onset of inhibitory neurotransmission in developing auditory brainstem and hippocampal neurons. Eur.J Neurosci 2008; 28(12):2371–80.

[131] Heinemann M. Das Hörvermögen bei Hyothyreosen. Z.Laryngol.Rhinol.Otol 1968; 47:806–13.

[132] Kemp WR. Deafness in Myxoedema. Br.Med.J 1907; 1:375.

[133] King JW. Deafness in myxoedema. Br.Med.J 1907; 1:562–3.

[134] Hilger JA. Otolaryngologic aspects of hypometabolism. Ann.Otol.Rhinol.Laryngol 1956; 65:395–413.

[135] Ritter FN, Lawrence M. Reversible hearing loss in human hypothyroidism and correlated changes in the chick inner ear. Laryngoscope 1960; 70:393–407.

[136] Yan-You W, Shu-Hua Y. Improvement in hearing among otherwise normal schoolchildren in iodine-deficient areas of Guizhou, China, following use of iodised salt. The Lancet 1985; September 7:518–20.

[137] Post JT. Hypothyroid deafness. A clinical study of sensori-neural deafness associated with hypothyroidism. Laryngoscope 1964; 74:221–32.

[138] Mra Z, Wax MK. Effects of acute thyroxin depletion on hearing in humans. Laryngoscope 1999; 109:343–50.

[139] Katz J. Effects of thyroxine depletion on hearing. Seminars in Hearing 1993; 14:265–70.

[140] Kohonen A, Jauhiainen T, Liewendahl K, Tarkkanen J, Kaimio M. Deafness in experimental hypo- and hyperthyroidism. Laryngoscope 1971; 81:947–56.

[141] Withers BT, Reuter SH, Janeke JB. The effects of hypothyroidism on the ears of cats and squirrel monkeys: a pilot study. Laryngoscope 1972; 82:779–84.

[142] Ruiz-Marcos A, Salas J, Sanchez-Toscano F, Escobar del Rey F, Morreale Escobar G de. Effect of neonatal and adult-onset hypothyroidism on pyramidal cells of the rat auditory cortex. Dev.Brain Res 1983; 9:205–13.

[143] Vanasse M, Fischer C, Berthezène F, Roux Y, Volman G, Mornex R. Normal brainstem auditory evoked potentials in adult hypothyroidism. Laryngoscope 1989; 99:302–6.

[144] Nemni R, Bottacchi E, Fazio R, Mamoli A, Corbo M, Camerlingo M et al. Polyneuropathy in hypothyroidism: clinical, electrophysiological and morphological findings in four cases. J.Neurol.Neurosurg.Psychiatr 1987; 50:1454–60.

[145] Rizzo V, Crupi D, Bagnato S, Quartarone A, Benvenga S, Bartolone L et al. Neural response to transcranial magnetic stimulation in adult hypothyroidism and effect of replacement treatment. J Neurol.Sci 2008; 266(1-2):38–43. Available from: URL:PM:17900624.

[146] Song T, Kim S, Kim GS, Choi Y, Kim W. The prevalence of thyrotoxicosis-related seizures. Thyroid 2010; 20(9):955–8.

[147] Schriefl S, Steinberg TA, Matiasek K, Ossig A, Fenske N, Fischer A. Etiologic classification of seizures, signalment, clinical signs, and outcome in cats with seizure disorders: 91 cases (2000-2004). J Am.Vet.Med.Assoc 2008; 233(10):1591–7.

[148] Seyfried TN, Glaser GH, Yu RK. Thyroid hormone influence on the susceptibility of mice to audiogenic seizures. Science 1979; 205(4406):598–600.

[149] Gould E, Allan MD, McEwen BS. Dendritic spine density of adult hippocampal pyramidal cells is sensitive to thyroid hormone. Brain Res 1990; 525:327–9.

[150] Ruiz-Marcos A, Cartagena Abella P, García García A, Escobar del Rey F, Morreale Escobar G de. Rapid effects of adult-onset hypothyroidism on dendritic spines of pyramidal cells of the rat cerebral cortex. Exp.Brain Res 1988; 73:583–8.

[151] Madeira MD, Sousa N, Lima-Andrade MT, Calheiros F, Cadete-Leite A, Paula-Barbosa MM. Selective vulnerability of the hippocampal pyramidal neurons to hypothyroidism in male and female rats. J.Comp.Neurol 1992; 322:501–18.

[152] Hun H, Prudden TM. Myxodema, four cases with two autopsies. Am.J.Med.Sci 1888; 96:140–56.

[153] Uyematsu S. A case of myxedematous psychosis. Clinical and pathologic report. Arch.Neurol.Psychiat 1920; 3:252–76.

[154] Johnstone EC, Owens DGC, Crow TJ, Colter N, Lawton CA, Jagoe R et al. Hypothyroidism as a correlate of lateral ventricular enlargement in manic-depressive and neurotic illness. Br.J.Psychiat 1986; 148:317–21.

[155] del Ser T, Iriarte I, Pondal M, Molina JA. Trastornos neuropsicológicos de la demencia hipotiroidea. Descripcíon de un caso. Neurología 1990; 5:246–50.

[156] Oh JD, Butcher LL, Woolf NJ. Thyroid hormone modulates the development of cholinergic terminal fields in the rat forebrain: relation to nerve growth factor receptor. Dev.Brain Res 1991; 59:133–42.

[157] Landa ME, González Burgos G, Cardinali DP. In vitro effect of thyroxine on cholinergic neurotransmission in rat sympathetic superior cervical ganglion. Neuroendocrinol 1991; 54:552–8.

[158] Salvati S, Attorri L, Campeggi LM, Olivieri A, Sorcini M, Fortuna S et al. Effect of propylthiouracil-induced hypothyroidism on cerebral cortex of young and aged rats: Lipid composition of synaptosomes, muscarinic receptor sites, and acetylcholinesterase activity. Neurochem.Res 1994; 19:1181–6.

[159] Riekkinen P, Buzsaki G, Riekkinen P, JR, Soininen H, Partanen J. The cholinergic system and EEG slow waves. EEG clin.Neurophysiol 1991; 78:89–96.

[160] Walker P, Weichsel ME, JR, Fisher DA, Gou SM. Thyroxine increases nerve growth factor concentration in adult mouse brain. Science 1979; 204:427–9.

[161] Rastogi RB, Singhal RL. Influence of neonatal and adult hyperthyroidism on behavior and biosynthetic capacity for norepinephrine, dopamine and 5-hydroxytryptamine in rat brain. J.Pharmacol.Exp.Therapeutics 1976; 198:609–18.

[162] Ito JM, Valcana T, Timiras PS. Effect of hypo- and hyperthyroidism on regional monoamine metabolism in the adult rat brain. Neuroendocrinol 1977; 24:55–64.

[163] Klawans HL, JR, Shenker DM. Observations on the dopaminergic nature of hyperthyroid chorea. J.Neural Transm 1972; 33:73–81.

[164] Henley WN, Chen X, Klettner C, Bellush LL, Notestine MA. Hypothyroidism increases serotonin turnover and sympathetic activity in the adult rat. Can.J.Physiol.Pharmacol 1991; 69:205–10.
[165] Sandrini M, Vitale G, Vergoni AV, Ottani A, Bertolini A. Effect of acute and chronic treatment with triiodothyronine on serotonin levels and serotonergic receptor subtypes in the rat brain. Life Sci 1996; 18:1551–9.
[166] Gross G, Brodde O, Schümann H. Decreased number of ß-adrenoceptors in cerebral cortex of hypothyroid rats. Eur.J.Pharmacol 1980; 61:191–4.
[167] Whybrow PC, Prange AJ. A hypothesis of thyroid-catecholamine-receptor interaction. Arch.Gen.Psychiat 1981; 38:106–13.
[168] Sandrini M, Marrama D, Vergoni AV, Bertolini A. Effects of thyroid status on the characteristics of alpha1-, alpha2-, beta, imipramine and GABA receptors in the rat brain. Life Sci 1991; 48:659–66.
[169] Dratman MB, Gordon JT. Thyroid hormones as neurotransmitters. Thyroid 1996; 6:639–47.
[170] Kragie L. Neuropsychiatric implications of thyroid hormone and benzodiazepine interactions. Endocrine Res 1993; 19:1–32.
[171] Davidoff RA, Ruskin HM. The effects of microelectrophoretically applied thyroid hormone on single cat central nervous system neurons. Neurology 1972; 22:467–72.
[172] Bergh JJ, Lin HY, Lansing L, Mohamed SN, Davis FB, Mousa S et al. Integrin alphaVbeta3 contains a cell surface receptor site for thyroid hormone that is linked to activation of mitogen-activated protein kinase and induction of angiogenesis. Endocrinol 2005; 146(7):2864–71.
[173] Martin JV, Williams DB, Fitzgerald RM, Im HK, Vonvoigtlander PF. Thyroid hormonal modulation of the binding and activity of the GABAA receptor complex of brain. Neurosci 1996; 73:705–13.
[174] Puia G, Losi G. Thyroid hormones modulate GABA(A) receptor-mediated currents in hippocampal neurons. Neuropharmacology 2011; 60(7-8):1254–61.
[175] Makii EA, Nerush PA, Rodinskii AG, Myakoushko VA. Evoked activity of afferent and efferent fibers of the sciatic nerve in rats under conditions of experimental hyperthyroidism. Neurophysiology 2002; 34:44–51.
[176] Bernal J. Thyroid hormones and brain development. Vitam.Horm 2005; 71:95–122.
[177] Short MJ, Wilson WP, Gills JP, JR. Thyroid hormone and brain function. IV. Effect of triiodothyronine on visual evoked potentials and electroretinogram in man. EEG clin.Neurophysiol 1968; 25:123–7.
[178] Takahashi K, Fujitani Y. Somatosensory and visual evoked potentials in hyperthyroidism. EEG clin.Neurophysiol 1970; 29:551–6.
[179] Hodgkin A. The optimum density of sodium channels in an unmyelinated nerve. Phil.Trans.R.Soc.Lond.B 1975; 270:297–300.
[180] Kopell BS, Wittner WK, Lunde D, Warrick G, Edwards D. Influence of triiodothyronine on selective attention in man as measured by the visual averaged evoked potential. Psychosomatic Med 1970; 32:495–502.
[181] Felzen B, Sweed Y, Binah O. Electrophysiological effects of thyroid hormones in guinea-pig ventricular muscle: time course and relationships to blood levels. J Mol.Cell Cardiol 1989; 21:1151–61.

[182] Di Meo S, Martino Rosaroll P de, Piro MC, Leo T de. Ventricular electrophysiological properties in normal and congenitally hypothyroid neonatal rats. Arch Int.Physiol.Biochim.Biophys 1994; 102:129–34.
[183] Bosch RF, Wang Z, Li GR, Nattel S. Electrophysiological mechanisms by which hypothyroidism delays repolarization in guinea pig hearts. Am.J Physiol 1999; 277(1 Pt 2):H211.
[184] Valcavi R, Menozzi C, Roti E, Zini M, Lolli G, Roti S et al. Sinus node function in hyperthyroid patients. J Clin.Endocrinol.Metab 1992; 75:239–42.
[185] Craelius W, Green WL, Harris DR. Acute effects of thyroid hormone on sodium currents in neonatal myocytes. Biosci.Rep 1990; 10:309–15.
[186] Harris DR, Green WL, Craelius W. Acute thyroid hormone promotes slow inactivation of sodium current in neonatal cardiac myocytes. Biochem.Biophys.Acta 1991; 1045:175–81.
[187] Wang YG, Dedkova EN, Fiening JP, Ojamaa K, Blatter LA, Lipsius SL. Acute exposure to thyroid hormone increases Na+ current and intracellular Ca2+ in cat atrial myocytes. J Physiol 2003; 546(Pt 2):491–9.
[188] Dudley SCJ, Baumgarten CM. Bursting of cardiac sodium channels after acute exposure to 3,5,3'-triiodo-L-thyronine. Circ.Res 1993; 73:301–13.
[189] Sen L, Sakaguchi Y, Cui G. G protein modulates thyroid hormone-induced Na(+) channel activation in ventricular myocytes. Am.J Physiol Heart Circ.Physiol 2002; 283(5):H2119.
[190] Schmidt BM, Martin N, Georgens AC, Tillmann HC, Feuring M, Christ M et al. Nongenomic cardiovascular effects of triiodothyronine in euthyroid male volunteers. J Clin.Endocrinol.Metab 2002; 87(4):1681–6.
[191] Sunagawa M, Yamakawa M, Shimabukuro M, Higa N, Takasu N, Kosugi T. Electrophysiologic characteristics of atrial myocytes in levo-thyroxine-treated rats. Thyroid 2005; 15(1):3–11.
[192] Potthoff O, Dietzel ID. Thyroid hormone regulates Na+ currents in cultured hippocampal neurons from postnatal rats. Proc.R.Soc.Lond.B 1997; 264:367–73.
[193] Hoffmann G, Dietzel ID. Thyroid hormone regulates excitability in central neurons from postnatal rats. Neurosci 2004; 125(2):369–79.
[194] Benvenuti S, Luciani P, Cellai I, Deledda C, Baglioni S, Saccardi R et al. Thyroid hormones promote cell differentiation and up-regulate the expression of the seladin-1 gene in in vitro models of human neuronal precursors. J Endocrinol 2008; 197(2):437–46.
[195] Sanchez-Alonso JL, Munoz-Cuevas J, Vicente-Torres MA, Colino A. Role of low-voltage-activated calcium current on the firing pattern alterations induced by hypothyroidism in the rat hippocampus. Neuroscience 2010; 171(4):993–1005.
[196] Sanchez-Alonso JL, Sanchez-Aguilera A, Vicente-Torres MA, Colino A. Intrinsic excitability is altered by hypothyroidism in the developing hippocampal CA1 pyramidal cells. Neuroscience 2012; 207:37–51.
[197] Yonkers MA, Ribera AB. Sensory neuron sodium current requires nongenomic actions of thyroid hormone during development. J Neurophysiol 2008; 100(5):2719–25.
[198] Yonkers MA, Ribera AB. Molecular components underlying nongenomic thyroid hormone signaling in embryonic zebrafish neurons. Neural Dev 2009; 4:20.
[199] Hines ML, Carnevale NT. The NEURON simulation environment. Neural Comput 1997; 9:1179–209.

[200] Deisz RA. A tetrodotoxin-insensitive [corrected] sodium current initiates burst firing of neocortical neurons. Neuroscience 1996; 70(2):341–51.
[201] Hartmann HA, Colom LV, Sutherland ML, Noebels JL. Selective localization of cardiac SCN5A sodium channels in limbic regions of rat brain. Nat. Neurosci 1999; 2(7):593–5.
[202] Donahue LM, Coates PW, Lee VH, Ippensen DC, Arze SE, Poduslo SE. The cardiac sodium channel mRNA is expressed in the developing and adult rat and human brain. Brain Res 2000; 887(2):335–43.
[203] Perrild H, Hansen JM, Arnung K, Olsen PZ, Danielsen U. Intellectual impairment after hyperthyroidism. Acta Endocrinol 1986; 112:185–91.
[204] Zander Olsen P, Stoier M, Siersbaek-Nielsen K, Molholm Hansen J, Schioler M, Kristensen M. Electroencephalographic findings in hyperthyroidism. EEG clin.Neurophysiol 1972; 32:171–7.
[205] Dunleavy DLF, Oswald I, Brown P, Strong JA. Hyperthyroidism, sleep and growth hormone. EEG clin.Neurophysiol 1974; 36:259–63.
[206] Tauboll E, Lindstrom S, Stokke KT, Gjerstad L. Triiodothyronine and brain excitability. Epilepsia 1990; 31(6):713–7.
[207] Niederkinkhaus V, Marx R, Hoffmann G, Dietzel ID. Thyroid hormone (T3)-induced up-regulation of voltage-activated sodium current in cultured postnatal hippocampal neurons requires secretion of soluble factors from glial cells. Mol.Endocrinol 2009; 23(9):1494–504.
[208] Gavaret JM, Toru-Delbauffe D, Baghdassarian-Chalaye D, Pomerance M, Pierre M. Thyroid hormone action: induction of morphological changes and protein secretion in astroglial cell cultures. Brain Res.Dev.Brain Res 1991; 58(1):43–9.
[209] Trentin AG, Alvarez-Silva M, Moura Neto V. Thyroid hormone induces cerebellar astrocytes and C6 glioma cells to secrete mitogenic growth factors. Am.J Physiol Endocrinol.Metab 2001; 281(5):E1088.
[210] Gomes FCA, Maia CG, Menezes JRL de, Moura Neto V. Cerebellar astrocytes treated by thyroid hormone modulate neuronal proliferation. Glia 1999; 25(3):247–55.
[211] Giordano T, Pan JB, Casuto D, Watanabe S, Arneric SP. Thyroid hormone regulation of NGF, NT-3 and BDNF RNA in the adult rat brain. Mol.Brain Res 1992; 16:239–45.
[212] Clauss W, Hoffmann B, Krattenmacher R, van Driessche W. Current-noise analysis of Na absorption in the embryonic coprodeum: stimulation by aldosterone and thyroxine. Am J Physiol 1993; 265:R1100.
[213] Mata M, Fink DJ, Gainer H, Smith CB, Davidsen L, Savaki H et al. Activity-dependent energy metabolism in rat posterior pituitary primarily reflects sodium pump activity. J. Neurochem 1980; 34(1):213–5.
[214] Kaplan JH. Biochemistry of Na,K-ATPase. Annu. Rev. Biochem 2002; 71:511–35.
[215] Orlowski J, Lingrel JB. Tissue-specific and developmental regulation of rat Na,K-ATPase catalytic alpha isoform and beta subunit mRNAs. J. Biol. Chem 1988; 263(21):10436–42.
[216] Huguenard JR, Hamill OP, Prince DA. Developmental changes in Na+conductances in rat neocortical neurons: Appearance of a slowly inactivating component. J.Neurophysiol 1988; 59:778–95.

[217] Kamitani T, Ikeda U, Muto S, Kawakami K, Nagano K, Tsuruya Y et al. Regulation of Na,K-ATPase gene expression by thyroid hormone in rat cardiocytes. Circ. Res 1992; 71(6):1457–64.

[218] Gick GG, Ismail-Beigi F, Edelman IS. Thyroidal regulation of rat renal and hepatic Na,K-ATPase gene expression. J. Biol. Chem 1988; 263(32):16610–8.

[219] Lindholm DB. Thyroxine regulates the activity and the concentration of synaptic plasma membrane Na,K-ATPase in the developing rat brain cortex. Dev.Brain Res 1984; 15:83–8.

[220] Schmitt CA, McDonough AA. Thyroid hormone regulates alpha and alpha + isoforms of Na,K-ATPase during development in neonatal rat brain. J Biol.Chem 1988; 263(33):17643–9.

[221] Pacheco-Rosado J, Arias-Citalán G, Ortiz-Butrón R, Rodríquez-Páez L. Selective decrease of Na+/k+ -ATPase activity in the brain of hypothyroid rats. Proc. West. Pharmacol. Soc 2005; 48:52–4.

[222] Carageorgiou H, Pantos C, Zarros A, Stolakis V, Mourouzis I, Cokkinos D et al. Changes in acetylcholinesterase, Na+, K+-ATPase, and Mg2+-ATPase activities in the frontal cortex and the hippocampus of hyper- and hypothyroid adult rats. Metabolism-Clinical and Experimental 2007; 56(8):1104–10.

[223] Chaudhury S, Bajpai M, Bhattacharya S. Differential effects of hypothyroidism on Na-K-ATPase mRNA alpha isoforms in the developing rat brain. J. Mol. Neurosci 1996; 7(3):229–34.

[224] Banerjee B, Chaudhury S. Thyroidal regulation of different isoforms of NaKATPase in the primary cultures of neurons derived from fetal rat brain. Life Sci 2002; 71(14):1643–54.

[225] Banerjee B, Chaudhury S. Thyroidal regulation of different isoforms of NaKATPase in glial cells of developing rat brain. Life Sci 2001; 69(20):2409–17.

[226] Bajpai M, Mandal SK, Chaudhury S. Identification of thyroid regulatory elements in the Na-K-ATPase alpha 3 gene promoter. Molecular Biology Reports 2001; 28(1):1–7.

[227] Brodie C, Sampson SR. Characterization of thyroid hormone effects on Na-K pump and membrane potential of cultured rat skeletal myotubes. Endocrinol 1988; 123:891–7.

[228] Harrison AP, Clausen T. Thyroid hormone-induced upregulation of Na+ channels and Na+-K+ pumps: implications for contractility. Am J Physiol 1998; 274:R864.

[229] Wolitzky BA, Fambrough DM. Regulation of the (Na^+ + K^+)-Atpase in Cultured Chick Skeletal-Muscle - Modulation of Expression by the Demand for Ion-Transport. Journal of Biological Chemistry 1986; 261(21):9990–9.

[230] Westerholz S, Lima AD de, Voigt T. Regulation of early spontaneous network activity and GABAergic neurons development by thyroid hormone. Neuroscience 2010; 168(2):573–89.

Chapter 3

"Quo Vadis?" Deciphering the Code of Nongenomic Action of Thyroid Hormones in Mature Mammalian Brain

Pradip K. Sarkar

Additional information is available at the end of the chapter

1. Introduction

Thyroid hormones (TH) have major well-known actions on the growth and development of the maturing tissues including mammalian brain via activation of specific nuclear receptors leading to gene expression and subsequent target protein synthesis. Deficiency of THs has serious issues on the development on all types of tissues including brain leading to severe thyroid disorders and as a result imposes overall metabolic malfunctioning of all system organs. Endemic goiter was probably first described with cretinism by Paracelsus (1493 -1541) and by other physicians of the Alps and Central Europe. However, the relationship between cretinism and involvement of thyroid gland was lacking over centuries. Thyroid gland was literally described by Wharton in 1656. Since then the progress of research on thyroid gland gained attention particularly for its most observed pleiotypic action in number of species from aquatic animals to humans. Developments of new scientific technologies and the progress in the area of molecular biology from time to time are continually changing our concepts of the regulation of the functions of THs at the subcellular level [1,2].

Immunocytochemical localization studies revealed that TH receptors (TR) in adult vertebrates are highly concentrated within choroids plexus, dentate gyrus, hippocampus, amygdaloid complex, pyriform cortex, granular layer of cerebellum, mammillary bodies and medial geniculate bodies. Although specific nuclear receptors for THs in adult brain have been identified, their functions are unclear about target gene expression. Imunohistochemical mapping further documented that locus coeruleus norepinephrine stimulates active conversion of L-tetraiodothyronine (L-T4) to L-triiodothyronine (L-T3). A morphologic linking between central thyronergic and noradrenergic systems has been established. This changes in TH ontogeny gradually started drawing attention that possible

TH action in mature brain switches its role which may be different from its classical action mediated through nuclear receptors. As the brain approaches adulthood, nuclear levels of iodothyronines decline gradually reaching a plateau and maintain it, and the TH levels increase within nerve terminals of adult vertebrates [1]. In particular, it showed decrease in nuclear L-T3 receptor binding in adult brain compared to developing brain. These switching differences in TH ontogeny between developing and adult vertebrate brain has gradually interested investigators to search for new functional role and mechanism of action of TH. Nevertheless, the action of THs remained limitedly judged in mature mammalian central nervous system (CNS) [3,4].

Recent research highlights about the nonconventional nongenomic action of THs and its metabolites. Adult mammalian CNS is of specific interest. Clinical observations specifically have shown that the adult-onset thyroid disorders lead to several neuropsychological diseases including but not limited to anxiety, depression, mood disorders etc. in humans. These complications can be improved with appropriate adjustment of circulatory THs [5-8]. However, the defined mechanism to explain this is inadequate. The involvement of TH nuclear receptors in ameliorating these neuropsychiatric dysfunctions in mature CNS is controversial. Current knowledge about the TH-responsive gene expression in adult mammalian CNS is largely unavailable except some few discrete reports with differential effects in certain brain areas. Indication of new rapid nongenomic effects of THs and its metabolites, within seconds to minutes, poses special significance.

The interest about the action of TH in brain originated because like the classical neurotransmitters, catecholamines, THs are also derived from the amino acid, tyrosine. Tyrosine is decarboxylased by specific aromatic amino acid decarboxylase to produce catecholamines. There are possibilities that THs can also undergo decarboxylation and form biogenic amine-like neuroactive compounds, such as thyronamines or iodothyronamines as hypothesized. However recent experiment challenges this initial hypothesis since aromatic amino acid decarboxylase failed to produce this and thus presence of TH specific decarboxylase is speculated [9]. For example, L-T4 and L-T3 can be decarboxylated to produce L-T4-amine and L-T3-amine respectively (Figure 1). L-T3-amine can further be deiodinated to form L-T2-amine and then further deiodination can generate L-T1-amine. Important deaminated metabolites of L-T4 and L-T3 are tetraiodothyroacetic acid (TETRAC) and triiodothyroacetic acid (TRIAC) respectively [9,10]. Thyronamines may have neurotransmitter-like actions. However, no evidence is present to-date to identify physiologic formation of thyronamines that describe their physiologic functions, except one new report which identified 3-iodo-thyronamine in adult brain including other tissue homogenates in sub-picomolar concentrations [10]. Few pharmacologic actions for these synthetically prepared iodothyronamines are known in other tissues. This theory of action of thyroid hormones could be like classical neurotransmission led to search for the nongenomic mechanism of action of THs.

Thus, besides the genomic concepts, a parallel idea of nongenomic of TH action was emerging with demonstration of direct plasma membrane-TH interaction and expression of some hormonal effects in a variety of cells. These studies include activation on Ca^{2+}-ATPase

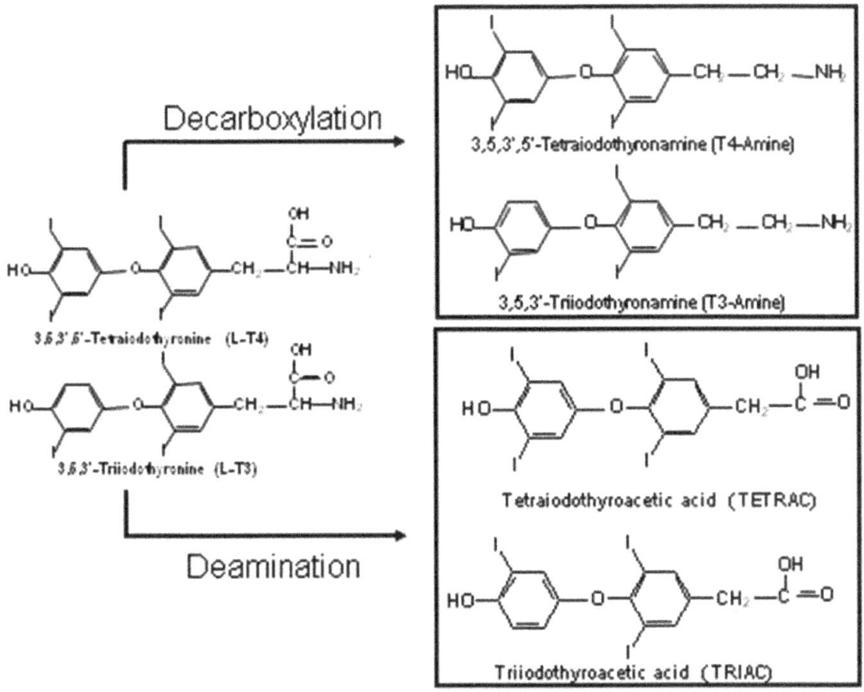

Figure 1. Thyroid hormones and their deaminated and decarboxylated products of interest.

in red blood cells, acetylcholinesterase in neuronal plasma membrane, inhibition of synaptosomal membrane Na^+-K^+-ATPase (NKA), rapid action of L-T3 on synaptosomal Ca^{2+}-influx, identification of specific L-T3-binding sites in rat thymocyte membrane, synaptosomal membrane, depolarization of actin filaments in cultured astrocytes by TH, and changes in second messengers and their corresponding regulatory systems following TH treatment [1,11,12].

Selective uptakes of THs have also been documented within the nerve terminals. Intravenous administration of [^{125}I]-L-T4 in rats followed by thaw mount autoradiography has described selective distribution of L-T4 in specific adult rat brain areas particularly within the nerve terminals. Within the nerve terminal this was concentrated as L-T3 [10]. Other reports about the transportation of TH in adult brain also indicated role of transthyretin as a major serum binding protein for TH required for its transportation in cerebrospinal fluids and ultimately enable crossing of TH of the blood brain barrier directing to the brain. A role of monocarboxylate anion transporter protein-8 (MCT-8) also has been found to play a major role in TH transportation across the plasma membrane [10]. Three important enzymes called monodeiodinase are involved in TH metabolism. These are 5′-deiodinase type I (D-I), 5′-deiodinase type II (D-II) and 5′-deiodinase type III (D-III). D-I and D-II catalyzes conversion of the L-T4 to L-T3. D-I is the major deiodinating enzyme in the peripheral tissues. In brain D-II is predominantly localized in glial cells, astrocytes, and in the tanycytes lining the lower part of the third ventricles. D-III catalyzes the conversion of L-T3 to L-T2. Concentration of L-T3 within the nervous system has been attributed to the brain D-II which has major functions in regulating the overall neuronal homeostasis for TH. Expression of D-II in nervous tissue is implicated in the neuronal uptake of the circulatory L-T4 and its conversion to L-T3 followed by its supply to the neuronal targets. Expression of D-II is an important protective mechanism against hypothyroidism. This prevalence of TH homeostasis is a preventive measure and thought to be neuroprotective [1,13-16].

Interest also materializes to explore further the nongenomic mechanism of action of THs in adult mammalian CNS. In this context TH-mediated signal transduction pathways are also being investigated. Particularly the regulation of the activation of the second messenger systems and subsequent protein phosphorylation are of much awareness. Understanding of the mechanism of action of TH in adult mammalian brain has key implications in the higher mental functions, learning and memory, and in the regulation of several neuropsychiatric disorders developed during adult-onset thyroid dysfunctions in humans.

2. Aim of the article

The major goal of this article is to search, discuss and review the nongenomic rapid actions of THs in mature mammalian CNS. This article aims to begin with observations describing subcellular distribution, and concentrations of THs within the brain and its biochemical and physiologic consequences, specific binding of THs onto the neuronal plasma membrane to examine for specific plasma membrane receptors of THs and correlate the receptor-binding followed by a specific cellular function. Next, the molecular basis of the TH and plasma membrane receptor interaction-mediated signals are evaluated via possible activation of G-protein signaling pathway, second messenger systems, and subsequent target protein phosphorylation.

3. Hypothesis

Thyroid hormones exercise a nongenomic action on the adult mammalian brain possibly by binding to neuronal membrane receptors followed by activation of second messenger cascade systems leading to substrate level protein phosphorylation and dephosphorylation by protein kinases and protein phosphatases (Figure 2).

4. Experimental tissue of interest

Author's experiments and results reported in this manuscript are obtained from the purified synaptosomes prepared from young adult rat brain cerebral cortex. Synaptosomes are subcellular nucleus-free preparation purified through density gradient centrifugation [17]. The question may arise why synaptosome? Synapses are the ultimate routes of communications in neurons where electrical impulses are normally translated to chemical signals from one neuron to the other leading to subsequent biochemical and physiologic events. This preparation is a fragment of neurons containing the neuronal membrane,

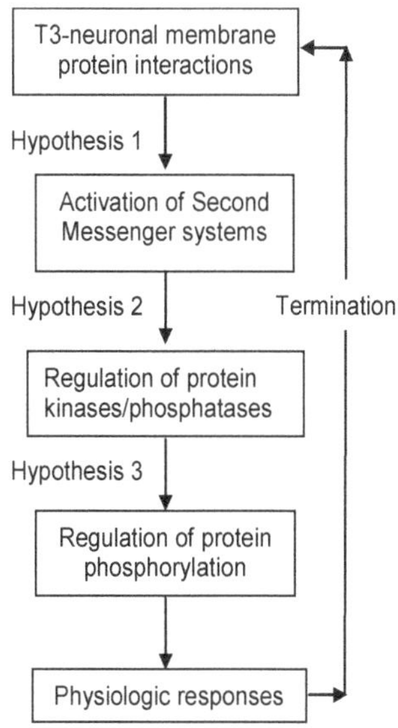

Figure 2. Hypothesis: Proposed nongenomic action of thyroid hormones in adult mammalian brain.

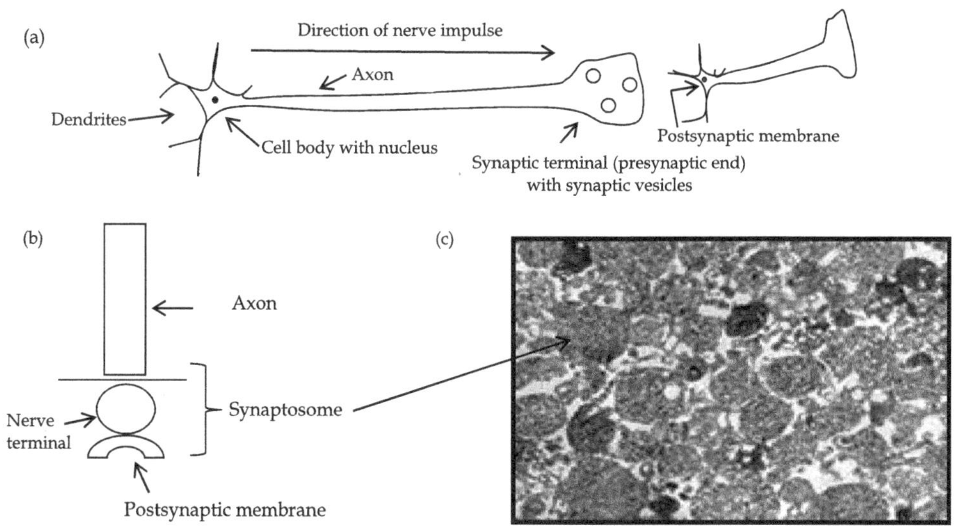

Figure 3. (a) A typical neuron. (b) Cartoon of a neuron showing synaptosome. (c) Scanning electron microscopic image of synaptosome.

Synaptic vesicles, and the other intracellular components (Figure 3). Synaptosomes can be considered as isolated nerve terminals. Synaptosomes are obtained after homogenization and fractionation of nerve tissue. The fractionation step involves several centrifugations steps to separate various organelles from the synaptosomes. Synaptosomes are formed from the phospholipid layer of the cell membrane and synaptic proteins such as receptors.

Synaptosomes are frequently used to study synaptic signal transduction pathways because they contain almost the entire molecular machinery necessary known for the uptake, storage, release of neurotransmitters, receptor properties, and enzyme actions etc.

5. Subcellular levels of L-triiodothyronine (L-T3) and L-thyroxine (L-T4) in adult rat brain cerebral cortex

As the brain approaches adulthood, nuclear iodothyronine concentrations gradually decreases reaching a plateau and maintains it, and the TH levels increase within nerve terminals of adult vertebrates [1,18-21]. It also demonstrated decrease in L-T3-binding in adult brain compared to developing brain.

Although, evidence of transportation ^{125}I-L-T3 and ^{125}I-L-T4 within the nerve terminal was demonstrated following intravenous injection in adult rat brain [10,18,19,22], its euthyroid concentrations and subcellular distribution was never been evaluated until recently [13,23]. Intravenous administration of [^{125}I]-L-T4 in rats followed by thaw mount autoradiography showed distribution of L-T4 in selective areas of adult brain in a saturable manner. Gradually L-T4 was concentrated more within nerve terminals fractions, where L-T4 was monodeiodinated to produce L-T3, the active form of TH [10]. L-T4 and L-T3 transportation within neurons are shown to occur by two different mechanisms. L-T3 is actively taken up in a saturable manner, while L-T4 transportation occurs by diffusion and in a non-saturable way. L-T4-transporation within the neuron is dependent upon L-T4-concentration gradient between extracellular and intracellular compartments and is maintained by high deiodination rate of L-T4 to L-T3 [24]. Role of transthyretin has also been described as a major binding protein in cerebrospinal fluid. Transthyretin has been implicated to facilitate L-T4 transportation across the blood-brain-barrier and finally into the brain. Recently MCT-8 has been ascribed to be the most effective TH transporter [25]. These MCT-8 are 12 transmembrane spanning proteins, and in particular plays a major role for very specific transportation of L-T3 within the neurons followed by the active conversion of the prohormone L-T4 to L-T3 by the D-II within the CNS [26]. D-II is essentially important for the conversion of the prohormone L-T4 into the active L-T3 within the CNS. However, understandings of the levels of THs within the neurons are imperative. This information is crucial to explore the role of L-T3 in neural signal transmission in mature brain. To help meet this requirement the following study was performed to quantify and compare the levels of THs in adult rat brain cerebral cortex.

5.1. Comparison of the levels of L-tetraiodothyronine (L-T4) and L-triiodothyronine (L-T3) in subcellular fractions

While serm levels of L-T4 (~ 41 ng/ml) and L-T3 (~ 0.7 ng/ml) were found consistent with the normal peripheral results, this assay system could not detect L-T4 in either synaptosomal or non-synaptic mitochondrial fractions. However, the L-T3 levels in synaptosomes (0.45±0.06 ng/mg synaptosomal protein), and non-synaptic mitochondria (1.44±0.12 ng/mg mitochondrial protein) were significant. The levels of L-T3 in non-synaptic mitochondria were ~3.2-fold higher compared to synaptosomal values in cerebral cortices [13,16]. The finding of undetectable levels of synaptosomal L-T4 was consistent with other studies [14,27,28]. A higher fractional rate of D-II activity that converts L-T4 to L-T3 is attributed [29,30].

This study quantifies the TH concentrations from adult rat brain synaptosomal and non-synaptic mitochondria. Although L-T4 levels could not be detected in synaptosomal and non-synaptic mitochondrial fractions, fair amounts of L-T3 were detected in these fractions purified from adult rat brain cerebral cortex [13,16]. Undetectable levels of synaptosomal L-T4 levels were also supported within synaptosomal fractions obtained from adult rat brain [27].

Despite very low levels of TH in hypothyroid condition as determined by serum levels of TH, previous report has shown that L-T3 production in brain is pretty high in stress situations like hypothyroidism [13]. D-II has also been shown to be activated in other stressful conditions and indicated to have a protective role in stressed brain [31]. Stimulated levels of D-II have been described during hypothyroidism. This supports the first initial report [13] of elevation of brain L-T3 levels during n-propylthiouracil (PTU)-induced hypothyroid conditions [14,15,32]. In brain, approximately 80% of the L-T3 is produced locally from L-T4 by D-II. The fractional rate of conversion of L-T4 to L-T3 is remarkably high in brain [29]. This might be a possible reason for undetectable L-T4 levels due to rapid conversion of L-T4 to L-T3 in these fractions. To detect the endogenous TH levels the subcellular fractions were ruptured hypo-osmotically. The use of 8-anilinonaphtho-sulfonic acid in the radioimmunoassay medium excluded the possibility of the non-detectable protein bound form of the hormone by releasing the endogenously bound form of the hormones [13].

Comparatively higher levels of L-T3 in the mitochondria may have implications on the mitochondrial bioenergetics such as, cellular oxygen consumption, oxidative phosphorylation and ATP synthesis, mitochondrial gene expression. These are few of the major regulatory functions of TH. THs also have been shown to affect mitochondrial genome mediated through imported isoforms of nuclear TH receptors and influence various mitochondrial transcription factors [3,33]. Concentration and localization of radiolabeled L-T3 within the nerve terminal was the first landmark research described in adult rat brain. This further followed with the immunohistochemical mapping demonstrating locus ceruleus norepinephrine stimulating active conversion of L-T4 to L-T3. This established a morphologic co-localization of central thyronergic and noradrenergic systems. Overall TH levels within different compartment of brain may have discrete, differential and potential regulatory function for neurotransmission in adult mammalian brain [10].

5.1.1. Thyroid hormone levels in hypothyroid rat cerebrocortical synaptosomes

Synaptosomal levels of L-T3 were also studied in different thyroidal conditions. Serum levels of L-T3 and L-T4 confirmed establishment of peripheral hypothyroidism induced by 14 days of intra-peritoneal (i. p.) injections of PTU (2 mg/g BW). However, surprisingly hypothyroid rat brain showed ~9.5-fold higher amount of L-T3 (126 nM) in synaptosomes compared to euthyroid control values. A single i. p. injection of L-T3 (2 μg/g BW) to the hypothyroid rats decreased the synaptosomal levels of L-T3 by ~1.6-fold compared to the hypothyroid rats and was still ~6-fold higher than the euthyroid value. An increase in ~2.5-fold of the L-T3 levels was noticed in euthyroid plus L-T3 (2 μg/g BW) group (Figure 4) [13]. Although the levels of L-T3 in whole rat brain homogenate was found to be in low nanomolar ranges [22], two concurrent reports estimated synaptosomal levels of L-T3 to be ~14.6 nM [23], and ~13 nM [13] in adult rat brain synaptosomes. Observation of high levels of synaptosomal L-T3 were also supportive [15] in hypothyroid rat cerebral cortex by ~1.7-fold compared to the control values maximally at day 4 of induction of hypothyroidism while the serum levels of L-T3 remained at the hypothyroid levels.

Hypothyroid condition shows an appreciable decline in both serum L-T4 and L-T3 level in rats in a usual way as found by other investigators [34]. Although it has been shown earlier that in hypothyroid condition, the whole brain, or different regions of the brain, maintain similar levels of L-T3 compared to the euthyroid control rats through increased activity of D-II, and corresponding high fractional rate of L-T4 to L-T3 conversion [35,36], insufficient evidence is available except for a few recent reports to quantitate the synaptosomal concentration of thyroid hormones. Approximately 8-fold higher concentration of L-T3 has been found in synaptosome compared to the whole brain in euthyroid rats. Our observation of approximately 9.5-fold higher L-T3 content in synaptosome of hypothyroid rats compared to the euthyroid controls may be the result of a higher fractional rate of L-T3 production by increased activity of D-II, and a correspondingly higher selective uptake and concentration of L-T3 molecules in the synaptosomes to cope up with the physiological need of THs in this tissue at this condition [13,23,37,38].

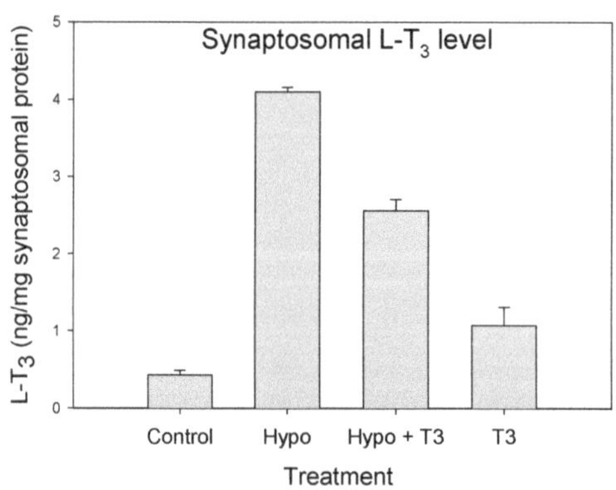

Figure 4. L-T3 levels in rat cerebrocortical synaptosomes in various thyroid states. (Ref. Sarkar and Ray 1994, Neuropsychopharmacology 11: 151-155 acknowledged [13]).

In euthyroid rat brain, selective uptake of ^{125}I-L-T3 and its concentration in synaptosomal compartment have been demonstrated [10]. In addition, the use of hypothyroid animals only after 14 days of PTU treatment, where some adaptive mechanisms still unknown in nature prevail, do not reach the equilibrium as compared to the animals kept in chronic hypothyroid condition for a much longer duration as used by other workers. This may be one of the reasons for maintaining a high level of synaptosomal L-T3 in our hypothyroid rats. Expression of the data in different forms such as per gram organ (brain) basis, or per mg compartmental (synaptosomal) protein basis, as presented in our experiment, also becomes an additive factor for discrepancies among different groups of workers regarding the quantitative aspects of L-T3 or L-T4 in the brain [23,34,38,39]. The fall in L-T3 concentration in synaptosomes prepared from L-T3-treated hypothyroid rat cerebral cortex may be the result of inhibition of D-II activity after 24 hours of the L-T3 administration, in the presence of the considerable amount of exogenous L-T3. An inhibition in the activity of D-II has been noticed within 4 hours of L-T3 treatment to the thyroidectomized rats. A rise in the synaptosomal L-T3 level in the hypothyroid rats, and a fall in the same in the L-T3-treated hypothyroid animals after 24 hours of L-T3-treatment, also reflects the tendency for a compensatory regulatory mechanism of thyroid hormone metabolism in the adult rat brain in altered thyroid conditions, although the nature of the mechanism remains unknown. L-T3-treated control rats have shown higher levels of synaptosomal L-T3, compared to the control values. This may be a result of the extra L-T3 transport influenced by a high dose of exogenously administered L-T3 (2 μg/g) [18,19,24].

Observation of undetected levels of L-T4 within cerebrocortical synaptosomes may reflect a state of rapid conversion of L-T4 to L-T3 in the brain by D-II enzyme. Other researchers have already shown that after intravenous administration of radiolabeled L-T4 and L-T3, the hormone is concentrated as L-T3 in a synaptosomal fraction of the whole rat brain, and L-T4 to L-T3 conversion occurs very rapidly within the nerve cells. L-T3 formed in the neuronal cell body then may be translocated down the axon to the synaptic ends. Saturable and nonsaturable uptake of L-T3 and L-T4 in isolated synaptosomes in an *in vitro* model also indicated two-component L-T3-uptake system [18,19,24,37,38].

The prediction of a role of D-II as suggested [13] is further supported by few other studies [15,31]. Increased D-II activity is suggested in hypothyroid brain. This is attributed to the maintenance of normal brain concentrations of L-T3 even under low peripheral levels of L-T4 [31]. The high level of L-T3 as observed by us is supported and suggested for maintenance of brain homeostasis. This demonstrated onset of a central homeostasis for THs in adult hypothyroid brain between the 1st and 2nd day, its maintenance for about 16-18 days and thereafter declined between the 18-20th day [15]. This report also confirms and confers higher activity of D-II (~ 1.6-fold higher compared to control) within the cerebrocortical synaptosomal fraction during short-term brain-hypothyroidsm. It is described as a protective mechanism of brain by raising the brain L-T3 levels. Another study also documents an increase in D-II activity within various brain regions and decrease in D-III activity, except in cerebrellum and medulla where specific D-III activity remained undetected [40]. However, controversially, although these investigation did observe higher D-II activity within various areas of adult brain during hypothyroidism, the changes in L-T3 levels remained lower than normal values as was noticed in case of serum levels of hypothyroidism. This investigation could not explain this high D-II activity and lower L-T3 levels in brain regions. The levels of THs measured in this study also were shown to be lower than found by other investigators. Some assay in brain regions was also performed in tissue homogenates instead of particular subcellular fractions. Possibly differences in the concentrations of THs could be due to a different method of severe extraction procedure employed to extract brain tissue THs resulting in loss of it.

The data emerged from our study reveal the quantitative aspects of involvement of L-T3 in synaptosomes in different thyroid states, and favors its role in neuronal functions as formerly described [10,41]. A stimulation of synthesis of synapsin-1 protein (related to neurotransmission) by L-T3 in the developing brain has been reported [42]. Although, the synaptosomal L-T3 levels varied widely with different treatments, our result illustrates a unique, but unknown regulatory mechanism of the TH metabolism in the mature mammalian brain.

5.2. Modulation of neuronal plasma membrane Na^+-K^+-ATPase specific activity as a function of specific binding of L-triiodothyronine in adult rat brain cerebrocortical synaptosomes

Subsequently the idea of concentration, distribution and metabolism of THs within the mature brain generated interest to search for potential role of TH and its nongenomic interaction, if any, with neuronal plasma membrane. TH is well known for its regulation of energy metabolism in developing tissues including brain. However, adult brain has not shown this effect on energy metabolism under the influence of TH until recently. Maintenance of ionic gradients by plasma membrane Na^+-K^+-ATPase (NKA) is one of the important cellular events by which TH regulate energy metabolism. NKA is an ion pump responsible for maintaining Na^+ and K^+ ion gradients across the cellular plasma membrane in eukaryotic cells. The Na^+ and K^+ ion gradients are important for establishment of resting membrane potentials as well as for transport of certain molecules. NKA has special significance in maintaining membrane potentials in neurons. Inhibition of NKA has been shown to release acetylcholine [43] and norepinephrine [44] from rat cortical synaptosomes, presumably as a result of depolarizing effects of lowered K^+ gradients. The level of NKA activity could therefore have consequence for the regulation of the neurotransmitter release and uptake across the synaptic membrane [43].

5.2.1. In vivo and in vitro actions of L-T3 on synaptosomal Na^+-K^+-ATPase activity

A dose-dependent inhibition of synaptosomal NKA activity by L-T3 both in *in vivo* [45], and in *in vitro* [46] conditions have been shown. This may be related to the differences in L-T3 status in adult rat cerebrocortical synaptosomes. L-T3 administration in a single i.p. injection showed inhibition of synaptosomal NKA specific activity maximally at 24 hours post-injection by ~ 44% compared to respective control euthyroid values. A range of L-T3 concentration (0.1 to 4.0 μg/g BW, single i. p. injection) administered *in vivo* showed dose-dependent inhibition of the synaptosomal NKA activity. In contrast PTU-treated hypothyroid animals showed ~ 38% increase in the NKA activity compared to the control values. This increase in NKA activity was abolished by injection of a single L-T3 injection

(2μg/g BW) to almost close to the euthyroid levels. However, this study could not distinguish between the genomic and nongenomic effects of L-T3. TH has also been reported to influence K^+-evoked release of [^{3}H]-GABA in adult rat cerebrocortical synaptosomes. Such evidence indicates a possible role of TH in neurotransmission in adult mammalian brain. A functional correlation between L-T3 binding and the corresponding inhibition of NKA activity under *in vitro* conditions in the synaptosomes of adult rat cerebral cortex were established [46]. To further test the hypothesis of nongenomic action of TH we investigated NKA activity in isolated synaptosomes which is devoid of nucleus to avoid the chances of nuclear activation [46]. In fact, *in vitro* addition of L-T3 ($1x10^{-12}$ M to $10x10^{-8}$ M) within 10 minutes of incubation indicated a dose-dependent inhibitory response to NKA activity. Such immediate action of L-T3 added in *in vitro* in synaptosomes was concluded as rapid nongenomic action of L-T3 on synaptosomal membrane NKA [46]. Further inhibition of NKA activity was corroborated with gradual binding of [^{125}I]-L-T3 to specific L-T3-binding sites in synaptosomes. Thus a physiologic response tied to the specific L-T3-binding in the synaptosomal membrane was demonstrated.

The presence of high affinity low capacity nuclear TH receptors in adult rat brain has been reported. Further evidence shows selective uptake of [^{125}I]-L-T3 and rapid conversion of L-T4 to L-T3 in synaptosomal fraction of adult rat brain. Specific [^{125}I]-L-T3 binding sites have also been demonstrated in the synaptosomes of adult rat brain [47] and chick embryo [48]. However, no functional relationship could be established due to the interaction of TH and its membrane receptor so far in adult brain.

Scatchard plot analysis demonstrated two sets of specific L-T3 binding sites: one with high affinity (K_{d1}: 12 pM; B_{max1}: 3.73±0.07 fmols/mg protein), and the other with low affinity (K_{d2}: 1.4±0.05 nM; B_{max2}: 349±7 fmols/mg protein). K_d represents dissociation constant. B_{max} represents maximum binding capacity. Rationale between gradual L-T3 binding and the corresponding dose-dependent L-T3-induced inhibition of synaptosomal NKA was established *in vitro* [46].

The relative order of potencies of binding affinities for the synaptosomal L-T3 binding sites and relative inhibition of NKA activity in the presence of different L-T3 analogues were as follows: L-T3>L-T3-amine>L-T4=L-TRIAC>r-T3>L-T2, and L-T3>L-T3-amine>L-T4>L-TRIAC>r-T3>L-T2, respectively. The concentrations of TH analogues required to displace 50% specific binding (ED_{50} value) of ^{125}I-L-T3 to its synaptosomal binding sites were 10-, 63-, 63-, 1000- and 6250 nM, respectively. This study showed the nature of inhibition of synaptosomal NKA activity as a function of L-T3 occupancy of synaptosomal receptor sites in mature rat brain [46].

This investigation demonstrates a novel action of TH in mature rat brain. This is the first report presenting a relationship between the inhibitions of synaptosomal NKA as a functional effect of L-T3 binding to its synaptosomal receptor in the cerebral cortex of adult rat. Occupancy of specific high affinity L-T3 binding sites demonstrated a concentration-dependent inhibition of the NKA activity with a maximum of 59%. At $1x10^{-10}$ M L-T3 concentration the enzyme inhibition was ~35% and the saturation of the L-T3 binding sites was ~74%. This appears to be physiological. Further inhibition of NKA activity as found with higher concentrations of L-T3 ($5x10^{-10}$ – $1x10^{-7}$ M), corresponds to the increase in the occupancy of the L-T3 binding sites (maximum of ~80%) at the low affinity binding range. However, this site was not saturated by 15.4 μM L-T3 used for determining non-specific binding. Hence, it is possible that this low affinity binding is due to non-specific effects of several other proteins located in synaptosomes. The relationship between the binding of L-T3 to its synaptosomal binding sites and the concentration dependent inhibition of the enzyme activity appears to hold good only with the occupancy of high affinity sites up to 5 x 10^{-10} M L-T3 [46]. Synaptosomes prepared from chick embryo cortex were also reported to have two sets of L-T3 binding sites [48]. Their properties and ontogeny showed a marked difference from those of nuclear receptors. Even though NKA activity was suppressed beyond the saturating concentration of L-T3 at high affinity binding sites, this may be non-specific and non-physiological. The relative order of binding affinities for TH analogues to the L-T3 binding sites and the inhibitory potencies for NKA activity were also correlated in the synaptosomes. L-T3-amine was used to examine its potency to inhibit specific [^{125}I]-L-T3 binding in synaptosomes with the idea that it may be a decarboxylated product of L-T3 and may have actions like L-T3. The ED_{50} value for L-T3-amine was determined as 10 nM. At this dose, L-T3-amine also inhibited the synaptosomal NKA activity by ~51% compared with L-T3. This result is also in good agreement with earlier studies, in which L-T3-amine was shown to be ~71% as effective as L-T3 in stimulating Ca^{2+}-ATPase activity at a dose of 10 nM in human RBC [49]. In earlier studies, L-T3-induced increase in NKA activity in the developing brain [50] and kidney cortex [51] of rat was reported to be due to an increase in the mRNA levels of α, α+ and β-subunits of the enzyme, while the NKA in adult was not responsive to L-T3. However, a dose-dependent inhibition and regulation of synaptosomal NKA activity in different *in vivo* situations was noticed. The immediate effect of added L-T3 on the synaptosomes appears to be nongenomic as synaptosomes do not have nuclei. This may exclude the possibility of involvement of nuclear receptors as reported earlier by us. One possible effect of L-T3 may be mediated through membrane receptors. Recently, membrane binding proteins for iodothyronines has been described in plasma membranes of most cells [52]. This protein has been designated as an integrin αVβ3. Also a role of MCT-8, a membrane spanning protein, has been ascribed as a very active and specific transporter of THs and some of its metabolites across the membrane [25,53]. However, its action through cytoplasmic L-T3-responsive proteins cannot be ruled out.

In conclusion this study demonstrates, for the first time, a correlation between the binding of TH to its putative receptors and inhibition of NKA activity in the synaptosomes of adult rat brain [46]. This may have implications in the involvement of thyroid hormone on important mental functions in adult mammalian brain.

5.3. In search for possible second messenger mediated events in synaptosomal L-T3-induced signaling

The evidence of L-T3-synaptosomal membrane interaction in association with the inhibition of the synaptosomal membrane NKA activity led us to search for if the L-T3-induced action is mediated via activation or regulation of the second messenger cascade systems. Besides the cyclic nucleotide cyclase systems calcium (Ca^{2+}) also plays an important role in cellular signal transmission. Ca^{2+}-influx is a major event in neurotransmission. Keeping such visions we further intended to explore the role of Ca^{2+} in L-T3-induction.

5.3.1. Effect of L-T3 on synaptosomal Ca^{2+}-influx: A comparison between euthyroid and hypothyroid brain

Metabotropic events are often initiated at the membrane level, mediated and amplified through G-protein coupled receptors (GPCR) and/or ion channels followed by activation of second messenger system and subsequent substrate protein phosphorylation. Ca^{2+}-influx is an important physiological function in brain, following which cascades of membrane events occur finally leading to neurosignaling. Disruption in this crucial membrane phenomenon may lead to variety of Ca^{2+}-dependent neuropsychological disorders. Although TH-mediated Ca^{2+} entry in adult rat brain synaptosomes [54,55], and in hypothyroid mouse cerebral cortex [56] have been reported, it's synaptic functions in adult neurons in dysthyroidism is unclear. Keeping in mind the role of Ca^{2+} ions as a messenger in the signaling pathway the effect of L-T3 on intracellular Ca^{2+}-influx, *in vitro*, was studied.

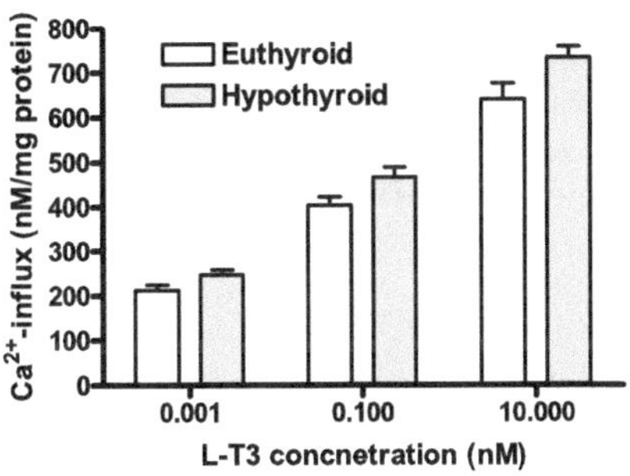

Figure 5. Effect of L-T3 on intrasynaptosomal Ca^{2+}-concentration in euthyroid and PTU-induced hypothyroid rat cerebral cortex *in vitro* (Ref. Modified from Sarkar and Ray 2003, Hormone and Metabolic Research 35: 562-564 acknowledged [57])).

Our study demonstrates a regulation and homeostatic mechanism of Ca^{2+} accumulation within cerebrocortical synaptosomes of hypothyroid adult rat [57]. Application of brain physiologic concentrations of L-T3 (0.001 nM to 10 nM), *in vitro*, significantly triggered Ca^{2+}-sequestration both in the euthyroid and hypothyroid rat brain synaptosomes in a dose-dependent manner (Figure 5). Unexpectedly, PTU-induced hypothyroid synaptosomes showed significant levels of increase in Ca^{2+}-influx compared to euthyroid controls between 0.1 nM and 10 nM doses of L-T3. However, 0.001 nM dose of L-T3 did not show significant changes between euthyroid and hypothyroid values.

Present study validates the role of Ca^{2+} ions under the influence of L-T3 in the synaptosomes from adult rat brain cerebral cortex. L-T3-induced dose-dependent Ca^{2+}-entry both in euthyroid and PTU-induced hypothyroid rat brain synaptosomes at low L-T3 doses (0.001

nM to 10 nM). This evidence indicates role of Ca^{2+} as a second messenger in synaptic functions. L-T3 also has been documented to increase ^{45}Ca uptake and Ca^{2+}-influx in adult euthyroid rat synaptosomes, and in hypothyroid mouse cortex. An enhancement of nitric oxide synthase (NOS) activity in adult rat cerebrocortical synaptosomes was shown [55]. This present study demonstrated a significant increase in Ca^{2+} accumulation in hypothyroid rat brain cerebrocortical synaptosomes compared to euthyroid control at below (0.1 nM) and at about brain physiologic concentrations (10 nM) of L-T3. At present clear understanding for the L-T3-induced release of intracellular calcium is not known; however possibility for L-T3-induced action in neuronal cells cannot be left out. Use of sodium azide blocked any mitochondrial accumulation of calcium. Our earlier studies have shown that 10 nM and 100 nM dose of L-T3 could saturate the specific synaptosomal L-T3-binding sites by ~69% and ~74% respectively. L-T3-mediated physiological increase in synaptosomal Ca^{2+} accumulation could be attributed to receptor-mediated physiological response having its maximal effect at 10 nM dose of L-T3. The differences in the observation of increased rate of Ca^{2+} accumulation in hypothyroid synaptosomes compared to the euthyroid values reflected an adaptive mechanism. This could be credited to homeostatic mechanism to overcome PTU-induced stress conditions persisted in the adult neuron. High intrasynaptosomal L-T3 level (~9.5-fold higher; 2.56 ng/mg synaptosomal protein ≅126 nM L-T3) could be one of the reasons. Although hypothyroid condition showed an appreciable decrease in both serum levels of L-T4 and L-T3 as predicted, supportive studies showed maintenance of similar levels of brain L-T3 in hypothyroid conditions through increased activity of D-II suggesting high fractional rate of L-T4 to L-T3 conversion. In brain approximately ~80% of L-T3 is produced locally from L-T4 by D-II. This data supports thyroid hormone-Ca^{2+}-ion interaction for normal functioning of adult brain during different neuropsychological conditions.

The important functional role of Ca^{2+} and several calcium-dependent proteins in neuronal signal transduction are well recognized. Ca^{2+} has been shown to inhibit neuronal NKA activity. Ca^{2+}-influx also lead to Ca^{2+}-dependent activation of protein kinase C and/or Ca^{2+}/CaM-dependent protein kinases followed by direct or indirect activation of phosphorylation of several target proteins. This indicated a rapid nongenomic action of L-T3.

5.3.2. Is thyroid hormone-membrane interaction is linked to G-protein coupled receptors (GPCR)?

5.3.2.1. Association of G proteins with membrane receptors

G proteins are GTP-binding proteins that couple activation of seven-helix receptors by neurotransmitters at the cell surface for the activation of the effector enzymes-adenylate cyclase (AC) or guanylate cyclase (GC), which synthesize the corresponding cyclic nucleotides, cAMP or cGMP respectively and regulate protein kinases., such as protein kinase A (PKA), protein kinase C (PKC) etc. Metabotropic events are often initiated at the membrane level, mediated and amplified through GPCR followed by activation of second messenger system and subsequent substrate protein phosphorylation. Phospholipase C (PLC), another effector enzyme, generates inositol triphosphate (IP_3) and diacylglycerol (DAG), the latter of which releases intracellular stores of calcium. The cAMP, cGMP, Ca^{2+}, DAG and IP_3 act as second messengers and activate protein kinases with broad substrate specificity. The kinases phosphorylate key intracellular proteins, including ion channels, enzymes, and transcription factors which modulate cellular biological processes [58,59]. Guanine nucleotides are known to have dual effects on most hormone-sensitive AC systems. This modulates activation of AC and binding of hormone to receptor. In neuronal membranes guanylate nucleotides has been shown to be required for the stimulation of AC. However, no modulation of TH binding at appropriate guanylate nucleotide concentrations has been reported. It is well established that cholera toxin enhances the activity of $G_{s\alpha}$ (stimulatory G protein α-subunit) by ADP-ribosylating $G_{s\alpha}$ subunit and inhibiting GTPase activity associated with the protein. This increases cAMP production.

The activity of NKA is regulated by various catecholamines [45,46,60] as well as by L-T3 [45,46]. Inhibition of NKA has been demonstrated in intact cell preparations by phorbol esters, dibutyryl cAMP, and phospho-DRPP-32 (dopamine- and cAMP-regulated phosphoprotein of molecular weight 32 kD), a protein phosphatase inhibitor [61-63].

Some information focuses to effect of TH or its metabolites on noradrenergic like responses. This idea develops since TH has possibility to produce a family of biogenic amine-like neurotransmitter compounds catalyzed by aromatic amino acid decarboxylase, such as iodothyronamines. Physiologic identification of these family of TH-derived iodothyronamines have not yet been discovered until recently in rat brain and in rat and human blood. These two compounds are monoiodothyronamine and thyronamine [10]. Thinking this could be a possibility before this identification of monoiodothyronamine and thyronamine were reported we studied the effect of L-T3 on synaptosomal NKA activity using various β- and α-adrenergic agonists and antagonists known to regulate G_s and G_i proteins of the neuronal signal transduction system, *in vitro*.

Our studies showed that although both L-T3 and isoproterenol (β-adrenergic receptor [ADR] agonist and activator of G_s-protein) similarly inhibited synaptosomal NKA activity, propranolol (β-ADR antagonist) could only block the effect of isoproterenol, but not the effect of L-T3. Instead propranolol produced a dose-dependent potentiation of the inhibitory influence of L-T3 (Figure 6). The augmentation of L-T3-effect by propranolol appeared to be a type of synergistic action and it might be due to some changes in the pre-synaptic membrane properties, the mechanism of which is unclear at present. However, clonidine (α_2-ADR agonist, and G_i-protein activator) (Figure 7) and glutamate (acts through metabotropic glutamate receptors and activator of G_i protein) (Figure 8) attenuated L-T3-effect, suggesting its possible coupling with GPCR. Equimolar concentration of clonidine (1 nM – 100 nM) counteracted the inhibitory effect of L-T3 on the NKA activity (Figure 7). This counteraction by clonidine, α_2-ADR agonist, appears to be mediated through the inhibition of adenylate cyclase activity with the activation of inhibitory G protein (G_i) followed by inhibition of cAMP synthesis and protein phosphorylation cascade mechanism. It is known that α_2-adrenergic receptor agonist system act through G_i protein activation [64].

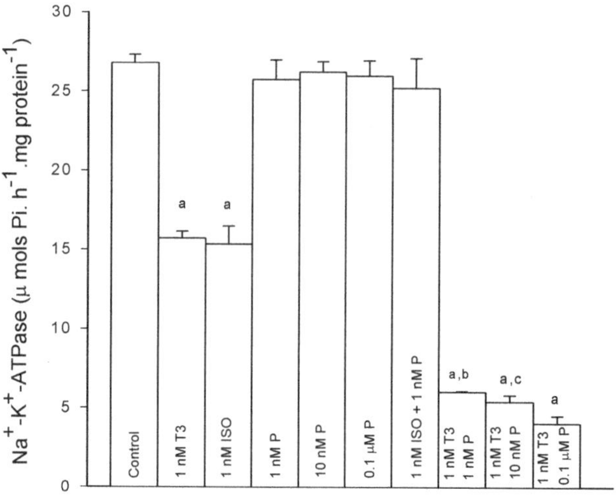

Figure 6. *In vitro* effect of L-T3, isoproterenol (ISO) and propranolol (P), on synaptosomal NKA activity.

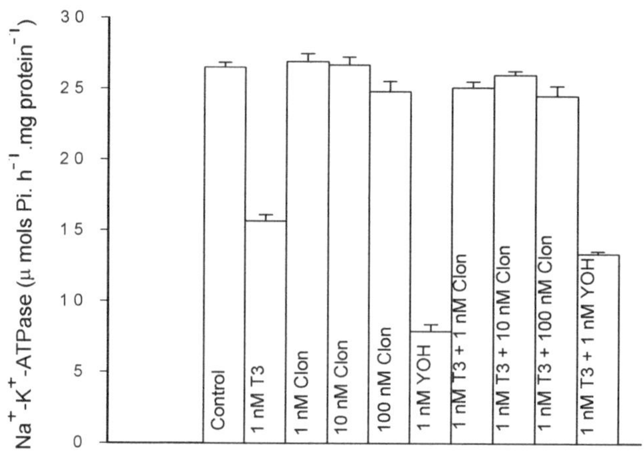

Figure 7. *In vitro* effect of L-T3, clonidine (CLON, and yohimbine (YOH, α_2-ADR antagonist) on synaptosomal NKA activity.

Thus it seems that the L-T3 action could be ascribed more to stimulate G_s protein during beta-blockade which might be directed to manage this adverse condition. The results also suggest that the L-T3-effect on the synaptosomal NKA activity was not mediated via the β-ADR-dependent systems, since it was not blocked by propranolol. Based on these results it was also hypothesized that L-T3-effect would alter adenylate cyclase activity. In cultured neuroblastoma plasma membrane increased adenylate cyclase activity was noticed followed by L-T3-treatment [65]. In fact, later, increased adenylate cyclase activity was noticed in brain hypothyroid condition which increases brain L-T3 levels. This observation was correlated well with increased D-II activity to the increased brain L-T3 levels in brain hypothyroid situations [15]. Guanosine 5'-O-(3-thiotriphosphate) or pertussis toxin also has been reported to inhibit TH-induced mitogen-activated protein kinase (MAPK) phosphorylation nongenomically in 293T cells which is consistent with a cell membrane mechanism mediated via a G-protein [66]. 3-iodothyronine (T_1AM), an endogenous and rapid-acting derivative of TH, is associated with G_s-protein coupled-trace amine receptor TAR1 in HEK cells. However, no modulation of TH binding at appropriate guanylate nucleotide concentrations in adult brain has been reported [67]. Determination of whether activation or inactivation of a specific type(s) of G-protein influences TH-effects on protein phosphorylation is crucial.

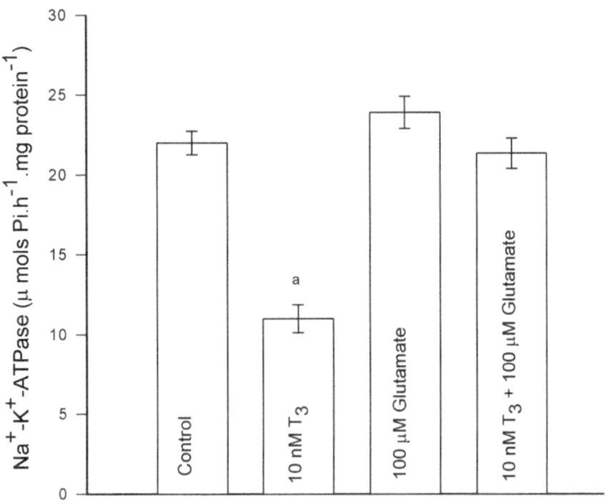

Figure 8. Attenuation of L-T3-effect on synaptosomal NKA activity by glutamate, *in vitro*.

A diverse nongenomic effect of TH has been observed in non-neural tissues including liver, heart, adipocytes, and blood [12,68]. Some possible nongenomic actions of THs include modulation of GABA uptake, regulation of NKA activity and increase of presynaptic Ca^{2+}-influx. In synaptoneurosomes TH inhibits the stimulation of chloride flux by GABA [69]. L-T4 has been shown to stimulate the MAPK pathway in a variety of cultured cell lines including HeLa and CV-1 cells which lack functional nuclear TH receptors [66,70-73], consistent with a cell membrane mediated mechanism via G-proteins. L-T4 and L-T3 were found to inhibit G_o-protein activities in synaptosomes from developing chick brain [48].

Direct interactions of G protein subunits with Ca^{2+}-channels are not well documented. However, increased evidences showed receptor activated G proteins modulate activities of ion channels by membrane-confined mechanisms [74]. Isoproterenol induced phosphorylation of ventricular Ca^{2+}-channels via PKA has been reported [75]. G_s protein also has been shown to regulate Ca^{2+}-channels both in a cAMP-independent membrane-confined mechanism [74] and in a cAMP-dependent phosphorylation of one of the subunits of L-type Ca^{2+}-channel [76]. Synaptosomal NKA has previously been described to be inhibited by cAMP in a dose-dependent manner suggesting a role of PKA. The activated form of this protein kinase was further phosphorylated a substrate protein which in turn depressed the total Na^+-dependent phosphorylation of the synaptosomal NKA [77]. Overall, our data indirectly support the involvement of second messenger system (cAMP and/or Ca^{2+}) mediated through G protein activation after specific L-T3-membrane receptor interaction. The membrane NKA has been implicated in several aspects of physiologic processes including its role in neurotransmitter release [43].

5.4. First evidence of rapid nongenomic action of thyroid hormone and its metabolites on the synaptosomal protein phosphorylation in adult rat brain, *in vitro*

Protein phosphorylation and dephosphorylation are now recognized to be major regulatory mechanisms by which neural activities are controlled by external physiological signals or stimuli. Several nongenomic mechanisms are coordinated by rapid post-transcriptional modifications, such as protein phosphorylation and dephosphorylation reactions, which act like a molecular switch to control intracellular signaling mechanisms. Abnormalities of these imperative regulatory signaling processes produce deleterious effects on the CNS. As a consequence, variety in unusual protein phosphorylation is the end result of many major neuropshychological dysfunctions leading to diseases [78]. Numerous second messenger molecules regulate cellular physiology by effects on protein kinases and phosphatases. Protein kinases catalyze the transfer of the terminal γ-phosphate group of ATP or GTP to the hydroxyl group of serine, threonine or tyrosine in substrate proteins. Their structure, subcellular localization and substrate specificity allow them to control cellular physiology. These proteins largely make up the cell signaling pathways that transmit, amplify and integrate signals from the extracellular environment. Protein phosphorylation promotes enzyme activation or deactivation. Phosphorylated proteins are substrates for protein phosphatases and dephosphorylation occur to serve as a molecular switch to fine tune a cellular response [79].

Variety of agents regulating the activity of NKA raises the possibility of the NKA as a substrate molecule that is subject to regulation by phosphorylation or dephosphorylation. Indeed, inhibition of NKA is associated with the phosphorylation of the enzyme by both PKA and PKC. This inhibition of NKA has been attributed to the phosphorylation of α_1-subunit of the NKA molecule at serine residues by PKA and PKC site-specifically. Isoproterenol (β-adrenergic agonist that activates adenylate cyclase to produce cAMP, an activator of PKA), forskolin (adenylate cyclase activator), and okadaic acid (an inhibitor of protein phosphatase-1 and -2A) have been reported to increase significantly the level of phosphorylation of wild-type α_1-subunit of the NKA in COS cells, accompanied by a significant inhibition of the enzyme activity [62,63]. Among nine distinct isoforms of adenylate cyclase (AC), three isoforms are Ca^{2+}/calmodulin-dependent, including type I-AC, III-AC [80,81], and VIII-AC. The Ca^{2+}/calmodulin-dependent AC is an integral membrane protein [82]. Hence, one possible role of Ca^{2+}/calmodulin may be to stimulate Ca^{2+}/calmodulin-dependent AC followed by cAMP production and phosphorylation of the NKA, exactly as β-adrenergic receptor agonists do.

While a direct effect of TH on protein kinase activity has not been formerly studied in tissues from mature brain, hypothyroidism has been linked with reduced levels of phosphorylated MAPK in the hippocampus [83]. Based on these observations, possibility of a metabotropic pathway for rapid actions of TH on protein phosphorylation in synaptosomes from adult rat brain was investigated.

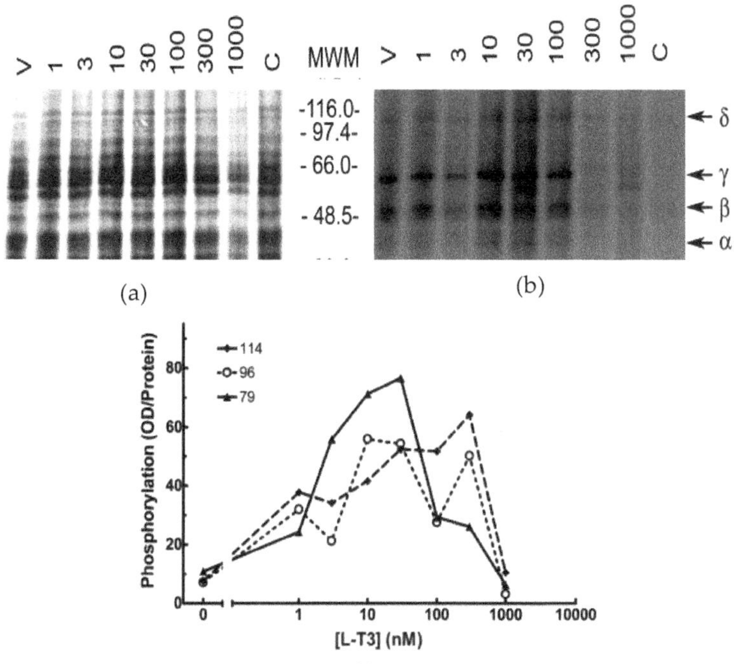

Figure 9. Representative autoradiogram of SDS-PAGE separation of proteins incorporating ^{32}P in the presence of L-T3. Lanes were loaded with synaptosomal lysates which had been preincubated at 0°C for 60 min and 37°C for 5 min with (from left): 1mM Na_3VO_4 (V), 1, 3, 10, 30, 100, 300, 1000, or 0 (C = control) nM L-T3 and then incubated with 20μM of [γ-^{32}P]-ATP (3 μCi) for 1 min at 37°C. Left panel (a): Silver-stained gel for visualization of protein bands. Right panel (b): Autoradiogram of same gel showing increased incorporation of ^{32}P in four prominent bands (α: 38±1 kD, β: 53±1 kD, γ: 63±1 kD, δ: 113±1 kD). (c) Normalized data showing effect of *in vitro* addition of graded doses of L-T3 on the levels of protein phosphorylation expressed as optical density (OD)/protein (Ref. Sarkar et al. 2006 *Neuroscience* 137: 125-132 acknowledged [11]).

Our observation demonstrated that TH induces rapid changes in synaptosomal protein phosphorylation. Incubation with L-T3 or L-T4 specifically showed significant biphasic dose-dependent effects on the phosphorylation of 38±1, 53±1, 62±1, and 113±1 kD proteins. *In vitro* brain physiologic concentrations of TH (1-30 nM) showed significant increase in the levels of protein phosphorylation rapidly within minutes (Figure 9). In contrast, incubations with similar doses of reverse-T3 (rT3) were without significant effect, indicating specificity for L-T3 and L-T4. The protein phosphorylation statuses of these four synaptosomal proteins were significantly increased followed by L-T3 and L-T4 treatment as well. Both L-T3 and L-T4 indicated bi-phasic nature of effect for each of these proteins phosphorylated. Maximum levels of phosphorylation were noticed at concentration range from 10-30 nM. However, no significant effect on protein phosphorylation was observed as an effect of rT3 on any of these proteins. This effect of rT3 clearly confirmed very structural and functional specificity of L-T3 on protein phosphorylation. Determination of time course of protein phosphorylation followed by one single *in vitro* dose of L-T3 showed it peaked rapidly between 180 seconds to 240 seconds and thereafter it decreased. This indicated a rapid action of THs and its metabolites [11].

Our next interest was to see which amino acids present in these phosphoyraled proteins are targets. Hence phospho-specifc antibodies for tyrosine and serine were used in western bolt analysis. Immunoblot analysis of synaptosomal lysates incubated with L-T3 (1 nM-1 μM) confirmed phosphorylation at the seryl residues of a ~112 kD protein and phosphorylation at tyrosyl residues of a distinct ~ 95 kD protein. These data support that THs have a diversity of rapid nongenomic pathways for regulation of protein phosphorylation in mature mammalian brain [11]. Especially, the α-subunit of NKA is a ~112 kD membrane protein. Indeed, inhibition of NKA is associated with the phosphorylation of its subunits by both PKA and PKC. This inhibition of NKA has been attributed to the site-specific phosphorylation of the α_1-subunit of the NKA at seryl residues by PKA and PKC [61-63]. In adult rat alveolar epithelial cell L-T3 induced translocation of NKA to plasma membrane. NKA stimulation by L-T3 was assigned to L-T3-induced stimulation of PI3K/PKB pathway via the Src family of tyrosine kinases nongenomically [84]. These data suggest possible involvement of membrane components in TH-induced protein phosphorylation.

Examples of nongenomic control of protein phosphorylation by L-T3 also have been reported in few other tissues. Nongenomic relationship of MAPK and MAPK-mediated protein phosphorylation at the seryl residue of nuclear TH receptor has been described in 293T cells [68]. This indicated a control of nongenomic mechanism on genomic mechanism. In developing brain, inhibition of PKA transcriptionally blocked L-T3-induced actin gene expression, whereas PKC and tyrosine kinase did not influence it significantly [85].

5.4.1. Thyroid hormones rapidly modulate synaptosomal protein phosphorylation via second messenger systems

In other studies, L-T3 induction has also been shown to nongenomically regulate Ca^{2+} influx and nitric oxide synthase activity within seconds in adult rat brain [57]. Thus, THs are likely to have numerous rapid nongenomic effects on signaling mechanisms in neural tissue, including alterations in the levels of intracellular second messengers (cAMP and Ca^{2+}) which regulate cAMP- and/or Ca^{2+}/calmodulin (CaM)-dependent protein kinases leading to protein phosphorylation. Effects of TH on Ca^{2+}-dependent activation of PKC and/or Ca^{2+}/CaM-dependent protein kinases are also possible, followed by direct or indirect activation of phosphorylation of the proteins. Thus further investigation demonstrated for the first time the rapid nongenomic second messenger mediated regulation of protein phosphorylation by

TH in mature mammalian brain and provided additional support for the contention that TH has a unique and complex signaling function in adult brain [12].

5.4.1.1. Role of calcium and calmodulin on synaptosomal protein phosphorylation, in vitro

Many nongenomic mechanisms are modulated by phosphorylation–dephosphorylation of substrate proteins. Multiple Ca^{2+}/calmodulin (CaM)-dependent protein kinases (CaM kinases) and Ca^{2+}/phospholipid-dependent protein kinases (PKCs) have been identified in brain. Among these, CaMPK-II is the most abundant Ca^{2+}/CaM-stimulated protein kinase in brain. CaMPK-II is important in several neuronal functions, including neurotransmitter release and the modulation of the functional properties of ion channels and receptors. CaMPK-II is differentially expressed in different brain regions of cells, exists in both cytosolic and membrane-associated forms and is especially concentrated in the postsynaptic density and synaptic vesicles. A distinct property of CaMPK-II is that autophosphorylation of its threonine residue near the calmodulin binding domain converts it to a Ca^{2+}-independent state. Further, it has been shown that calmodulin-dependent autophosphorylation of CaMPK-II induces a conformational changes in the region of the calmodulin binding domain that allows additional stabilizing interactions with calmodulin. This autophosphorylation may involve in extending the effects triggered by a transient calcium signal. PTU-induced mild hypothyroidism in chick brain during posthatch development has been shown to increase the level of Ca^{2+}/CaM-stimulated phosphorylation in cytosol, but lower it in the membrane, indicating a role of thyroid hormones in distributing CaMPK-II during developmental changes [78,86].

5.4.1.1.1. Effect of L-T3 on total protein phosphorylation

The effect of Ca^{2+} and calmodulin on TH-induced total protein phosphorylation and their regulation was explored. L-T3 significantly and dose-dependently (10 nM-1 μM) increased total ^{32}P- incorporation into synaptosomal proteins, *in vitro*, over the basal level of phosphorylation. Although L-T3 exerted its own independent effect on increase in overall total protein phosphorylation, specifically it established its role to be at least dependent on Ca^{2+} and calmodulin. Ca^{2+} also showed its independent influence on the basal L-T3-induced total protein phosphorylation in synaptosomal isolates. The dependency of L-T3-induced total synaptosomal protein phosphorylation was evaluated and finally confirmed using EGTA (Ca^{2+}-ion chelator) and KN-62 (a specific blocker of CaMK-II). *In vitro* addition of 10 nM and 100 nM doses of L-T3 alone did not alter significantly the basal levels of phosphorylation. However, the 1 μM dose of L-T3 significantly amplified the signal by ~1.3-fold compared to the basal level ($P<0.05$). Next, we wanted to determine whether Ca^{2+} augments protein phosphorylation in the presence of L-T3. Ca^{2+} (0.5 mM) were able to significantly increase the basal phosphorylation level. However, no further significant changes were noticed with additional 10 nM or 100 nM L-T3. However, 1 μM concentration of L-T3 augmented the signal significantly ($P<0.05$) by ~1.5-fold (0.2167 pmols/min/mg protein) as compared to the Ca^{2+}-treated baseline (0.1475 pmols/min/mg protein), and by ~2.2-fold over the basal phosphorylation (0.097 pmols/min/mg protein). In contrast, the effects of low physiological concentrations of L-T3 were dramatically enhanced when 2 μM CaM was added to the Ca^{2+}+ L-T3-treatment group. In the presence of Ca^{2+} and CaM, L-T3

(10 nM-1 μM) induced a dose-dependent increase in ^{32}P- incorporation into synaptosomal protein, by 47±8 , 74±13 and 52±11 % ($F = 6.77$, $P<0.0001$) rapidly within 1 min compared with the Ca^{2+}/CaM-treated control phosphorylation (0.189 pmols/min/mg protein) [87].

Physiological concentrations L-T3 in nerve terminals are difficult to measure. Predictable levels of L-T3 within the nerve terminals range from ~10 nM to 64 nM. PTU-induced peripheral hypothyroidism in adult rats showed endogenous synaptosomal level of L-T3 is about ~126 nM. Thus L-T3 (1 μM) is well above this range, and would be considered to have a more pharmacological type of action on ^{32}P- incorporation to synaptosomal phosphoproteins. Treatment with agents regulating Ca^{2+} could be a potential strategy for enhancing clinical treatment of conditions, such as certain affective disorders, which may be responsive to pharmacological doses of TH. In an earlier *in vitro* study, L-T3 doses (0.1 to 100 nM), have been shown to induce an increase in intrasynaptosomal Ca^{2+} levels with an optimum at 100 nM of L-T3. Although higher levels of L-T3 (1 μM) produced slight depression of intrasynaptosmal Ca^{2+} levels, picomolar levels of L-T3 were also shown to be able to significantly increase intrasynaptosomal Ca^{2+} levels *in vitro*. The synergistic effect of L-T3 and Ca^{2+}/CaM on protein phosphorylation would likely be further amplified by the effect of L-T3 to increase Ca^{2+} levels intracellularly in the physiological situation. In particular, this study demonstrated that of 10 nM dose of L-T3 (brain physiological concentration) and a ten times higher dose of L-T3 (as observed to be the brain levels of L-T3 in PTU-induced hypothyroid young adult rat brain synaptosomes alone or with Ca^{2+} did dramatically increased L-T3-induced total protein phosphorylation. Thus the present study demonstrated that Ca^{2+}/CaM-dependent mechanisms synergistically increase the rapid nongenomic effect of L-T3 on synaptosomal protein phosphorylation [87]. The Ca^{2+}/CaM-dependent effects could be due to an activation of an unknown CaM-dependent protein kinase(s), deactivation of protein phosphatase(s) or a combination of effects. However, it proved to be highly sensitive to L-T3 activation.

Numerous phosphoproteins are greatly influenced by PKA and PKC in a Ca^{2+}- and/or CaM-dependent way. Often Ca^{2+} also functions in combination with CaM or with phosphoinositides/diacylglycerol to induce additional signal transduction pathways within the synaptic network. Regulation of intracellular Ca^{2+}, CaM and subsequent protein phosphorylation are important for brain and cognitive functions affected by various psychiatric disorders. Membrane depolarization-induced Ca^{2+}-influx activates extracellularly regulated kinases/MAPK in a Ca^{2+}/CaM-dependent way in PC12 cells. THs also promote MAPK-mediated serine phosphorylation of the nuclear TH receptor β-1 isoform nongenomically in 293T cells. Ca^{2+} and CaM also differentially regulate of TH-induced neuronal protein phosphorylation [12,87].

5.4.1.1.2. L-T3-induced stimulation of phosphorylation of 63- and 53 kD proteins was regulated by Ca^{2+} and calmodulin

After getting an idea of L-T3-induced total protein phosphorylation within neuronal membrane it was an obvious interest to look for specific proteins phosphorylated under the influence of L-T3. *In vitro* addition of L-T3 (10 nM, brain physiologic concentrations of L-T3) demonstrated differential regulation of phosphorylation status of five different synaptosomal proteins (63-, 53-, 38-, 23-, and 16 kD) in both a Ca^{2+}/CaM-dependent and -independent manner in mature rat brain cortical synaptosomes. L-T3 increased the level of phosphorylation of all these five proteins. Ca^{2+}/CaM further stimulated phosphorylation of 63- and 53 kD proteins by L-T3, which were inhibited both specifically by EGTA (Ca^{2+}-chelator) or KN62 (Ca^{2+}/CaM kinase-II [CaMK-II] inhibitor), suggesting the role of CaMK-II. However, presence of Ca^{2+} significantly decreased L-T3-induced phosphorylation of 63-, 53 kD proteins (Figure 10).

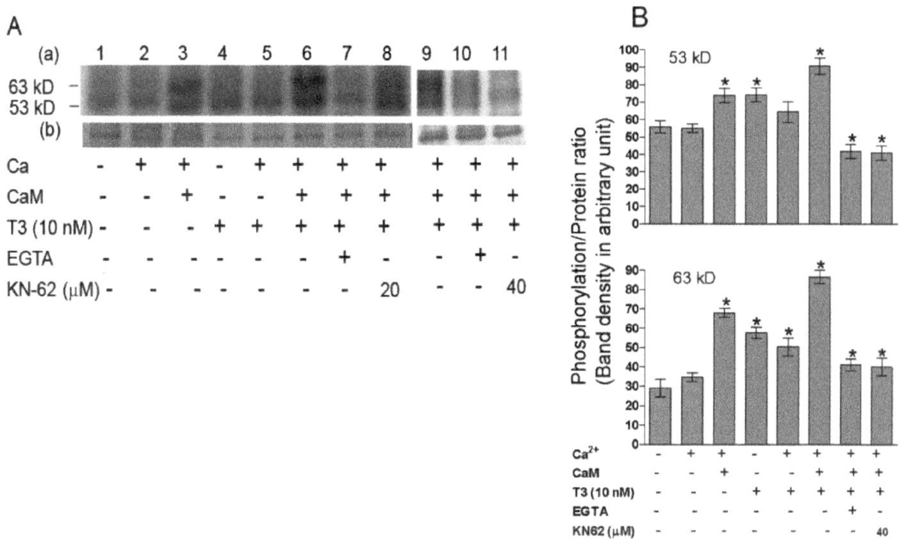

Figure 10. A. L-T3-stimulated phosphorylation of 63- and 53 kDa proteins are regulated by Ca^{2+}/CaM-dependent protein kinase II. (a) Representative autoradiogram of the 63- and 53 KD proteins followed by various treatment conditions as described. (b) Corresponding protein bands from silver stained gel used for normalization of the data and demonstrates comparable equal amounts of sample loading. B. The quantification of the L-T3 (10 nM)-induced phosphorylation presented as a graph of ratio of the band densities of the phosphorylated proteins in the autoradiogram (a) and the corresponding protein in the silver stained gel (b) at different treatment conditions as indicated. * represents the level of significance of $P<0.05$ compared to the corresponding basal level (control). The data presented are normalized results (mean ± S.E.M.) for an indicated protein band (Ref. Sarkar 2008 Life Sciences 82: 920-927 acknowledged [12]).

5.4.1.1.3. Inert action of Ca^{2+} and calmodulin on the independent effect of L-T3 on the phosphorylation of 38- and 23 kD proteins

L-T3 also increased the phosphorylation of 23- and 38 kD proteins. The effect was independent of EGTA or KN62. L-T3 only slightly enhanced the phosphorylation of the 38 kD protein ($p<0.05$, $F = 3.74$) by ~1.2-fold in the presence of Ca^{2+}/CaM compared to Ca^{2+}/CaM control group. Although addition of Ca^{2+} decreased the level of L-T3-induced phosphorylation of 38 kD protein (P = non-significant), it was significantly increased

(P<0.05) in the presence of CaM compared to Ca^{2+} + L-T3 treatment and only L-T3 effect. However, the presence of Ca^{2+} or the Ca^{2+}/CaM did not further affect the phosphorylation status of the 38 kD protein. This further suggested no involvement of Ca^{2+}/CaM-dependent pathways mediated through CaMK-II.

The study also described the phosphorylation status of a 23 kD protein. Phosphorylation level of 23 kD protein was highest among all the proteins. L-T3 significantly increased the phosphorylation level of 23 kD by ~2.2-fold compared to the basal level. Especially of interest, EGTA or KN62 did not show any more or less influence on the L-T3-induced increase in the phosphorylation status of the 23 kD protein suggesting lack of significant regulation by CaMK-II (Figure 11).

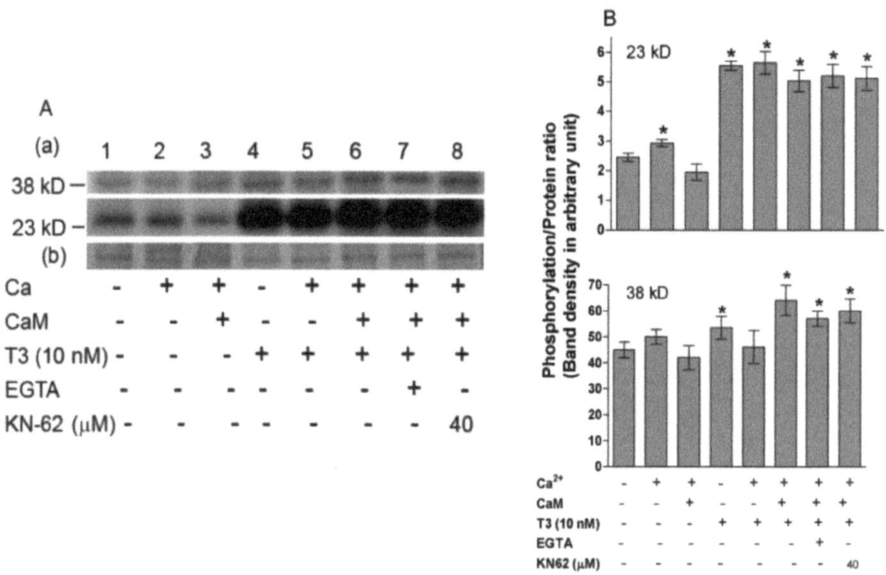

Figure 11. A. Ca^{2+}/CaM do not modulate L-T3-stimulated phosphorylation of 23- and 38 kD proteins. (a) A representative autoradiogram of the 23- and 38 kD protein separated by SDS-PAGE showing independent stimulatory action of L-T3 upon the phosphorylation of the 23- and 38 kD proteins. B. The quantification of the L-T3-induced phosphorylation presented as a graph of ratio of the band densities of the phosphorylated proteins in the autoradiogram (a) and the corresponding protein in the silver stained gel (b) at different treatment conditions as indicated. The data presented are normalized results (mean ± S.E.M.) for an indicated protein band. * Indicates levels of significance P<0.05 (Ref. Sarkar 2008 Life Sciences 82: 920-927 acknowledged [12]).

5.4.1.1.4. Calmodulin dephosphorylated 16 kD protein following L-T3-induction

In vitro addition of L-T3 (10 nM) significantly increased the level of phosphorylation of 16 kD protein by ~8-fold. The L-T3-induced phosphorylation of 16 kD protein was not further activated in the presence of Ca^{2+}. Surprisingly, L-T3-induced phosphorylation of 16 kD protein was not augmented further with Ca^{2+} or Ca^{2+}/CaM; instead, the presence of CaM abolished the L-T3-induced phosphorylation. EGTA or KN62 could not restore the effect of CaM-induced dephosphorylation of this protein (Figure 12).

Immunoblotting experiment with anti-phosphoserine antibodies also showed significant enhancement of seryl residue phosphorylation of this protein by Ca^{2+}/CaM (Figure 13). Abolition of this effect by EGTA and KN-62 further suggested an important role of CaMK-II. This study identified the role of Ca^{2+}/CaM in the regulation of L-T3-induced protein phosphorylation and supported a unique nongenomic mechanism of second messenger-mediated regulation of protein phosphorylation by TH in mature rat brain.

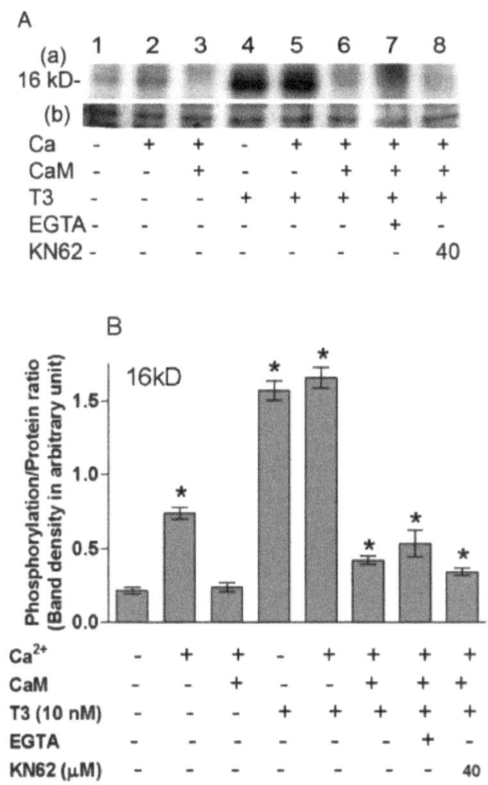

Figure 12. A. Phosphorylation of 16 kD protein by L-T3 was conquered by the dephosphorylation activity of CaM. (a) A representative autoradiogram of the 16 kD protein separated by SDS-PAGE is showing independent stimulatory action of L-T3 upon the phosphorylation of the 16 kD protein. (b). Corresponding protein bands of silver stained gel. B. The quantification of the L-T3 (10 nM)-induced phosphorylation and its dephosphorylation by CaM are presented as a graph of ratio of the band densities of the phosphorylated proteins in the autoradiogram (a) and the corresponding protein in the silver stained gel (b) at different treatment conditions as indicated. The data presented are normalized results (mean ± S.E.M.) for an indicated protein band. * Indicates levels of significance $P<0.05$, compared to the basal level (control group) (Ref. Sarkar 2008 Life Sciences 82: 920-927 acknowledged [12]).

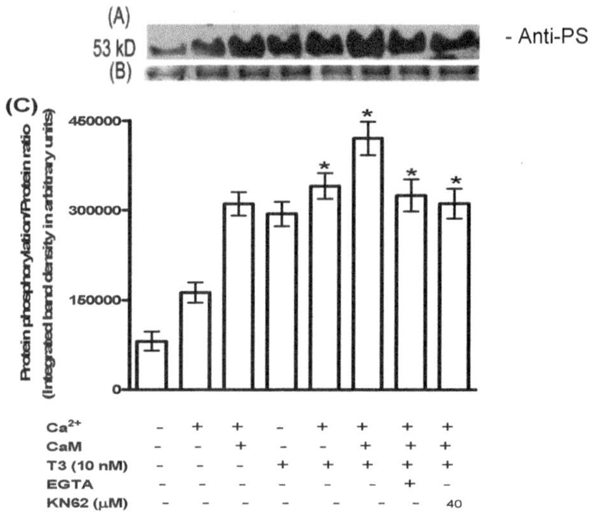

Figure 13. L-T3 induced phosphorylation of the 53 kD protein is regulated by Ca^{2+}/calmodulin protein kinase II: Serine residue phosphorylation. (A) Phosphorylation status of the 53 kD protein immunoblotted with anti-phosphoserine (PS) antibody. (B) Corresponding protein band of silver stained gel. (C) Graphical representation of the levels of phosphorylation of the 53 kD protein at various treatment conditions. The data presented are normalized results (mean ± S.E.M.) for an indicated protein band. * Indicates levels of significance $P<0.05$, compared to the basal level (control group).

5.4.1.2. Role of cAMP on synaptosomal protein phosphorylation, in vitro

After searching for whether Ca^{2+} plays a major role as second messenger following L-T3 induced protein phosphorylation, our next step was to examine for the role of cyclic AMP (cAMP) as another second messenger upon L-T3-induction, *in vitro,* to explore furthermore the nongenomic mechanism of TH. To search for any role of cAMP-dependent protein kinase (PKA) the effects of cAMP and H7 (a specific blocker of PKA) were studied. *In vitro* addition of H7 significantly diminished the effect of L-T3-induced increase in serine phosphorylation of two closely associated proteins with 51- and 53 kD by ~14-fold and ~11-fold respectively (Figure 14). This suggested prevalence of a PKA-mediated mechanism in L-T3-induced synaptosomal protein phosphorylation. To test further whether THs exert adrenergic-like actions by binding to or modulating adrenergic receptor activities another study was performed to test this hypothesis. The idea of formation of thyronamines and its possible binding to the ADR is considered here. Effect of clonidine was studied on the L-T3-induced protein phosphorylation and on the L-T3-binding to the synaptosomal membrane receptors. Scatchard plot analysis revealed clonidine and yohimbine (α_2-ADR antagonist) could not alter specific L-T3 binding at the high affinity L-T3 synaptosomal membrane binding sites. L-T3 induced phosphorylation of this 51-/53 kD protein was blocked by H7, a PKA inhibitor. Activation of α_2-ADR by clonidine normally decreases the levels of cAMP via inhibiting adenylate cyclase activity. Possibly in the absence of adequate cAMP levels during clonidine treatment, the phosphorylation status of the 51-/53 kD protein remained unchanged. This suggests L-T3-membrane interaction was independent of the activation of the α_2-ADR system. Overall these data implicate that PKA and CaMK-II both contribute for L-T3 regulated protein phosphorylation in adult mammalian brain and reveals a nongenomic mechanistic pathway in relation to higher mental functions.

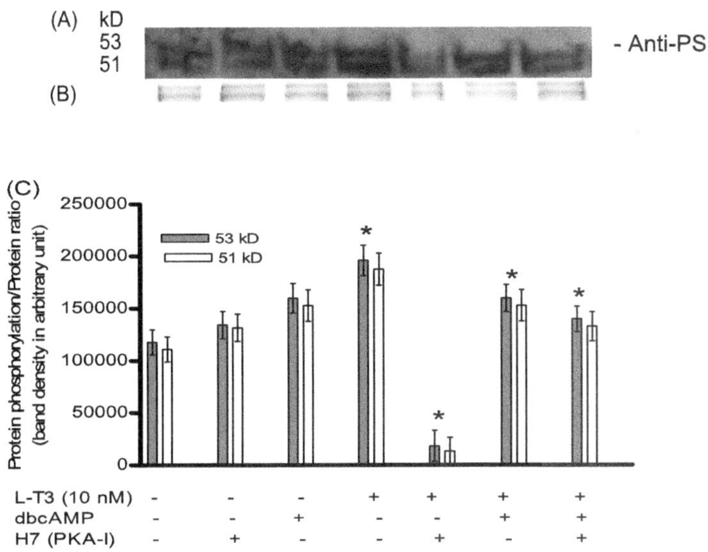

Figure 14. L-T3 induced phosphorylation of the 51-/53- kD proteins are abolished by Protein Kinase A Inhibitor (H7). (A) One representative phosphorylation status of the 51-/53-kD protein immunoblotted with anti-phosphoserine (PS) antibodies. (B) Corresponding protein band of silver stained gel. (C) Graphical representation of the levels of phosphorylation of the 51-/53-kD protein at various treatment conditions. dbcAMP is dibutyryl cyclic AMP. The data presented are normalized results (mean ± S.E.M.) for an indicated protein band. * Indicates levels of significance $p<0.05$, compared to the basal level (control group).

6. Conclusion

In conclusion the recent evidence-based information regarding the nongenomic mechanism of action of THs are opening new signal transduction clues to be studied and to reveal the underlying mechanism in mature mammalian brain. The results of the study conducted will advance our knowledge of the fundamental molecular mechanism of TH action in mature CNS, likely in future will lead to more rational and effective approach to the development of novel therapeutic agents, and thus will shed insights on to the neuropshychological manifestations of adult on-set thyroid disorders in humans, particularly in relation to higher mental functions.

7. Future research direction

Recent information regarding nongenomic mechanism of thyroid hormone action in various tissue types including mammalian CNS is interesting. These studies are diligently engaged in decoding the molecular consequences of thyroid hormone action from the specific gene expression to the nongenomic rapid actions of the hormone. Open-minded investigators are desperately searching for the truth and the relationship of thyroid hormone action explicated through its classical well-known doctrine which is mediated via activation of specific nuclear receptors to the newly emerging idea of rapid nongenomic actions of the hormone and an association to enlighten the both. In particular, adult mammalian brain are of best curiosity since clinical observations of numerous thyroid dysfunction related neuropsychological disorders produced during mature conditions in humans can be corrected with the adjustment of the thyroid hormone levels. However the mechanism of action is lacking. Nongenomic rapid events mediated by thyroid hormones could have connection to the long-term genomic actions. Deciphering the nongenomic molecular mechanism of action of thyroid hormones has future prospects to study its importance regulating higher mental functions in humans. This fundamental knowledge could be the basis to find novel strategies to treat adult-onset thyroid dysfunctions including neuropsychological diseases many of which are precisely controlled by demarcated cellular fine-tuning of the protein phosphorylation mechanisms related to neuronal signal transmission.

Author details

Pradip K. Sarkar
Department of Basic Sciences, Parker University, Dallas, Texas, USA

Acknowledgement

Financial support was provided by Parker University, Dallas, Texas, USA.

8. References

[1] Sarkar PK (2002) In quest of thyroid hormone function in mature mammalian brain. Indian J. Exp. Biol. 40(8): 865-873.
[2] Oetting A, Yen PM (2007) New insights into thyroid hormone action. Best Pract. Res. Clin. Endocrinol. Metab. 21:193-208.
[3] Cheng SY, Leonard JL, Davis PJ (2010) Molecular aspects of thyroid hormone actions. Endocr. Rev. 31: 139-170.
[4] Davis PJ, Davis FB (1996) Nongenomic actions of thyroid hormone. Thyroid 6: 497-504.
[5] Haggerty JJ, Jr., Prange AJ, Jr. (1995) Borderline hypothyroidism and depression. Annu. Rev. Med.46: 37-46.

[6] Bauer M, London ED, Silverman DH, Rasgon N, Kirchheiner J, Whybrow PC (2003) Thyroid, brain and mood modulation in affective disorder: insights from molecular research and functional brain imaging. Pharmacopsychiatry 36: S215-S221.

[7] Laurberg P (1990) Hypothyroidism In: Greer MA, editor. The Thyroid Gland. New York: Raven Press, p. 497-535.

[8] Utiger RD (1987) Hyperthyroidism. In: Green WL, editor. The Thyroid. New York: Elsevier, p. 157-218.

[9] Hoefig CS, Renko K, Piehl S, Scanlan TS, Bertoldi M, Opladen T, Hoffmann GF, Klein J, Blankenstein O, Schweizer U, Kohrle (2012) Does the aromatic L-amino acid decarboxylase contribute to thyronamine biosynthesis? Mol. Cell. Endocrinol. 349: 195-201.

[10] Gompf HS, Greenberg JH, Aston-Jones G, Ianculescu AG, Scanlan TS, Dratman MB (2010) 3-Monoiodothyronamine: the rationale for its action as an endogenous adrenergic-blocking neuromodulator. Brain Res. 1351:130-140.

[11] Sarkar PK, Durga ND, Morris JJ, Martin JV (2006) In vitro thyroid hormone rapidly modulates protein phosphorylation in cerebrocortical synaptosomes from adult rat brain. Neurosci. 137: 125-132.

[12] Sarkar PK (2008) L-triiodothyronine differentially and nongenomically regulates synaptosomal protein phosphorylation in adult rat brain cerebral cortex: role of calcium and calmodulin. Life Sci. 82: 920-927.

[13] Sarkar PK, Ray AK (1994) Synaptosomal T_3 content in cerebral cortex of adult rat in different thyroidal states. Neuropsychopharmacol. 11: 151-155.

[14] Kundu S, Pramanik M, Roy S, De J, Biswas A, Ray AK (2006) Maintenance of brain thyroid hormone level during peripheral hypothyroid condition in adult rat. Life Sci. 79: 1450-1455.

[15] Kundu S, Biswas A, Roy S, De J, Pramanik M, Ray AK (2009) Thyroid hormone homeostasis in brain: possible involvement of adrenergic phenomenon in adult rat. Neuroendocrinol.89: 140-151.

[16] Sarkar PK (2010) Subcellular levels of L-T3 and L-T4 in adult rat brain cerebral cortex. Thyroid Sci. 5: 1-4.

[17] Sarkar PK, Ray AK (1992) A simple biochemical approach to differentiate synaptosomes and non-synaptic mitochondria from rat brain. Methods Find. Exp. Clin. Pharmacol. 14: 493-497.

[18] Dratman MB, Crutchfield FL, Axelrod J, Colburn RW, Thoa N (1976) Localization of triiodothyronine in nerve ending fractions of rat brain. Proc. Natl. Acad. Sci. U S A 73: 941-944.

[19] Dratman MB, Crutchfield FL (1978) Synaptosomal [^{125}I]triiodothyronine after intravenous [^{125}I]thyroxine. Am. J. Physiol. 235: E638-E647.

[20] Dratman MB, Crutchfield FL, Futaesaku Y, Goldberger ME, Murray M (1987) [^{125}I]Triiodothyronine in the rat brain: Evidence for neural localization and axonal transport derived from thaw-mount film autoradiography. J. Comp. Neurol. 260: 392-408.

[21] Dratman MB, Futaesaku Y, Crutchfield FL, Berman N, Payne B, Stumpf WE, Sar M (1982) Iodine ^{125}-labeled triiodothyronine in rat brain: Evidence for localization in discrete neural systems. Science 215: 309-312.
[22] Dratman MB, Crutchfield FL, Gordon JT, Jennings AS (1983) Iodothyronine homeostasis in rat brain during hypo- and hyperthyroidism. Am. J. Physiol. 245: E189-E193.
[23] Mason GA, Walker CH, Prange AJ (1993) L-Triiodothyronine: Is this peripheral hormone a central neurotransmitter? Neuropsychopharmacol. 8: 253-258.
[24] Kastellakis A, Valcana T (1989) Characterization of thyroid hormone transport in synaptosomes of rat cerebral cortex. Mol. Cell. Endocrinol. 67: 231-241.
[25] Visser WE, Friesema EC, Visser TJ (2011) Minireview: thyroid hormone transporters: the knowns and the unknowns. Mol. Endocrinol. 25: 1-14.
[26] Kinne A, Schulein R, Krause G (2011) Primary and secondary thyroid hormone transporters. Thyroid Res. 4: S7.
[27] Constantinou C, Margarity M, Valcana T (2005) Region-specific effects of hypothyroidism on the relative expression of thyroid hormone receptors in adult rat brain. Mol. Cell. Biochem. 278: 93-100.
[28] Bolaris S, Constantinou C, Valcana T, Margarity M (2005) Pentylenetetrazole-induced convulsions affect cellular and molecular parameters of the mechanism of action of triiodothyronine in adult rat brain. Neuropharm 48: 894-902.
[29] Crantz FR, Silva JE, Larsen PR (1982) An analysis of the sources and quantity of 3,5,3'-triiodothyronine specifically bound to nuclear receptors in rat cerebral cortex and cerebellum. Endocrinol. 110: 367-375.
[30] Halperin Y, Shapiro LE, Surks MI (1994) Down-regulation of type II L-thyroxine, 5'-monodeiodinase in cultured GC cells: different pathways of regulation by L-triiodothyronine and 3,3',5'-triiodo-L-thyronine. Endocrinol. 135: 1464-1469.
[31] Guadano-Ferraz A, Escamez MJ, Bernal J (1999) Expression of type 2 iodothyronine deiodinase in hypothyroid rat brain indicatesan important role of thyroid hormone in the development of specific primary sensory systems. J. Neurosci. 19: 3430.
[32] Biswas A, Kundu S, Roy S, De J, Pramanik M, Ray AK (2006) Thyroid hormone profile during annual reproductive cycle of diploid and triploid catfish, Heteropneustes fossilis (Bloch). Gen. Comp. Endocrinol. 147: 126-132.
[33] Soboll S (1993) Thyroid hormone action on mitochondrial energy transfer. Biochim. Biophys. Acta 1144: 1-16.
[34] Leonard JL, Kaplan TJ, Visser JE, Silva JE, Larsen PR (1981) Cerebral cortex responds rapidly to thyroid hormone. Science 214: 571-573.
[35] Leonard JL, Silva JE, Kaplan MM, Mellen SA, Visser TJ, Larsen PR (1984) Acute posttranscriptional regulation of cerebrocortical and pituitary iodothyronine 5'-deiodinases by thyroid hormone. Endocrinol. 114: 998-1004.
[36] Serrano-Lozano A, Morata P, Montiel M, Perez-Aguilar JP, Morell M (1991) L-thyroxine and L-triiodothyronine in the cerebral tissues of the adult rat. Effect of hypothyroidism. Rev. Esp. Fisiol. 47: 141-145.

[37] Crantz FR, Larsen PR (1980) Rapid thyroxine to 3,5,3'-triiodothyronine conversion and nuclear 3,5,3'-triiodothyronine binding in rat cerebral cortex and cerebellum. J. Clin. Invest. 65: 935-938.

[38] Kaplan MM, Yaskoski KA (1980) Phenolic and tyrosyl ring deiodination of iodothyronines in rat brain homogenates. J. Clin. Invest. 66: 551-562.

[39] Morreale de Escobar G, Calvo R, Escobar del Rey F, Obregon MJ (1994) Thyroid hormones in tissues from fetal and adult rats. Endocrinol. 134: 2410-2415.

[40] Broedel O, Eravci M, Fuxius S, Smolarz T, Jeitner A, Grau H. Stoltenburg-Didinger G, Plueckhan H, Meinhold H, Baumgartner A (2003) Effects of hyper- and hypothyroidism on thyroid hormone concentrations in regions of the rat brain. Am. J. Physiol. Endocrinol. Metab. 285: E470-E480.

[41] Hashimoto H, Walker CH, Prange AJ, Jr., Mason GA (1991) The effects of thyroid hormones on potassium-stimulated release of ^{3}H-GABA by synaptosomes of rat cerebral cortex. Neuropsychopharmacol. 5: 49-54.

[42] Salemi G, Ferraro D, Savattieri G (1990) Triiodothyronine accelerates the synthesis of synapsin I in developing neurons from fetal rat brain cultured in a synthetic medium. Neurochem. Res. 15: 827-831.

[43] Stahl WL, Harris WE (1986) Na^+,K^+-ATPase: structure, function, and interactions with drugs. Adv. Neurol. 44: 681-693.

[44] Vatta M, Pena C, Fernandez B, Rodriguez de Lores AG (1999) A brain Na^+, K^+-ATPase inhibitor (endobain E) enhances norepinephrine release in rat hypothalamus. Neurosci. 90: 573-579.

[45] Sarkar PK, Ray AK (1993) Synaptosomal action of thyroid hormones: Changes in Na^+ -K^+-ATPase activity in adult rat cerebral cortex. Horm. Metab. Res. 25: 1-3.

[46] Sarkar PK, Ray AK (1998) Specific binding of L-triiodothyronine modulates Na^+-K^+-ATPase activity in adult rat cerebrocortical synaptosomes. NeuroReport 9: 1149-1152.

[47] Mashio Y, Inada M, Tanaka K, Ishii H, Naito K, Nishikawa M, Takahashi K, Imura H (1983). Synaptosomal T_3 binding sites in rat brain: their localization on synaptic membrane and regional distribution. Acta Endocrinol. 104: 134-138.

[48] Giguère A, Fortier S, Beaudry C, Gallo-Payet N, Bellabarba D (1996) Effect of thyroid hormones on G proteins in synaptosomes of chick embryo. Endocrinol. 137: 2558-2564.

[49] Davis FB, Cody V, Davis PJ, Borzynski LJ, Blas SD (1983) Stimulation by thyroid hormone analogues of red blood cellCa^{2+} ATPase activity in vitro. Correlations between hormone structure and biological activity in a human cell system. J. Biol. Chem. 258: 12373-12377.

[50] Schmitt CA, McDonough AA (1988) Thyroid hormone regulates alpha and alpha+ isoforms of Na,K-ATPase during development in neonatal rat brain. J. Biol. Chem. 263: 17643-17649.

[51] McDonough AA, Brown TA, Horowitz B, Chiu R, Schlotterbeck J, Bowen J, Schmitt CA (1988) Thyroid hormone coordinately regulates Na^+-K^+-ATPase alpha- and beta-subunit mRNA levels in kidney. Am. J. Physiol. 254: C323-C329.

[52] Davis PJ, Davis FB, Cody V (2005) Membrane receptors mediating thyroid hormone action. Trends Endocrinol. Metab. 16: 429-435.

[53] Friesema EC, Ganguly S, Abdalla A, Manning Fox JE, Halestrap AP, Visser TJ (2003) Identification of monocarboxylate transporter 8 as a specific thyroid hormone transporter. J. Biol. Chem. 278: 40128-40135.
[54] Mason GA, Walker CH, Prange AJ, Jr (1990) Depolarization-dependent ^{45}Ca uptake by synaptosomes of rat cerebral cortex is enhanced by L-triiodothyronine. Neuropsychopharmacol. 3: 291-295.
[55] Chakrabarti N, Ray AK (2000) Rise of intrasynaptosomal Ca^{2+} level and activation of nitric oxide synthase in adult rat cerebral cortex pretreated with 3-5-3'-L-triiodothyronine. Neuropsychopharmacol. 22: 36-41.
[56] Iqbal Z, Koenig H, Trout JJ (1984) Triiodothyronine (T3) stimulates calcium influx and membrane trasport processes in nerve cells and terminals of hypothyroid mouse cortex. Fed. Proc. 43: 735
[57] Sarkar PK, Ray AK (2003) Calcium mobilization within hypothyroid adult rat brain synaptosomes. Horm. Metab. Res. 35: 562-564.
[58] Divecha N, Irvine RF (1995) Phospholipid signaling. Cell 80: 269-278.
[59] Taussig R, Gilman AG (1995) Mammalian membrane-bound adenylyl cyclases. J. Biol. Chem. 270: 1-4.
[60] Beguin P, Beggah AT, Chibalin AV, Burgener-Kairuz P, Jaisser F, Mathews PM, Rossier BC, Cotecchia S, Geering K (1994) Phosphorylation of the Na,K-ATPase alpha-subunit by protein kinase A and C in vitro and in intact cells. Identification of a novel motif for PKC-mediated phosphorylation. J. Biol. Chem. 269: 24437-24445.
[61] Bertorello AM, Aperia A, Walaas SI, Nairn AC, Greengard P (1991) Phosphorylation of the catalytic subunit of Na^+,K^+-ATPase inhibits the activity of the enzyme. Proc. Natl. Acad. Sci. U S A 88: 11359-11362.
[62] Cheng XJ, Hoog JO, Nairn AC, Greengard P, Aperia A (1997) Regulation of rat Na(+)-K(+)-ATPase activity by PKC is modulated by state of phosphorylation of Ser-943 by PKA. Am. J. Physiol. 273: C1981-C1986.
[63] Cheng XJ, Fisone G, Aizman O, Aizman R, Levenson R, Greengard P, Aperia A (1997) PKA-mediated phosphorylation and inhibition of Na(+)-K(+)-ATPase in response to beta-adrenergic hormone. Am. J. Physiol. 273(3 Pt 1):C893-C901.
[64] Levitzki A (1988) Signal transduction in hormone-dependent adenylate cyclase. Cell. Biophys. 12: 133-143.
[65] Walz MA, Howlett AC (1987) Thyroid effects on adenosine 3',5'-monophosphate levels and adenylate cyclase in cultured neuroblastoma cells. Endocrinol. 120: 1265-1271.
[66] Lin HY, Shih A, Davis FB, Davis PJ (1999) Thyroid hormone promotes the phosphorylation of STAT3 and potentiates the action of epidermal growth factor in cultured cells. Biochem. J. 338: 427-432.
[67] Scanlan TS, Suchland KL, Hart ME, Chiellini G, Huang Y, Kruzich PJ, Frascarelli S, Crossley DA, Bunzow JR, Ronca-Testoni S, Lin ET, Hatton D, Zucci R, Grandy DK (2004) 3-Iodothyronamine is an endogenous and rapid-acting derivative of thyroid hormone. Nat. Med. 10: 638-642.
[68] Davis PJ, Leonard JL, Davis FB (2008) Mechanisms of nongenomic actions of thyroid hormone. Front. Neuroendocrinol. 29: 211-218.

[69] Martin JV, Williams DB, Fitzgerald RM, Im HK, VonVoigtlander PF (1996) Thyroid hormonal modulation of the binding and activity of the $GABA_A$ receptor complex of brain. Neurosci. 73: 705-713.
[70] Tang HY, Lin HY, Zhang S, Davis FB, Davis PJ (2004) Thyroid hormone causes mitogen-activated protein kinase-dependent phosphorylation of the nuclear estrogen receptor. Endocrinol. 145: 3265-3272.
[71] Lin HY, Zhang S, West BL, Tang HY, Passaretti T, Davis FB, Davis PJ (2003) Identification of the putative MAP kinase docking site in the thyroid hormone receptor-beta1 DNA-binding domain: functional consequences of mutations at the docking site. Biochemistry 42: 7571-7579.
[72] Storey NM, Gentile S, Ullah H, Russo A, Muessel M, Erxleben C. Armstrong DL (2006) Rapid signaling at the plasma membrane by a nuclear receptor for thyroid hormone. Proc. Natl. Acad. Sci. U S A 103: 5197-5201.
[73] Hiroi Y, Kim HH, Ying H, Furuya F, Huang Z, Simoncini T, Noma K, Ueki K, Nguyen NH, Scanlan TS, Moskowitz MA, Cheng SY, Liao, JK (2006) Rapid nongenomic actions of thyroid hormone. Proc. Natl. Acad. Sci. U S A 103: 14104-14109.
[74] Schultz G, Hescheler J (1993) Hormonal modulations of calcium channel activity. Arzneimittel-Forschung Drug Res. 43: 229-232.
[75] Kameyama M, Kameyama A, Kaibara M, Nakayama T, Irisawa H (1990) Intracellular mechanisms involved in "run-down" of calcium channels. Adv. Exp. Med. Biol. 255: 111-118.
[76] Dolphin AC (1995) Voltage-dependent calcium channels and their modulation by neurotransmitters and G proteins. Experimental Physiol. 80: 1-36.
[77] Lingham RB, Sen AK (1982) Regulation of rat brain (Na+ +K+)-ATPase activity by cyclic AMP. Biochim. Biophys. Acta 688: 475-485.
[78] Patwardhan P, Miller WT (2007) Processive phosphorylation: mechanism and biological importance. Cell. Signal. 19: 2218-2226.
[79] Manning G, Plowman GD, Hunter T, Sudarsanam S (2002) Evolution of protein kinase signaling from yeast to man. Trends Biochem. Sci. 27: 514-520.
[80] Choi EJ, Xia Z, Villacres EC, Storm DR (1993) The regulatory diversity of the mammalian adenylyl cyclases. Curr. Opin. Cell. Biol. 5: 269-273.
[81] Laurent-Demir C, Decorte L, Jaffard R, Mons N (2000) Differential regulation of Ca(2+)-calmodulin stimulated and Ca(2+) insensitive adenylyl cyclase messenger RNA in intact and denervated mouse hippocampus. Neurosci. 96: 267-274.
[82] Tang WJ, Iniguez-Lluhi JA, Mumby S, Gilman AG (1992) Regulation of mammalian adenylyl cyclases by G-protein alpha and beta gamma subunits. Cold Spring Harb. Symp. Quant. Biol. 57: 135-144.
[83] Gerges NZ, Alkadhi KA (2004) Hypothyroidism impairs late LTP in CA1 region but not in dentate gyrus of the intact rat hippocampus: MAPK involvement. Hippocampus 14: 40-45.
[84] Lei J, Mariash CN, Ingbar DH (2004) 3,3',5-Triiodo-L-thyronine up-regulation of Na,K-ATPase activity and cell surface expression in alveolar epithelial cells is Src kinase- and phosphoinositide 3-kinase-dependent. J. Biol. Chem. 279: 47589-47600.

[85] Sarkar S, Biswas SC, Chatterjee O, Sarkar PK (1999) Protein kinase A Linked phosphorylation mediates triiodothyronine induced actin gene expression in developing brain. Mol. Brain Res. 67: 158-164.

[86] Wang X, Rostas JAP (1996) Effect of hypothyroidism on the subcellular distribution of Ca^{2+}/ calmodulin-stimulated protein kinase II in chicken brain during posthatch development. J. Neurochem. 66: 1625-1632.

[87] Sarkar PK, Morris JJ, Martin JV (2011) Non-genomic effect of L-triiodothyronine on calmodulin-dependent synaptosomal protein phosphorylation in adult rat cerebral cortex. Indian J. Exp. Biol. 49: 169-176.

Chapter 4

Ecological Genetics of Thyroid Hormone Physiology in Humans and Wild Animals

Asano Ishikawa and Jun Kitano

Additional information is available at the end of the chapter

1. Introduction

Hormones are important mediators in the responses of a suite of phenotypic traits to environmental changes. Therefore, populations inhabiting different environments are expected to vary in several hormonal pathways. Such variation results from both plastic response to environments and genetic differences. Therefore, information about the genetic basis of hormonal variation is crucial to better understand the ecological and evolutionary mechanisms of phenotypic diversification in animals. Furthermore, information about the racial and geographical variation in hormone physiology is crucial for better diagnosis of hormone-related diseases in clinical fields. Thyroid hormones play key roles in regulation of many physiological and behavioral traits, such as metabolism, ion homeostasis, basal activity, and longevity. Therefore, thyroid hormone can play important roles in adaptation to external environments. In the present study, we review interspecies, racial, geographical, and interindividual variation in the thyroid hormone pathways in humans and other animals. The present review focuses on natural and subclinical variation in thyroid hormone physiology and will not cover the genetic basis for congenital hypothyroidism [1,2,3,4,5], congenital hyperthyroidism [6,7], autoimmune diseases [8], and thyroid cancers [9], for which a number of good review articles are already available. We also review what is known about the genetic basis for such variation. We found several shared features in the patterns of variation in thyroid hormone physiology in humans and other animals. This review demonstrates the importance of undertaking further integrative studies of human genetics and animal ecology for a better understanding of the ecological and genetic mechanisms of variation in thyroid hormone signaling pathways.

2. Variation in thyroid hormone physiology in humans

2.1. Interindividual, geographical, and racial variation

Geographical variation in the frequency of euthyroid endemic goiter has been extensively investigated [10,11,12]. In addition to iodine deficiency, other factors, such as smoking, age, sex, goitrogens, and body mass index, can also influence the etiology of euthyroid endemic goiter [13]. Although genetic predisposition to euthyroid goiter has been demonstrated [12,13,14], the molecular genetic mechanisms underlying the variation in susceptibility to goiter are not well understood. Polymorphism at the thyroglobulin (*TG*) [15,16] and Na^+/I^- symporter (*NIS*) loci [17] are reportedly associated with euthyroid goiter; however, linkage mapping in different families could not connect euthyroid goiter with such genetic variation [18,19].

Racial variation in the level of thyroid-stimulating hormone (TSH), one of the major hormones regulating synthesis and secretion of thyroid hormone, has been also found. Multiple studies have revealed that serum TSH levels are higher in whites and Mexican Americans than in blacks [20,21,22]. These results suggest that race-specific reference values of TSH are necessary for evaluation of thyroid hormone-related diseases. Currently, the genetic and ecological basis for the racial variation in TSH levels is not well understood. The serum levels of thyroxine-binding globulin (TBG), a major thyroid hormone-binding protein in plasma, are lower in Australian Aborigines than in Caucasians in Western Australia [23]. Aborigines have a TBG variant that has reduced affinity for thyroid hormone and is more susceptible to heat and acid denaturation [24,25,26]. Two amino acids are substituted in this variant, one of which is considered responsible for the low binding affinity for thyroid hormones [26]. Aborigines usually have lower T4 levels, but have normal TSH levels and normal or borderline T3 levels. Because Aborigines do not show any clinical symptoms of hypothyroidism, the homeostasis of thyroid hormone physiology in Aborigines differs from that in other human populations.

Although the adaptive significance of the variations remain elusive in the above cases, some interpopulation variation may result from adaptive evolution to divergent environments. Serum free T4 levels are higher in indigenous Evenki women than in nonindigenous Russian women living in the same communities in central Siberia [27]. The variation in free T4 levels was correlated with the variation in basal metabolic rate both in Evenki and Russian men and women [27]. Similar cases were also found for indigenous Nenets and nonindigenous Russians: both showed significant increases in total T4 levels during winter, but the magnitude of the increase was significantly greater in the Nenets than in the Russians [27]. Because thyroid hormones play important roles in regulating metabolic rate and adaptation to cold environments [28,29], human populations inhabiting colder environments may acquire genetic basis for more efficient thyroid hormone-induced thermogenesis and may therefore be genetically adapted to cold environments [30].

Interindividual differences in TSH levels are prevalent, and have been found to be associated with variation in life span. In Ashkenazi Jews and Northern Italians, healthy oldest-old people of around 100 years of age had higher TSH levels than elderly controls of around 70 years of age [31,32]. In addition, follow-up studies revealed that participants with abnormally high TSH levels had a lower mortality rate than those with normal or low TSH levels [33]. The offspring of Ashkenazi Jewish centenarians had significantly higher TSH levels, suggesting that higher TSH levels and longevity have heritable components [32]; however, the molecular mechanisms of this variation are unknown.

2.2. Genetic basis for variation

In addition to the case of TGB in Australian Aborigines [34], polymorphisms associated with variation in thyroid hormone physiology have been found in other populations [35]. Several studies have focused on candidate genes involved in thyroid hormone signaling pathways and revealed that single nucleotide polymorphisms (SNPs) of the TSH receptor (*TSHR*) [36], iodothyronine deiodinases (*DIO1*, *DIO2*, and *DIO3*) [36,37], thyroid hormone transporter and thyroid hormone receptor genes accounted for variation in serum TSH and thyroid hormone levels [38,39]. Genome-wide association studies have also identified several genes involved in thyroid hormone signaling. Three SNPs at intron 1 of the phosphodiesterase 8B (*PDE8B*) gene are significantly associated with serum TSH levels [40,41]. *PDE8B* encodes a high-affinity cAMP-specific phosphodiesterase catalyzing the hydrolysis and inactivation of cAMP. Because the *PDE8B* transcript is undetectable in the pituitary, it is thought that PDE8B may affect TSH levels through its effect on TSH-dependent thyroid hormone synthesis and secretion in the thyroid gland. Interestingly, other cAMP-specific phosphodiesterases have also been showed to be associated with variation in TSH levels [41]. Since there are only a few studies revealing the mechanisms by which SNPs modify thyroid hormone signaling [38], further studies are needed to confirm their actual contribution to the natural variation in thyroid hormone physiology.

If genes involved in thyroid hormone pathways were targets of natural selection, we would be able to find some signatures of natural selection in the human genome. When natural selection increases the frequency of a new beneficial mutation in a population, the neighboring regions will reduce the genetic variation and increase the level of linkage disequilibrium [42]. Two genes involved in the thyroid hormone pathway, thyroid hormone receptor interactor 4 (*TRIP4*) and iodotyrosine deiodinase (*IYD*), showed a signature of selection in the genome of African Pygmies [43]. Importantly, a low frequency (9.4%) of goiter was reported for an African Pygmy population, although they inhabit an iodine-deficient region [44]. Because another population in the same region had a much higher frequency of goiter (42.9%), López Herráez et al. (2010) concluded that the signatures of selection in these genes might reflect genetic adaptations of Pygmies to iodine-deficient diets. Another study tried to identify the genes whose allele frequencies were significantly correlated with climate. The frequency of an SNP in *TRIP6* showed strong correlation with latitude [45].

The high rate of nonsynonymous (amino acid–altering) changes compared with the rate of synonymous (silent) changes also indicates that the genes might be under positive selection

[42]. By comparing the synonymous and nonsynonymous substitutions in the human and chimp genomes, putatively positively selected genes were screened [46]. Genes expressed in the thyroid gland have an excess of rapidly evolving genes compared with other tissues, except testis, which has more putatively positively selected genes [46]. Changes in thyroid hormone physiology may contribute to some of the physiological and morphological divergence between humans and apes [47,48].

3. Inter-population and geographical variation in thyroid hormone physiology in animals

Anatomical studies conducted in the 1960s and 1970s showed interspecies morphological variation for fishes and amphibians [49,50]. Since then, natural variation in thyroid hormone physiology has been extensively investigated in diverse taxa of vertebrate (Table 1). Some of the variation results from environmental factors. For example, environmental contaminants can cause goiter. In salmon populations introduced into the Great Lakes in the late 1960s, the frequency of thyroid goiter increased in the mid-1970s [51,52,53]. In addition, herring gulls *Larus argentatus* from the Great Lakes also suffered from goiter in the 1980s [54]. It was demonstrated that laboratory rats fed with the salmons caught in the lakes exhibited hypothyroidism and goiter, suggesting the presence of goitrogenic substances in the Great Lakes fishes [55].

Species/Family	Phenotypic variation	Potential factors and functions	Reference
Intraspecific variation			
Coho salmon	Goiter, T_4, T_3	Goitrogen	[51,53,97]
Chinook salmon	Goiter	Goitrogen	[53]
Herring gull	Goiter	Goitrogen	[54]
American alligator	T_4	Goitrogen	[98]
Japanese pond frog	Morphology		[49]
Bottlenose dolphin	T_4 and T_3	Temperature	[62]
Northern cardinal	T_4 and T_3		[61]
Alaskan husky	T_4 and T_3	Temperature	[60]
Bonnethead shark	T_4 and T_3 in yolk	Temperature	[70]
Brook charr	T_4 and T_3	Migration	[87]
Stickleback	Goiter, TSHß, T_4,T_3	Migration, metabolism	[57,58,86]
Interspecific variation			
Poeciliidae	Morphology, tumor		[50,99,100]
Spadefoot toad	T_4, T_3, sensitivity	Dry environment, metamorphosis	[63]
Big-eared mouse	T4, T3, iodide	Low iodide concentration	[59]
Rodent	T_4	Life span	[101]

Table 1. Variation in thyroid hormone physiology in natural animal populations

Goiters were also observed in hatchery fishes and possibly resulted from iodine deficiency, because iodine treatment was able to cure the goiter [56]. In the case of the threespine stickleback *Gasterosteus aculeatus*, interpopulation variation in susceptibility to goiter when reared in fresh water was observed [57,58], although whether the goiter in the sticklebacks was caused by iodine deficiency is unknown. Interestingly, a mammalian species, *Auliscomys boliviensis*, inhabiting an environment severely depleted of iodine did not show goiter [59], suggesting that genetic variation in the susceptibility to endemic goiter exists among populations and species.

Latitudinal variation in plasma concentrations of thyroid hormone has been observed in both mammals and birds, and these variations might have evolved as adaptations to environments with divergent temperatures. Plasma total T4, free T4, and total T3 levels of sled dogs living in Alaska were higher than dogs in New York, especially in winter [60]. In addition, plasma T3 increased with increasing latitude in the northern cardinals *Cardinalis cardinalis*, whereas plasma T4 did not show a simple latitudinal cline: both southern and northern birds had higher T4 levels than birds living at an intermediate latitude [61]. In mammals, bottlenose dolphins *Tursiops truncatus* show variation in thyroid hormone concentrations between populations inhabiting different latitudes [62]: plasma total T3 and T4 were higher in dolphins from South Carolina with colder year-round temperatures than those from Florida with much warmer water temperatures. Since thyroid hormones play key roles in metabolism and heat generation, evolutionary adaptation to habitats with different temperatures may account for some of the latitudinal and geographical variation in thyroid hormone levels among natural populations. The genetic basis for the latitudinal variation is currently unknown.

Several studies have demonstrated that variation in thyroid hormone physiology correlates with other potentially adaptive traits. Interspecies variation in tissue thyroid hormone levels and tissue sensitivity to thyroid hormone may be correlated with variation in the duration of the larval period in spadefoot toads [63]. For example, the tadpole of the desert-dwelling toad *Scaphiopus couchii* has higher tail and liver levels of thyroid hormone, and the tail tip is more sensitive to thyroid hormone *in vitro* than tail tips of other closely related species [63]. Because frog metamorphosis is controlled by thyroid hormone, the higher thyroid hormone levels and the higher sensitivity may explain the short larval period in this species. Rapid metamorphosis (i.e., the short period of water-dwelling at the tadpole stage) observed in the desert toad is likely adaptive for survival in the deserts where water is scarce [64,65].

Thyroid hormones also play critical roles as yolk hormones in mammalian [66], bird [67], and teleost [68,69] development. In the bonnethead shark *Sphyrna tiburo*, the concentrations of T3 and T4 in the yolk from the Tampa Bay population were consistently higher than those in the yolk from the Florida Bay population [70]. The bonnethead shark in Tampa Bay develops faster and is larger at birth than that in Florida Bay [71]. Tampa Bay is located in a more northern region and is colder than Florida Bay. Because rapid growth is generally adaptive in colder environments [72,73], higher york thyroid hormone levels in the Tampa Bay population may be adaptive.

Thyroid hormone is also implicated in the regulation of longevity in animals [74,75]. Long-lived species of squirrels, deer mice, bats and mole-rats maintain low levels of thyroid hormone [76,77,78,79]. Hypothyroid Wister rats live longer than hyperthyroid rats [80]. Furthermore, investigations in the Ames and Snell dwarf mice have demonstrated that mutation at the *Prop-1* and *Pit-1* genes lead to defects in the generation of pituitary cells including thyrotrope and the dwarf mice have extended longevity [81,82,83,84,85]. Thus, it is possible that changes in the thyroid hormone pathway are involved in variation of life span among wild animals, as is observed among human races (see above). Further research on the genetic basis for the low thyroid hormone levels observed in the long-lived animals should be conducted.

Divergence in thyroid hormone physiology may also be important for adaptation of stickleback fishes to marine and freshwater environments [86]. Stream-resident populations of the threespine stickleback have repeatedly evolved from ancestral marine populations. First, Kitano et al. (2010) found plasma thyroid hormone levels and metabolic rate were lower in stream-resident populations than in ancestral marine populations [86]. Since thyroid hormones regulate metabolic rate in sticklebacks [86], it is likely that lower thyroid hormone in stream-resident sticklebacks is adaptive for permanent residency in small streams where oxygen and food are often scarce. In addition, the expression level of thyroid stimulating hormone *TSHß2* gene was significantly lower in the pituitary gland of stream-resident fish than in that of marine fish. Allele-specific expression analysis with F1 hybrids revealed that some of the differences in *TSHß2* expression levels were caused by *cis*-regulatory changes at the *TSHß2* locus. Importantly, a signature of natural selection was found at *TSHß2* locus: several SNPs within the *cis*-regulatory region exhibited marked differences in the allele frequency between marine and stream-resident populations. Thus, changes in the thyroid hormone pathways may play important roles in genetic adaptation to freshwater environments. In other fishes exhibiting alternate life history style, such as the brook charr *Salvelinus fontinalis* anadromous and resident forms show differences in thyroid hormone concentrations, although genetic factors seem to be of little importance in the interpopulation variation seen in the brook charr [87].

Other than the *TSH* loci in sticklebacks, there are few studies that have examined whether thyroid hormone-related genes are under selective pressure in wild animal populations. However, domestication seems to be a strong artificial selection on thyroid hormone-related genes. Very strong selective sweeps were found at the *TSHR* loci in chickens [88] and sheep [89]. Because TSH is found to regulate photoperiodic control of reproduction [90,91,92,93,94], artificial selection favoring continuous reproduction under domestication might act on the *TSH* locus.

4. Conclusions and future directions

We found similar features in the patterns of variation in thyroid hormone physiology in humans and other animals. First, genetic variation in the susceptibility to endemic goiter exists among populations and species. Second, some of the latitudinal and racial variation in thyroid hormone physiology likely results from adaptation to environments with divergent ambient temperatures. Third, variation in thyroid hormone physiology may be associated with variation in longevity. Fourth, genomic scan of signatures of selection have revealed that some thyroid hormone-related genes experience selective pressure during evolution or domestication.

In humans, it is very difficult to experimentally test the adaptive significance of such variation. However, ecological experiments can be conducted using animals. For example, reciprocal transplant experiments on divergent populations or species with different thyroid hormone physiology can test whether wild animals have higher fitness in native habitats than in foreign habitats [95,96]. We can also investigate whether the fitness is correlated with the thyroid hormone levels. In addition, hormonal manipulation would be able to directly test whether the higher or lower thyroid hormone levels can change the fitness in a variety of environments.

Until recently, it has been difficult to study the genetic basis for physiological differences between natural animal populations. However, it is now becoming increasingly easier to conduct genomic studies because of the recent progress in genomic technologies. Therefore, we can test whether candidate loci involved in thyroid hormone signaling pathways are correlated with fitness in natural environments or laboratory conditions. Furthermore, ecological and genomic studies of wild animal populations will help answer fundamental evolutionary questions, such as whether the same environmental variables are strong agents of natural selection on the thyroid hormone pathways and whether genetic variation in the same genes caused the adaptive divergence in thyroid hormone physiology across diverse taxa, including humans.

Author details

Asano Ishikawa and Jun Kitano*
Ecological Genetics Laboratory and JST PRESTO, National Institute of Genetics, Mishima, Japan

Acknowledgement

This research is supported by JST PRESTO program, the Naito Foundation, Grant-in-Aid for Scientific Research on Innovative Areas (23113007 and 23113001) from the Ministry of Education, Science, Sports, and Culture to JK. AI is a Fellow of the Japan Society of Promotion of Science.

5. References

[1] Park SM, Chatterjee VKK (2005) Genetics of congenital hypothyroidism. J Med Genet 42: 379-389.

---

* Corresponding Author

[2] Grasberger H, Refetoff S (2011) Genetic causes of congenital hypothyroidism due to dyshormonogenesis. Curr Opin Pediatr 23: 421-428.
[3] Rastogi MV, LaFranchi SH (2010) Congenital hypothyroidism. Orphanet J Rare Dis 5: 17.
[4] Grüters A, Krude H, Biebermann H (2004) Molecular genetic defects in congenital hypothyroidism. Eur J Endocrinol 151: U39-U44.
[5] Moreno JC, de Vijlder JJM, Vulsma T, Ris-Stalpers C (2003) Genetic basis of hypothyroidism: recent advances, gaps and strategies for future research. Trends Endocrinol Metab 14: 318-326.
[6] Hébrant A, van Staveren VCG, Maenhaut C, Dumont JE, Leclère J (2011) Genetic hyperthyroidism: hyperthyroidism due to activating TSHR mutations. Eur J Endocrinol 164: 1-9.
[7] Prummel MF, Strieder T, Wiersinga WM (2004) The environment and autoimmune thyroid diseases. Eur J Endocrinol 150: 605-618.
[8] Tomer Y (2010) Genetic susceptibility to autoimmune thyroid disease: past, present, and future. Thyroid 20: 715-725.
[9] Landa I, Robledo M (2011) Association studies in thyroid cancer susceptibility: are we on the right track? J Mol Endocrinol 47: R43-R58
[10] Selinus O, Alloway B, Centeno JA, Finkelman RB, Fiuge R, et al. (2005) Essentials of Medical Geology. Burlington: Elsevier.
[11] Koutras DA, Matovinovic J, Vought R (1985) The ecology of iodine. In: Stanbury JB, Hetzel BS, editors. Endemic Goitre and Cretinism, Iodine Nutrition in Health and Disease. New York: Wiley. pp. 185-195.
[12] Davenport CB (1932) The genetical factor in endemic goiter. Lancaster: Lancaster Press.
[13] Böttcher Y, Eszlinger M, Tönjes A, Paschke R (2005) The genetics of euthyroid familial goiter. Trends Endocrinol Metab 16: 314-319.
[14] Singer J, Eszlinger M, Wicht J, Paschke R (2011) Evidence for a more pronounced effect of genetic predisposition than environmental factors on goitrogenesis by a case control study in an area with low normal iodine supply. Horm Metab Res 43: 349-354.
[15] Perez-Centeno C, Gonzalez-Sarmiento R, Mories MT, Corrales JJ, Miralles-Garcia JM (1996) Thyroglobulin exon 10 gene point mutation in a patient with endemic goiter. Thyroid 6: 423-427.
[16] Corral J, Martin C, Pérez R, Sánchez I, González-Sarmiento R, et al. (1993) Thyroglobulin gene point mutation associated with non-endemic simple goitre. Lancet 341: 462-464.
[17] Matsuda A, Kosugi S (1997) A homozygous missense mutation of the sodium/iodide symporter gene causing iodide transport defect. J Clin Endocrinol Metab 82: 3966-3971.
[18] Neumann S, Bayer Y, Reske A, Tajtáková, Paschke R (2003) Further indications for genetic heterogeneity of euthyroid familial goiter. J Mol Med 81: 736-745.
[19] Neumann S, Willgerodt H, Ackermann F, Reske A, Jung M, et al. (1999) Linkage of familial euthyroid goiter to the multinodular goiter-1 locus and exclusion of the candidate genes thyroglobulin, thyroperoxidase, and Na^+/I^- symporter. J Clin Endocrinol Metab 84: 3750-3756

[20] Hollowell JG, Staehling CA, Flanders WD, Hannon WH, Gunter EW, et al. (2002) Serum TSH, T4, and thyroid antibodies in the United States population (1988 to 1994): National Health and Nutrition Examination Survey (NHANES III). J Clin Endocrinol Metab 87: 489–499.
[21] Walker JA, Illions EH, Huddleston JF, Smallridge RC (2005) Racial comparisons of thyroid function and autoimmunity during pregnancy and the postpartum period. Obstet Gynecol 106: 1365-1371.
[22] Surks MI, Boucai L (2010) Age- and race-based serum thyrotropin reference limits. J Clin Endocrinol Metab 95: 496-502.
[23] Dick M, Watson F (1980) Prevalent low serum thyroxine-binding globulin level in western Australian Aborigines. Med J Australia 1: 115-118.
[24] Dick M, Watson F (1981) A possible variant of thyroxine-binding globulin in Australian Aborigines. Clin Chim Acta 116: 361-367.
[25] Takeda K, Mori Y, Sobieszczyk S, Seo H, Dick M, et al. (1989) Sequence of the variant thyroxine-binding globulin of Australian aborigines. Only one of two amino acid replacements is responsible for its altered properties. J Clin Invest 83: 1344-1348.
[26] Murata Y, Refetoff S, Sarne DH, Dick M, Watson F (1985) Variant thyroxine-binding globulin in serum of Australian aborigines: its physical, chemical and biological properties. J Endocrinol Invest 8: 225-232.
[27] Leonard WR, Sorensen MV, Galloway VA, Spencer GJ, Mosher MJ, et al. (2002) Climatic influences on basal metabolic rates among circumpolar populations. Am J Hum Biol 14: 609-620.
[28] Laurberg P, Andersen S, Karmisholt J (2005) Cold adaptation and thyroid hormone metabolism. Thieme eJournal 37: 545-549.
[29] Launay J-C, Savourey G (2009) Cold adaptations. Ind Health 47: 221-227.
[30] Leonard WR, Snodgrass JJ, Sorensen MV (2005) Metaolic adaptation in indigenous Siberian populations. Ann Rev Anthropol 34: 451-471.
[31] Ravaglia G, Forti P, Maioli F, Nesi B, Pratelli L, et al. (2000) Blood micronutrient and thyroid hormone concentrations in the oldest-old. J Clin Endocrinol Metab 85: 2260-2265.
[32] Atzmon G, Barzilai N, Hollowell JG, Surks MI, Gabriely I (2009) Extreme longevity is associated with increased serum thyrotropin. J Clin Endocrinol Metab 94: 1251-1254.
[33] Gussekloo J, van Exel E, de Craen AJ, Meinders AE, Frolich M, et al. (2004) Thyroid status, disability and cognitive function, and survival in old age. JAMA - J Am Med Assoc 292: 2591-2599.
[34] Murata Y, Refetof S, Same DH, Dick M, Watson F Variant thyroxine-binding globulin in serum of Australian Aborigines-its physical, chemical and biological properties. J Endocrinol Invest 8: 225-232.
[35] Peeters RP, van der Deure WM, Visser TJ (2006) Genetic variation in thyroid hormone pathway genes; polymorphisms in the TSH receptor and the iodothyronine deiodinases. Eur J Endocrinol 155: 655-662.

[36] Peeters RP, van Toor H, Klootwijk W, de Rijke YB, Kuiper GG, et al. (2003) Polymorphism in thryoid hormone pathway genes are associated with plasma TSH and iodothyronine levels in healthy subjects. J Clin Endocrinol Metab 88: 2880-2888.
[37] Panicker V, Cluett C, Shields B, Murray A, Parnell KS, et al. (2008) A common variation in deiodinase 1 gene DIO1 is associated with the relative levels of free thyroxine and triiodothyronine. J Clin Endocrinol Metab 93: 3075-3081.
[38] Alberobello AT, Congedo V, Liu H, Cochran C, Skarulis MC, et al. (2011) An intronic SNP in the thyroid hormone receptor beta gene is associated with pituitary cell-specific over-expression of a mutant thyroid hormone receptor beta2 (R338W) in the index case of pituitary-selective resistance to thyroid hormone. J Transl Med 9: 144.
[39] Dayan CM, Panicker V (2009) Novel insights into thyroid hormones from the study of common genetic variation. Nat Rev Endocrinol 5: 211-218.
[40] Horvath A, Faucz F, Finkielstain GP, Nikita ME, Rothenbuhler A, et al. (2010) Haplotypeanalysis of the promoter region of phosphodiesterase type 8B (PDE8B) in correlation with inactivating PDE8B mutation and the serum thyroid-stimulating hormone Levels. Thyroid 20.
[41] Arnaud-Lopez L, Usala G, Ceresini G, Mitchell BD, Pilia MG, et al. (2008) Phosphodiesterase 8B gene variants are associated with serum TSH levels and thyroid function. Am J Hum Genet 82: 1270-1280.
[42] Sabeti PC, Schaffner SF, Fry B, Lohmueller J, Varilly P, et al. (2006) Positive natural selection in the human lineage. Science 312: 1614-1620.
[43] López Herráez D, Bauchet M, Tang K, Theunert C, Pugach I, et al. (2010) Genetic variation and recent positive selection in worldwide human populations: evidence from nearly 1 million SNPs. PLoS One 4: e7888.
[44] Dormitzer PR, Ellison PT, Bode HH (1989) Anomalously low endemic goiter prevalence among Efe pygmies. Am J Phys Anthropol 78: 527–531.
[45] Hancock AM, Witonsky DB, Alkorta-Aranburu G, Beall CM, Gebremedhin A, et al. (2011) Adaptations to climate-mediated selective pressures in humans. PLoS Genet 7: e1001375.
[46] Nielsen R, Bustamante C, Clark AG, Glanowski S, Sackton TB, et al. (2005) A scan for positively selected genes in the genomes of humans and chimpanzees. PLoS Biol 3: e170.
[47] Gagneux P, Amess B, Diaz S, Moore S, Patel T, et al. (2001) Proteomic comparison of human and great ape blood plasma reveals conserved glycosylation and differences in thyroid hormone metabolism. Am J Phys Anthropol 115: 99-109.
[48] Newton P (1996) Hypothyroid nails and evolution. Lancet 347: 1832-1833.
[49] Iwasawa H (1960) On the local variation of the thyroid gland in the Japanese pond frog, *Rana nigromaculata*. Doubutsugaku zasshi 69: 125-128.
[50] Woodhead AD, Scully PM (1977) A comparative study of the Pretumorous thyroid gland of the gynogenetic teleost, *Poecilia formosa,* and that of other Poeciliid fishes. Cancer Res 37: 3751-3755.
[51] Moccia RD, Leatherland JF, Sonstegard RA (1977) Increasing frequency of thyroid goiters in Coho salmon (*Oncorhynchus kisutch*) in the Great Lakes. Science 198: 425-426.

[52] Sonstegard RA (1976) Studies of the etiology and epizootiology of lymphosarcoma in Esox (*Esox lucius* L. and *Esox masquinongy*). Prog Exp Tumor Res 20: 141-155.
[53] Moccia RD, Leatherland JF, Sonstegard RA (1981) Quantitative interlake comparison of thyroid pathology in Great Lakes coho (*Oncorhynchus kisutch*) and chinook (*Oncorhynchus tschawytscha*) salmon. Cancer Res 41: 2200-2210.
[54] Moccia RD, Fox GA, Britton A (1986) A quantitative assessment of thyroid histopathology of herring gulls (*Larus argentatus*) from the Great Lakes and a hypothesis on the causal role of environmental contaminants. J Wildlife Dis 22: 60-70.
[55] Sonstegard RA, Leatherland JF (1979) Hypothyroidism in rats fed Great Lakes coho salmon. Bull Environ Contam Toxicol 22: 779-784.
[56] Schlumberger HG (1955) Spontaneous goiter and cancer of the thyroid in animals. Ohio J Sci 55: 23-43.
[57] Honma Y, Shioda S, Yoshie S (1977) Changes in the thyroid gland associated with the diadromous migration of the threespine stickleback, *Gasterosteus aculeatus*. Jpn J Ichthyol 24: 17-25.
[58] Hamada K (1975) Excessively enlarged thyroid follicles of the threespine stickleback, *Gasterosteus aculeatus aculeatus*, reared in freshwater. Jpn J Ichthyol 21: 183–190
[59] Cabello G, Vilaxa A, Spotorno AE, Valladares JP, Pickard M, et al. (2003) Evolutionary adaptation of a mammalian species to an environment severely depleted of iodide. Pflug Arch Eur J Phy 446: 42-45.
[60] Dunlap KL, Reynolds AJ, Refsal KR, Kerr WW, Duffy LK (2008) Cross-latitudinal, seasonal and diurnal comparisons in thyroid hormone concentrations in sled dogs. Am J Anim Vet Sci 3: 96-103.
[61] Burger MF, Denver RJ (2001) Plasma thyroid hormone concentrations in a wintering passerine bird: their relationship to geographic variation, environmental factors, metabolic rate, and body fat. Physiol Biochem Zool 75: 187-199.
[62] Fair PA, Montie E, Balthis L, Reif JS, Bossart GD (2011) Influences of biological variables and geographic location on circulating concentrations of thyroid hormones in wild bottlenose dolphins (*Tursiops truncatus*). Gen Comp Endocrinol 174: 184-194.
[63] Buchholz DR, Hayes TB (2005) Variation in thyroid hormone action and tissue content underlies species differences in the timing of metamorphosis in desert frogs. Evol Dev 7: 458-467.
[64] Bragg AN (1945) The spadefoot toads in Oklahoma with a summary of our knowledge of the group. II. Am Nat 79: 52-72.
[65] Newman RA (1988) Genetic variation for larval anuran (*Scaphiopus couchii*) development time in an uncertain environment. Evolution 42: 763-773.
[66] Pickard MR, Sinha AK, Ogilvie LM, Leonard AJ, Edwards PR, et al. (1999) Maternal hypothyroxinemia influences glucose transporter expression in fetal brain and placenta. J Endocrinol 163: 385-394.
[67] Wilson CM, McNabb FM (1997) Maternal thyroid hormones in Japanese quail eggs and their influence on embryonic development. Gen Comp Endocrinol 107: 153-165.
[68] Brown DD (1997) The role of thyroid hormone in zebrafish and axolotl development. Proc Natl Acad Sci USA 94: 13011-13016.

[69] Tagawa M, Hirano T (1987) Presence of thyroxine in eggs and changes in its content during early development of chum salmon, *Oncorhynchus keta*. Gen Comp Endocrinol 68: 129-135.

[70] McComb DM, Gelsleichter J, Manire CA, Brinn R, Brown CL (2005) Comparative thyroid hormone concentration in maternal serum and yolk of the bonnethead shark (*Sphyrna tiburo*) from two sites along the coast of Florida. Gen Comp Endocrinol 144: 167-173.

[71] Parsons GR (1993) Geographic variation in reproduction between two populations of the bonnethead shark, *Sphyma tiburo*. Environ Biol Fish 38: 25-35.

[72] Arendt JD (1997) Adaptive intrinsic growth rates: an integration across taxa. Q Rev Biol 72: 149-177.

[73] Conover DO (1990) The relationship between capacity for growth and length of growing season: evidence for and implications of countergradient variation. Trans Am Fish Soc 119: 416-430.

[74] Habra M, Sarlis NJ (2005) Thyroid and aging. Rev Endocr Metab Disord 6: 145-154.

[75] Brown-Borg HM (2007) Hormonal regulation of longevity in mammals. Ageing Res Rev 6: 28-45.

[76] Hulbert AJ, Hinds DS, MacMillen RE (1985) Minimal metabolism, summit metabolism and plasma thyroxine in rodents from different environments. Comp Biochem Phys A 81: 687-693.

[77] Kwiecinski GG, Damassa DA, Gustafson AW (1986) Control of sex steroid-binding protein (SBP) in the male little brown bat: relationship of plasma thyroxine levels to the induction of plasma SBP in immature males. J Endocrinol 110: 271-278.

[78] Buffenstein R (2005) The naked mole-rat: a new long-living model for human aging research. J Gerontol A Biol Sci Med Sci 60: 1369-1377.

[79] Buffenstein R, Woodley R, Thomadakis C, Daly TJ, Gray DA (2001) Cold-induced changes in thyroid function in a poikilothermic mammal, the naked mole-rat. Am J Physiol-Reg I 280: R149-155.

[80] Ooka H, Shinkai T (1986) Effects of chronic hyperthyroidism on the lifespan of the rat. Mech Ageing Dev 33: 275-282.

[81] Lin SC, Li S, Drolet DW, Rosenfeld MG (1994) Pituitary ontogeny of the Snell dwarf mouse reveals Pit-1-independent and Pit-1-dependent origins of the thyrotrope. Development 120: 515-522.

[82] Sornson MW, Wu W, Dasen JS, Flynn SE, Norman DJ, et al. (1996) Pituitary lineage determination by the Prophet of Pit-1 homeodomain factor defective in Ames dwarfism. Nature 384: 327-333.

[83] Boylston WH, DeFord JH, Papaconstantinou J (2006) Identification of longevity-associated genes in long-lived Snell and Ames dwarf mice. Age 28: 125-144.

[84] Vergara M, Smith-Wheelock M, Harper JM, Sigler R, Miller RA (2004) Hormone-treated snell dwarf mice regain fertility but remain long lived and disease resistant. J Gerontol A Biol Sci Med Sci 59: 1244-1250.

[85] Hauck SJ, Hunter WS, Danilovich N, Kopchick JJ, Bartke A (2001) Reduced levels of thyroid hormones, insulin, and glucose, and lower body core temperature in the growth hormone receptor/binding protein knockout mouse. Exp Biol Med 226: 552-558.
[86] Kitano J, Lema SC, Luckenbach JA, Mori S, Kawagishi Y, et al. (2010) Adaptive divergence in the thyroid hormone signaling pathway in the stickleback radiation. Curr Biol 20: 2124-2130.
[87] Boura D, Castric V, Bernatchez L, Audet C (2002) Physiological, endocrine, and genetic bases of anadromy in the brook charr, *Salvelinus fontinalis*, of the Laval River (Quebec, Canada). Environ Biol Fish 64: 229-242.
[88] Rubin CJ, Zody MC, Eriksson J, Meadows JR, Sherwood E, et al. (2010) Whole-genome resequencing reveals loci under selection during chicken domestication. Nature 464: 587–591.
[89] Kijas JW, Lenstra JA, Hayes B, Boitard S, Porto Neto LR, et al. (2012) Genome-wide analysis of the world's sheep breeds reveals high levels of historic mixture and strong recent selection. PLoS Biol 10: e1001258.
[90] Nakao N, Ono H, Yamamura T, Anraku T, Takagi T, et al. (2008) Thyrotrophin in the pars tuberalis triggers photoperiodic response. Nature 452: 317-322.
[91] Ono H, Hoshino Y, Yasuo S, Watanabe M, Nakane Y, et al. (2008) Involvement of thyrotropin in photoperiodic signal transduction in mice. Proc Natl Acad Sci U S A 105: 18238-18242.
[92] Hanon EA, Lincoln GA, Fustin JM, Dardente H, Masson-Pevet M, et al. (2008) Ancestral TSH mechanism signals summer in a photoperiodic mammal. Curr Biol 18: 1147-1152.
[93] Masumoto K, Ukai-Tadenuma M, Kasukawa T, Nagano M, Uno KD, et al. (2010) Acute induction of Eya3 by late-night light stimulation triggers TSHβ expression in photoperiodism. Curr Biol 20: 2199 - 2206
[94] Dardente H, Wyse CA, Birnie MJ, Dupré SM, Loudon ASI, et al. (2010) A molecular switch for photoperiod responsiveness in mammals. Cur Biol 20: 1193 - 2198
[95] Schluter D (2000) The Ecology of Adaptive Radiation. New York: Oxford University Press.
[96] Barrett RDH, Hoekstra HE (2011) Molecular spandrels: tests of adaptation at the genetic level. Nat Rev Genet 12: 767-780.
[97] Sonstegard R, Leatherland JF (1976) The epizootiology and pathogenesis of thyroid hyperplasia in coho salmon (*Oncorhynchus kisutch*) in Lake Ontario. Cancer Res 36: 4467-4475.
[98] Hewitt EA, Crain DA, Gunderson MP, Guillette LJJ (2002) Thyroid status in juvenile alligators (*Alligator mississippiensis*) from contaminated and reference sites on Lake Okeechobee, Florida, USA. Chemosphere 47: 1129-1135.
[99] Gorbman A, Gordon M (1951) Spontaneous thyroidal tumors in the swordtail *Xiphophorus montezumae*. Cancer Res 11: 184-187.
[100] Berg O, Gordon M, Gorbman A (1954) Comparative effects of thyroidal stimulants and inhibitors of normal and tumorous thyroids in Xiphophorin fishes. Cancer Res 14: 527-533.

[101] Buffernstein R, Pinto M (2009) Endocrine function in naturally long-living small mammals. Mol Cell Endocrinol 299: 101-111.

Section 2

Developmental Physiology

Chapter 5

Maternal-Fetal Thyroid Interactions

R.G. Ahmed

Additional information is available at the end of the chapter

1. Introduction

Life is getting complicated in the world of local thyroid hormones (THs) regulation. On account of TH action can be controlled in individual cells through selective TH uptake and intracellular TH metabolism, the placenta is an important link in the maternal-fetal communication network for THs which are essential for the normal development and differentiation of the fetus [1-3]. Generally, intracellular activation or inactivation of L-thyroxine (T4) and 3,5,3'-triiodothyronine (T3) in turn is determined by three types of iodothyronine deiodinases (Ds), namely DI, DII, and DIII [4-7]. The placenta transports and metabolizes maternal THs, and mainly expresses DIII, which inactivates T4 and other iodothyronines and thus limits the transfer of maternal active THs to the fetus in the late pregnancy [8]. DII is also active in the placenta and locally provides active T3 from the maternal prohormone T4 for placental metabolic functions [1,2]. The placental expression of DI, which also activates T4 to T3, is still controversial. Because of the lipophilic nature of THs, it was thought that they traversed the plasma membrane by simple diffusion [9,10]. The transport of T4 and T3 in and out of cells is controlled by several classes of transmembrane TH-transporters (THTs) [11], including members of the organic anion transporter family (OATP), L-type amino acid transporters (LATs), Na^+/Taurocholate cotransporting polypeptide (NTCP), and monocarboxylate transporters (MCTs) [10,12]. Particularly, monocarboxylate transporter 8 (MCT8) has recently been identified as an active and specific TH transporter. Also, placental membranes are also involved in 4'-OH-sulfation reactions of iodothyronines [8]. Sulfation (S) plays a role in TH metabolism by interacting between the deiodination and sulfation pathways of TH [13]. Interestingly, placental cells express high affinity, stereo-specific, energy-dependent uptake systems for T4 and T3. On the other hand, the cellular activity of THs is usually classified as genomic (nuclear) and non-genomic (initiated either at cytoplasm or at membrane TH receptors) [14-21]. Binding of T3 to its nuclear thyroid receptors (TRs) directly affects transcription of many genes that are important in development [22].

In general, pregnancy is accompanied by profound alterations in the thyroidal economy (hypo- or hyper-thyroidism), resulting from a complex combination of factors specific to the pregnant state, which together concur to stimulate the maternal thyroid machinery [1,23]. Also, clinical studies showed that maternal TH deficiency during the first trimester of pregnancy can affect the outcome of human neurodevelopment [24,25]. Experiments in rats showed that early maternal TH deficiency affects neuronal migration in the cortex [26], while maternal hyperthyroidism too can disturb fetal brain development [27]. Experimental data on the mechanisms regulating intracellular TH availability and action prior to the onset of fetal TH secretion, however, remain scarce. Thus, in this chapter will be aware about the significant roles of THs, their metabolism by Ds and sulfotransferases, their transport by THTs and their binding to TRs from the mother via the placenta to the fetal compartment especially during the gestation period in both human and animals.

2. Placental transport of thyroid hormones

2.1. By thyroid hormone-deiodinases (Table 1 and Figure 1)

The synthesis of THs is regulated through the hypothalamus–pituitary–thyroid (HPT) axis [28] and the follicular cells of the thyroid gland synthesize and secrete T4 and T3 [1,2,21]. This process is under the control of the circulating TH levels through negative feedback loops of this axis [28]. The availability of the active ligand T3 within tissues is locally determined by the action of the iodothyronine deiodinases (Ds) [29]. There are three selenocysteine monodeiodinase subtypes (DI, DII and DIII) [30]. Whilst T3 is generated by the activity of DI and DII, via 5'- reductive or outer ring deiodination (ORD) of the T4 [31], DIII activity (and to a lesser extent that of DI) convert T4 to 3,3',5'-tri-iodothyronine (reverse T3; rT3) and T3 into 3,3'-T2 via inner ring deiodination (IRD), in effect acting as a deactivating enzyme for THs [13,32].

Activities of all three iodothyronine deiodinase subtypes have been demonstrated in most rat placenta [33]. However, in contrast to man, rodent total serum T3 and T4 increase with gestation [34] and the predominant subtype expressed appears to be DIII [35], although DII is also present with significant activity [36]. Placental DIII activity is much greater (approx. 200 times) than DII activity; however, the activity and expression of both DII and DIII fall as gestation progresses [37-40]. Placental DII provides T3 for 'housekeeping' processes, and as indicated above, its activity is much less than that of D3 [40]. DII has been localized to the villous cytotrophoblasts in the first trimester and syncytiotrophoblasts in the third trimester, whereas DIII has been localized to the villous syncytiotrophoblasts in both the first and third trimesters of pregnancy [39]. Both DIII mRNA and activity are present at the implantation site in rodents, as early as gestational day 9 (GD 9), being expressed in mesometrial and antimesometrial decidual tissue [41]. Also, in rabbit [42] and pig [43], the placenta appears to express DIII activity predominantly. The positioning of the deiodinases, particularly DIII, suggests that they might regulate the amount of maternal TH reaching fetal circulation [40]. Interestingly, however, fetuses with total thyroid agenesis but with evidence of circulating maternal TH have normal placental DIII activity, suggesting that there might be other factors modulating T4 access to the deiodinases, such as intracellular protection of TH by TH-binding protein (THBP) [40,44]. Collectively, express placental Ds (II, III) may play a critical role in delivery of TH to the fetus as summarized in figure1 [2,45-47] and table 1 [1,2,31,48].

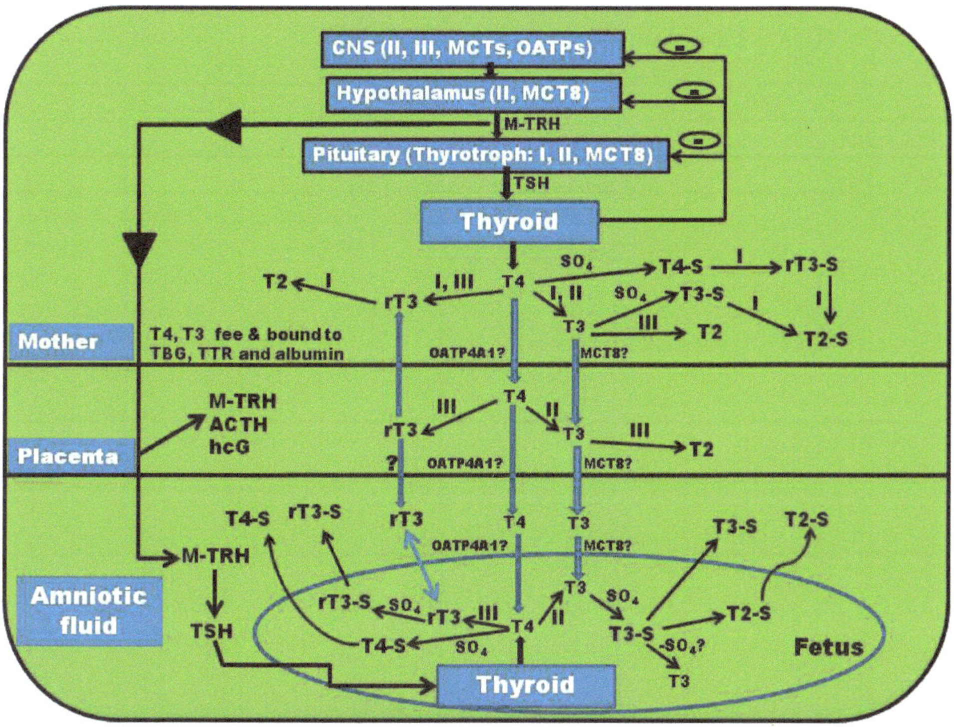

Figure 1. Summary about the interactions of maternal, placental and fetal thyroid metabolism. I, II and III denote deiodinases type 1 (DI), type two (DII) and type three (DIII). SO_4 is a sulfation pathway and $-SO_4$ is a desulfation pathway. CNS is central nervous system, TRH is thyroid releasing hormone, M-TRH is maternal thyroid releasing hormone, TSH is thyrotrophin, T2 is diiodothyronine, T3 is triiodothyronine, rT3 is reverse triiodothyronine, T4 is thyroxine, T2S is diiodothyronine sulfate, T3S is triiodothyronine sulfate, T4S is thyroxine sulfate, rT3S is reverse triiodothyronine sulfate, MCT8 is monocarboxylate transporter 8, OATP4A1 is organic anion transporter 4A1, TBG is thyroxin binding globulin, TTR is transthyretin, ACTH is adrenocorticotrophin and hCG is human chorionic gonadotrophin.

Characteristic	DI	DII	DIII
Reaction kinetics	Ping-pong	Sequential	
Reaction catalyzed (Deiodination)	5 or 5' (ORD+IRD)	5' (ORD)	5 (IRD)
Main form	T4-T3, rT3- T2	- T4- rT3, T3- T2	- T4- rT3- T2
Substrate preference	5: T4S>T3S>>T3, T4 5': rT3, rT3S>T2S>>T4	T4>rT3	T3>T4
Sulfation of substrates	Stimulation	Inhibition	
Substrate limiting *KM*	0.5 mM	1–2 nM	5–20 mM
In vitro cofactor limiting *KM*	1–10 Mm DTT	>10 mM DTT	=70 mM DTT
Molecular mass (kDa)	29	30	32
Selenocysteine	present		
Homodimer	Yes		
Location	- Liver, kidney, thyroid and pituitary.	- Pituitary, brain, BAT, thyroid[a], heart[a] and skeletal muscle[a].	- Brain, skin, uterus, placenta, fetus and in other sites of the maternal- fetal interface, such as the umbilical arteries and veins.
Subcellular location	- Liver: endoplasmic reticulum. - kidney: basolateral plasma membrane	- Microsomal membranes	
Functions	- Production serum T3 and the clearance of serum rT3.	- Catalyzes the outer ring deiodination of T4 to T3 and is thus important for the local production of T3.	- Catalyzes the inner ring deiodination of T4 to rT3 and of T3 to 3,3'-T2.
Activity in hypothyroidism	- Decrease in liver and kidney. - increase in thyroid.	- Increase in all tissues.	- Decrease in brain.
Activity in hyperthyroidism	- Unknown in liver and kidney. - Increase in thyroid.	- Decrease in most tissues. - Increase in thyroid[a].	- Increase in brain.
Low-T3 syndrome	- Decrease	- No change	

Active site residues	- Selenocysteine histidine and phenylalanine.	- (Seleno-)cysteine?	- Selenocysteine
Human gene structure and location	- 1p32-p33, 17.5 kb and 4 exons.	- 14q24.3, 2 exons, and 7.4-kb intron.	- 14q32
Promoter elements	- TRE, RXR, no CAAT or TATA box.	--	
Propylthiouracil inhibitor	++++	+	+/-
Aurothioglucose inhibitor		++	
Iopanoic acid inhibitor	+++	++++	+++
Thiouracils	++++	-/+	-
iodoacetate		+	?
flavonoids	+	+++	

[a] Humans only. T2 is diiodothyronine, T3 is triiodothyronine, rT3 is reverse triiodothyronine, T4 is thyroxine, T2S is diiodothyronine sulfate, T3S is triiodothyronine sulfate, T4S is thyroxine sulfate, rT3S is reverse triiodothyronine sulfate, ORD is outer ring deiodination, IRD is inner ring deiodination, TRE is T3-responsive element, RXR is retinoid X receptors and DDT is dithiols.

Table 1. General characteristics of the iodothyronine deiodinases.

2.2. By thyroid hormone-transporters (THTs) (Tables 2 & 3 and Figure 1)

Membrane transporters mediate cellular uptake and efflux of TH [12,40,49]. The ability to transport TH has been described in members of different transporter groups including the monocarboxylate transporters (MCT), L-type amino acid transporters (LAT), Na^+/Taurocholate cotransporting polypeptide (NTCP), and organic anion transporting polypeptides (OATP) [50]. With the exception of MCT8, these transporters do not exclusively transport TH and they all have slightly different affinities for specific forms of TH. To date six different THTs are known to be present in the placenta: MCT8, MCT10, LAT1, LAT2, OATP1A2 and OATP4A1 but their relative contributions to placental TH transport are unknown [50-55]. Also, their anatomical localization, ontogeny in the human placenta and relative affinity for the TH and thyronines are very complex. MCT8, MCT10, OATP1A2, OATP4A1 and LAT1 are expressed in villous syncytiotrophoblasts, and MCT8, MCT10 and OATP1A2 in cytotrophoblasts [50]. Although transporters in the apical syncytiotrophoblast membrane are well placed to maximize maternal cellular TH uptake early in gestation, the large numbers and variety of THTs are intriguing [51,53,55]. Moreover, the expression of MCT8 mRNA increased with advancing gestation [55] but there is limited information regarding the ontogeny of the other THTs. In addition, it is likely that the lower expression of MCT8, MCT10, OATP1A2 and LAT1 before 14 week compared to term, as well as the nadir in OATP4A1 expression in the late 1st and early 2nd trimester, may play a role in the necessary limitation of maternal-fetal TH transfer, particularly around the time of onset of endogenous fetal TH production in the early 2nd trimester [56]. Increased expression of THTs in late gestation is consistent with the proposal that there is continued/ increased maternal to fetal supply of TH in the 3rd trimester despite increasing fetal TH production [57]. It is also likely that increased expression of these transporters with gestation may also fulfil the increased need for other biological substances for fetal growth and development, such as amino acids. The most factors regulating the placental expression of these transporters are unknown until now. There are suggestions in rodents that the activity of system-L and the expression of MCT8 in non-placental tissues are influenced by thyroid status [58] suggesting that TH may be a regulator of its own transporters [50]. During the passage of THs from the maternal circulation to the fetal circulation, each THT is likely to have a specific role in each different plasma membrane layer, which might include cellular influx, efflux, or both [59]. To sum, THTs of the various placental cell types serve as channels that help to maintain the differences in the composition of THs and their metabolites between maternal and fetal circulations (figure1 [2,45-47] and tables 2 & 3 [51,52,55,59,60,61]). The relative contributions of these THTs to the transplacental transport of thyroid hormones are still a subject for research.

Transporter[a]	Iodothyronine derivates	Specificity[b]
MCT8	T3, T4, rT3, T2	+++
MCT10	T3, T4	++
OATP1A1	T3, T4, rT3, T2, T4S, T3S, rT3S, T2S	+
OATP1A2	T4, T3, rT3	
OATP1A3	T4, T3	
OATP1A4		
OATP1A5		
OATP1B1	T4, T3, T3S, T4S, rT3S	
OATP1B2	T3, T4	
OATP1B3	rT3, T4S, T3S, rT3S	
OATP1C1	T4, rT3, T3, T4S	++
OATP2B1	T4	+
OATP3A1 (V1/V2)		++
OATP4A1	T3, T4, rT3	+
OATP4C1	T3, T4	
OATP6B1		
OATP6C1		
LAT1	T3, T4, rT3, T2	
LAT2		
NTCP	T4, T3, T4S, T3S	++

[a] The human protein symbol is presented, if TH transport has been demonstrated in different species including humans. [b] If a transporter only transports iodothyronine derivatives, specificity is high (+++). If fewer than five other ligands are known, specificity is moderate (++). If more than five ligands are known, the transporter is denoted as multispecific (+).

Table 2. Types of thyroid hormone transporters and their iodothyronine derivates.

Transporter family	Monocarboxylate transporters		System L amino acidtransporters		Organic anion transporting polypeptides	
	MCT8	MCT10	LAT1	LAT2	OATP1A2	OATP4A1
Heterodimer	N/A		4F2hc		N/A	
Additional molecules transported	N/A	Aromatic amino acids	Large neutral amino acids		Amphipathic organic compounds	
Localization in first and second trimester[a]	ST, CT, EVT	N/A				
Localization in third trimester[b]	ST	N/A	ST^{ap}	N/A		ST^{ap}
Km T4 (μM)	4.7[c]	>Km T3[d]	7.9		8.0	>Km T3
Km T3 (μM)	4.0[c]	≤4.0[d]	0.8		6.5	0.9
Km rT3 (μM)	2.2[c]	N/A	12.5		N/A	
Km T2 (μM)	N/A		7.9	N/A		

[a]Only MCT8 has been localized in the placenta in all three trimesters of pregnancy. [b]LAT1 and OATP4A1 have been localized only at term. [c] These Km values were determined for the rat MCT8 protein expressed in Xenopus laevis oocytes. The other Km values shown are mainly from studies using the human gene expressed in X. laevis oocytes. [d]Human MCT8 or MCT10 transporters expressed in COS1 cells both showed a greater preference for T3 than T4 uptake. Whereas MCT10 showed a greater capacity than MCT8 to transport T3, MCT8 was found to be a more active transporter of T4.

Abbreviations: CT is cytotrophoblast cells, EVT is extravillous trophoblast cells, N/A is no data available, rT3 is reverse T3, ST is syncytiotrophoblast layer and ST^{ap} is predominantly at apical surface of the ST.

Table 3. Expression of the thyroid hormone transporters in human placenta.

2.3. By thyroid hormone-sulfotransferases (Figure 1)

Sulfation (S) appears to be an important pathway for the reversible inactivation of THs during fetal development [2,13,45-47]. Monique Kester and the group from Erasmus University have used a rat model to study the regulation of fetal TH status and have also extended their studies to human pregnancy [62]. The sulfotransferases catalyze the sulfation of the hydroxyl group of compounds, using 3'-phosphoadenosine-5'-phosphsulfate (PAPS) as the universal sulfate donor [63]. This co-factor PAPS is synthesized from two ATP molecules and inorganic sulfate. Neither the DII or DIII iodothyronines catalyze the deiodination of sulfated iodothyronines nor sulfation strongly facilitates the inner ring deiodination of T4 and T3 by DI, but blocks the outer ring deiodination of T4 (activation) [13,64]. The outer ring deiodination of rT3 by DI is not affected by sulfation [64]. Sulfation thus induces the irreversible degradation of TH. Thus, rapid inner ring deiodinations of T4S, T3S and out ring deiodination of rT3S lead to high concentrations of these sulfates in plasma of adult humans [13,65].

High concentrations of the different iodothyronine sulfates, T4S (thyroxine sulfate), T3S (triiodothyronine sulfate), rT3S (reverse triiodothyronine sulfate) and T2S (diiodothyronine sulfate), have been documented in human fetal and neonatal plasma as well as in amniotic fluid [65,66], and similar findings have been reported for sheep [67]. This has classically been explained by the low hepatic DI expression in the human fetus until the postnatal period [68] and lack of hepatic DI expression until birth in rats [69]. Also, in the rat placenta, where there are insignificant sulfotransferases activities but high DIII activity, irreversible inactivation of DIII appears to be the predominant pathway of iodothyronine metabolism [13]. In the rat fetal liver, sulfotransferase activity is present from the end of the third trimester (GD 17), a time when DI activity is relatively absent [69]. The TH-sulfates may accumulate under such circumstances to form a 'reservoir' of inactive TH from which active hormone may be liberated, in a tissue specific and gestational dependent manner by the action of arylsulfases [13]. To date, six members of this family (ARSAeARSF) have been identified in humans [13,70]. It is interesting that DIII is abundantly expressed in the human placenta [39] and deiodinates T4 and T3 to 3,3'-T2 and rT3, respectively, thus providing substrates for these actions. In the human fetal circulation, T4S and in particular T3S, may represent a reservoir of inactive TH, from which active hormone may be liberated as required (vide supra) [13]. The iodothyronine sulfates in human fetal circulation and amniotic fluid may be derived, at least in part, from sulfation of THs by thermostabile phenol sulfotransferases in the uterus and placenta [13,45]. This may provide a route for the supply of maternal TH to the fetus in addition to placental transfer. Alternatively, iodothyronine sulfates may accumulate in the fetal circulation because of the absence of hepatic transporters which mediate their removal from plasma. It has been demonstrated recently that hepatic uptake of the different iodothyronine sulfates in rats is mediated at least in part through the NTCP and OATP families [71]. Thus, the TH-sulfation mechanism might be useful for non-invasive prenatal diagnostics of fetal thyroid function which is autonomously regulated. The overviews presented here are consistent with the evolving view that sulfation is a major chemical defense system in the maternal-fetal thyroid axis and will hopefully provide a basis for understanding more about these enzymes.

2.4. By thyroid hormone-genomic and non-genomic actions (Tables 4 & 5 and Figure 2)

Although the thyroid gland predominantly secretes T4, T3 is the most active TH, since it has a higher affinity by the nuclear thyroid hormone receptors (TRs; α, β) (Figure 2A) [75], which mediate most actions of these hormones [72,73]. THs are released by the thyroid gland to the circulation where they are carried bound to proteins such as thyroxin binding globulin (TBG), transthyretin (TTR) or serum albumin (Table 4) [74]. The level of albumin, which has the lowest T4 affinity and enables a fast release of T4 [76], gradually decreases during pregnancy [77]. TBG is an active carrier and has a possibility to switch between the high-affinity and the low-affinity form [78]. TBG levels are the highest in the second and third trimester of pregnancy [79,80] and the same holds true for TH-binding ratio [81] and thyroid-binding capacity [82], which decreases as soon as 3-4 days after delivery.

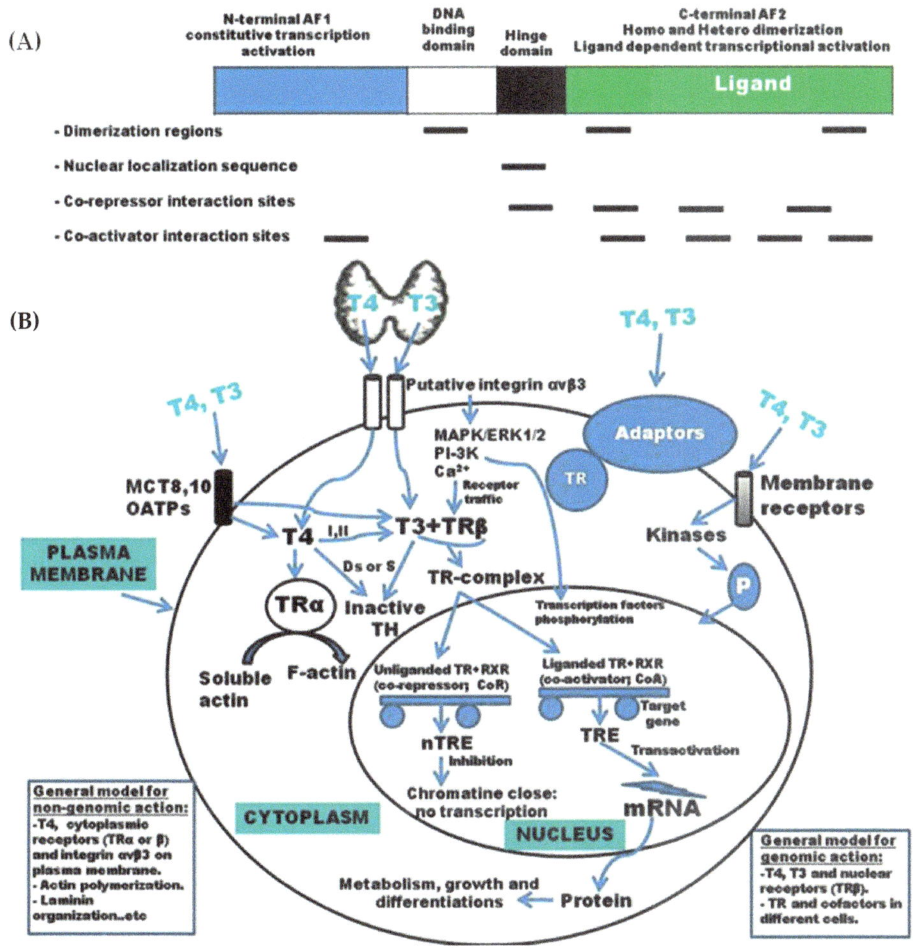

Abbreviations: T3 is triiodothyronine, T4 is thyroxine, TR is thyroid hormone receptor, RXR is retinoid X receptors, TRE is T3-responsive element, nTRE is none T3-responsive element, Ds is deiodonases, S is sulfotransferases, MCT is monocarboxylate transporter, OATP is organic anion transporter, MAPK/ERK1/2 is mitogen-activated protein kinase, P is phosphorylation and PI-3K is phosphatidylinositol 3-kinase.

Figure 2. (A) Schematic representation of major thyroid hormone receptors (TRα, β) domains and functional sub-regions. (B) General model for genomic and non-genomic actions of TH in both adult and fetus; Schematic representation of thyroid hormones (THs; T4 and T3) genomic actions, initiated at the nuclear receptors (TRβ), and non-genomic actions, initiated at cytoplasmatic receptors (TRβ, TRα) and at the plasma membrane on the membrane receptors, particularly integrin $\alpha v\beta 3$ receptor. T4 binding (but not T3) to cytoplasmic TRα may cause a change of state of actin. T3 binding (but not T4) to cytoplasmic TRβ activates the phosphatidylinositol 3-kinase (PI-3K) pathway leading to alteration in membrane ion pumps and to transcription of specific genes. TH binding to the integrin receptor results in activation of mitogen-activated protein kinase (MAPK/ERK1/2). Phosphorylated MAPK (pMAPK) translocates to the nucleus where it phosphorylates transcription factors including thyroid receptors (TRβ), estrogen receptor (ER) and signal transducer activators of transcription (STAT). Generally, activity is regulated by an exchange of corepressor (CoR) and coactivator (CoA) complexes.

TH-binding protein	Cellular location
Transthyretin	Plasma
T4-binding globulin	
Serum albumin	
Lipoproteins	
Myosin light chain kinase	Cytoplasmic
Pyruvate kinase, subtype M1	
Pyruvate kinase, subtype M2	
Prolyl 4-hydroxylase, b-subunit	
Aldehyde dehydrogenase	

Table 4. Types of thyroid hormone-binding proteins.

2.4.1. General genomic action (Table 5 and Figure 2)

T4 and T3 enter the cell through transporter proteins such as MCT8 and 10 or OATPs. Inside the cells, deiodinases (DI, II) convert T4, the major form of thyroid hormone in the blood, to the more active form T3. DIII produces rT3 and T2 from T4 and T3, respectively [1,73,83]. T3 binds to nuclear TRs, TRα and TRβ, that activate transcription by binding, generally as heterodimers with the retinoid X receptor (RXR) (Table 5) [87], to thyroid hormone response elements (TREs) located in regulatory regions of target genes [84]. Activity is regulated by an exchange of corepressor (CoR) and coactivator (CoA) complexes. Negative TREs (nTRE) can mediate ligand-dependent transcriptional repression, although in this case the role of coactivators and corepressors is not well defined [73,85]. TRs can also regulate the activity of genes that do not contain a TRE through "cross-talk" with other transcription factors (TF) that stimulate target gene expression [28,86]. Both receptors and coregulators are targets for phosphorylation (P) by signal transduction pathways stimulated by hormones and growth factors [84,85]. Thus, the nuclear actions of T3 are sensitive to inhibitors of transcription and translation and have a latency of hours to days [9,73]. Thus, the genomic action will play a critical role in the cellular proliferations and differentiations.

2.4.2. General non-genomic action (Table 5 and Figure 2)

Although T3 is known to exert many of its actions through the classical genomic regulation of gene transcription, a number of T3 effects occur rapidly and are unaffected by inhibitors of transcription and protein synthesis [88,89]. However, the levels of circulating THs are tightly regulated and stable and thus rapidly mediated responses must involve regulation of pre-receptor ligand metabolism, ligand membrane transport or receptor availability leading to local cell type specific variation in thyroid hormone signaling [87]. Non-genomic actions of THs have been described at the plasma membrane, in the cytoplasm and in cellular organelles [15,21,83,90,91]. They have included the modulation of Na^+, K^+, Ca^{2+} and glucose transport, activation of protein kinase C (PKC), protein kinase A (PKA) and mitogen-activated protein kinase (ERK/MAPK) and regulation of phospholipid metabolism by activation of phospholipase C (PLC) and D (PLD) [92-94]. Generally, binding of T3 to a subpopulation of receptors located outside the nuclei can also cause rapid "non-genomic" effects through interaction with adaptor proteins, leading to stimulation of signaling pathways. T4 can also bind to putative membrane receptors such as integrin receptor (αVβ3) inducing MAPK activity [18,73,95,96]. Thus, several observations suggest that the rapid nongenomic effects of TH are widespread and may be involved in multiple physiological processes in many different cell types [87]. However, no specific membrane associated TR isoform or thyroid hormone binding G protein-coupled receptors (GPCR) have been identified or cloned and thus the area remains controversial.

Compare face	Ligand	Receptor	Dimerization partners	Associated factors or signalling pathways	Actions
Classical, genomic actions (hours to days)					
Nuclear transcription	T3	TRα and TRβ	RXR and TRs	- NCoR/SMRT Basal	- Transcriptional repression
				- SRC/p160/TRAPs	- Transcriptional activation and repression
Non-classical non-genomic actions (seconds to minutes)					
Cell surface receptor	T4/T3	Putative GPCR		Raf1/MEK/MAPK	TR phosphorylation and altered transcriptional activity p53 phosphorylation and general transcriptional activity
				MEK/STATs	Increased STAT mediated transcription
Mitochondrial gene transcription	T3	TRαp43	mtRXR and mtPPAR	Co-factors?	Increased mitochondrial gene expression
Mitochondrial oxidation	T3	TRαp28		ANT, UCPs	Increased thermogenesis
	T2	Cytochrome -*c* Va			Increased oxidative phosphorylation

Abbreviations: T4 is Thyroxine, T3 is triiodothyronine, T2 is diiodothyronine, RXR is retinoid X receptor, TR is thyroid hormone receptor, GPCR is G protein coupled receptor, mtRXR is mitochondrial retinoid X receptor α isoform, mtPPAR is mitochondrial peroxisome proliferator activator receptor γ2 isoform, NCoR is nuclear receptor co-repressor, SMRT is silencing mediator of RAR and TR, SRC is steroid receptor cooactivator, TRAPs is thyroid receptor associated protein, Raf1 is Raf serine/threonine kinase, MEK is mitogen activated protein kinase kinase, MAPK is mitogen activated protein kinase, STAT is signal transducers and activators of transcription, ANT is adenine nucleotide translocase and UCP is uncoupling protein.

Table 5. General thyroid hormone actions.

There also are reports of nongenomic effects on cell structure proteins by THs. Actin depolymerization blocks DII inactivation by T4 in cAMP-stimulated glial cells, suggesting that an intact actin cytoskeleton is important for this downregulation of deiodinase activity [9,97]. Interestingly, T4, but not T3, can promote actin polymerization in astrocytes [98] and thus may influence the downregulation of DII activity by a secondary mechanism, perhaps by targeting to lysosomes [9,99]. Moreover, the regulation of actin polymerization and F-actin contents also could contribute to the effects of TH on arborization, axonal transport, and cell-cell contacts during brain development, where the regulation of these factors is fundamental for the organization of guidance molecules such as laminin on the astrocyte plasma membrane and modulates integrin–laminin interactions [3]. T4 was required for integrin clustering and attachment to laminin by integrin in astrocytes [100]. These data suggest that the non-genomic action may play an important role in promoting the normal development.

3. Maternal-fetal thyroid in normal state

THs are essential for normal neonatal development in both humans and rodents [3,23,101-104] and the experimental work indicated that THs are transported from the mother to the fetus, albeit in limited amounts, and that the fetal brain is exposed to THs before initiation of fetal TH synthesis [1]. In addition, the maternal TH regulates early fetal brain development in human and animal models [2]. The TH of maternal origin can cross the placenta and reach the fetus [2,105,106] and that TRs are expressed in the fetal rat brain before the onset of fetal thyroid function [107]. Thus, the THs are essential for brain maturation from early embryonic stages onward [103,104,108]. However, TH-dependent stages of fetal brain development remain to be characterized. Notably, the maternal thyroid is the only source of T4 and T3 for the brain of the fetus because its thyroid gland does not start contributing to fetal requirements until midgestation in man, and days 17.5–18 in rats [109]. Therefore, the amount of maternal T4 that the fetus receives early in pregnancy will determine TH action in its brain because it depends on maternal T4 for its intracellular supply of the active form of the hormone, T3. However, fetal brain total T3 levels are low (ca. 100 pM) at this time [1], but receptor occupancy approximates 25% since free T3 concentrations are high in the nucleus relative to the cytosol [110]. In general, materno-fetal transfer of THs has been demonstrated in early fetal stages [111] and continues, at least in the case of fetal inability, to produce sufficient TH until term [44]. Actually, brain cells can protect themselves against higher fetal T4 and T3 values by decreasing DII and increasing DIII activity [2]. Taken together, thyroid activity undergoes many changes during normal pregnancy including [1,112-115]: (a) a significant increase in serum thyroxine-binding globulin, thyroglobulin, total T4, and total T3; (b) an increase in renal iodide clearance; and (c) stimulation of the thyroid by human chorionic gonadotropin (hCG). These changes can make diagnosis of thyroid dysfunction during pregnancy difficult.

4. Maternal-fetal thyroid in hypothyroid state

THs are important for growth and differentiation of a variety of organs, including the brain. In developing brain, THs stimulate and coordinate processes such as neuronal proliferation, migration, growth of axons and dendrites, synapse formation and myelination [1,2].

Disturbance of these processes leads to abnormalities in the neuronal network and may result in mental retardation and other neurological defects, including impaired motor skills and visual processing [115]. If TH deficiency occurs at the perinatal stage, such as in congenital hypothyroidism, timely treatment may rescue most of the symptoms. A shortage of THs starting at the early stages of pregnancy, such as in cretinism, results in neurological deficits that cannot be rescued by exogenous TH addition at later stages [25].

The role of THs in brain development has been studied most extensively in the cerebellum [23,116]. The cellular proliferation and migration processes are disturbed by TH deficiency as investigated predominantly in rodents, where most of cerebellar maturation occurs in the early postnatal period [2]. In the hypothyroid cerebellum, the number and length of Purkinje cell dendrites is severely reduced [1]. At the same time the granule cell parallel fiber growth is reduced, leading to a reduction in axodendritic connections between the Purkinje cells and the granule neurons [117]. Additionally, other cell types such as astrocytes, Golgi epithelial cells, basket cells, and oligodendrocytes show abnormalities under hypothyroid conditions [116]. Several TH target genes have been identified over the years, including genes coding for myelin proteins, cytoskeletal proteins, neurotrophins and their receptors, transcription factors, and intracellular signaling proteins [118] and recent transcriptome analyses continue to increase their number [119-121]. Some of these genes only respond to thyroid status for a short and specific period during development, a feature that is typical for many TH target genes in brain [122]. Interestingly, a reduction or absence of TH during brain maturation yields molecular, morphological and functional alterations in the cerebral cortex, hippocampus and cerebellum [123-132].

5. Maternal-fetal thyroid in hyperthyroid state (Figure 3)

Neonatal hyperthyroidism was described as a critical disease marked mainly by cardiac symptoms, poor weight gain and severe neurological manifestations [1,133-137]. Fetal thyrotoxicosis is the result of thyroid-stimulating antibody transfer to the fetus in the setting of maternal Grave's disease [2,138]. It may present with a variety of clinical features, which include persistent sinus tachycardia, fetal hydrops, intrauterine growth restriction, goiter and fetal demise [1,139]. The vast majority of cases of excessive serum TH concentration seen in pregnancy are due to the overproduction of THs (Graves' disease, toxic nodular goiter); in the postpartum period, thyrotoxicosis may be due to exacerbation of Graves' hyperthyroidism or to the release of thyroid hormone due to an acute autoimmune injury to the thyroid tissue (postpartum thyroiditis-PPT) [2,140].

The management of hyperthyroidism in pregnancy, which most often is caused by Graves' disease, has been reviewed recently [141,142]. Hyperthyroidism occurs in about 0.2–0.4% of all pregnancies. Hyperthyroidism should be distinguished from gestational transient thyrotoxicosis, which is due to the TSH-receptor stimulating effects of hCG [143,144]. This hCG-induced hyperthyroidism is mostly mild and need not be treated. Only rare cases with extremely high hCG (i.e. due to a hydatidiform mole) might induce severe thyrotoxicosis [145]. The signs and symptoms of hyperthyroidism due to Graves' disease may aggravate in the first trimester and thereafter may become mild. Untreated hyperthyroidism is associated with severe effects on maternal and neonatal outcome. The risk for premature fetal loss, preeclampsia, preterm delivery, intrauterine growth retardation and low birth weight is significantly increased [144]. It has to be considered that the transfer of stimulating receptor antibodies (TSAbs) are transferred from the mother to the child, and therefore the fetus is at risk to develop Graves' disease. Close monitoring of the fetus is, therefore, strictly recommended, even in mothers treated by thyroidectomy before pregnancy but have still elevated TSAbs [142].

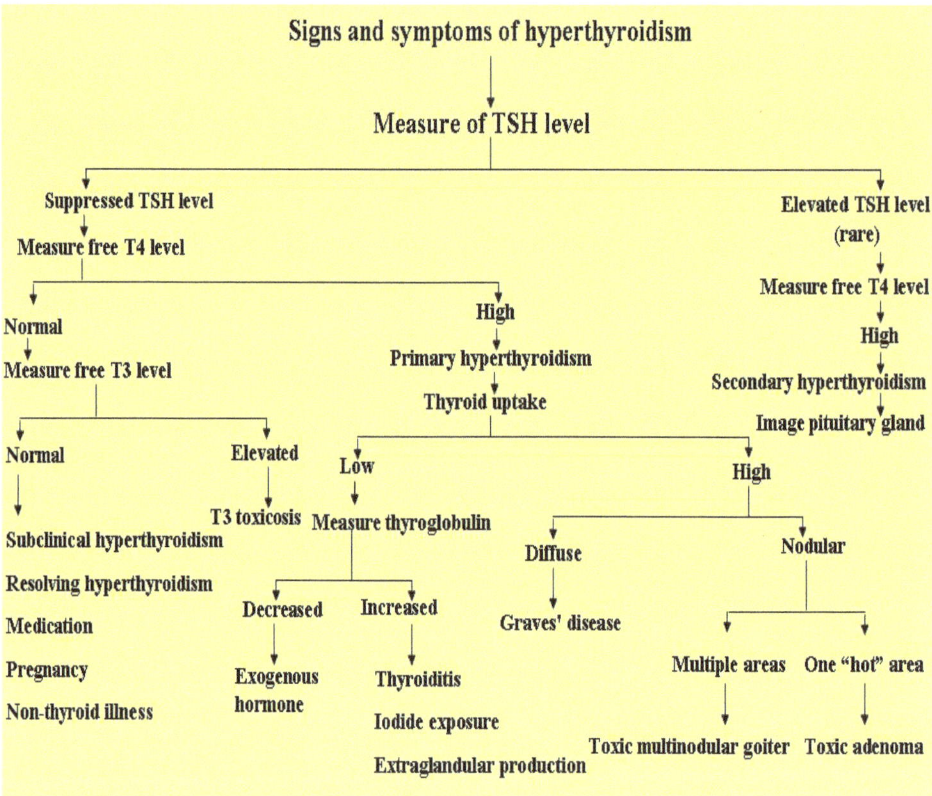

Figure 3. Different cases of hyperthyroidism.

Taken together, there are two known causes of central hyperthyroidism [1,146]; (1) TSH-producing pituitary tumors (TSHomas) and (2) the syndrome of pituitary resistance to thyroid hormone (PRTH). In general, thyrotoxicosis is the syndrome resulting from an excess of circulating free T4 and/or free T3 [147,148]. Babies likely to become hyperthyroid have the highest TSH receptor antibody titer whereas if TSH receptor antibodies are not detectable, the baby is most unlikely to become hyperthyroid (Figure 3) [1,2,149]. In the latter case, it can be anticipated that the baby will be euthyroid, have transient hypothalamic-pituitary suppression or have a transiently elevated TSH, depending on the relative contribution of maternal hyperthyroidism versus the effects of maternal antithyroid medication, respectively [150].

6. Summary

about the developmental thyroid hormone mechanisms (deiodinases, transporters, sulfotransferases and receptors) in human [1,2,50,52,127,130,151-154], rat [1,2,41,60,135,154-156] and chicken [7,157-170]. Note that the chicken is born early compared to the rat and human, as well as the rat is born early compared to the human (Table 6).

Human		Rodent (rat)		Chicken	
Week post conception		Day post conception		Incubation day	
1 W	- DIII is detected in uterine wall.	1 GD	DII and DIII are observed in uterine wall.	5 h (blastula stage)	- TRα mRNA is noticed and the levels markedly increased during neurulation.
3 W	- Thyroid gland begins.	7 -8.5 GD	- Time of implantation process. - Very high DIII activity is detected in decidual tissue.	24 h	- mRNA levels of DI, DII and DIII are detected in whole embryos.
4-6 W	- TBG is observed in thyroid follicle cells at GD 29. - TRH is detected in fetal whole-brain at 4.5 weeks of gestation. - T4 is transferred *via* the placenta and has been found in the gestational fluid sac from 4 to 6 W.	9 GD	- Thyroid gland is first visible as an endodermal thickening in the primitive buccal cavity. - TH is detected in rat embryotrophobl asts	48 h	- OATP1c1 expression appears.
5-11 W	- Maternal-embryo transfer of THs has been detected in embryonic coelomic fluid and amniotic fluid. - All the mRNAs encoding THTs are expressed in placenta from 6 W and throughout pregnancy.				

8 W	- T4, T3 and rT3 are detected in coelomic/amniotic fluids. - TRs, DII and DIII are noticed in fetal brain.	10 GD	- T4, T3 and TRβ are detected in embryo/trophoblast unit.	E2-E4	- T3, THTs, Ds and TRs are expressed in whole embryos.
10 W	- TSH is first detected in the fetal pituitary.			E4	- OATP1c1 expression is more than 10-fold higher in the telencephalon and diencephalon compared to the mesencephalon and rhombencephalon. - DII mRNA levels are highest in the diencephalon.
8-10 W	- The fetus is able to produce THs during this period, but prior to that time, is totally dependent on maternal THs.			E5	- TRα mRNA is widely distributed in fore-, mid- and hind-brain.
11 W	- TBG levels are detected in fetal serum and increased through gestation.			E6	- T4 and T3 are detected in embryonic brain.
8-11 W	- TRH is detected in fetal hypothalamus.			E7	- DII activity is observed in the brain before the onset of thyroid function and increases significantly.
12 W	- T4 and T3 are observed in serum and brain. - Total serum T4 and T3 are low, free T4 is relatively high. - rT3 is noticed in serum relatively high. - TH synthesis begins in fetal thyroid.	13 GD	- Placental circulation established. - TRs and TH are observed in fetal brain. - DIII and DII are detected in uterus and placenta.	E8	- DII mRNA is noticed in cell clusters throughout the brain, particularly in rhombencephalon. - OATP1c1 levels are declined substantially in all brain regions.

	- Decreased mRNA expression of OATP1A2 but no change for OATP4A1 at 9–12 W compared to term.				
14 W	- Expressions of mRNAs encoding MCT8, MCT10, OATP1A2 and LAT1 are significantly lower prior to 14 W compared to term	14 GD	- TRH mRNA is detected in neurons of the fetal hypothalamus.	E4-E8	- DIII mRNA levels are markedly different in the telencephalon and diencephalon but remain stable, while the levels in mesencephalon and rhombencephalon show a sharp decrease and increase, respectively, during these days.
		15 GD	- Pituitary TSH mRNA expression begins. - TRH mRNA is detected in the developing paraventricular nuclei of the hypothalamus.	E9-10	- Several elements of the TH action cascade are present in the brain of embryos long before their own thyroid gland starts hormone secretion.
16 W	- DIII is observed in placenta and fetal epithelial cells. - DIII and TRs are detected in fetal liver. - DI is noticed in heart and lung. - Significant fetal TH secretion begins.	16-19.5 GD	- TRs are observed in liver, heart and lung. - DI and DII are noticed in fetal tissues. - TRH is produced in low levels in hypothalamus and increases approximately threefold by GDI9.5.	E10	- The thyroid gland is fully functional.
16-20 W	- Duplication of TBG concentrations.	17 GD	- TH synthesis begins in fetal thyroid	E13	- Brain DII is elevated at the peak of neuroblast proliferation.

			- TSH protein and Sulfotransferase are observed.		
		18 -22 GD	- The total T4 and T3 concentrations in fetuses are increased drama-tically because of maturation of hormone synthesis of the fetal thyroid gland. - The coordination between THTs and Ds is regulated both transplacental TH passage from mother to fetus and the development of the placenta itself through the progress of gestation.	E14	- The strong increase in intracellular T3 has been observed.
20 W	- A steady increase in serum TH levels begins and continues to term.	19 GD	- Significant fetal TH secretion begins. - Marked rise in serum TH but levels at birth still below those in adult.	E15	- Plasma T4 levels start rising markedly around this day.
22-32 W	- Serum total and free T4 and T3 near and below adult levels, respectively. - The HPT axis begins to mature during the second half of gestation.	22 GD	- Birth state. - Thyroid system is less developed. - As much as 17.5% of THs found in the newborn are of maternal origin.	E16	- The decrease in DI activity in gonads is combined with the relatively high DIII activity. - A significant increase in T3 production and in DII-activity and -mRNA expression are combined with a decreased in DIII activity.

	- LAT1 and OATP4A1 have been localized only during the third trimester.				
40 W	- Birth state. - Complete maturation of thyroid system. - MCT8 has been localized in the placenta in all three trimesters of pregnancy. - High concentrations of the different iodothyronine sulfates, T4S, T3S, rT3S and T2S, have been documented in human fetal and neonatal plasma as well as in amniotic fluid during the pregnancy.	10 PND	- Brain development equivalent to human birth.	E13/14–E17 (synaptogenesis)	- Brain DII activity is moderately elevated, whereas DIII activity and mRNA expression are highest between these days, followed by a dramatic decrease thereafter.
		10-20 PND	- Serum TH levels continue to rise and are higher than adult levels between these days.	E18	- DI and DIII are expressed in the granule cells, whereas DII is found mostly in the molecular layer and the Purkinje cells at that time.
		14-50 PND	- The levels of pituitary and serum TSH slowly decrease from PND 14–16 until reaching adult levels at PND 40. - TRH levels increase to adult levels by PNDI7–29, then decrease transiently between PND 31–41; adult levels are once again reached at PND 50. - Adult TRH mRNA expression patterns are present at PND 22.	E19	- The increase in brain T3 production correlates with the appearance of TRβ expression in the cerebellum, telencephalon and optic lobes.
				E20 (at the moment of pipping)	- The brain is quite well developed at the time of hatching. - The gradual increases in plasma T4 and hepatic DI are detected. - DIII levels are decreased in spleen and increased in skin and the lungs towards hatching. - T3 production seems to be elevated markedly in liver. - The rise of T4 is much more pronounced than in plasma. - Diminished T4 sulfation is detected.

		30 PND	Complete maturation of thyroid gland.	E14-E19/20	- The T3 breakdown capacity by DIII is high in liver but low in kidney.
				E15/16-E20	- T4 levels in plasma increase gradually during these days. - In contrast to TRα expression which increases gradually towards hatching, expression of TRβ shows an abrupt elevation in late development, especially in the cerebellum. - The majority of tissues express DIII together with either DI or DII.
				E17-E20	- The levels of DIII activity present in liver are rapidly drop by more than 90%. - DI levels in testis and ovary strongly decrease around hatching.
				E18–E20	- Brain DII activity is moderately decreased, whereas DIII activity is low.
				E19-E20	- The low T3/T4 ratio is associated with high T3 breakdown in liver and with high T4 inactivation or T3 secretion in kidney.
				E20-C0	- DI activity gradually increases, reaching a maximum around these period, and decreases slowly to posthatch levels thereafter.
				C1 (first day post-hatch)	- The expression of DI is limited to the mature granule cells and that of DIII to the Purkinje cells exclusively, whereas DII remains clearly present in the molecular layer.

				C2	- Highest DI-activities and -mRNA expressions are detected in the liver, kidney, and intestine.
				C1-C7	- The circulating T3/T4 ratio started to increase gradually during the first week after hatching.

Abbreviations: W is week, GD is gestation day, E is incubation day, PND is postnatal day, C is posthatch day, THs is thyroid hormones, TRH is thyroid releasing hormone, TSH is thyroid stimulating hormone, THTs is thyroid hormone transporters, MCT is monocarboxylate transporter, OATP is organic anion transporter, Ds is deiodinases (DI, II, III), TRs is thyroid hormone receptors (TRα, β), T4 is Thyroxine, T3 is triiodothyronine, rT3 is reverse triiodothyronine, T2S is diiodothyronine sulfate, T3S is triiodothyronine sulfate, T4S is thyroxine sulfate, rT3S is reverse triiodothyronine sulfate, HPT is hypothalamic-pituitary-thyroid axis and TBG is thyroxin binding globulin.

Table 6. Summary about the developmental thyroid hormone mechanisms (deiodinases, transporters, sulfotransferases and receptors) in human, rat and chicken.

7. Conclusion

The actions of THs are highly pleiotropic, affecting many tissues at different developmental stages. As a consequence, their effects on proliferation and differentiation are highly heterogeneous depending on the cell type, the cellular context, and the developmental or transformation status.

Maternal THs are important in promoting normal fetal development especially the placental and CNS development. Clinical epidemiological and basic findings clearly show that maintaining normal TH regulation from the beginning of pregnancy is important to reduce the risk of obstetric complications and to ensure optimal neurodevelopment of the offspring.

In normal pregnancy, transplacental TH passage is modulated by plasma membrane THTs, Ds, sulfotransferases, TRs and several different proteins within placental cells.

In pathological/abnormal pregnancies with either maternal or fetal THs disturbances (hypo- or hyper-thyroidism), the placenta lacks the full compensatory mechanisms necessary to optimize the maternal–fetal transfer of THs to achieve the normality of TH levels in the fetus.

8. Future challenges

Further studies are still needed to improve our understanding of the mechanisms mediating the transplacental transport of THs in both human and animals, particularly the role of the different THTs, and the mechanisms that ensure that sufficient amounts of THs are protected from D3 inactivation during their transit across the placenta. Such knowledge would facilitate the development of interventions to increase TH passage in pathological situations, in order to ensure normal fetal development. A better understanding of these mechanisms would also permit us to refine the timing and dosage of the increase in levothyroxine therapy in hypothyroid pregnant women and to establish whether thyroxine on its own is indeed the best form of TH replacement in pregnancy.

Elucidation of tissue-, cell-, and sex-specific expression of individual Ds and THTs during the development of both human and animals, in the adult, during aging and when sick.

I hope that new insights into the complex actions by which the THs and their receptors control cell proliferation and differentiation will be provided in the near future.

Author details

R.G. Ahmed

Division of Anatomy and Embryology, Zoology Department, Faculty of Science, Beni-Suef University, Egypt

9. References

[1] Ahmed OM, El-Gareib AW, El-bakry AM, Abd El-Tawab SM, Ahmed RG. Thyroid hormones states and brain development interactions. Int. J. Dev. Neurosci. 2008;26 (2):147–209. Review.

[2] Ahmed RG. Effects of experimentally-induced hypothyroidism and hyperthyroidism in pregnant albino rats on the development of their offspring. PhD. Thesis, Fac. of Sci., Beni-Suef Univ., Egypt 2009.

[3] Scapin S, Leoni S, Spagnuolo S, Gnocchi D, De Vito P, Luly P, Pedersen JZ, Incerpi S. Short-term effects of thyroid hormones during development: Focus on signal transduction. Steroids 2010;75:576–584.

[4] Incerpi S, Scapin S, D'Arezzo S, Spagnuolo S, Leoni S. Short-term effect of thyroid hormone in prenatal development and cell differentiation. Steroids 2005;70:434-443.

[5] Gereben B, Zeold A, Dentice M, Salvatore D, Bianco AC. Activation and inactivation of thyroid hormone by deiodinases: local action with general consequences. Cell. Mol. Life Sci. 2008;65:570–590.

[6] Horn S, Heuer H 2010. Thyroid hormone action during brain development: more questions than answers. Mol. and Cell. Endocrinol. 2010;315:19–26.

[7] Van Herck SLJ, Geysens S, Delbaere J, Tylzanowski P, Darras VM. Expression profile and thyroid hormone responsiveness of transporters and deiodinases in early embryonic chicken brain development. Mol. and Cell. Endocrinol. 2012;349(2):289-297.

[8] Köhrle J. Transfer and metabolism of thyroid gland hormones in the placenta. Acta Med. Austriaca 1997;24(4):138-143.

[9] Yen PM. Physiological and molecular basis of thyroid hormone action. Physiol. Rev. 2001;81(3):1097-1126.

[10] Suzuki T, Abe T. Thyroid hormone transporters in the brain. Cerebellum 2008;75–83.

[11] Incerpi S, De Vito P, Luly P, Spagnuolo S, Leoni S. Short-term effects of thyroid hormones and 3,5-diiodothyronine on membrane transport systems in chick embryo hepatocytes. Endocrinol. 2002;143:1660-1668.

[12] Visser WE, Friesema EC, Jansen J, Visser TJ. Thyroid hormone transport in and out of cells. Trends Endocrinol. Metab. 2008;19:50–56.
[13] Kilby MD, Barber K, Hobbs E, Franklyn JA. Thyroid Hormone Action in the Placenta. Placenta 2005;26:105-113.
[14] D'Arezzo S, Incerpi S, Davis FB, Acconcia F, Marino M, Farías RN, Davis PJ. Rapid nongenomic effects of 3,5,3'-triiodo L-thyronine on the intracellular pH of L-6 myoblasts are mediated by intracellular calcium mobilization and kinase pathways. Endocrinol. 2004;145:5694-5703.
[15] Incerpi S 2005. Editorial. Thyroid hormones: rapid reply by surface delivery only. Endocrinol. 2005;146 (7):2861–2863.
[16] Farias NR, Fiore AM, Pedersen JZ, Incerpi S. Nongenomic actions of thyroid hormones: Focus on membrane transport systems. Immun. Endocr. Metab. Agents in Med. Chem. 2006;6:241-254.
[17] Pinto M, Soares P, Ribatti D. Thyroid hormone as a regulator of tumor induced angiogenesis. Cancer Letters 2011;301:119–126. Mini-review
[18] Incerpi S. Abstract: at the 90th annual Meeting of the Endocrine Society, San Francisco 2008.
[19] Incerpi S, Davis PJ, De Vito P, Farias RN, Lin H-Y, Davis FB. Nongenomic actions of thyroid hormones and intracellular calcium metabolism. Clin. Rev. Bone & Miner. Metab. 2008;6(1-2):53-61.
[20] Incerpi S, De Vito P, Pedersen JZ, Luly P. Extranuclear Effects of Thyroid Hormones in Skeletal Muscle. Immun. Endocr. Metab. Agents Med. Chem. 2011;11:188-198.
[21] Incerpi S. Editorial. Nongenomic effects of thyroid hormones in skeletal muscle and central nervous system: from zebrafish to man. Immun. Endocr. Metab. Agents Med. Chem. 2011;11:150-151.
[22] Harvey CB, Williams GR. Mechanism of thyroid hormone action. Thyroid 2002;12:441-446.
[23] Ahmed RG. Perinatal 2,3,7,8-tetrachlorodibenzo-p-dioxin exposure alters developmental neuroendocrine system. J. of Food and Chemical Toxicol. 2011;49:1276-1284.
[24] Pop VJ, Kuijpens JL, van Baar AL, Verkerk G, van Son MM, de Vijlder JJ, Vulsma T, Wiersinga WM, Drexhage HA, Vader HL. Low maternal free thyroxine concentrations during early pregnancy are associated with impaired psychomotor development in infancy. Clin. Endocrinol. (Oxf) 1999;50:149-155.
[25] Pop VJ, Brouwers EP, Vader HL, Vulsma T, van Baar AL, de Vijlder JJ. Maternal hypothyroxinaemia during early pregnancy and subsequent child development: a 3-year follow-up study. Clin. Endocrinol. 2003;59:282-288.
[26] Lavado-Autric R, Auso E, Garcia-Velasco JV, Arufe Mdel C, Escobar del Rey F, Berbel P, Morreale de Escobar G. Early maternal hypothyroxinemia alters histogenesis and cerebral cortex cytoarchitecture of the progeny. J. Clin. Invest. 2003;111:1073–1082.
[27] Evans IM, Pickard MR, Sinha AK, Leonard AJ, Sampson DC, Ekins RP. Influence of maternal hyperthyroidism in the rat on the expression of neuronal and astrocytic cytoskeletal proteins in fetal brain. Endocrinol. 2002;175:597-604.

[28] Sirakov M, Plateroti M. The thyroid hormones and their nuclear receptors in the gut: From developmental biology to cancer. Biochimica et Biophysica Acta 2011;1812:938-946.
[29] Berry MJ, Banu L, Larsen PR. Type 1 iodothyronine deiodinase is a selenocysteine-containing enzyme. Nature 1991;349(6308):438-440.
[30] St. Germain DL, Galton VA. The deiodinase family of selenoproteins. Thyroid 1997;7(4):655-668.
[31] Köhrle J. Local activation and inactivation of thyroid hormones: the deiodinase family. Mol. and Cell. Endocrinol. 1999;15:103–119.
[32] Visser TJ, Schoenmakers CH. Characteristics of type III iodothyronine deiodinases. Acta Medica Austriaca 1992;19:18-21.
[33] Bates JM, St. Germain DL, Galton VA. Expression profiles of the three iodothyronine deiodinases, D1, D2 and D3, in the developing rat. Endocrinol. 1999;140(2):844-851.
[34] Obregon MJ, Mallol J, Morreale de Escobar G, Escobar del Rey F. The presence of thyroxine and tri-iodothyronine in tissues of thyroidectomised rats. Endocrinol. 1981;109:908-913.
[35] Roti E, Fang SL, Braverman LE, Emerson CH. Rat placenta is an active site of inner ring deiodination of thyroxine and 3,3',5-triiodothyronine. Endocrinol. 1982;110:34-37.
[36] Kaplan MM, Shaw EA. Type II iodothyronine 5'-deiodination by human and rat placentas in vitro. J. of Clin. Endocrinol. and Metab. 1984;59:253-257.
[37] Koopdonk-Kool JM, de Vijlder JJ, Veenboer GJ, Ris-Stalpers C, Kok JH, Vulsma T, Boer K, Visser TJ. Type II and type III deiodinase activity in human placenta as a function of gestational age. J. Clin. Endocrinol. Metab. 1996;81:2154–2158.
[38] Stulp MR, Vijlder JJ, Ris-Stalpers C.. Placental iodothyronine deiodinase III and II ratios, mRNA expression compared to enzyme activity. Mol. Cell. Endocrinol. 1998;142:67–73.
[39] Chan S, Kachilele S, Hobbs E, Bulmer JN. Iodothyronine deiodinase expression and activity in human placenta: the effects of intrauterine growth restriction. J. Clin. Endocrinol. Metab. 2003;88:4488-4495.
[40] Patel J, Landers K, Li H, Mortimer RH, Richard K. Delivery of maternal thyroid hormones to the fetus. Trends in Endocrinol. & Metab. 2011;22(5):164-170.
[41] Galton VA, Martinez E, Hernandez A, St. Germain EA, Bates JM, St. Germain DL. Pregnant rat uterus expresses high levels of the type 3 iodothyronine deiodinase. J. Clin. Invest. 1999;103:979-987.
[42] Brzezinska-Slebodzinska E, Slebodzinski AB, Krysin E. Placental outer and inner ring monodeiodination of thyroxine and triiodothyronines in the rabbit. J. of Dev. Physiol. 1989;11(6):351-353.
[43] Krysin E, Brzezinska-Slebodinska E, Slebodzinski AB. Divergent deiodination of thyroid hormones in the separated parts of the fetal and maternal placenta in pigs. Endocrinol. 1997;155(2):295-303.
[44] Vulsma T, Gons M, de Vijlder JJM. Materno-fetal transfer of thyroxine in congenital hypothyroidism due to a total organification defect or thyroid agenesis. N. Engl. J. Med. 1989;321:13-16.

[45] Burrow GN, Fisher DA, Larsen PR. Maternal and fetal thyroid function. N. Engl. J. Med. 1994;331:1072-1078.
[46] Bianco, AC, Salvatore D, Gereben B, Berry MJ, Larsen PR. Biochemistry, Cellular and Molecular Biology, and Physiological Roles of the Iodothyronine Selenodeiodinases. Endocr. Rev. 2002;23:38–89.
[47] James SR, Franklyn JA, Kilby MD. Placental transport of thyroid hormone. Best Pract. & Res. Clin. Endocrinol. & Metab. 2007;21(2):253–264.
[48] St. Germain DL, Galton VA, Hernandez A. Minireview: Defining the Roles of the Iodothyronine Deiodinases: Current Concepts and Challenges. Endocrinol. 2009;150:1097-1107.
[49] Hennemann G, Docter R, Friesema EC, de Jong M, Krenning EP, Visser TJ. Plasma membrane transport of thyroid hormones and its role in thyroid hormone metabolism and bioavailability. Endocr. Rev. 2001;22:451–476.
[50] Loubière LS, Vasilopoulou E, Bulmer JN, Taylor PM, Stieger B, Verrey F, McCabe CJ, Franklyn JA, Kilby MD, Chan S-Y. Expression of thyroid hormone transporters in the human placenta and changes associated with intrauterine growth restriction. Placenta 2010;31: 295-304.
[51] Ritchie JW, Taylor PM. Role of the System L permease LAT1 in amino acid and iodothyronine transport in placenta. Biochem. J. 2001;356:719–725.
[52] Patel P, Weerasekera N, Hitchins M, Boyd CA, Johnston DG, Williamson C. Semi quantitative expression analysis of MDR3, FIC1, BSEP, OATP-A, OATP-C, OATP-D, OATP-E and NTCP gene transcripts in 1st and 3rd trimester human placenta. Placenta 2003;24:39–44.
[53] Sato K, Sugawara J, Sato T, Mizutamari H, Suzuki T, Ito A. Expression of organic anion transporting polypeptide E (OATP-E) in human placenta. Placenta 2003;24:144–148.
[54] Park SY, Kim J-K, Kim IJ, Choi BK, Jung KY, Lee S. Reabsorption of neutral amino acids mediated by amino acid transporter LAT2 and TAT1 in the basolateral membrane of proximal tubule. Arch Pharm. Res. 2005;28: 421-432.
[55] Chan SY, Franklyn JA, Pemberton HN, Bulmer JN, Visser TJ, McCabe CJ. Monocarboxylate transporter 8 expression in the human placenta: the effects of severe intrauterine growth restriction. Endocrinol. 2006;189:465–471.
[56] de Escobar GM, Obregon MJ, del Rey FE. Maternal thyroid hormones early in pregnancy and fetal brain development. Best Pract. Res. Clin. Endocrinol. Metab. 2004;18:225–248.
[57] Fisher DA. Fetal thyroid function: diagnosis and management of fetal thyroid disorders. Clin. Obstet. Gynecol. 1997;40:16–31.
[58] Capelo LP, Beber EH, Fonseca TL, Gouveia CH. The monocarboxylate transporter 8 and L-type amino acid transporters 1 and 2 are expressed in mouse skeletons and in osteoblastic MC3T3-E1 cells. Thyroid 2009;19:171–180.
[59] Chan SY, Vasilopoulou E, Kilby MD. The role of the placenta in thyroid hormone delivery to the fetus. Nature clin. Pract. Endocrinol. & Metab. 2009;5(1):45-54.
[60] Visser WE, Friesema ECH, Visser TJ. Minireview: Thyroid Hormone Transporters: The Knowns and the Unknowns. Mol. Endocrinol. 2011;25:1–14.

[61] Friesema EC, Jansen J, Jachtenberg JW, Visser WE, Kester MH, Visser TJ. Effective cellular uptake and efflux of thyroid hormone by human monocarboxylate transporter 10. Mol. Endocrinol. 2008;22:1357–1369.
[62] Kester MH. The importance of thyroid hormone sulfation during fetal development. PhD Thesis, University of Erasmus, Netherlands; 2001. ISBN 90-9015010-2.
[63] Farooqui AA. 3'-Phosphoadenosine-5'-phosphosulfate metabolism in mammalian tissue. Int. J. of Biochem.1980;12:529-536.
[64] Visser TJ. The role of sulfation in thyroid hormone metabolism. Chemico-Biological Interactions 1994;92:292-303.
[65] Chopra IJ, Wu SY, Chua Teco GN, Santini F. A radioimmunoassay of 3,5,3'-triiodothyronine sulfate: studies in thyroidal and nonthyroidal diseases, pregnancy, and neonatal life. J. Clin. Endocrinol. Metab. 1992;75:189–194.
[66] Santini F, Cortelazzi D, Baggiani AM, Marconi AM, Beck-Peccoz P, Chopra IJ. A study of the serum 3,5,3'-triiodothyronine sulfate concentration in normal and hypothyroid fetuses at various gestational stages. J. Clin. Endocrinol. Metab. 1993;76:1583-1587.
[67] Polk DH, Reviczky A, Wu SY, Huang WS, Fisher DA. Metabolism of sulfoconjugated thyroid hormone derivatives in developin sheep. Am. J. Physiol. 1994;266:E892–E898.
[68] Wu SY, Huang WS, Polk D, Chopra IJ. The development of a radioimmunoassay for reverse triiodothyronine sulfate in human serum and amniotic fluid. J. of Clin. Endocrinol.and Metab. 1993;76:1625-1630.
[69] Kester MHA, Kaptein E, Roest TJ, Hume R, Visser TJ. Characterisation of human iodothyronine sulfotransferases. J. of Clin. Endocrinol. and Metab. 1999;84:1357-1364.
[70] Parenti G, Meroni G, Ballabio A. The sulfatase gene family. Curr. Opin. in Gen. Dev. 1997;7:386-391.
[71] Friesema ECH, Docter R, Moerings EPCM, Stieger B, Hagenbuch B, Meier PJ, Krenning EP, Hennemann G, Visser TJ. Identification of thyroid hormone transporters. Biochem. Biophys. Res. Commun. 1999;254:497–501.
[72] Flamant F, Baxter JD, Forrest D, Refetoff S, Samuels H, Scanlan TS, Vennstrom B, Samarut J. International Union of Pharmacology. LIX. The pharmacology and classification of the nuclear receptor superfamily: thyroid hormone receptors. Pharmacol. Rev. 2006;58:705–711.
[73] Pascual A, Aranda A. Thyroid hormone receptors, cell growth and differentiation. Biochimica et Biophysica Acta 2012 xxx–xxx.
[74] Shi Y-B, Ritchieb JWA, Taylor PM. Complex regulation of thyroid hormone action: multiple opportunities for pharmacological intervention. Pharmacol. & Therapeutics 2002;94:235– 251.
[75] Oetting A, Yen PM. New insights into thyroid hormone action. Best Pract. & Res. Clin. Endocrinol. & Metab. 2007;21(2):193-208.
[76] Schussler GC. The thyroxine-binding proteins. Thyroid 2000;10(2):141-149.
[77] Larsson A, Palm M, Hansson LO, Axelsson O. Reference values for clinical chemistry tests during normal pregnancy. BJOG 2008;115(7):874–881.
[78] Zhou A, Wei Z, Read RJ, Carrell RW. Structural mechanism for the carriage and release of thyroxine in the blood. Proc. Natl Acad. Sci. USA 2006;103(36):13321-13326.

[79] Glinoer D. The regulation of thyroid function in pregnancy: pathways of endocrine adaptation from physiology to pathology. Endocr. Rev. 1997;18(3):404–433.
[80] Glinoer D, De Nayer P, Bourdoux P. Regulation of maternal thyroid during pregnancy. J. Clin. Endocrinol. Metab. 1990;71(2):276–287.
[81] Lee RH, Spencer CA, Mestman JH. Free T4 immunoassays are flawed during pregnancy. Am. J. Obstet. Gynecol. 2009;200(3):e1–e6.
[82] Kurioka H, Takahashi K, Miyazaki K. Maternal thyroid function during pregnancy and puerperal period. Endocr. J. 2005;52(5):587–591.
[83] De Vito P, Incerpi S, Pedersen JZ, Luly P, Davis FB, Davis PJ. Thyroid hormones as modulators of immune activities at the cellular level. Thyroid 2011;21:879-890.
[84] Chen C, Zhou Z, Zhong M, Li M, Yang X, Zhang Y, Wang Y, Wei A, Qu M, Zhang L, Xu S, Chen S, Yu Z. Excess thyroid hormone inhibits embryonic neural stem/progenitor cells proliferation and maintenance through STAT3 signalling pathway. Neurotox. Res. 2011;20:15-25.
[85] Contreras-Jurado C, Garcia-Serrano L, Gomez-Ferreria M, Costa C, Paramio JM, Aranda A. The thyroid hormone receptors as modulators of skin proliferation and inflammation. J. Biol. Chem. 2011;286:24079–24088.
[86] Blair AS, Hajduch E, Litherland GJ, Hundal HS. Regulation of glucose transport and glycogen synthesis in L6 muscle cells during oxidative stress. Evidence for cross-talk between the insulin and SAPK2/p38 mitogen-activated protein kinase signaling pathways. J. Biol. Chem. 1999;274:36293–36299.
[87] Bassett JHD, Harvey CB, Williams GR. Mechanisms of thyroid hormone receptor-specific nuclear and extra nuclear actions. Mol. and Cell. Endocrinol. 2003;213:1–11.
[88] Davis PJ, Shih A, Lin HY, Martino LJ, Davis FB. Thyroxine promotes association of mitogen-activated protein kinase and nuclear thyroid hormone receptor (TR) and causes serine phosphorylation of TR. J. Biol. Chem. 2000;275:38032–38039.
[89] Wrutniak-Cabello C, Casas F, Cabello G. Thyroid hormone action in mitochondria. J. Mol. Endocrinol. 2001;26:67–77.
[90] Incerpi S, Luly P, De Vito P, Farias RN. Short - term effects of thyroid hormones on the Na/H antiport in L-6 myoblasts: high molecular specificity for 3,3′,5-triiodothyronine. Endocrinol. 1999;140:683 - 689.
[91] De Vito P, Balducci V, Leone S, Percario Z, Mangino G, Davis FB, Davis PJ, Affabris E, Luly P, Pedersen JZ, Incerpi S. Nongenomic effects of thyroid hormones on the immune system cells: new targets, old players. Steroids 2012 xxx-xxx.
[92] Kavok NS, Krasilnikova, OA, Babenko, NA. Thyroxine signal transduction in liver cells involves phospholipase C and phospholipase D activation genomic independent action of thyroid hormone. BMC Cell. Biol. 2001;2:5.
[93] Incerpi S. Actions of thyroid hormones on ion transport. Curr. Op. Endocrinol. Diab. 2002;9:381-386.
[94] Lin HY, Sun M, Tang HY, Lin C, Luidens MK, Mousa SA, Incerpi S, Drusano GL, Davis FB, Davis PJ. L-Thyroxine vs. 3,5,3'-triiodo-L-thyronine and cell proliferation: activation of mitogen-activated protein kinase and phosphatidylinositol 3-kinase. Am. J. Physiol. Cell. Physiol. 2009;296:C980–991.

[95] Bergh JJ, Lin HY, Lansing L, Mohamed SN, Davis FB, Mousa S, Davis PJ. Integrin alphaVbeta3 contains a cell surface receptor site for thyroid hormone that is linked to activation of mitogen-activated protein kinase and induction of angiogenesis. Endocrinol. 2005;146:2864–2871.
[96] Gnocchi D, Leoni S, Incerpi S, Bruscalupi G. 3,5,3′-Triiodothyronine (T_3) stimulates cell proliferation through activation of PI3K/Akt pathway and Reactive Oxygen Species (ROS) production in chick embryo hepatocytes. Steroids 2012 xxx-xxxx.
[97] Farwell AP, Dibenedetto DJ, Leonard JL. Thyroxine targets different pathways of internalization of type II iodothyronine 5'-deiodinase in astrocytes. J. Biol. Chem. 1993;268:50–55.
[98] Siegrist-Kaiser CA, Juge-Aubry, Tranter MP, Ekenbarger DM, Leonard JL. Thyroxine-dependent modulation of actin polymerization in cultured astrocytes: a novel extranuclear action of thyroid hormone. J. Biol. Chem. 1990;26:5296–5302.
[99] Farwell AP, Safran M, Dubord S, Leonard JL. Degradation and recycling of the substrate-binding subunit of type II iodothyronine 5'-deiodonase in astrocytes. J. Biol. Chem. 1996;271:16369–16374.
[100] Farwell AP, Tranter MP, Leonard JL. Thyroxine-dependent regulation of integrin-laminin interactions in astrocytes. Endocrinol. 1995;136:3909–3915.
[101] Wang QW, Yu B, Huang RP, Cao F, Zhu ZQ, Sun DC, Zhou H. Assessment of thyroid function during pregnancy: the advantage of self-sequential longitudinal reference intervals. Arch Med. Sci. 2011;7(4):679-684.
[102] Brent GA. The debate over thyroid-function screening in pregnancy. N Engl J Med. 2012;366(6):562-563.
[103] Heather N, Hall K, Neas K, Potter H, Wiltshire E. Growth and development in a child with resistance to thyroid hormone and ectopic thyroid gland. Pediatr. 2012;129(3):e817-e820.
[104] Lazarus JH, Bestwick JP, Channon S, Paradice R, Maina A, Rees R, Chiusano E, John R, Guaraldo V, George LM, Perona M, Dall'Amico D, Parkes AB,Joomun M, Wald NJ. Antenatal thyroid screening and childhood cognitive function. N. Engl. J. Med. 2012;366(6):493-501.
[105] Morreale de Escobar G, Pastor R, Obregón MJ, Escobar del Rey F. Effects of maternal hypothyroidism on the weight and thyroid hormone content of rat embryonic tissues before and after onset of fetal thyroid function. Endocrinol. 1985;117:1890–1901.
[106] Morreale de Escobar G, Obregón MJ, Ruiz de Oña C, Escobar del Rey F. Transfer of thyroxine from the mother to the rat fetus near term: effects on brain 3,5,3'-triiodothyronine deficiency. Endocrinol. 1988;122(4):1521–1531.
[107] Falcone M, Miyamoto T, Fierro-Renoy F, Macchia E, DeGroot LJ. Evaluation of the ontogeny of thyroid hormone isotypes in rat brain and liver using an immunohistochemical technique. Eur. J. Endocrinol. 1994;130:97–106.
[108] Morreale de Escobar G, Obregón MJ, Escobar del Rey F. Is neuropsychological development related to maternal hypothyroidism or to maternal hypothyroxinemia? J. Clin. Endocrinol. Metab. 2000;85:3975–3987.

[109] Ausó E, Lavado-Autric R, Cuevas E, Escobar del Rey F, Morreale de Escobar G, Berbel P. A moderate and transient deficiency of maternal thyroid function at the beginning of fetal neocorticogenesis alters neuronal migration. Endocrinol. 2004;145:4037-4047.
[110] Ferreiro B, Bernal J, Morreale de Escobar G, Potter BJ. Preferential saturation of brain T3 receptor during development in fetal lambs. Endocrinol. 1988;122:438–443.
[111] Chan S, Kilby MD. Thyroid hormone and central nervous system development. Endocrinol. 2000;165:1-8.
[112] Fantz CR, Dagogo-Jack S, Ladenson JH, Gronowski AM. Thyroid function during pregnancy. Clin. Chem. 1999;45:2250–2258.
[113] Zoeller RT. Editorial: Local control of the timing of thyroid hormone action in the developing human brain. J. Clin. Endocrinol. Metab. 2004;89(7):3114–3116.
[114] Zoeller RT, Crofton KM. Thyroid hormone action in fetal brain development and potential for disruption by environmental chemicals. Neurotoxicol. 2000;21(6):1–11.
[115] Zoeller RT, Rovett J. Timing of thyroid hormone action in the developing brain: Clinical observations and experimental findings. Neuroendocrinol. 2004;16:809-818.
[116] Anderson GW. Thyroid hormone and cerebellar development. Cerebellum 2008;7:60-74.
[117] Nicholson JL, Altman J. The effects of early hypo- and hyperthyroidism on the development of the rat cerebellar cortex. II. Synaptogenesis in the molecular layer. Brain Res. 1972;44:25-36.
[118] Bernal J. In "Hormones, Brain and Behavior", Eds Arnold AP et al. Academic Press, 2002;4:543-587.
[119] Quignodon L, Grijota-Martinez C, Compe E, Guyot R, Allioli N, Laperrière D, Walker R, Meltzer P, Mader S, Samarut J, Flamant F. A combined approach identifies a limited number of new thyroid hormone target genes in post-natal mouse cerebellum. J. Mol. Endocrinol. 2007;39:17-28.
[120] Takahashi M, Negishi T, Tashiro T. Identification of genes mediating thyroid hormone action in the developing mouse cerebellum. J. Neurochem. 2008;104:640-652.
[121] Dong H, Yauk CL, Rowan-Carroll A, You SH, Zoeller RT, Lambert I, Wade MG. Identification of thyroid hormone receptor binding sites and target genes using ChIP-on-chip in developing mouse cerebellum. PLoS ONE 2009;4:e4610.
[122] Anderson GW, Schoonover CM, Jones SA. Control of thyroid hormone action in the developing rat brain. Thyroid 2003;13:1039-1056.
[123] Lee PR, Brady D, Koenig JI. Thyroid hormone regulation of Nmethyl-D-aspartic acid receptor subunit mRNA expression in adult brain. J. Neuroendocrinol. 2003;15(1):87–92.
[124] Agrawal A, Diwan SK. Pituitary hyperplasia resulting from primary hypothyroidism. Asian J. Neurosurg. 2011;6(2):99-100.
[125] Burman KD. Thyroid function: Gestational hypothyroidism-a need for universal screening? Nat. Rev. Endocrinol. 2012 xxx-xxx.
[126] Celik C, Abali R, Tasdemir N, Guzel S, Yuksel A, Aksu E, Yılmaz M. Is subclinical hypothyroidism contributing dyslipidemia and insulin resistance in women with polycystic ovary syndrome? Gynecol. Endocrinol. 2012 xxx-xxx.

[127] Danzi S, Klein I. Subclinical hypothyroidism and the heart: the beat goes on. Thyroid. 2012;22(3):235-236.

[128] Hashemipour M, Abari SS, Mostofizadeh N, Haghjooy-Javanmard S, Esmail N, Hovsepian S, Masoud A, Kelishadi R, Hasanzadeh A, Mirouliaei M. The role of maternal thyroid stimulating hormone receptor blocking antibodies in the etiology of congenital hypothyroidism in isfahan, iran. Int. J. Prev. Med. 2012;3(2):128-133.

[129] McCoy SS, Crowson CS, Gabriel SE, Matteson EL. Hypothyroidism as a Risk Factor for Development of Cardiovascular Disease in Patients with Rheumatoid Arthritis. J. Rheumatol. 2012 xxx-xxx.

[130] Perry KD, Hope J, Yang J. Dyshormonogenetic goiter-like changes in a child with congenital hypothyroidism and a euthyroid adult. Diagn. Cytopathol. 2012 xxx-xxx.

[131] Resta F, Triggiani V, Barile G, Benigno M, Suppressa P, Giagulli VA, Guastamacchia E, Sabbà C. Subclinical Hypothyroidism and Cognitive Dysfunction in the Elderly. Endocr. Metab. Immune Disord Drug Targets. 2012 xxx-xxx.

[132] Shamshiri AR, Yarahmadi S, Forouzanfar MH, Haghdoost AA, Hamzehloo G, Holakouie Naieni K. Evaluation of Current Guthrie TSH Cut-off Point in Iran Congenital Hypothyroidism Screening Program: A Cost-Effectiveness Analysis. Arch Iran Med. 2012;15(3):136-141.

[133] Péter F, Muzsnai A. Congenital disorders of the thyroid: hypo/hyper. Pediatr. Clin. North Am. 2011;58(5):1099-1115.

[134] Rugge B, Balshem H, Sehgal R, Relevo R, Gorman P, Helfand M. Screening and Treatment of Subclinical Hypothyroidism or Hyperthyroidism [Internet]. Agency for Healthcare Research and Quality (US); 2011;11(12)-EHC033-EF.

[135] Czyzewska U, Tylicki A, Siemieniuk M, Strumilo S. Changes of activity and kinetics of certain liver and heart enzymes of hypothyroid and T(3)-treated rats. J. Physiol. Biochem. 2012 xxx-xxx.

[136] Pearce EN. Iodine-induced thyroid dysfunction: comment on "association between iodinated contrast media exposure and incident hyperthyroidism and hypothyroidism". Arch Intern. Med. 2012;172(2):159-161.

[137] Rhee CM. Association between iodinated contrast media exposure and incident hyperthyroidism andhypothyroidism. Arch Intern. Med. 2012;172(2):153-159.

[138] Jaeggi ET, Roman KS. Maternal autoimmune disease and its impact on the fetal heart: management and prognosis. Prog. Pediatr. Cardiol. 2006;22:85–93.

[139] Zimmerman D. Fetal and neonatal hyperthyroidism. Thyroid 1999;9:727–733.

[140] Momotani N, Noh J, Ishikawa N, Ito K. Relationship between silent thyroiditis and recurrent Graves' disease in the postpartum period. J. Clin. Endocrinol. Metab. 1994;79:285–289.

[141] Marx H, Amin P, Lazarus JH. Hyperthyroidism in pregnancy. BMJ 2008;336:663–667.

[142] Laurberg P, Bournaud C, Karmisholt J, Orgiazzi J. Management of Graves' hyperthyroidism in pregnancy: focus on both maternal and foetal thyroid function, and caution against surgical thyroidectomy in pregnancy. Eur. J. Endocrinol. 2009;160:1–8.

[143] Mestman JH. Hyperthyroidism in pregnancy. Best Pract. Clin. Endocrinol. Metab. 2004;18:267–288.

[144] Gärtner R. Thyroid diseases in pregnancy. Curr. Opin. Obstet. Gynecol. 2009;21:501–507.
[145] Chiniwala NU, Woolf PD, Bruno CP. Thyroid storm caused by a partial hydatidiform mole. Thyroid 2008;18:479–481.
[146] McDermott MT, Ridgway EC. Central hyperthyroidism. Endocrinol. Metab. Clin. North Am. 1998;27(1):187–203.
[147] Cooper DS 2003. Hyperthyroidism. Lancet 2003;362:459-468.
[148] Panzer C, Beazley R, Braverman L. Rapid preoperative preparation for severe hyperthyroid Graves' disease. J. Clin. Endocrinol. Metab. 2004;89: 2142–2144.
[149] Reid JR, Wheeler SF. Hyperthyroidism: Diagnosis and treatment. Am. Fam. Phys. 2005;72(4):623-630.
[150] Matsuura N, Konishi J, Fujeda K, Iida Y, Fujimoto S, Kasagi K, Hagisawa M, Fukushi M, Takasugi N. TSH-receptor antibodies in mothers with Graves' disease and outcome in their offspring. Lancet 1988;2:14.
[151] Legrand J. Thyroid hormone effects on growth and development. In: Hennemann G (ed) Thyroid Hormone Metabolism. Marcel Dekker, Inc., New York, 1986; 503–534.
[152] Shambaugh GE. Biologic and cellular effects. In: Ingbar SH, Braverman LE (eds) Werner's The Thyroid: A Fundamental and Clinical Text, 5th ed. J.B. Lippincott Co., Philadelphia, 1986; 201–218.
[153] Visser TJ. Metabolism of thyroid hormones. In: Cooke BA, King RJB, van der Molen HJ (eds) Hormones and their Action, Part 1. Elsevier Science Publishers, New York, 1988; 81–103.
[154] Galton VA. The Roles of the Iodothyronine Deiodinases in Mammalian Development. Thyroid 2005;15(8):832-834.
[155] Leonard JL, Visser TJ. Biochemistry of deiodination. In: Hennemann G (ed) Thyroid Hormone Metabolism. Marcel Dekker, New York, 1986;189–229.
[156] Porterfield SP, Hendrich CE. The role of thyroid hormones in prenatal and neonatal neurological development-Current perspectives. Endocr. Rev. 1993;14:94–106.
[157] Valverde RC, Aceves C, Reyes ZE. Ontogenesis of iodothyronine deiodinase activities in brain and liver of the chick embryo. Endocrinol. 1993;132:867–872.
[158] Darras VM, Visser TJ, Berghman LR, Kühn ER. Ontogeny of type I and type III deiodinase activities in embryonic and posthatch chicks: Relationship with changes in plasma triiodothyronine and growth hormone levels. Comp. Biochem. Physiol. 1992;103A:131–136.
[159] Darras VM, Robert H, Visser TJ. Regulation of thyroid hormone metabolism during fetal development. Mol. & Cell. Endocrinol. 1999;151:37–47.
[160] Darras VM, Verhoelst CHJ, Reyns GE, Kühn ER, Van der Geyten S. Thyroid Hormone Deiodination in Birds. Thyroid 2006;16(1):25-35.
[161] Darras VM, Van Herck SLJ, Geysens S, Reyns GE. Involvement of thyroid hormones in chicken embryonic brain development. Gen. and Comp. Endocrinol. 2009;163:58–62.
[162] Darras VM, Van Herck SLJ, Heijlen M, De Groef B. Thyroid Hormone Receptors in Two model Species for Vertebrate Embryonic Development: Chicken and Zebrafish. J. Thyroid Res. 2011;1-8.

[163] Van der Geyten S, Segers I, Gereben B, Bartha T, Rudas P, Larsen PR, Kühn PR, Darras VM. Transcriptional regulation of iodothyronine deiodinases during embryonic development. Mol. & Cell. Endocrinol. 2001;183:1–9.

[164] Van der Geyten S, Van den Eynde I, Segers IB, Kühn ER, Darras VM. Differential expression of iodothyronine deiodinases in chicken tissues during the last week of embryonic development. Gen. and Comp. Endocrinol. 2002;128:65–73.

[165] Verhoelst CHJ, Vandenborne K, Severi T, Bakker O, Zandieh Doulabi B, Leonard JL, Kühn ER, Van der Geyten S, Darras VM. Specific detection of type III iodothyronine deiodinases protein in chicken cerebellar Purkinje cells. Endocrinol. 2002;143:2700–2707.

[166] Verhoelst CHJ, Darras VM, Zandieh Doulabi B, Reyns G, Kühn ER, Van der Geyten S. Type I iodothyronine deiodinases in euthyroid and hypothyroid chicken cerebellum. Mol. and Cell. Endocrinol. 2004;214:97–105.

[167] Verhoelst CHJ, Roelens SA, Darras VM. Role of spatiotemporal expression of iodothyronine deiodinase proteins in cerebellar cell organization. Brain Res. Bulletin 2005;67:196–202.

[168] Reyns GE, Venken K, Morreale de Escobar G, Kühn ER, Darras VM. Dynamics and regulation of intracellular thyroid hormone concentrations in embryonic chicken liver, kidney, brain, and blood. Gen. and Comp. Endocrinol. 2003;134:80–87.

[169] Scapin S, Leoni S, Spagnuolo S, Fiore AM, Incerpi S. Short-term effects of thyroid hormones on the Na^+-K^+ATPase activity of chick embryo hepatocytes during development: Focus on signal transduction. Am. J. Physiol. Cell. Physiol. 2009;296:C4-C12.

[170] Grommen SV, Iwasawa A, Beck V, Darras VM, De Groef B. Ontogenic expression profiles of thyroid-specific genes in embryonic and hatching chicks. Domest. Anim. Endocrinol. 2011;40(1):10-18.

Section 3

Thyroid Hormone Excess

Chapter 6

Thyroid Hormone Excess: Graves' Disease

N.K. Agrawal, Ved Prakash and Manuj Sharma

Additional information is available at the end of the chapter

1. Introduction

Thyroid hormone excess due to any cause is state of thyrotoxicosis, whereas hyperthyroidism is a state of thyroid hormone excess due to hyperfunctioning of thyroid gland. The major causes of thyrotoxicosis include Graves' disease, solitary toxic adenoma, and toxic multinodular goiter. In thyrotoxicosis, free hormone levels are invariably increased. The reverse is not true in that increased free thyroid hormone levels do not always point to thyrotoxicosis. In illness or resistance to thyroid hormones increased free hormone levels are present while the patients are clinically euthyroid or even sometimes hypothyroid. Subclinical thyrotoxicosis is defined as a state in which free thyroid homones (FT4 & FT3) are within normal limit, but serum TSH level is low. The most common cause of subclinical thyrotoxicosis is exogenous administration of thyroid hormone rather than Graves' disease. Patients of subclinical thyrotoxicosis either have no symptoms or have mild non specific symptoms.

The various causes of thyrotoxicosis are listed below in table 1

1.1. Clinical features

Clinical manifestations of the thyrotoxicosis are similar for various causes of thyrotoxicosis. However certain features provide some clues about specific cause of throtoxicosis. These features include the duration and mode of onset of thyrotoxicosis, size and shape of the thyroid gland, presence or absence of the extra-thyroidal manifestations like Graves' eye sign, pre-tibial myxoedema, acropachy. Patient presenting with toxic features can be because of thyroiditis or Graves' disease, but the symptoms are of few weeks duration in former while in later condition, it is for several months, most of the time. The common clinical features of thyrotoxicosis are listed below in table 2.

A. Thyroid hormone excess with hyperthyroidism
   a. Primary Hyperthyroidism
      i. Graves' Disease
      ii. Toxic Thyroid adenoma
      iii. Toxic Multinodular Goiter
      iv. Metastases from Thyroid carcinoma
      v. Mutations of TSH receptor, Gsα (Mc Cune Albright Syndrome)
      vi. Struma Ovarii
      vii. Iodine ingestion (jod-Basedow phenomenon)
   b. Secondary hyperthyroidism
      i. TSH secreting pituitary tumours
      ii. Pituitary Thyroid hormone resistance
B. Thyroid hormone excess without hyperthyroidism
   a. Throiditis: subacute, silent
   b. Ingestion of thyroid tissue, thyroid hormone
   c. Thyroid gland destruction by amiodarone, radiotherapy, infarction in thyroid adenoma

Table 1. Causes of thyroid hormone excess

Symptoms	Signs
Irritability, Hyperactivity, Dysphoria	Tachycardia, Lone Atrial Fibrillation
Heat Intolerance	Fine tremor
Palpitation, Nervousness	Warm moist skin, Goiter
Fatigue, lethargy	Proximal Myopathy
Dyspnoea	Hyperreflexia
Weight loss despite polyphagia	Lid lag, Lid tremors
Hyperdefecation, Polyuria	Gynaecomastia
Oligomenorrhoea	Loss of libido

Table 2. Common clinical features

2. Graves' disease

Diffuse toxic goitre is commonly known as Graves' disease. Classically it is characterized by hyperthyroidism and diffuse goiter. Graves' disease may be associated with an infiltrative orbitopathy and ophthalmopathy and less commonly with an infiltrative dermopathy. Infiltrative orbitopathy is an unique manifestation of Graves' disease.

2.1. Historical perspective

Robert James Graves, an Irish physician, first described 3 females with this disease in 1835[1] and for his contribution, this disease is known as Graves' disease in most part of the world. Although a similar syndrome was described by Caleb Hiller Parry, a physician from Bath,

England, in 1825.[2] Carl A. Von Basedow from Germany first described the triad of exophthalmos, goiter and palpitation.[3] In most non English speaking European countries the disease is still known as Basedow's disease.

2.2. Epidemiology

Graves' disease is the most common cause of thyrotoxicosis and it accounts for 60-80% cases of thyrotoxicosis. Prevalence of Graves' disease varies with the degree of iodine sufficiency, and it is the most common cause of thyrotoxicosis in iodine sufficient countries.[4] High dietary iodine intake is associated with an increased prevalence of Graves' disease. Prevalence of Graves' disease is about 0.4% in USA,[5] 0.6% in Italy,[6] and 1.1% in UK.[7] A recent meta-analysis of various studies showed that prevalence of the Graves' disease is about 1% in general population.[7] Prevalence of Graves' disease is 1-2% in women, and it is about 10 fold more prevalent in women than men. Peak age of onset of Graves' disease is in fourth to sixth decade of life,[8] but it can occur in children and elderly.

2.3. Risk Factors for Graves' disease

Graves' disease is a multifactorial disease in which genetic ,environmental, and hormonal factors play their role.

2.3.1. Genetic factors for Graves' disease

High prevalence of Graves' disease in family members and relatives of Graves' disease and Hashimoto's thyroiditis support that genetic factors are involved in causation of Graves' disease. There is also evidence that occurrence rate of Graves' disease is higher in monozygotic twins than dizygotic twins. The concordance rate in monozygotic twins is only 17-35% which indicate low penentrance of genes.

Graves' disease is a polygenic disease. Polymorphism in HLA-DR, CTLA-4 and PTPN-22 genes are associated with increased risk of Graves' disease. HLA-DR3 (HLA-DRB1*03), HLA-DQA1*0501 and HLA-B8 gives a risk ratio of three fold to fourfold in white population. HLA-DQ3 is involved in patients with African descent whereas HLA-BW46 is involved in patients with Asian descent. The other genes involved in pathogenesis of Graves' disease are CD40 gene, thyroglobulin gene, TSHR gene, immunoglobulin genes, GD-1 gene (on chromosome 14q13), GD-2 gene (on chromosome 20) and GD-3 gene (on chromosome Xq21-22).

2.3.2. Environmental Factors for Graves' disease

Infection

From very early it has been suggested that Graves' disease is associated with infectious agents, but this hypothesis has not been confirmed. Incidence of recent viral infections are high in patients with Graves' disease. The association of Graves' disease with infectious agents can be explained by molecular mimicry. Molecular mimicry implies structural similarity between infectious agent with a self antigen. Circulating antibody against Yersinia enterocolitica has been found in high percentage of patients with Graves' disease. Furthermore, serum from some patients recovering from Yersinia infections block the binding of TSH to its receptor. Low affinity binding sites for TSH have also been found with Leishmania and Mycoplasma species. However, no studies proved that infections agents have causative role in Graves' disease.

Stress

In different studies, it has been found that stressful life events precedes the onset of Graves' disease. Severe emotional and physical stress, like separation from the loved one or following road traffic accident, cause release of cortisol ad corticotrophin releasing hormone. So, stress is a relatively immune suppression state. Immune system overcompensates once stress is over which can precipitate disease similar to postpartum period. In conclusion there is limited but significant evidence that stressful life events can precipitate the onset of Graves' disease in genetically susceptible individuals.

Gender

Typically Graves' disease is more prevalent in females than males. It is about 5-10 times more common in females at any age. [6,7] In children this difference is smaller. The exact cause for female preponderance is not known, but it is similar to other autoimmune disorders. In experimental animal models of autoimmune thyroiditis it has been seen that androgens appear to down regulate the immune system.[8,9] Other possible explanation for female preponderance is female sex steroids. But Graves' disease also occurs in men and postmenopausal women. These observations have suggested that it is the X-chromosome, not the sex steroids, which is responsible. But most of the x-linked disorders are only present in man, it has been thought that a gene with dose dependent effect on X-chromosome is responsible.

Pregnancy

Postpartum period is an important risk factor for both the onset and relapse of Graves' disease. Postpartum period is associated with a fourfold to eightfold increased risk for the onset of Graves' disease. Rebound immunity is the likely explanation for this increased risk. Graves' disease is associated with low pregnancy rate because thyrotoxicosis decreases the fertility rate. However in women with Graves' disease who became pregnant, successful pregnancy outcome is low because Graves' disease causes increased pregnancy loss and its complications. Graves' disease exacerbates during the first trimester of pregnancy and postpartum period, while it improves during the second and third trimester of pregnancy.

Smoking

Smoking is a minor risk factor for Graves' disease; however it is a major risk factor for Graves' ophthalmopathy. There are number of studies showing relationship between Graves' disease, Graves' ophthalmopathy and smoking. [11,12]

Other risk factors:

Direct trauma to the thyroid gland, ethanol injection for the treatment of autonomously functioning thyroid nodules, or thyroid injury following radio-iodine treatment for toxic adenoma or toxic multinodular goiter are associated with an increased risk of Graves' disease. Radio-iodine treatment may also cause onset or worsening of ophthalmopathy. Possible explanation is that thyroid injury by any means cause massive release of thyroid antigens, which in turn stimulate an autoimmune reaction to TSHR in susceptible individuals.

Graves' disease onset and recurrence is also associated with iodine and iodine containing drugs like amiodarone and radio-contrast media especially in iodine deficient population.

3. Pathogenesis

Graves' disease is an example of organ specific autoimmune disorder in which both humoral and cell mediated immunity directed against different thyroid antigens are involved. TSHR is the primary autoantigen of Graves' disease, while other autoantigens like thyroglobulin and thyroid peroxidase are secondarily involved.

3.1. Humoral immunity

TSHR is a member of GPCR super family and involves cAMP and phosphoinositol pathways for signal transduction. TSHR has large intracellular domain (subgroup B). It is a glycoprotein consisting of 744 amino acids and having molecular weight of 84 kd. Gene for TSHR is located on chromosome 14q31 and is formed by 10 exons. Circulating autoantibody directed against the TSHR is the primary factor responsible for Graves' disease. TSHR antibodies (TSHR-Ab) are of three types- namely stimulating antibody, blocking antibody and neutral antibody. Stimulating antibodies are those who after binding to TSHR activate adenylate cyclase and cause increased thyroid growth and vascularity, and increases the production of thyroid hormones. Blocking antibodies are those who after binding to TSHR act as an antagonist, whereas neutral antibodies does not have any functional activity.

Almost 50 years ago(in 1956) long acting thyroid stimulators (LATS) was discovered by Adams and Purves during a search for thyroid stimulating activity in patients with Graves' disease. [13] Later on it was found that LATS are nothing but immunoglobulin of IgG1 subclass.

Transplacental transfer of TSHR stimulating antibodies (TSAb) from TSAb positive pregnant mother to fetus causes transient neonatal thyrotoxicasis that improves spontaneously after the disappearance of TSAb. [14] This provides the definite role of TSAb in the causation of Graves' disease. TSAb are oligoclonal.

TSAb are produced mainly by the lymphocytes infiltrating the thyroid gland and lymphocytes present in the draining lymph nodes, and partly by the circulating blood lymphocytes.[15,16] There is a positive correlation exists between the TSAb level and serum triiodothyronine level, serum thyroglobulin level and goiter size. TSAb are found in 90-100% of untreated Graves' disease patients.[17, 18] Level of TSAb decreases after treatment with anti- thyroid drugs and radio-iodine.[19, 20]

3.2. Assays for TSHR-Ab

Two types of assays are used for TSHR-Ab-Radioreceptor assays and invitro bioassays.

3.2.1. Radioreceptor assay

Radioreceptor assay is most readily available and most widely used in clinical practice. Basic principle of radioreceptor assay is displacement of labeled TSH from solubilized TSHR from patient's serum. This TSH- binding inhibitory immunoglobulins (TBII) assay does not provide information regarding the functionality of TSHR-Ab. TBII assays are cheaper and having good precision. The first generation TBII assays have sensitivity of 75-95% in untreated Graves' disease patients. Most recently a monoclonal human antibody to TSHR is used. This second generation radio-receptor assay has sensitivity of 99% and very high specificity. [21]

3.2.2. In vitro bioassays

In vitro bioassays are based on the ability of patients serum to stimulate adenylate cyclase and produce cAMP from cultured hamster ovary cells transfected with human TSHR (CHO-R),[23] or rat thyroid cell strain (FRTL-5)[24] or human thyroid follicular cells [25] are used as a source for functional TSHR. CHO-R system is slightly more sensitive, and requires an easier culture condition than other systems. Advantages of bioassays are that it gives information about the functional property of TSHR-Ab, but bioassays are more expensive, not widely available, having poor precision and sensitivity of more than 90%. These problems have been solved in newer bioassays.

3.2.3. Cellular immunity

The thyroid gland in Graves' disease is characterized by non-homogenous lymphocytic infiltration. Majority of the intrathyroidal lymphocytes are T lymphocytes. B-lymphocytes are much less common than Hashimoto's thyroiditis. Cytokine profile produced by intrathyroidal T lymphocytes suggested that both TH1 & TH2 cells are present in thyroid. Majority of the T-lymphocytes are of TH1 subtype.[26,27]

TH1 cells are mainly involved in delayed type of hypersensitivity reactions, and it produces the cytokines like TNF-B, IFN-Y, IL-2, IL-10 and IL-17. TH1 cells are implicated in the pathogenesis of organ specific autoimmune diseases that is mediated mainly by TNF-β subtype, which uniquely produces IL-17. TH 2 cells are mainly responsible for humoral immune responses and they produce cytokines like IL-4, IL-5, IL-6 and IL-13.TH1 cells may also induce antibody formation through secretion of IL-10 [28]. IgG1 subclass of antibody are selectively induced by TH1 cells. Most of the intrathyroidal T cells are of memory ($CD4^+$, $CD29^+$) subtype. Concentration of cytotoxic T cells ($CD8^+$) are much less in Graves' disease patients than patients of Hashimoto's thyroiditis. So the functional role of T cells in Graves' disease is primarily a helper than a suppressor or cytotoxic role.

4. Pathogenic mechanisms

4.1. Molecular mimicry or specificity crossover

Structural or conformational similarity between different antigens like infectious agent with a self antigen can lead to crossover of specificity or molecular mimicry. Molecular mimicry has been reported between Reoviral antigen and a tissue antigen expressed in multiple endocrine tissues, Yersinia enterocolitica and TSHR, Retroviral sequences and TSHR & Borrelia and TSHR.

4.2. Bystander effect

There is evidence that bystander activation of local resident antigen specific and nonspecific T- cells by a local viral infection would induce an inflammatory reaction and stimulates the production of cytokines induce autoimmunity. This bystander activation can also occur in any infections and antigens unrelated to the thyroid gland.

4.3. Aberrant expression of class II HLA Antigens

MHC class II molecules (HLA-DP, DQ, and DR) are not expressed on the normal thyroid epithelial cells but they are expressed on thyroid epithelial cells in patients of autoimmune thyroid disease. This aberrant expression of class II HLA antigens on thyroid epithelia cells can be induced by local thyroid insult which causes production of interferon γ and other cytokines. Interferon γ is able to over express HLA class I molecule and induce the expression of class II molecule on thyroid epithelial cells.

4.4. Cryptic antigens

Autoimmunity results from the loss of tolerance or the ability to differentiate between self and non self. Tolerance induction is a staged process that initiates in the thymus during T-cell maturation. This process depends in part on the presence of peripheral antigens in the thymus. Peripheral antigens are antigens normally expressed in tissues outside of the immune system which are expressed at low levels in thymus. T cells that react strongly to these peripheral molecules in the context of MHC are deleted in thymus. T cells that react with peripheral antigens that are not expressed in the thymus have a greater opportunity to escape tolerance.

4.5. Hygiene hypothesis

Hygiene hypothesis implies that infection may protect form autoimmune diseases rather than precipitating it. Decreased exposure to antigens due to improved living standards can lead to increased risk of autoimmune disorder.

4.6. Super antigens

Super antigens are endogenous or exogenous proteins such as microbial proteins, capable of stimulating a strong immune response through molecular interactions with non-variant parts of the T- cell repertoire and the HLA class II proteins.

5. Pathology

Grossly the thyroid gland is diffusely enlarged with smooth and hyperemic surface. Rarely the gland is grossly nodular. Consistency of the gland varies from soft to firm. Pyramidal lobe is often prominent.

Microscopically both hypertrophy and hyperplasia are seen. Follicles are small with scanty colloid, and lined by hyperplasic columnar epithelium which can give a pseudopapillary appearance. Vascularity of the gland is increased. There is varying degree of infiltration by lymphocytes and plasma cells. T cells predominate in the interstitium, whereas B cells and plasma cells predominate in lymphoid follicles.

On electron microscopy there is increased golgi reticulum and mitochondria, and it is also characterized by presence of prominent microvilli.

After treatment with antithyroid drugs and radioiodine, the vascularity of the gland decreases, follicles enlarges and filled with colloid, and papillary projection regresses.

6. Clinical features

Graves' disease is the most common cause of thyrotoxicosis. Most common age of onset is third to fourth decade of life but it can occur in children and elderly. The hallmark of Graves' disease is signs and symptoms of thyrotoxicosis along with diffuse goiter and typical Graves' orbitopathy. Most of the signs and symptoms are similar to other causes of thyrotoxicosis, but some of the signs and symptoms like orbitopathy, dermopathy or pretibial myxedema and thyroid acropachy are unique to Graves' disease.

Onset of Graves' disease is usually gradual. Signs and symptoms are presents months before the diagnosis, and usually patients do not remember the exact date of onset of symptoms. Onset can be abrupt in some cases. The signs and symptoms are usually more severe than other causes of thyrotoxicosis.

6.1. Thyroid gland

Thyroid gland is diffusely enlarged in Graves' disease, but it can be nodular especially in areas of iodine deficiency where nodular goiter preexists before the onset of Graves' disease. Goiter size is variable. It can range from normal size thyroid gland to massively enlarged thyroid. Usually size of goiter is two to three times that of normal. Normal size thyroid gland can the seen in as many as 20% of patients and most of them are elderly. The consistency of the goiter varies from soft to firm but softer than the goiter of Hashimoto's thyroiditis. Thrill and bruit can be present over goiter in severe cases and it is due to increased vascularity of the gland. Thrill and bruit are present usually on upper or lower pole and continuos in nature, but sometimes can present only in systole. Large goiter with intrathoracic extension can be associated with facial swelling and flushing, and neck vein distension upon raising the arm above the head. This is known as Pemberton sign.

6.2. Graves' ophthalmopathy

Graves' ophthalmopathy is one of the distinctive manifestations of Graves' disease. Overall clinical ophthalmopathy is present in about 50% of Graves' disease patients,[29] however CT or MRI reveals extraocular muscle enlargement in about 70% of patients without overt clinical ophthamopathy.[30,31] Bimodal age distribution was noted for ophthalmopathy in both men and women. Peak age is 40 to 44 years and 60 to 64 years in women, whereas in men it is 45 to 49 years and 65 to 69 years.

6.2.1. Risk factors for Graves' ophthalmopathy

There is no specific genetic predisposition for graves' ophthalmopathy. Environmental factors are more important for ophthalmopathy.

Smoking

Smoking is a major risk factor for ophthalmopathy. Smoking also increases the risk for worsening of ophthalmopathy after radioiodine treatment. Possible contributors are orbital hypoxia and free radical present is smoke. [32,33]

Gender

Graves' disease is predominantly a disease of females (F: M= 8-10:1). In comparison to Graves' disease, ophthalmopathy is relatively more common in males (F: M= 1:1.8-2.8) than females. [34,35]

Radioiodine

Graves' disease patients treated with radioiodine are at increased risk for onset and worsening of eye disease, as compared to antithyroid drugs alone. [36,37] This risk can be decreased by concurrent use of corticosterodis.[38,39]

6.2.2. Pathogenesis

Current evidence support an autoimmune pathogenesis with important environmental influences, particularly smoking. Orbital muscles, connective tissues, and adipose tissues are infiltrated by lymphocytes and macrophages. TH1 mediated immune response predominates in early stage of disease while TH2 response predominates in late stage. [40] In response to cytokines secreted by the infiltrating immune cells, orbital fibroblasts start synthesizing and secreting hydrophilic glycosaminoglycans, resulting in edema of orbital tissues. Additionally adipocytes present in orbit become active and results in expansion of orbital adipose tissues. Both these factors are responsible for expansion of orbital tissues.

6.2.3. Natural history

Onset of eye disease usually coincides with that of thyrotoxicosis in 40% of cases, follow it in 40%, and precedes it in 20%.[41,42] Even when the onset of the two disorders does not coincide, each occurs within 18 months from the onset of the first manifestation. Eye disease usually shows a progressive deterioration lasting for several months followed by a phase of spontaneous improvement lasting upto a year and longer and quiescent stage when inflammatory signs disappear and clinical features stabilizes.

6.2.4. Sings and symptoms

The earliest manifestations of ophthalmopathy are usually a sensation of grittiness, eye discomfort, and excess tearing. Other common symptoms are spontaneous retroorbital pain, pain on ocular movement and diplopia. Diplopia is most common in upgaze or in extremes of lateral gaze, because of the involvement of inferior or lateral rectus muscle. About one third of patients have proptosis which can best be detected by visualization of the sclera between the lower border of iris and the lower eyelid when the eyes are kept in primary position.

In severe cases proptosis can cause exposure keratitis and corneal ulcerations. Proptosis is frequently assymetrical. Retraction of the upper eyelid and less commonly of lower eyelid results in lid lag, globe lag, and lagophthalmos. Movements of the lids are jerky, and also there is tremor of lightly closed eyes. These are the non specific manifestations of thyrotoxicosis. Other signs and symptoms are photophobia, swelling of the eyelids, blurring of vision, conjunctival injection and chemosis, periorbital edema.

Decreased visual acuity and color vision, corneal ulceration, and subluxation of globe are present in most severe cases. Blindness may result from corneal ulceration and compression of the optic nerve at the orbital apex due to increased orbital pressure and venous congestion.

Graves' ophthalmopathy can occur in absence of Graves' disease in 10% cases, that's why it is also known as thyroid associated ophthalmopathy, or euthyroid Graves' opthalmopathy. Graves' ophthalmopathy is usually bilateral but it can be unilateral in upto 10% cases.

6.2.5. Staging severity of ophthalmopathy

The acronym NO SPECS was given by American Thyroid Association for severity of ophthalmopathy, where no indicates absence or mild ophthalmopathy, and SPECS indicates more severe degree of involvement, but NO SPECS scheme is inadequate and patients do not necessarily progress from one class to other.

Classes	Ocular symptoms and signs
0	No signs and symptoms
1	Only signs (lid retraction, lid lag, proptosis upto 22 mm)
2	Soft tissue involvement (periorbital edema)
3	Proptosis (>22 mm)
4	Extraocular muscle involvement (diplopia)
5	Corneal involvement
6	Sight loss (optic nerve involvement)

Table 3.

6.2.6. Clinical activity of ophthalmopathy

To know the clinical activity of ophthalmopathy is important, because active disease is more likely to respond to immunosuppressive therapy. Clinical Activity Score (CAS) is used to know the clinical activity. Seven parameters are used in the clinical activity scoring which include spontaneous retrobulbar pain, pain on eye movement, eyelid erythema, conjuctival injection, swelling of the eyelids, inflammation of the caruncle and conjunctival edema or chemosis. Each parameter is assigned 1 point. CAS of more than or equal to 3/7 indicates active ophthalmopathy.

6.3. Thyroid dermopathy

Thyroid dermopathy presents in less than 5% of patients with Graves' disease. It is almost always accompanied by moderate to severe ophthalmopathy. Most commonly it is present over anterior and lateral aspects of leg, hence it is also known as pretibial myxoedema. Less commonly it can present over dorsa of the feet, dorsa of the hands, forearm, face and elbows, particularly after trauma. The typical lesion is a noninflamed, indurated plaque with a deep pink or purple color and an orange skin appearance. Nodular form is the intermediate while elephantiasis is the most severe form of thyroid dermopathy. Thyroid dermopathy occurs due to accumulation of glycosaminoglycans in the dermis and subcutaneous tissues.

6.4. Thyroid acropachy

Thyroid acropachy is the least common manifestation of Graves' disease. It is a form of clubbing, and presents in less than 1 percent of patients of Graves' disease. It is almost always associated with the severe and long standing ophthalmopathy and dermopathy. An alternate diagnosis should be considered in the absence of ophthalmopathy and dermopathy. Deposition of glycosaminoglycans in skin is responsible for thyroid acropachy.

7. Laboratory diagnosis

Diagnosis of Graves' disease can be confirmed by measurement of serum TSH and total thyroxine (TT_4) and triiodothyronine (TT_3). Serum TSH level is suppressed or undetectable with increased TT_4 and TT_3 level in patients of Graves' disease. Serum TSH level is the most sensitive test. The free T_4 (FT_4) and free T_3 (FT_3) levels are increased more than that of TT_4 and TT_3. Measurement of FT_4 and FT_3 are expensive, and there is more chance of laboratory errors. FT_4 and FT_3 can be measured in conditions associated with high serum TBG level like pregnancy, oral contraceptive use and chronic liver disease. In patients of Graves' disease serum T_3 level is proportionately more elevated than the serum T_4 level. In upto 12% of patients, especially in the iodine deficient areas, only TT_3 or FT_3 is elevated with a normal TT_4 or FT_4 level, a condition known as T_3 toxicosis. Conversely in some patients (iodine induced hyperthyroidism, drugs like amiodarone and propronolol which block the conversion of T_4 to T_3), only TT_4 or FT_4 is elevated with normal TT_3 and FT_3 (T_4 toxicosis). Serum thyroglobulin level is high in all cases of thyrotoxicosis except factitious thyrotoxicosis.

Anti TPO antibody can be detected in upto 90%[43,44] of patients with Graves' disease whereas anti-thyroglobulin antibody is present in 50-80% cases.[45,46] They are useful in confirming the presence of thyroid autoimmunity but they are of limited diagnostic value. TSHR-Ab assay is very sensitive and specific (upto 98%) for the diagnosis of Graves' disease. But TSHR-Ab assay is quite expensive and not widely available. TSHR-Ab assay is indicated only when clinical and laboratory diagnosis are not clear. Indications for TSHR-Ab assay are:

- Euthyroid Graves' disease, especially when it is unilateral
- Pregnant women with Graves' disease to predict the likelihood of neonatal thyrotoxicosis
- Nodular variant of Graves' disease

TSHR-Ab assay is also a useful indicator of the degree of disease activity. It can also predict the prognosis of Graves' disease. There is more chance of relapse in patients with persistently high TSHR-Ab level after cessation of antithyroid drug.[47]

Associated hematological abnormalities include increased RBC mass, leucopenia with relative lymphocytosis, monocytosis and eosinophilia, increased factor VIII level. Other associated abnormalities include elevated liver enzymes, bilirubin and ferritin.

7.1. Radioactive iodine uptake (RAIU)

RAIU is not required in each and every case of Graves' disease, but it is useful in excluding thyrotoxicosis caused by thyroiditis, factitious thyrotoxicosis, and type II amiodarone induces thyrotoxicosis. RAIU is absolutely contraindicated in pregnancy. In Graves' disease RAIU is diffusely increased.

7.2. Thyroid ultrasound

In Graves' disease thyroid tissue typically become hypoechoic because of reduction in colloid content, increase in thyroid vascularity and lymhocytic infiltration. In colour flow doppler there is a distinct pattern characterized by markedly increased signals, inferior thyroid artery and itrathyroidal artery velocities more than 40 cm/s. This pattern, in conjunction with a hypoechoic pattern allows distinction from Hashimoto's thyroiditis.

7.3. Differential diagnosis

If a patient presented with diffuse goiter with clinical and biochemical thyrotoxicosis, ophthalmopathy and positive autoimmune markers like anti TPO antibody or TSHR-Ab, diagnosis of Graves' disease is straight forward. In absence of these classical features radionuclide scan (I^{123}, I^{131}, Tc^{99m}) in the most reliable distinguishing test. In case of Graves' disease there is diffuse and high uptake, whereas in patients with toxic adenoma or toxic multinodular goiter there is patchy uptake. In patients with thyroiditis and factitious thyrotoxicosis there is decreased uptake. In patients with TSH producing adenoma, there is also a diffuse goiter, but TSH is inappropriately normal or increased instead of suppress TSH of graves' disease. Panic attacks, mania, pheochromocytoma and malignancy can be easily ruled out by thyroid function test.

8. Treatment

There is no ideal treatment option present targeting the basic pathogenic mechanisms of Graves' disease. Available treatment options target the increased synthesis of thyroid hormones by antithyroid drugs, or ablation of thyroid tissue by surgery or radioiodine. Antithyroid drugs are the predominant therapy in Europe and Japan whereas radioiodine is first line of treatment in USA. No single treatment is optimal and patients often require multiple treatment.

8.1. Antithyroid drugs

Thionamides are the main antithyroid drugs which includes propylthiouracil, carbimazole and methimazole. Thionamides act by inhibiting the enzyme thyroid peroxidase, reducing the oxidation and organification of iodide and coupling of iodotyrosines. Carbimazole is not an active drug, and in body it is converted to active metabolite methimazole. Proylthiouracil, in addition to inhibit thyroid hormone synthesis, also inhibits the peripheral conversion of T_4 to T_3. Methimazole is ten times more potent than prophylthiouracil. Half life of methimazole is about 6 hours while that of prophylthiouracil is about 90 minutes. Duration of action of methimazole is more than 24 hours while that of propylthiouracil is 12-24 hours. Transplacental transfer of prophylthiouracil is lowest. Antithyroid drugs do not block the release of preformed hormones, so euthyroidism is not obtained until intrathyroidal hormone store is depleted. These drugs also reduce thyroid antibody level.

Antithyroid drugs can be used as a primary treatment or as a preparatory treatment before radioiodine or surgery. The antithyroid drugs are usually started in higher doses. The starting dose of methiomazole or carbimazole is 10-20 mg every 8-12 hours and that of propylthiouracil is 100-200 mg every 6-8 hours. Once euthyroidism is achieved which usually takes 4-5 weeks, methimazole can be given in single daily dose while propylthiouracil is given in multiple daily doses throughout the treatment. There are two treatment strategies for using antithyroid drugs. In titration regimen, antithyroid drugs are started in high doses and dose can be gradually decreased to maintain euthyroid state. In Block and Replace regimen, the antithyroid drugs are maintained in high doses and subsequently levothyroxine is added to maintain the euthyroid status. At present there is no proven advantage of block and replace regimen over titration regimen.

Patient should be reviewed clinically and biochemically after every 3-4 weeks. Dose of antithyroid drugs is adjusted based on the TT_4 or FT_4 level, as TSH level often remain suppressed for several months. The usual daily maintenance dose of carbimazole or methimazole is 2.5 – 10 mg and that of propylthiouracil is 50-100 mg. When TSH level become normal, it can also be used to monitor therapy. Size of the goiter decreases in about 30-50% of patients during treatment. In remaining patients it may remain unchanged or even enlarge. Increase in goiter size is one of the earliest manifestations of iatrogenic hypothyroidism. The other features are weight gain, lethargy, fatigue and other signs of mild hypothyroidism.

Maximum remission rate with antithyroid drugs is 30-50%, which can be achieved by continuation of the drug for 6-18 months or even longer. Most of the relapses occur within first 3-6 months after discontinuation of drug. Suppressed TSH level below the normal limit is the first signal of relapse even in the presence of a normal serum T_4 level. In most of the studies, the relapse rate is 50-80%.[48,49] Most important predictor of relapse is goiter size.[50] Other factors influencing recurrence of Graves' disease include high TSHR-Ab concentration, large iodine intake, marked residual goiter, short duration of antithyroid drug treatment and previous recurrence. Factors which favor long term remission after therapy include the initial presence of T_3 toxicosis, a small goiter, decrease in the size of goiter, and return of TSH to normal during treatment, the return of serum thyroglobulin to normal, and low iodine diet.

Most common side effects of thionamides are pruritus, skin rash, urticaria, fever and arthralgia. These may resolve spontaneously or after substituting another drug. Rare but major side effects are hepatitis, cholestasis, SLE like syndrome, ANCA positive vasculitis and most importantly agranulocytosis. Major side effects occur in less than 1% of patients.Antithyroid drugs should be stopped and not restarted if patient develop major side effects.

8.2. Iodine and iodine containing components

Inorganic iodine acts in many ways in thyrotoxicosis. Iodine blocks its own transport in thyroid, inhibits iodine organification and inhibits the release of hormone. Inhibition of iodine organification by inorganic iodide is known as Wolf-Chaikoff effect. Major action of iodine is inhibition of hormone release. Iodine also decreases the vascularity of thyroid gland. All of these effects of iodine are transient and lasts only for a few days or weeks. Now a days iodine is used only for preoperative preparation for Graves' disease and in the management of thyrotoxic crisis. The usual dose of Lugol's solution is 3-5 drops three times per day and that of SSKI is 2-3 drops twice daily. Iodine decreases the effect of subsequently administad thionamides and radioiodine for severe weeks.

Iodinated radio contrast agents like iopanoic acid, and sodium ipodate acts by blocking the peripheral conversion of T4 to T3 and inhibition of hormone release. They are ideally used in emergency situations when rapid control of thyrotoxicosis is needed or in preoperative preparation or while awaiting the response of radioiodine.

8.3. Thiocyanate and perchlorate

They act by intititing the transport of iodine to thyroid gland.

8.4. Lithium

Lithium also acts as a thyroid constipating agent (block the release of thyroid hormones). Lithium also potentiates the beneficial effect of radioiodine. The usual dose of lithium is 450-900 mg per day in divided doses. Serum lithium concentration should be maintained at 1meEq/L. No adverse effects are reported with this dose of lithium.

8.5. Glucocorticoids

Dexamethasone in high doses (8mg/day) decreases the T4 secretion by the thyroid gland, inhibit the peripheral conversion of T4 to T3, and has immunosuppressive effect. Effect on peripheral conversion of T4 to T3 is additive to propylthiouracil. Glucocorticaids are indicated for the treatment of ophthalmopathy, dermopathy and in thyrotoxic crisis.

8.6. β- blockers

β- blockers do not affect the synthesis or secretion of thyroid hormones. Many of the symptoms & signs of thyrotoxicosis are due to hypersensitivity of the sympathetic nervous system to thyroid hormones. Thus use of β- blockers in thyrotoxicosis, improve the signs and symptoms mediated by the sympathetic nervous system. Tachycardia, palpitation, tremor, anxiety, excess sweating, lid retraction improves with β- blockers. Propranolol has additional advantage over other β- blockers. It inhibits the peripheral conversion of T4 to T3. β- blockers reduce cardiac output without altering oxygen consumption, can have adverse effect in liver, where the arteriovenous oxygen difference is already elevated in the hyperthyroid state. Propranolol is most commonly used agent but other β- blockers can also be used. It is used in a dose of 20-60 mg every 6-8 hours. Short acting agents like esmolol is used for intravenous purpose. Long acting agents like atenolol or metoprolol are used for prolonged treatment. β- blockers should be rapidly tapered and discontinued once stable euthyroidism it achieved.

8.7. Radioiodine

Radioiodine is one of the first line therapy for the Graves' disease. Among different isotopes of radioiodine, I^{131} is the agent of choice. I^{131} is a β-emitter isotope. After oral administration, $I^{131}$is completely absorbed and rapidly concentrated in thyroid follicular cells. β- particles, which are emitted by I^{131}, destroy the thyroid follicular cells that results in reduced thyroid hormone synthesis. Initially destruction of thyroid follicular cells results in release of preformed hormones that can precipitate the thyortoxic crisis. Weeks to months are required for control of thyrotoxicosis. Long term effects of radioiodine include atrophy and fibrosis, and a chromic inflammatory response resembling Hashimoto's thyroiditis.

Radioiodine is given as single oral dose. Three outcomes of radioiodine treatment are possible- patients become euthyroid or remain thyrotoxic or become permanently hypothyroid. Dose of radioiodine depends on the size of gland, the uptake of I^{131} and its subsequent rate of release. Dose of radioiodine ranges from 80-200 μCi/gm of thyroid tissues. A total dose of 20 mCi achieves thyroid ablation in almost all patients and results in permanent hypothyroidisms in 75-90% of patients. [51] The incidence of post radioiodine hypothyroidism in first year is 25% and steadily increases thereafter at a rate of 5% per year. When required, the second dose of radioiodine should be given at least 6 months after the first dose. Failure of radioiodine treatment is more common in patients with large goiter, rapid iodine turnover and adjunctive antithyroid drugs too soon after radioiodine. Prior use of antithyorid drugs decreases the risk of thyrotoxic crisis. Chance of worsening ophthalmopathy can also be reduced by antithyroid drugs. Antithyroid drugs should be stopped 3 to 8 days prior to radioiodine treatment and should be restarted after 7 days when required. Propylthiouracil may cause radio-resistance, but it not a major concern. Short term side effects of radioiodine include transient exacerbation of thyrotoxicosis in the first few months, transient worsening of ophthalompathy, acute radiation thyroids in the first week. Radiation thyroidits may lead to transient worsening of thyrotoxicosis and ophthalmopathy. Presence of mild to moderate ophthalmopathy is not a contraindication for radioiodine treatment. Concomitant use of oral glucocorticoids, decreases the risk of worsening ophthalmopathy. Long term side effect of radioiodine is permanent hypothyroidism. Initially there was a concern regarding possible carcinogenic effect and risk of genetic damage after radioiodine treatment. But now it is proven that there is no association between radioiodine treatment and thyroid carcinoma, leukemia, solid tumors and genetic damage.[52] Thyroid cancer is associated with low dose of I^{131} rather than higher dose of I^{131} in children. [53] Some centers uses radioiodine even in children of 10 years of age or younger, but still there is no consensus regarding use of radioiodine for persons younger than 16 to 18 years.

8.8. Surgery

Surgery is a form of ablative therapy. Enough thyroid tissue is removed by surgery to reduce the synthesis of thyroid hormones and prevent recurrence. Two type of thyoid surgery are used for Graves' disease. In subtotal thyroidectomy, bulk of the thyroid gland is removed and only about 2 gm (0.5%) of thyroid tissue is left in both lobes. In near total thyroidectomy, most of the thyroid gland is removed, with only subcentimeter fragment are left around recurrent laryngeal nerve and parathyroid glands. Subtotal thyroidectomy was the procedure of choice in past, but it is associated with higher recurrence rate. Now-a-days near total thyroidectomy is used most often. Near total thyroidectomy is associated with more chance of permanent hypothyroidism but less chance of recurrence than subtotal thyroidectomy.

Complications of thyroid surgery depends on the skill and experience of operating surgeon. In specialized hands, complication rate is as low as 2%, whereas complication rate increases up to 10-15% in non specialized centers. Post Operative bleeding is the most serious complication. It can be fatal by producing asphyxia, if it is not evacuated immediately. Other complications like thyroid storm, injury to recurrent laryngeal nerve and hypoparathyroidism are specific to thyroid surgery. Thyroid storm is rare now-a-days. Injury to recurrent laryngeal nerve causes dysphonia, that usually improves with time, but that may leave the patient slightly hoarse. Hypoparathyroidism can be transient or permanent. Transient hypoparathyroidism is due to removal of the some parathyroid and impairment of blood supply to parathyroid glands, whereas permanent hypoparathyroidism is due to inadvertent removal of all 4 glands. Transient hypoparathyroidism usually occur on day 1-7 postoperatively. Severe symptomatic hypoparathyroidism should be treated by intravenous calcium gluconate. Oral calcium (upto 3 gm/day) is sufficient for milder cases. Immediate postoperative hypocalcemia is due to hungry bone syndrome. Recurrence of hyperthyroidism and permanent hypothyroidism are inversely related and depends on the amount of thyroid tissue left. In case of recurrence, radioiodine should be used as treatment, as second surgery is technically difficult.

Preoperative preparation

Preoperative use of thionamides is associated with lesser morbidity and mortality. Preoperative thionamides are recommended to achieve euthyroidism and to deplete. The hormone store. Preoperative use of inorganic iodine decreases the gland size and vcascularity. In case of emergency surgery oral cholecystographic agents are the fastest way to obtain euthyroidism. The goal of preoperative management is to maintain euthyroid states by thionamides and then to induce involution of the gland by the inorganic iodine. β blockers can be used in preoperative preparation.

Choice of therapy

Choice of therapy depends on the patient preference, personal experience of the treating doctor and availability of the treatment options. All the three treatment options (antithyroid drugs, radioiodine, surgery) can be used as first line therapy. In most of the Europe, antithyroid drugs are the preferred treatment whereas in USA, radioiodine is the preferred treatment. Primary choice of treatment in children and young adults upto 18 years of age is antithyroid drugs, although radioiodine is not associated with any adverse events. Pregnancy should be delayed for 6-12 months after radioiodine treatment. Presence of severe ophthalmopathy is a contraindication for radioiodine treatment. Surgery is the preferred treatment for patients with large goiter, especially if compressive symptoms are present, endemic goiter with multiple cold nodules, and suspected malignancy.

Thyroid ophthalmopathy

Mild to moderate ophthalmopathy does not require any specific treatment. General measures include control of thyrotoxicosis, smoking cessation, dark glasses with side frame for photophobia and sensitivity to air, artificial tear (1% methyl cellulose) or eye ointment for eye discomfort and dry eye, eye patches or taping during sleep for lagophthalmos, elevation of the head end for periorbital edema, prism for correction of mild diplopia.

Other patients with more severe signs and symptoms affecting daily lives to a significant extent may benefit from immunosuppressive therapy in active disease or surgical decompression in case of inactive disease. Severe ophthalmopathy with optic neuropathy and corneal ulcer is an emergency.

Glucocorticoids

Oral glucocorticoids is initiated at a relatively high dose, such as 40-80 mg of prednisolone per day. After 2-4 weeks, the daily dose is tapered by 2.5-10 mg every 2-4 weeks. Improvement in soft tissue inflammation begins within 1-2 days. Intravenous methylprednisolone pulse therapy is more effective and better tolerated than oral prednisolone.[54] 500 mg of methylprednisolone per week for 6 weeks followed by 250 mg of methylprednisolone per week for 6 weeks is most commonly used regimen. Cyclosporine can also be used either as a single therapy or in combination with oral prednisolone. Combination therapy of cyclosporine with prednisolone is more effective than either drug alone.[55]

Orbital Radiotherapy

Orbital radiotherapy is well tolerated and provide benefit in approximately two third of patients. This treatment is steroid sparing rather than steroid replacing therapy.

Other immunomodulatory therapy

Rituximab, azathioprine, cyclophosphamide, ciamexon, pentoxifylline and intravenous immunoglobulins have some benefit and are currently under trial.

Orbital decompression

Indications for orbital decompression include optic neuropathy, severe proptosis, vision threatening ocular exposure, debilitating retrobulbar and periorbital pain and intolerable corticosteroid side effects. Transantral orbital decompression with removal of a portion of medial wall and the orbital floor is most commonly used procedure. Upto 5 mm reduction in proptosis can be achieved by orbital decompression. Orbital decompression can cause onset or worsening of diplopia.

Thyroid storm

Thyroid storm or thyrotoxic crisis is a life threatening exacerbation of hyperthyroidism. Most of the cases of thyroid storm are associated with Graves' disease, but it can also occur with toxic multinodular goitre. Precipitating factor for thyroid storm include infection, trauma, thyroid surgery, radioiodine, diabetic ketoacidosis, stroke etc. It can present with fever, tachycardia, arrhythmias, profuse sweating, diarrhea and vomiting, confusion, delirium, seizures, jaundice, coma, congestive heart failure, hypotension. Thyroid storm is associated with very high mortality rate (upto 30%, even with treatment).

Treatment of thyroid storm requires strict monitoring and proper care. Precipitating factors should be identified and treated. Supportive treatment include cooling blankets and drugs like acetaminophen, chlorpromazine or meperidine for hyperthermia, oxygen inhalation, intravenous fluids. Antithyroid drug of choice is prophylthiouracil but carbimazole can also be used. Prophylthiouracil 600 mg is given as loading dose by mouth or nasogastric tube or per rectum followed by 200-300 mg every 6-8 hourly. One hour after the first dose of propylthiouracil, stable iodide is given in the form of SSKI (3 drops twice daily) or Lugol's iodine (10 drops twice daily). Propranolol should also be given in a dose of 40-80 mg orally every 6 hours or 2 mg intravenously every 4 hours. If β blockers are contraindicated, calcium channel blockers like diltiazem can be used to control tachycardia. Large dose of dexamethasone (8 mg) by oral or intravenous route should be given to block the release of hormone from gland and peripheral conversion of T4 to T3.

Author details

N.K. Agrawal and Ved Prakash
Department of Endocrinology and Metabolism, Institute of Medical Sciences, Banaras Hindu University, Varanasi, India

Manuj Sharma
Department of Medicine, Gandhi Medical College, Bhopal

9. References

[1] Graves RJ: Newly observed affection of the thyroid. *London Med Surg J* 1835; 7:515-523.

[2] Parry CH: *Collections from the Unpublished Medical Writings of the Late Caleb Hillier Parry*. London, Underwood, 1825.

[3] von Basedow KA: Exophthalmos durch hypertrophie des zellgewebes in der Augenhole. *Wochenschr Ges Heilk Berl* 1840; 6:197.

[4] Laurberg P, Pedersen KM, Vestergaard H, et al: High incidence of multinodular toxic goitre in the elderly population in a low iodine intake area vs. high incidence of Graves' disease in the young in a high iodine intake area: comparative surveys of thyrotoxicosis epidemiology in East-Jutland Denmark and Iceland. *J Intern Med* 1991; 229:415-420.

[5] Furszyfer J, Kurland LT, McConahey WM, et al: Epidemiologic aspects of Hashimoto's thyroiditis and Graves' disease in Rochester Minnesota (1935–1967), with special reference to temporal trends. *Metabolism* 1972; 21:197-204.

[6] Aghini-Lombardi F, Antonangeli L, Martino E, et al: The spectrum of thyroid disorders in an iodine-deficient community: the Pescopagano survey. *J Clin Endocrinol Metab* 1999; 84:561-566

[7] Aghini-Lombardi F, Antonangeli L, Martino E, et al: The spectrum of thyroid disorders in an iodine-deficient community: the Pescopagano survey. *J Clin Endocrinol Metab* 1999; 84:561-566
[8] Bülow Pedersen I, Laurberg P, Knudsen N, et al: Increase in incidence of hyperthyroidism predominantly occurs in young people after iodine fortification of salt in Denmark. *J Clin Endocrinol Metab* 2006; 91:3830-3834,2006.
[9] Chiovato L, Lapi P, Fiore E, et al: Thyroid autoimmunity and female gender. *J Endocrinol Invest* 1993; 16:384-391.
[10] Amino N, Tada H, Hidaka Y: Postpartum autoimmune thyroid syndrome: a model of aggravation of autoimmune disease. *Thyroid* 1999; 9:705-713.
[11] Bartalena L: Smoking and Graves' disease. *J Endocrinol Invest* 2002; 25:402.
[12] Holm IA, Manson JE, Michels KB, et al: Smoking and other lifestyle factors and the risk of Graves' hyperthyroidism. *Arch Intern Med* 2005; 165:1606-1611.
[13] Adams DD, Purves HD: Abnormal responses in the assay of thyrotropin. *Proc Univ Otago Med Sch* 1956; 34:11-12.
[14] McKenzie JM, Zakarija M: Fetal and neonatal hyperthyroidism and hypothyroidism due to maternal TSH receptor antibodies. *Thyroid* 1992; 2:155-159.
[15] McLachlan SM, Dickinson AM, Malcolm A, et al: Thyroid autoantibody synthesis by cultures of thyroid and peripheral blood lymphocytes. I: Lymphocyte markers and response to pokeweed mitogen. *Isr J Med Sci* 1983; 52:45-53.
[16] Okuda J, Akamizu T, Sugawa H, et al: Preparation and characterization of monoclonal antithyrotropin receptor antibodies obtained from peripheral lymphocytes of hypothyroid patients with primary myxedema. *J Clin Endocrinol Metab* 1994; 79:1600-1604.
[17] Bolton J,Sanders J,Oda Y,et al.Measurment of thyroid stimulating hormone receptor autoantibodies by ELISA.Clin Chem 1999;45:2285-2287.
[18] CostagliolaS,Morgenthaler NG,Hoermann R,et al.Second generation assay for thyrotropin receptor antibodies has superior diagnostic sensitivity for Graves disease.J Clin Endocrinol Metab 1999;84:90-97.
[19] Pinchera A, Liberti P, Martino E, et al: Effects of antithyroid therapy on the long-acting thyroid stimulator and the antithyroglobulin antibodies. *J Clin Endocrinol* 1969; 29:231-289.
[20] Fenzi GF, Hashizume K, Roudeboush CP, et al: Changes in thyroid-stimulating immunoglobulins during antithyroid therapy. *J Clin Endocrinol Metab* 1979; 48:572-576.
[21] Costagliola S, Morgenthaler NG, Hoermann R, et al: Second generation assay for thyrotropin receptor antibodies has superior diagnostic sensitivity for Graves' disease. *J Clin Endocrinol Metab* 1999; 84:90-97.
[22] Schott M, Scherbaum WA, Morgenthaler NG: Thyrotropin receptor autoantibodies in Graves' disease. *Trends Endocrinol Metab* 2005; 16:243-248.
[23] Ludgate M, Perret J, Parmentier M, et al: Use of the recombinant human thyrotropin receptor (TSH-R) expressed in mammalian cell lines to assay TSH-R autoantibodies. *Mol Cell Endocrinol* 1990; 73:R13-R18.

[24] Vitti P, Valente WA, Ambesi-Impiombato FS, et al: Graves' IgG stimulation of continuously cultured rat thyroid cells: a sensitive and potentially useful clinical assay. *J Endocrinol Invest* 1982; 5:179-182.
[25] Rapoport B, Greenspan FS, Filetti S, et al: Clinical experience with a human thyroid cell bioassay for thyroid-stimulating immunoglobulin. *J Clin Endocrinol Metab* 1984; 58:332-338.
[26] Mariotti S, del Prete GF, Mastromauro C, et al: The autoimmune infiltrate of Basedow's disease: analysis of clonal level and comparison with Hashimoto's thyroiditis. *Exp Clin Endocrinol* 1991; 97:139-146.
[27] Watson PF, Pickerill AP, Davies R, et al: Analysis of cytokine gene expression in Graves' disease and multinodular goiter. *J Clin Endocrinol Metab* 1994; 79:355-360.
[28] Leovey A, Nagy E, Balazs G, et al: Lymphocytes resided in the thyroid are the main source of TSH-receptor antibodies in Basedow's-Graves' disease?. *Exp Clin Endocrinol* 1992; 99:147-150.
[29] Burch HB, Wartofsky L: Graves' ophthalmopathy: current concepts regarding pathogenesis and management. *Endocr Rev* 1993; 14:747-793.
[30] Forbes G, Gorman CA, Brennan MD, et al: Ophthalmopathy of Graves' disease: computerized volume measurements of the orbital fat and muscle. *Am J Neuroradiol* 1986; 7:651-656
[31] Villadolid MC, Nagataki S, Uetani M, et al: Untreated Graves' disease patients without clinical ophthalmopathy demonstrate a high frequency of extraocular muscle (EOM) enlargement by magnetic resonance. *J Clin Endocrinol Metab* 1995; 80:2830-2833.
[32] Metcalfe RA, Weetman AP: Stimulation of extraocular muscle fibroblasts by cytokines and hypoxia: possible role in thyroid-associated ophthalmopathy. *Clin Endocrinol (Oxf)* 1994; 40:67-72.
[33] Burch HB, Lahiri S, Bahn R, et al: Superoxide radical production stimulates human retroocular fibroblast proliferation in Graves' ophthalmopathy. *Exp Eye Res* 1997; 65:311-316.
[34] Vanderpump MP, Tunbridge WM, French JM, et al: The incidence of thyroid disorders in the community: A twenty-year follow-up of the Whickham survey. *Clin Endocrinol (Oxf)* 1995; 43:55-68.
[35] Perros P, Kendall-Taylor P: Pathogenetic mechanisms in thyroid-associated ophthalmopathy. *J Intern Med* 1992; 231:205-211.
[36] Fernandez-Sanchez JR, Vara-Thorbeck R, Garbin-Fuentes I, et al: Graves' ophthalmopathy after subtotal thyroidectomy and radioiodine therapy. *Br J Surg* 1993; 80:1134-1136.
[37] Bartalena L, Pinchera A, Martino E, et al: Relation between therapy for hyperthyroidism and the course of Graves' ophthalmopathy. *N Engl J Med* 1998; 338:73-78.
[38] Bartalena L, Marcocci C, Bogazzi F, et al: Use of corticosteroids to prevent progression of Graves' ophthalmopathy after radioiodine therapy for hyperthyroidism. *N Engl J Med* 1989; 321:1349-1352..
[39] Weetman AP, Wiersinga WM: Current management of thyroid-associated ophthalmopathy in Europe: results of an international survey. *Clin Endocrinol (Oxf)* 1998; 49:21-28.

[40] Aniszewski JP, Valyasevi RW, Bahn RS: Relationship between disease duration and predominant orbital T cell subset in Graves' ophthalmopathy. *J Clin Endocrinol Metab* 2000; 85:776-780.
[41] Bartalena L, Pinchera A, Marcocci C: Management of Graves' ophthalmopathy: reality and perspectives. *Endocr Rev* 2000; 21:168-199.
[42] Bartalena L, Wiersinga WM, Pinchera A: Graves' ophthalmopathy: state of the art and perspectives. *J Endocrinol Invest* 2004; 27:295-301.
[43] Mariotti S, Caturegli P, Piccolo P, et al: Antithyroid peroxidase autoantibodies in thyroid diseases. *J Clin Endocrinol Metab* 1990; 71:661-669.
[44] McLachlan SM, Rapoport B: Thyroid peroxidase as an autoantigen. *Thyroid* 2007; 17:939-994.
[45] McLachlan SM, Rapoport B: Why measure thyroglobulin autoantibodies rather than thyroid peroxidase autoantibodies?. *Thyroid* 2004; 14:510-520.
[46] Mariotti S, Barbesino G, Caturegli P, et al: Assay of thyroglobulin in serum with thyroglobulin autoantibodies: an unobtainable goal?. *J Clin Endocrinol Metab* 1995; 80:468-472.
[47] Davis TF.Thyroid stimulating antibodies predict hyperthyroidism.J Clin Endocrinol Metab 1998;83:3777-3781.
[48] Hedley AJ, Young RE, Jones SJ, et al: Antithyroid drugs in the treatment of hyperthyroidism of Graves' disease: long-term follow-up of 434 patients. Scottish Automated Follow-Up Register Group. *Clin Endocrinol (Oxf)* 1989; 31:209-218.
[49] Schleusener H, Schwander J, Fischer C, et al: Prospective multicentre study on the prediction of relapse after antithyroid drug treatment in patients with Graves' disease [published erratum appears in Acta Endocrinol (Copenh) 1989 Aug;121(2):304]. *Acta Endocrinol (Copenh)* 1989; 120:689-701.
[50] Vitti P, Rago T, Chiovato L, et al: Clinical features of patients with Graves' disease undergoing remission after antithyroid drug treatment. *Thyroid* 1997; 7:369-375.
[51] Razvi S,Basu A,McIntyre EA,et al.Low failure rate of fixed administered activity of 400 MBq of I131 with pre-treatment with carbimazole for thyrotoxicosis:the Gateshead Protocol.Nucl Med Commun 2004;25:675-682.
[52] Franklyn JA, Daykin J, Drolc Z, et al: Long-term follow-up of treatment of thyrotoxicosis by three different methods. *Clin Endocrinol (Oxf)* 1991; 34:71-76.
[53] Dobyns BM, Sheline GE, Workman JB, et al: Malignant and benign neoplasms of the thyroid in patients treated for hyperthyroidism: a report of the Cooperative Thyrotoxicosis Therapy Follow-Up Study. *J Clin Endocrinol Metab* 1974; 38:976-998.
[54] Kahaly GJ, Pitz S, Hommel G, et al: Randomized, single blind trial of intravenous versus oral steroid monotherapy in Graves' orbitopathy. *J Clin Endocrinol Metab* 2005 Sep; 90(9):5234-5240.
[55] Prummel MF, Mourits MP, Berghout A, et al: Prednisone and cyclosporine in the treatment of severe Graves' ophthalmopathy. *N Engl J Med* 1989; 321:1353-1359.

Section 4

Thyroid Hormone Deficiency

Chapter 7

Mild Thyroid Deficiency in the Elderly

Giuseppe Pasqualetti, Angela Dardano, Sara Tognini,
Antonio Polini and Fabio Monzani

Additional information is available at the end of the chapter

1. Introduction

Subclinical hypothyroidism (sHT) is defined as serum thyrotropin-stimulating hormone (TSH) concentration above the statistically defined upper limit of the reference range in the face of serum free T_4 (FT_4) and free T_3 (FT_3) concentrations within the normal range (Ross, 2004). sHT is a frequent condition among the general population, especially middle-aged and elderly women (Canaris et al., 2000). Depending on the degree of TSH elevation, sHT has been associated with hyperlipidemia, intermediary metabolism alterations, arterial hypertension and cardiovascular disease (CVD) as well as neuropsychiatric features, including cognitive impairment (Ashizawa et al., 2010; Biondi & Cooper., 2008; Cappola et al., 2006; Ceresini et al., 2010; Mitrou et al., 2011; Monzani et al., 2006; Rodondi et al., 2010; Tan et al., 2008; Tappy, 1987). Interestingly, the analysis of variation in thyroid function tests in healthy volunteers has shown that the physiological individual reference ranges for test results are narrow compared with laboratory references (Andersen et al., 2002). This finding suggests that a test result within laboratory reference limits is not necessarily normal for an individual. Giving that serum TSH responds with logarithmically amplified degree to minor changes in serum T_4 and T_3, abnormal serum TSH may indicate that T_4 and T_3 are not normal for an individual although still within the laboratory references. These data point out that the distinction between subclinical and overt thyroid failure (elevated serum TSH and low T_4 and/or T_3) is somewhat arbitrary. Indeed, for the same degree of thyroid function abnormality, the diagnosis depends to a considerable extent on the position of the patient's normal set point for T_4 and T_3 within the laboratory reference range.

Because sHT is mainly detected as a biochemical TSH abnormality, the definition of the TSH reference range represents a critical point, especially in the elderly (Baloch et al., 2003; Olsen, 1978; Dayan et al., 2001). In the past, the upper normal limit of TSH was considered about 10 mIU/L with the first-generation TSH RIA assay while, the current normal reference range of serum TSH concentration is around 0.45 to 4.5 mIU/L (Biondi & Cooper, 2008; Surks et al.,

2004). Considering that serum TSH concentrations in a healthy population have a skewed distribution with a "tail" toward higher TSH values, the use of age specific reference limits for TSH has been suggested (Surks et al., 2004). This is especially proper in the elderly, in whom normal TSH is often shifted to a higher level (Mariotti, 1995) and the clinical presentation may differ from that in their younger counterparts (Mohandas, 2003). These considerations outline how making a correct diagnosis of sHT is challenging in the elderly but crucial to avoid significant misclassification of patients with abnormal TSH, who may or may not have thyroid dysfunction and may receive unnecessary or even harmful therapy (Laurberg, 2011). Indeed, the clinical significance of sHT in the elderly should be ascertained also in relation to the physiological changes of thyroid function with ageing (Biondi & Cooper, 2008; Carlè, 2007; Ceresini, 2010; Helfand, 2004; Surks et al., 2004). Therefore, the fundamental clinical question regarding these patients is on the clinical significance of sHT and the actual need of hormone replacement therapy (Villar, 2007).

2. Epidemiology

Several population-based studies have reported that sHT is common in the general population, with a prevalence that increases with increasing age (Gharib et al., 2005a,b; Hollowell et al., 2002; Samuels, 1998; Tunbridge et al., 1977). In interpreting epidemiologic data, it should be taken into account that the ability to identify people with sHT varies by TSH assay and cut-off value, which ranged from >3 to >7 mIU/L (Kanaya et al., 2002; Rivolta et al., 1999). In this setting, it is noteworthy that some investigators suggest that the upper limit of normal for serum TSH level should be 2.5 mIU/L (Spencer et al., 1993). In support of this position is a higher prevalence of anti-thyroid antibodies in subjects with serum TSH levels >2.5 mIU/L (Vanderpump et al., 1995). Reasoning about these considerations, it is not astonishing that the reported prevalence of sHT in the general population ranges widely from 1.3% to 21%, depending on age, gender, and iodine intake (Kanaya et al., 2002; Rivolta et al., 1999; Samuels, 1998; Sawin et al., 1985; Tunbridge et al., 1977; Wang et al., 1997).

In the Wickham survey, the prevalence of sHT (TSH > 6 mIU/L) was 7.5% in women and 2.8% in men (Wickham study). An age dependent increase in serum TSH concentrations was found only when women with high serum anti-thyroid antibody values were included in the analysis; with 17.4% prevalence of sHT in women older than 75 years (Wickham study). Accordingly, in a Dutch study the prevalence of sHT in a group of middle-aged women (mean age 55 years) was 4%, the rate rising to 7.3% 10 years later (Geul et al., 1993). The higher prevalence of sHT in older people was confirmed by data from the Framingham Study, which reported a prevalence of sHT of 8.2% in men and 16.9% in women, older than 60 years and, the Colorado study (16% in men and 21% in women older than 74 yrs) (Sawin et al., 1979, Canaris et al., 2000). Overall these findings demonstrate that ageing is associated with an increased prevalence of positive anti-thyroid antibody titers and mild hypothyroidism (Mariotti et al., 1995). The prevalence of sHT varies also according to iodine intake; being higher in areas with elevated intake with respect to areas with low-normal or deficient intake (Biondi & Cooper, 2012). In this setting, the occurrence of sHT among nursing home elderly residents was 4.2% in an iodine-deficient area (urinary iodine 72 micrograms/g creatinine), 10.4% in region of obligatory iodinated salt prophylaxis (urinary iodine 100 micrograms/g creatinine) and 23.9% in an abundant iodine intake area (urinary iodine 513 micrograms/g creatinine) (Szabolcs et al., 1997).

Overall, these data show that sHT is a very frequent condition and raise the question of the opportunity for general population screening programs, although a consensus is still lacking on this topic (Biondi & Cooper, 2012). The above notwithstanding, screening older people for thyroid disorders is still suggested by some authorities, aiming at the discovery of previously undiagnosed cases of overt hypothyroidism and the monitoring of cases with subclinical dysfunction (Ladenson et al., 2000; Surks et al., 2004).

3. Subclinical hypothyrodism: Clinical features and etiology

Hypothyroidism is a graded phenomenon that encompasses a wide variety of clinical conditions from full blown myxedema to sHT, which is characterized by elevated serum TSH concentrations in the face of normal free thyroid hormone levels (Cooper, 2001). Currently, the most widely accepted interpretation of these biochemical findings is that increased TSH is an indication of slightly reduced peripheral thyroid hormone effect, leading to mild hypothyroidism instead of a new steady state of euthyroidism (Karmisholt et al., 2011, Ross, 2004). In a consensus statement of the American Association of Clinical Endocrinologists, sHT was classified in two categories according to TSH level: mildly increased serum TSH levels (4.5–10 mIU/liter), and more severely increased serum TSH value (>10 mIU/liter) (Gharib et al., 2005a,b). However, this classification was not adopted in all clinical investigations, thus making the comparison of different trials quite difficult.

There is scientific consensus that sHT is caused by the same etiology of overt hypothyroidism (Biondi & Cooper, 2008), the most frequent one being Hashimoto's thyroiditis. This is an autoimmune, inflammatory disorder of the thyroid gland, whose prevalence increases with increasing age, being higher in women (Canaris et al., 2000; Surks et al., 1996). Other causes of primary hypothyroidism may result from therapies that destroy the thyroid tissue such as radioactive iodine treatment, external radiation therapy or partial thyroidectomy (Cooper, 2001). Chemotherapy also was associated to hypothyroidism in patients with cancer or lymphoma (Hancock et al., 2001; Kumar et al., 2004). Moreover, both subclinical and overt hypothyroidism could be induced by many drugs such as amiodarone, lithium carbonate, type I interferons, sulfonamides and several other toxic molecules (Basaria & Cooper, 2004; Caraccio et al., 2005).

Patients with sHT have a different rate of progression to clinically overt hypothyroidism in the presence or not of autoimmunity: 2.6% each year if thyroperoxidase (TPO) antibodies are absent and 4.3% if they are present (Vanderpump et al., 1995). However, a significant number of sHT subjects do not show progression and some experiences normalization. One of the most predictive markers of progression to overt hypothyroidism is serum TSH level higher than 10 mIU/L, by contrast a level less than 6 mIU/L depicts a lower likelihood of progression (Fatourechi, 2009). Accordingly, a clinical study, enrolling men and women older than 55 years with mean follow-up of 32 months, indicated that serum TSH levels normalized in 52% of those with serum TSH value less than 10 mIU/L (Díez & Iglesias, 2004).

The most common symptoms reported by sHT patients are the same although less evident than those observed in overt hypothyroidism: dry skin, poor memory, slow thinking, muscle weakness, fatigue, muscle cramp, cold intolerance, puffy eyes, constipation, and hoarseness (Canaris et al., 2000; Canaris et al., 1997). It is conceivable that clinical symptoms of hypothyroidism are related to the degree of thyroid failure, disease duration, and individual sensitivity to thyroid hormone deficiency (Biondi & Cooper, 2008). However, the presence of typical symptoms in patients with sHT remains controversial considering that many of them are non-specific and shared with many clinical conditions, especially in the elderly. Therefore, it is difficult to distinguish euthyroid subjects from sHT patients only by using clinical symptoms (Biondi & Cooper, 2008). Baseline data from a randomized clinical study confirmed a significant prevalence of hypothyroid symptoms among individuals with sHT (Cooper et al., 1984). Moreover, Canaris et al., (2000) reported fewer symptoms related to hypothyroidism in subclinical than in overt hypothyroid patients, but more frequently than in euthyroid controls. However, this study did not distinguish between treated or untreated subclinical and overt hypothyroid patients. By contrast, other cross-sectional and case-control studies did not confirm these observations, but they were conducted among selected or referred populations often involving old hospitalized patients (Bemben et al., 1994; Zulewski et al., 1997). Age represents a confounding factor that may hinder the identification of symptoms of mild hypothyroidism: the typical findings of hypothyroidism are less common in the elderly and, if present, often either resemble or are attributed to chronic illnesses, drugs, depression or ageing *per se* (Billewitc et al., 1969; Samuels, 1998). Therefore, clinical signs and symptoms are poor predictors of sHT especially in the elderly; this fact may explain why the diagnosis of sHT, and sometime overt disease yet, may be delayed in older people (Biondi & Cooper, 2008).

4. Thyroid function and ageing

The relationship between thyroid function and ageing has been hypothesized more than one decade ago (Mariotti et al., 1995). Human ageing is associated with an increased prevalence of serum anti-thyroid antibodies and overt or mild thyroid dysfunction (Hollowell et al., 2002; Gharib et al., 2005a,b; Samuels, 1998; Tunbridge et al., 1977). Several clinical studies confirmed an age-dependent decrease of thyroid function including iodine uptake and thyroid hormone production (Hollowell et al., 2002; Gharib et al., 2005a,b; Samuels, 1998; Sawin et al., 2009; Tunbridge et al., 1977). Although there is a consensus on the detrimental effects of overt hypothyroidism in older patients, the clinical relevance of mild to moderate thyroid failure remains an uncertain area (Surks et al., 2004) and, animal models indicated that low thyroid hormones are associated to increased life span (Ooka et al., 1983). The relative small number of epidemiological studies with inappropriate statistical power, and the lack of large prospective randomized trials directed to evaluate the therapeutic effect and impact on survival of hormonal therapy in mild thyroid impairment, does not allow to conclude whether mild thyroid impairment is a favorable phenotype or a negative clinical condition, especially in older people. An age-dependent thyroid dysfunction (particularly hypothyroidism) has been well documented in the elderly, including the oldest-old population (>85 yr) (Helfand et al., 2004; Mariotti et al., 1993). An interesting study focused on thyroid function during physiological ageing was carried out by Mariotti et al. (1993). In this study thyroid status was assessed in 41 healthy centenarians and 33 healthy elderly subjects as compared to two control groups: 98 healthy normal adult subjects and 52 patients with miscellaneous non-thyroidal illness. Healthy centenarians showed a lower prevalence of positive anti-thyroid autoantibody titer than elderly controls with a relatively low (7%) prevalence of sHT although the median serum FT_3 level was lower than in each other group. Interestingly, median serum TSH level of centenarians was lower than in healthy elderly subjects, in whom however, was significantly lower than in young controls (Mariotti et al., 1993). This study did not resolve the question whether the decreased FT_3 and TSH value observed in healthy centenarians, represents an adaptive mechanism to reduced metabolic homeostasis or a protective condition in ageing. At partial odds with these data, a population based survey and one large cross-sectional study (Atzmon et al., 2009; Surks et al., 2007) showed a progressive shift of the normal serum TSH range towards higher values from healthy young individuals up to centenarians. Overall these data seem to suggest that ageing is associated with a certain degree of down regulation of the hypothalamus-pituitary-thyroid-peripheral axis, although the clinical significance of such condition is far to be elucidated. To this regard, Rozing et al. (2010) reported that the offspring of nonagenarian siblings presented a lower thyroidal sensitivity to TSH and a paradoxical beneficial cardiometabolic profile as compared to their partners. The authors concluded that the favorable role of low thyroid hormone metabolism on health and longevity, already observed in animal models, might be applicable to humans as well. However, the study by Rozing et al. (2010) enrolled a specific population in order to identify familial determinants of healthy longevity in nonagenarian siblings. The results might, therefore, be affected by some bias and cannot be extended to the general population. On the other hand, a cross-sectional study by Corsonello et al. (2010) carried out in 604 home-dwelling subjects born in Calabria (southern Italy), with ancestry in the region ascertained up to the grandparents, confirms a declining of serum thyroid hormone levels with ageing. Moreover, lower levels of FT_3, FT_4 and TSH were found in centenarians' children and nieces/nephews with respect to age-matched controls. Indeed, the authors conclude that an age-related subtle decline of thyroid function (either due to a familial component or due to a reset of the thyroid function occurring between the sixth and the eighth decade of life) seems to be related to longevity. Two other studies support the hypothesis that mild hypothyroidism in elderly might be associated to a better survival and performance status. In the first, Gussekloo et al. (2006) found lower all-cause and cardiovascular mortality in hypothyroid subjects aged more than 85 years followed for 4 years, when compared with euthyroid individuals. In the second, van den Beld et al. (2005) showed that low-serum T_3 (with normal rT_3) concentrations were associated with a better survival and physical performance, while subjects with low-serum T_3 and high rT_3 concentrations ("low T_3 syndrome") did not show any survival advantage and had lower baseline physical activity. The authors suggested that higher serum rT_3 concentrations may result from a decreased peripheral metabolism of thyroid hormones due to the ageing process itself and/or disease and may reflect a catabolic state although, a certain degree of lower activity of the thyroid hormone axis might be beneficial during the aging process.

All together, these findings might support the idea that mild physiologically decline of thyroid activity at the tissue level might have favorable effects in the oldest-old subjects. However, the interpretation of the predictive value of thyroid failure in old subjects has to be considered with caution, carefully defining the context and the criteria of analyzed populations. In this setting, the comparison of observational trials is not so easy and the different population analyzed should be taken into account. Indeed, there is not a unique definition of TSH limits for patient classification in the clinical studies or statistical analysis, and the population of published trials is very heterogeneous differing for the age of enrolled patients, life styles, comorbidities, treatments, ethnics etc. Although in some selected elderly subjects (specific ethnic population or very old subjects) (subtle) thyroid failure might be a beneficial factor or a longevity associated character, one of the most debated issues regarding the health consequences of (subclinical) hypothyroidism in the elderly is represented by the potential increase of ischemic heart disease (IHD) or other CVDs as well as cognitive impairment (Mariotti et al., 2005).

5. Subclinical hypothyroidism and cardiovascular diseases

5.1. Pathophysiology

The most characteristic and common symptoms and signs, experienced by patients with thyroid disease, are those related to the cardiovascular (CV) system (Klein & Ojamaa, 2001). Both hyperthyroidism and hypothyroidism produce changes in cardiac contractility, myocardial oxygen consumption, cardiac output, blood pressure, and systemic vascular resistances (SVR) (Dillmann, 2002). Indeed, either hyper or hypothyroidism can produce heart arrhythmias, although it is less well recognized that hypothyroidism may predispose to specific dysrhythmias (Klein & Danzi., 2007). Cardiovascular signs and symptoms of hypothyroidism include bradycardia, mild (diastolic) hypertension, narrowed pulse pressure, cold intolerance, and fatigue (Klein & Ojamaa, 2001).

Subclinical hypothyroidism might be interpreted as an intermediate alteration between overt dysfunction and euthyroidism, consequently, the modifications of CV system observed in sHT qualitatively resemble those produced by overt hypothyroidism even if less evident. Accordingly, several evidences indicated that there is a direct association between serum TSH value and CV alterations as well as blood pressure, cholesterol level etc. (Biondi & Cooper, 2008; Asvold et al., 2007). There are many evidences that, in major part of the cases of thyroid patients, cardiovascular changes are reversible when the underlying thyroid disorder is recognized and treated (Kahaly et al., 2005). Moreover, there is substantial evidence that overt hypothyroidism and also sHT, although to a lesser extent, may alter several of the traditional risk factors for ischemic CVD.

The effects of thyroid hormone deficiency on the cardiovascular system have been evaluated from many points of view as heart diastolic and systolic dysfunction, endothelial dysfunction, hypertension, metabolic alterations and impaired exercise performance (Biondi & Cooper, 2008). To understand well the impact of sHT on CV system and the consequent increased risk of cardiovascular events, it is necessary to review the molecular effects of T_3 and T_4, and the modifications that they exert in myocytes, endothelium, vascular muscle cells, intermediate metabolism etc. The decrease of cardiac output associated with hypothyroidism results, in part, from changes in cardiac gene expression, specifically reduced expression of the sarcoplasmic reticulum Ca2-ATPase, and increased expression of its inhibitor, phospholamban (Belke et al., 2007). In addition, these molecular changes explain the prolonged isovolumic relaxation phase of the hypothyroid myocardium and early reversible diastolic impairment (Klein & Danzi, 2007). Interestingly, this mechanism functionally resembles the progressive age related myocardium modification, in which increased fibrosis, myocyte hypertrophy and myocyte loss result in increased myocardial stiffness leading to diastolic heart failure (Biondi & Cooper, 2008).

Triiodothyronine produces a decrease in systemic vascular resistance enhancing arteriole dilatation of the peripheral circulation (Klein & Ojamaa, 2001). The endothelium and smooth muscle cells are biological targets of action of T_3 with a vasodilatation effect, also in coronary arteries (Ojamaa et al., 1996). As stated by Klein & Ojamaa (2001), T_3 induces in vitro relaxation of smooth muscle cells with a non-genomic effect and independently of nitric oxide production (Klein & Ojamaa, 2001). Indeed, Ojamaa et al. (1996) found that the exposure of primary cultures vascular smooth muscle cells to T_3 resulted in cellular relaxation within 10 min while, the exposure of primary cultures of vascular endothelial cells to the same hormone did not induce nitric oxide production, suggesting a direct effect of T_3 on vascular smooth muscle cells. By contrast, Colantuoni et al. (2005) showed that *in vivo* thyroid hormone induced vasodilatation is delayed and mainly dependent to nitric oxide. The aim of their study was to assess the effects of topically applied T_3 and T_4 on the arterioles of hamster cheek pouch microcirculation *in vivo* by visualizing microvessels through a fluorescent microscopy technique. Topical application of both T_3 and T_4 consistently induced a dose-dependent dilation of arterioles within few minutes. However, T_3-induced dilation was countered by the inhibition of nitric oxide synthase with specific *i*Nos inhibitors. These discrepancies between *in vitro* and *in vivo* findings might be related to differences in experimental procedures and to the fact that *in vivo* conditions are more complex than *in vitro* insolated cell cultures (Galli et al., 2010). The vascular action of T_3 and T_4 has been also reported to be associated with the modulation of gene expression related to endothelial homeostasis like angiotensin receptors (Fukuyama et al., 2003), reinforcing the hypothesis that thyroid hormones mainly target the vasculature. Accordingly, a cross-sectional study on 30728 patients without previous known thyroid diseases revealed a linear positive association between TSH level and systolic and diastolic blood pressure (Asvold et al., 2007). In this setting, Fommei et al. (2002) reported the physiological relationships between blood pressure and neuro-humoral modifications induced by acute hypothyroidism [levothyroxine (LT_4) withdrawal] in normotensive subjects. During the hypothyroid state daytime arterial blood pressure (mainly diastolic) significantly increased along with noradrenaline and adrenaline levels. By contrast, plasma renin activity remained unchanged. These data, besides confirming the role of thyroid hormones in systemic arterial blood pressure homeostasis, suggest that sympathetic and adrenal reversible activation may contribute to the development of arterial hypertension in human hypothyroidism (Fommei et al., 2002).

Arterial hypertension related to thyroid hormone deficiency may result in aortic stiffness and early atherosclerosis. In this setting, aortic stiffness was studied in 30 patients who never received treatment for hypertension or hypothyroidism, 15 patients with normal blood pressure and hypothyroidism, and 15 patients with hypertension and normal thyroid function. Aortic diameter, evaluated by M-mode echocardiography and blood pressure measured by sphygmomanometer, were assessed to calculate the aortic stiffness index. Patients with hypertension and hypothyroidism have increased aortic stiffness, which was decreased in all patients by hormone replacement therapy, although hypertension resulted completely reversible in 50% of the patients (Dernellis et al., 2002). In addition, it has been hypothesized that thyroid hormone deficiency might be related to endothelial dysfunction. In this area, Lekakis et al. (1997) enrolled 35 subjects with various serum TSH levels to assess endothelial and smooth muscle responses of the brachial artery by high-resolution ultrasound imaging. Results of this study showed that flow-mediated, endothelium-dependent (FMD) vasodilatation progressively impaired with increasing serum TSH value; the phenomenon appearing still in patients with TSH value within the normal reference range (2.01-4.00 microIU/mL) (Lekakis et al., 1997). Furthermore, in order to assess vascular reactivity and NO availability in patients with sHT and its relation to the serum lipid profile, Taddei et al. (2003) evaluated, by strain-gauge plethysmography, the forearm blood flow response to intrabrachial acetylcoline, an endothelium-dependent vasodilator, at baseline and during infusion of the *e*NO synthase inhibitor Ng-monomethyl-L-arginine (L-NMMA). Results from sHT patients were compared with two groups of euthyroid control subjects, one with normal lipid profile and one with mildly elevated serum TC levels, comparable to those of sHT patients. They found that vasodilation in response to acetylcholine of patients affected by sHT was reduced as compared to that of both groups of euthyroid control subjects. Similarly, L-NMMA blunted the vasodilation in response to acetylcholine either in normolipemic or in mildly hypercholesterolemic controls, whereas it was ineffective in sHT patients, thus suggesting a reduced NO availability due to impaired NO synthase induced by sHT *per se*. Interestingly, six months of euthyroidism induced by LT_4 replacement increased acetylcholine vasodilation and restored L-NMMA inhibition. Subsequently, the same group (Taddei et al. 2006) demonstrated that endothelial dysfunction of a cohort of sHT patients with autoimmune thyroiditis was, at least partially, related to oxidative stress and low-grade systemic inflammation. Indeed, sHT patients had higher plasma C-reactive protein (CRP) levels as compared to euthyroid controls, and endothelium dysfunction was significantly improved after either local infusion of vitamin C or systemic administration of indomethacin, a non-selective cyclo-oxygenase (COX) inhibitor. Comparable results were obtained after administration of celecoxib, a selective COX-2 inhibitor, thus suggesting that an association between thyroid function and low-grade systemic inflammation could be postulated. Accordingly, several studies (Kvetny et al., 2004; Luboshitzky et al., 2004; Christ-crain et al., 2003; Lee et al., 2004) investigated the possible relationship between TH deficiency and serum CRP level, that was mostly found higher in hypothyroid patients, although unaffected by LT_4 therapy (Christ-crain, 2003).

Another concurring factor for developing early atherosclerosis in hypothyroidism is represented by the metabolic alterations induced by hormone deficiency. Hypothyroidism is characterized by hypercholesterolaemia with elevation of low-density lipoprotein cholesterol (LDLc) levels because of decreased fractional clearance of LDLc by a reduced number of the receptors in the liver (Duntas et al., 2002; Staub et al., 1992). Early studies in hypothyroid humans, using isotopically labeled LDLc, demonstrated a prolonged half-life of LDLc due to a decreased catabolism; this effect was reversible with LT_4 therapy (Walton et al., 1965). Accordingly, the addition of T_3 to human fibroblast cultures induced a higher LDLc degradation, through an increase in LDLc receptor number, without any receptor affinity change (Chait et al., 1979). Molecular mapping has revealed functional thyroid response elements in the promoter region of the LDLc receptor. Indeed, specific stimulation by T_3 of a chimeric gene resulting from the LDLc receptor promoter linked to a reporter gene, cotransfected with the isoform of the thyroid hormone receptor into a hepatic cell line, has been reported (Bakker et al., 2001). Moreover, the deletion of the upstream thyroid response elements in the LDLc receptor promoter inhibited T_3-mediated reporter gene activity (Cappola et al., 2003). Although the relationship between thyroid function and altered lipid profile is well documented in overt hypothyroidism it is still controversial in sHT (Biondi & Cooper, 2012). The conflicting results about lipid profile and sHT might reflect differences in study design as well as in age, gender, and ethnicity of the study cohorts (Palmieri et al., 2002).

Various changes in the coagulation-fibrinolytic system have been described in patients with thyroid dysfunction although, data regarding the association between thyroid failure and modifications of the coagulation-fibrinolytic system are still controversial (Chadarevian et al., 2001; Canturk et al., 2003; Muller et al., 2001). The influence of thyroid hormone on the coagulation fibrinolytic system is mainly mediated by the interaction between the hormone and its receptors (Shih et al., 2004). Various abnormalities have been described, ranging from subclinical laboratory abnormalities to major hemorrhages or fatal thromboembolic events (Squizzato et al. 2007). The relationship between thyroid hormones and the coagulation system is, however, often ignored. One of the reasons could be that, although several in vivo abnormalities have been reported in patients with hypothyroidism and hyperthyroidism, most published studies focus on laboratory measurements, and good studies on the relationship between thyroid dysfunction and clinically manifest bleeding or thrombosis are lacking. However, most studies confirm that both overt hyper- and hypothyroidism modify the coagulation-fibrinolytic balance. Thyroid hormone excess or deficit is the probable main pathophysiological mechanism and, patients with overt hypo- and hyperthyroidism appear to have an increased risk of bleeding and of thrombosis, respectively (Squizzato et al. 2007).

Overall, these findings support a biologically plausible role for hypothyroidism in increasing the risk of atherosclerotic CV disease, via the increase in circulating levels of LDLc, systemic (diastolic) hypertension, diastolic dysfunction and heart failure as well as an imbalance of the coagulation system and direct effects on vascular smooth muscle (Cappola et al., 2003). However, the actual relationship between sHT and increased cardiovascular risk is still unresolved and represents one of the most common topics in endocrinology, leading to several controversies concerning the clinical management of sHT patients (Turemen et al., 2011).

5.2. Clinical evidences

As above described, thyroid hormone deficiency is associated to several cardiovascular and metabolic abnormalities (Biondi & Cooper, 2008; Caraccio et al., 2003; Dardano & Monzani, 2008). Indeed, thyroid failure may favour the onset of several CV risks like diastolic hypertension, hyperlipidemia, vascular stiffness, heart failure etc. However, although the relationship between overt hypothyroidism and coronary heart disease (CHD) as well as increased CHD mortality is widely recognized (Klein, 2004), the clinical significance of sHT is still controversial and conflicting opinions remain on the association between sHT and CVD or mortality, especially in older people (Biondi & Cooper, 2008; Monzani et al., 2006). Indeed, data regarding the association between sHT and CHD or total mortality are contradictory among various population based, observational studies (Aho et al., 1984; Cappola et al., 2004; Hak et al., 2000; Walsh et al., 2005).

One of the first large study (Whickham Survey) that evaluated vascular events over 20 years in community-dwelling subjects stratified by thyroid function and thyroid autoantibody status did not show any association between CHD and sHT (Vanderpump et al., 1995). This result appeared at odds with the findings of other subsequent cohort studies (Hak et al., 2000; Imaizumi et al., 2004; Walsh et al., 2005). However, while reanalyzing incident CHD events and mortality in Whickham participants including LT_4 replacement during follow-up as covariate, a significant increment of incident CHD events and mortality was found in individuals with baseline sHT (Razvi et al., 2010). Based on the results of this analysis, it would appear that treatment of sHT might be associated with reduced mortality as well as CHD events. However, besides the small total number of events in each group of sHT participants, there is a potential for bias in this retrospective observational analysis (i.e. sHT patients who were treated may have been more health conscious leading to a healthy user bias). Therefore, these results need to be interpreted with caution until a large prospective, randomized controlled trial will be available. The inconsistency in results among several studies (Aho et al., 1984; Hak et al., 2000; Cappola et al., 2004; Razvi et al., 2010; Walsh et al., 2005) may be due to differences in the enrolled populations as well as the duration either of tissues exposure to sHT or of follow-up of the various studies. Nonetheless, meta-analyses of CHD events and sHT have shown that such an association probably exists (Razvi et al., 2008; Rodondi et al., 2006), especially in younger cohorts. In this regard, to assess the risks of CHD and total mortality for adults with sHT, Rodondi et al. (2010) carried out a large meta-analysis on 11 prospective cohorts, enrolling a total of 55,287 participants. The risk of CHD events was examined in 25,977 participants from 7 cohorts with available data. Among 55,287 adults, 3450 had sHT (6.2%) and 51,837 were euthyroid. The Authors found that the risk of CHD events and mortality increased with higher TSH concentrations. Results were similar after adjustment for traditional cardiovascular risk factors. Moreover, this pooled analysis showed a higher rate of CHD events in sHT patients with higher TSH levels (>10 mIU/L). These data are consistent with most previous meta-analysis and several naturalistic studies, showing an increased risk of CHD events associated with sHT (Hak et al., 2000; Singh et al., 2007; Walsh et al., 2005).

These studies, however, did not accurately explore potential differences related to participant characteristics like age, even if older people represented large a share of the population. In this setting, the pooled analysis of large cohort of patients may be affected by hypothetical bias and may not investigate specific classes of patients like very old people versus moderate elderly patients or other specific conditions affecting the clinical outcome. Ochs et al. (2008) analysed in a meta-analysis the effect of ageing on sHT associated CV events and total mortality. Similar to previous meta-analysis, they found a pattern of modestly increased risk for CHD and mortality associated with sHT. A weak evidence for statistical heterogeneity among individual study findings was found, and age explained part of the heterogeneity for the association between sHT and CHD, with an increased risk for CHD only in cohorts with a younger mean age. Accordingly, Cappola et al. (2006), in a large population-based, longitudinal study of coronary heart disease and stroke in adults aged 65 years and older, concluded that the results did not support the hypothesis of an association between unrecognized sHT and increased CV events or mortality. On the other hand, one cross-sectional study with subgroup analyses by age found that increased risk for CHD was present in younger sHT participants only (<50 years old) (Kvetny et al. 2004). In this regard, a prospective, observational, population-based follow-up study carried out on 599 participants followed up from age 85 years through age 89 years showed no association between serum TSH and FT_4 levels and disability in daily life, depressive symptoms, and cognitive impairment at baseline or during follow-up. Moreover, increasing serum TSH levels were associated with a lower mortality rate that remained after adjustments for baseline disability and health status (Gusseklo et al. 2004). Overall, these data support the hypothesis that in the oldest old population, individuals with abnormally high levels of TSH do not experience adverse effects and may have a prolonged life span. The study focused on a specific class of patients (very older people), for this reason, the results should be rigorously interpreted, also considering the weakness of observational studies. However, these data together with the results obtained by Rozing et al., (2010) that demonstrated a possible genetic predisposition of nonagenarians to a decrease function of hypothalamus-pituitary-thyroid axis, suggest that the oldest old may represent a different population respect to moderate old people or young adults. Potential explanations for these age differences might be competing mortality among older adults (for example, due to cancer) or more competing risk factors for CHD among older adults (for example, age or sex). However, the above reported substantial age differences should be interpreted with caution, given the possibility of ecological fallacy without individual patient data and, should be confirmed by stratified analyses in future prospective cohort studies with a wide age range (Egger et al., 2001).

There are few clinical studies evaluating the effects of hormone replacement in sHT subjects and none aimed to determine the impact of therapy on total mortality especially in older people. Previous research in this area has shown contradictory results, with some randomized, controlled trials (number of patients ranging from 45 to 63) showing an improvement in the atherogenic lipid profile as well as surrogate endpoints of atherosclerosis (Meier et al., 2001; Caraccio et al., 2002; Monzani et al., 2004) but others (number of patients ranging from 17 to 35) showing no difference (Cooper et al., 1984; Jaeschke et al., 1996; Kong et al., 2002; Nystrom et al., 1988). Recently, Razvi et al. (2007)

conducted a randomized, double-blind, crossover study to determine the short-term (12 weeks) effect of LT_4 replacement therapy in 100 sHT patients (age range 18-80 yrs, mean 53.8) with serum TSH level>4.0 mIU/L. Primary end points included: serum cholesterol level variations along with improvement in flow-mediated dilation (FMD) as a marker of vascular endothelial function. LT_4 treatment significantly reduced either TC or LDLc concentrations, and improved FMD, as compared to placebo group. Moreover, multivariate analysis showed that increased serum FT_4 level was the most significant variable predicting reduction in TC or FMD improvement. The Authors hypothesized that if the reduction of LDLc level would be long term sustained, this would result in a relative reduction in 10-yr CV mortality of about 10%, thus supporting the use of LT_4 replacement therapy also in patients with slightly elevated TSH value. Long-term studies are nonetheless required to confirm whether these apparent short-term benefits will translate into reduction in CV mortality and morbidity. Moreover, notwithstanding the wide age range of the studied patients, these results cannot directly transfer to the elderly, especially the oldest old population.

In summary, conflicting results among large prospective cohort studies regarding the relationship between sHT and cardiovascular disease might reflect differences in participants such as age, gender, TSH value, or pre-existing cardiovascular disease. However, as demonstrated by some meta-analyses, the negative effect of sHT on cardiovascular risk is well established in younger people while in moderately old population (>65 and <85 years) it appears no longer evident. Moreover, in the oldest old people (>85 years) one study suggested that high levels of TSH not only do not exert adverse effects but also may favor a prolonged life span (Fig. 1). In this regard, elderly population can be interpreted as a heterogeneous group, nonagenarians representing a genetically selected cluster. Indeed, these subjects may have a genetic background that protects from CVD and/or thyroid hormone deficiency, thus suggesting an intriguing link between gene, thyroid status and longevity.

6. Thyroid function and cognitive impairment

Thyroid hormones are crucial for brain development and function: thyroid failure at any age causes cognition to deteriorate because thyroid hormones are essential for adequately sustaining the energy (glucose)-consuming processes needed for neurotransmission, memory, and other higher brain functions (Herholz, 2010; Patel et al., 2011). Low brain uptake of glucose is commonly associated with deteriorating cognition and Alzheimer's disease and can be present decades before clinical evidence of Alzheimer's disease occurs (Herholz, 2010). Brain hypometabolism therefore appears to be a precursor lesion increasing the risk of at least some forms of cognitive decline. Elevated TSH levels in the range found in patients with overt hypothyroidism have been described to be associated with impaired function in many cognitive domains, but the association between sHT and cognition is less clear (Graham et al., 1997; Gardner, 2004; Chavanne et al., 2011). On the other hand, several cross-sectional studies have observed that high or low TSH levels, still within the normal range (clinically euthyroid), are each related to poor cognitive performance, although some other investigations failed to demonstrate these findings (Prinz et al., 1999; Volpato et al.,

2002). It should be underlined, however, that different cognitive deficits possibly related to thyroid failure do not necessarily follow a consistent pattern, and LT_4 treatment may not always completely restore normal functioning in patients with hypothyroidism. Giving these premises, we summarize here the growing, conflicting literature on the relationship between cognitive performance and thyroid function from an ageing perspective.

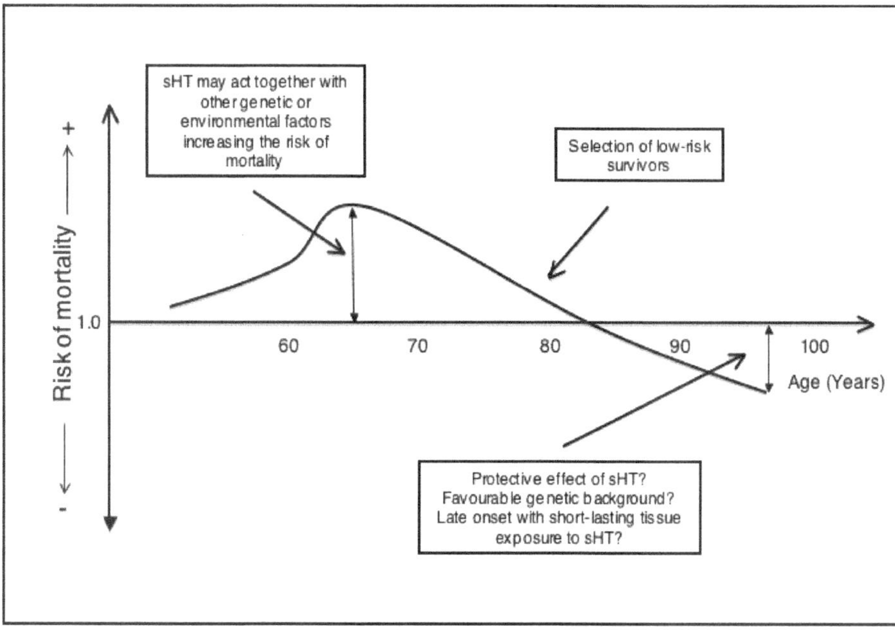

Figure 1. Hypothetical relationship between risk of total mortality and age in patients with subclinical hypothyroidism (sHT) (Modified from Mariotti, 2005).

Subclinical hypothyroidism and cognitive function have been investigated in several preclinical experiments and clinical trials. To date, the actual relationship between mild thyroid hormone deficiency and cognitive impairment in the elderly is not well understood. In fact, there are several contrasting data resulting from cross-sectional and clinical experiments (Gussekloo et al., 2004; Roberts et al., 2006; Tan et al., 2008; Ceresini et al., 2009). Moreover, the available published data, in many cases, are not easily comparable considering the differences in inclusion criteria of each clinical study. Several small observational and interventional studies have reported an association,, although not homogeneously, between cognitive impairment and sHT and, in some cases, it was described a cognitive performance improvement after LT_4 replacement (Etgen et al., 2011; Monzani et al., 1993; Osterweil et al., 1992; St. John et al., 2009; Volpato et al., 2002). Moreover, Hogervost et al. (2008) studied the association between TSH and FT_4 levels and cognition at baseline and after 2 years of follow-up in 1047 participants over 64 years of age, without physical frailty or severe cognitive impairment. The study showed that elevated TSH levels were associated with lower MMSE performance at baseline, independently of

FT_4 value, age, sex, education and mood. Interestingly, epidemiological surveys using the revised Wechsler Adult Intelligence Scale (WAIS-R) and the Mini-Mental State Examination (MMSE) showed a relationship between plasma thyroid hormone levels and cognitive status in subjects with thyroid function still within the upper limit of the normal range (Prinz et al., 1999; Volpato et al., 2002). Accordingly, altered plasma thyroid hormone concentrations have been recognized as a risk factor for cognitive impairment or dementia (Bulens, 1981; Kalmijn et al., 2000; Tan et al., 2008). More specifically, with the increasing sensitivity of neuropsychological tools, it has become evident that thyroid hormone deficiency might produce measurable deficits in very specific neuropsychological functions (Zoeller & Rovet 2004). In this regard, in a recent prospective, open-labeled interventional study, cognitive impairment associated with (mild) thyroid failure appeared predominantly mnemonic in nature, suggesting that the etiology is not indicative of general cognitive slowing (Correia et al., 2009).

Conflicting data were obtained by large, population-based studies, leading to uncertain conclusions regarding the association between (mild) thyroid failure and cognition (Gussekloo et al., 2004; Roberts et al., 2006; Tan et al., 2008; Ceresini et al., 2009). In this setting, one critical point that could affect the results of these studies is the diverse age groups of the enrolled patients (moderate or very old) as well as the presence of comorbidity. Cognitive impairment observed in older sHT individuals might be also an epiphenomenon of the increased risk for atherosclerosis or the effect of thyroid hormone on vasculature. Indeed, arterial stiffness is a potential mechanism of advancing cognitive decline in sHT (Yamamoto et al., 2012) and elevated TSH values might negatively affect vascular function through systemic low-grade inflammation (Taddei et al., 2006). Moreover, whereas in moderate older people sHT might produce a detrimental effect on cognitive performance, in very old individuals (mild) thyroid failure might be not associated to a negative outcome (Gussekloo et al., 2004; Tan et al., 2008). To determine whether subclinical thyroid dysfunction should be treated in old age and the long-term impact of thyroid dysfunction on performance and survival in the elderly, a prospective, observational, population-based survey was carried out within the Leiden 85-Plus Study. A total of 599 participants were followed up from age 85 years through age 89 years. Plasma levels of TSH and FT_4 were not associated with disability in daily life, depressive symptoms, and cognitive impairment at baseline or during follow-up. Conversely, increasing levels of TSH were associated with a lower mortality rate that remained after adjustments were made for baseline disability and health status (Gussekloo et al., 2004). It is noteworthy, however, that similarly to CHD risk, these results should be confirmed by stratified analyses in future prospective large cohort studies with a wide age range.

Another important aspect is the possible relationship between sHT and the risk to develop Alzheimer disease (AD). On this basis, many studies investigated a possible association between AD and thyroid dysfunction. Increasing evidence supports an extensive interrelationship between thyroid hormones and the cholinergic system, which is selectively and early affected in AD. Thyroid hormones negatively regulate expression of the amyloid-beta protein precursor, which plays a key role in the development of AD (Belakavadi et al.,

2011). In a study aimed to examine the feasibility of using thyroid hormone as a therapeutic agent for AD, mice were injected intra-hippocampally with aggregated amyloid beta-peptide (Abeta) to produce AD animal model. Intraperitoneal administration of LT_4 into Abeta-induced AD model mice prevented their cognitive impairment and improved their memory function. The authors suggested that the mechanisms of LT_4 treating AD might be associated with regulating cholinergic function, protecting the brains of AD model mice against damage and rescuing hippocampal neurons from apoptosis. The results of this study seem indicate that the use of thyroid hormone may have some therapeutic potential in AD (Fu et al., 2010). Accordingly, in a post mortem study it was evaluated the brain thyroid hormone levels in AD measured with radioimmunoassay (RIA) samples of prefrontal cortex of patients with pathologically confirmed AD and controls without any primary neurological disease. Thyroxine levels did not differ between groups while T_3 levels were significantly lower in Alzheimer's brains respect to controls. These results suggest that the conversion of T_4 to T_3 may be altered in advanced AD, perhaps due to modifications in deiodinase activity, and the reduced hormone conversion might be associated with both AD pathology and the clinical presentation of dementia (Davis et al., 2008). Moreover, Tan et al. (2008) related serum TSH concentrations to the risk of Alzheimer disease in 1864 cognitively intact, euthyroid participants of the Framingham original cohort (mean age 71 years). During a mean follow-up of 12.7 years, 209 participants (142 women) developed AD. Women in the lowest (<1.0 mIU/L) and highest (>2.1 mIU/L) tertiles of serum TSH concentration were at increased risk for AD compared with those in the middle tertile while, TSH levels were not related to AD risk in men. On the other hand, at odds with these findings, the InChianti study showed an association between subclinical hyperthyroidism and cognitive impairment without any correlation with mild thyroid failure in a large cohort of older people (Ceresini et al., 2009).

In conclusion, a certain degree of cognitive (mnemonic) impairment is generally recognized in case of overt hypothyroidism while, the relationship between cognition and sHT is still a disputed field, and it remains unclear whether to treat or not this kind of patients. In particular, there is little or no consensus in the literature whether thyroid failure is associated with impaired cognitive performance in the elderly, especially in the oldest old population. While interpreting the above reported conflicting results it should be outlined, however, that thyroid hormone concentrations change with age and cognitive decline is often concomitant with ageing; therefore, a reciprocal relationship could exist between changes of thyroid function and cognitive decline during normal ageing.

7. Conclusions

Levothyroxine replacement therapy for reducing sHT associated CV risk factors is still controversial, especially in the elderly. The lack of specific randomized trials, enrolling either old or very old subjects, aimed to evaluate the efficacy of hormonal replacement on overall survival and cardiovascular risk reduction as well as the possible negative effects of LT_4 supplementation, makes the decision to treat elderly people very difficult. Generally,

LT_4 replacement therapy should be considered for three main reasons: i) to prevent progression of sHT to overt hypothyroidism which, however, is much more important in young patients; ii) to reduce the symptoms associated with mild thyroid failure, which are especially scarce in the elderly; iii) to improve the lipid profile and other risk factors that may contribute to atherosclerosis progression and CV events.

Subclinical thyroid failure causes changes in cardiac function similar to, but less marked than, those occurring in patients with overt hypothyroidism. Diastolic dysfunction both at rest and upon effort is the most consistent cardiac abnormality in patients with sHT, even in those with slightly elevated TSH levels (>6 mIU/L) (Arem et al., 1996; Biondi & Cooper, 2012;). Mild thyroid failure may also increase diastolic blood pressure as a result of increased systemic vascular resistances (Faber et al., 2002; Kahaly, 2000; Luboshitzky et al., 2002). Interestingly, restoration of euthyroidism by LT_4 replacement is able to reduce systemic hypertension as well as improve left ventricular myocardial function (Brenta et al., 2003). Moreover, sHT has been claimed to be a risk factor for atherosclerosis and ischemic CVD, therefore, it is appropriate to consider whether treatment confers some protection from such a risk. Although a consensus is still lacking, the strongest evidence for a beneficial effect of levothyroxine replacement therapy is the substantial demonstration that restoration of euthyroidism can lower TC and LDLc levels in most patients with sHT. Besides hypercholesterolemia several emerging risk factors for CHD have been claimed to be associated with sHT. Among them, altered coagulation parameters, endothelial dysfunction, and elevated CRP levels are consistently regarded to combine with the raised LDLc levels of untreated patients with sHT to enhance the cardiovascular risk.

As a whole, these findings suggest that the decision to treat patients with sHT should depend on the presence of risk factors, rather than on a TSH threshold. International organizations and guidelines suggest starting replacement therapy in patients who have TSH concentrations greater than 10 mIU/liter and in those with evidence of autoimmunity, and in symptomatic patients with TSH levels between 4.5 and 10 mIU/L (Gharib et al., 2005a,b; Surks et al., 2004). However, the treatment of sHT patients, especially the elderly, must be individualized once any underlying coexisting morbidity or pharmacologic interference has been excluded. Generally LT_4 replacement results effective and safe in young patients, providing that excessive dosing is avoided by monitoring serum TSH level. Indeed, LT_4 replacement therapy can always be discontinued if there is no apparent benefit. It is noteworthy that, once a stable, elevated TSH value is detected, the costs of annual follow-up with clinical assessment and laboratory testing are relatively similar whether or not a patient is treated with LT_4 (Cooper et al., 2001). On the other hand, the possibility that restoring euthyroidism may be harmful in the older population has been raised, and should be taken into account in making the decision of treating such patients, especially those older than 85 years. In this setting, hormonal replacement might be considered in old patients on the base of a specific evaluation of the possible thyroid dysfunction causes, pre-existent cardiovascular risk including cholesterol level, hearth failure as well as the presence of comorbidities or frailty and the level of TSH. However, until adequate data are accumulated, clinicians should consider each patient a unique situation, and best clinical practice continues to be a combination of clinical judgment and the patient's preference.

Author details

Giuseppe Pasqualetti, Angela Dardano, Sara Tognini, Antonio Polini and Fabio Monzani
Geriatrics Unit, Department of Internal Medicine, University of Pisa, Italy

8. References

Aho, K., Gordin, A., Palosuo, T., Punsar, S., Valkeila, E., Karvonen, M., Inkovaara, J., Pasternack, A. (1984). Thyroid autoimmunity and cardiovascular diseases. Eur Heart J, Vol. 5, No. 1 (Jan 1984), pp. 43-46, issn 0195-668X (Print) 0195-668X (Linking).

Andersen, S., Pedersen, K.M., Bruun, N.H., Laurberg, P. (2002). Narrow individual variations in serum T(4) and T(3) in normal subjects: a clue to the understanding of subclinical thyroid disease. J Clin Endocrinol Metab, Vol. 87, No. 3 (Mar 2002), pp. 1068-1072, issn 0021-972X (Print) 0021-972X (Linking).

Arem, R., Rokey, R., Kiefe, C., Escalante, D.A., Rodriguez, A. (1996). Cardiac systolic and diastolic function at rest and exercise in subclinical hypothyroidism: effect of thyroid hormone therapy. Thyroid, Vol. 6, No. 5 (Oct 1996), pp. 397-402, issn 1050-7256 (Print) 1050-7256 (Linking).

Ashizawa, K., Imaizumi, M., Usa, T., Tominaga, T., Sera, N., Hida, A., Ejima, E., Neriishi, K., Soda, M., Ichimaru, S., Nakashima, E., Fujiwara, S., Maeda, R., Nagataki, S., Eguchi, K., Akahoshi, M. (2010). Metabolic cardiovascular disease risk factors and their clustering in subclinical hypothyroidism. Clin Endocrinol (Oxf), Vol. 72, No. 5 (May 2010), pp. 689-695, issn 1365-2265 (Electronic) 0300-0664 (Linking).

Asvold, B.O., Bjoro, T., Nilsen, T.I., Vatten, L.J. (2007). Association between blood pressure and serum thyroid-stimulating hormone concentration within the reference range: a population-based study. J Clin Endocrinol Metab, Vol. 92, No. 3 (Mar 2007), pp. 841-845, issn 0021-972X (Print) 0021-972X (Linking).

Atzmon, G., Barzilai, N., Hollowell, J.G., Surks, M.I., Gabriely, I. (2009). Extreme longevity is associated with increased serum thyrotropin. J Clin Endocrinol Metab, Vol. 94, No. 4 (Apr 2009), pp. 1251-1254, issn 1945-7197 (Electronic) 0021-972X (Linking).

Bakker, S.J., ter Maaten, J.C., Popp-Snijders, C., Slaets, J.P., Heine, R.J., Gans, R.O. (2001). The relationship between thyrotropin and low density lipoprotein cholesterol is modified by insulin sensitivity in healthy euthyroid subjects. J Clin Endocrinol Metab, Vol. 86, No. 3 (Mar 2001), pp. 1206-1211, issn 0021-972X (Print) 0021-972X (Linking).

Baloch, Z., Carayon, P., Conte-Devolx, B., Demers, L.M., Feldt-Rasmussen, U., Henry, J.F., LiVosli, V.A., Niccoli-Sire, P., John, R., Ruf, J., Smyth, P.P., Spencer, C.A., Stockigt, J.R. (2003). Laboratory medicine practice guidelines. Laboratory support for the diagnosis and monitoring of thyroid disease. Thyroid, Vol. 13, No. 1 (Jan 2003), pp. 3-126, issn 1050-7256 (Print) 1050-7256 (Linking).

Basaria, S., Cooper, D.S. (2005). Amiodarone and the thyroid. Am J Med, Vol. 118, No. 7 (Jul 2005), pp. 706-714, issn 0002-9343 (Print) 0002-9343 (Linking).

Belakavadi, M., Dell, J., Grover, G.J., Fondell, J.D. (2011). Thyroid hormone suppression of beta-amyloid precursor protein gene expression in the brain involves multiple epigenetic regulatory events. Mol Cell Endocrinol, Vol. 339, No. 1-2 (Jun 6 2011), pp. 72-80, issn 1872-8057 (Electronic) 0303-7207 (Linking).

Belke, D.D., Gloss, B., Swanson, E.A., Dillmann, W.H. (2007). Adeno-associated virus-mediated expression of thyroid hormone receptor isoforms-alpha1 and -beta1 improves contractile function in pressure overload-induced cardiac hypertrophy. Endocrinology, Vol. 148, No. 6 (Jun 2007), pp. 2870-2877, issn 0013-7227 (Print) 0013-7227 (Linking).

Bemben, D.A., Winn, P., Hamm, R.M., Morgan, L., Davis, A., Barton, E. (1994). Thyroid disease in the elderly. Part 1. Prevalence of undiagnosed hypothyroidism. J Fam Pract, Vol. 38, No. 6 (Jun 1994), pp. 577-582, issn 0094-3509 (Print) 0094-3509 (Linking).

Billewicz, W.Z., Chapman, R.S., Crooks, J., Day, M.E., Gossage, J., Wayne, E., Young, J.A. (1969). Statistical methods applied to the diagnosis of hypothyroidism. Q J Med, Vol. 38, No. 150 (Apr 1969), pp. 255-266, issn 0033-5622 (Print) 0033-5622 (Linking).

Biondi, B., Cooper, D.S. (2008). The clinical significance of subclinical thyroid dysfunction. Endocr Rev, Vol. 29, No. 1 (Feb 2008), pp. 76-131, issn 0163-769X (Print) 0163-769X (Linking).

Biondi B., Cooper, D.S. (2012). Subclinical thyroid disease. Lancet, (Jan 20 2012). [Epub ahead of print] PubMed PMID: 22273398. 0140-6736 (Linking)

Brenta, G., Mutti, L.A., Schnitman, M., Fretes, O., Perrone, A., Matute, M.L. (2003). Assessment of left ventricular diastolic function by radionuclide ventriculography at rest and exercise in subclinical hypothyroidism, and its response to L-thyroxine therapy. Am J Cardiol, Vol. 91, No. 11 (Jun 1 2003), pp. 1327-1330, issn 0002-9149 (Print) 0002-9149 (Linking).

Bulens, C. (1981). Neurologic complications of hyperthyroidism: remission of spastic paraplegia, dementia, and optic neuropathy. Arch Neurol, Vol. 38, No. 10 (Oct 1981), pp. 669-670, issn 0003-9942 (Print) 0003-9942 (Linking).

Canaris, G.J., Manowitz, N.R., Mayor, G., Ridgway, E.C. (2000). The Colorado thyroid disease prevalence study. Arch Intern Med, Vol. 160, No. 4 (Feb 28 2000), pp. 526-534, issn 0003-9926 (Print) 0003-9926 (Linking).

Canaris, G.J., Steiner, J.F., Ridgway, E.C. (1997). Do traditional symptoms of hypothyroidism correlate with biochemical disease? J Gen Intern Med, Vol. 12, No. 9 (Sep 1997), pp. 544-550, issn 0884-8734 (Print) 0884-8734 (Linking).

Canturk, Z., Cetinarslan, B., Tarkun, I., Canturk, N.Z., Ozden, M. (2003). Lipid profile and lipoprotein (a) as a risk factor for cardiovascular disease in women with subclinical hypothyroidism. Endocr Res, Vol. 29, No. 3 (Aug 2003), pp. 307-316, issn 0743-5800 (Print) 0743-5800 (Linking).

Cappola, A.R., Fried, L.P., Arnold, A.M., Danese, M.D., Kuller, L.H., Burke, G.L., Tracy, R.P., Ladenson, P.W. (2006). Thyroid status, cardiovascular risk, and mortality in older adults. JAMA, Vol. 295, No. 9 (Mar 1 2006), pp. 1033-1041, issn 1538-3598 (Electronic) 0098-7484 (Linking).

Cappola, A.R., Ladenson, P.W. (2003). Hypothyroidism and atherosclerosis. J Clin Endocrinol Metab, Vol. 88, No. 6 (Jun 2003), pp. 2438-2444, issn 0021-972X (Print) 0021-972X (Linking).

Caraccio, N., Dardano, A., Manfredonia, F., Manca, L., Pasquali, L., Iudice, A., Murri, L., Ferrannini, E., Monzani, F. (2005). Long-term follow-up of 106 multiple sclerosis patients undergoing interferon-beta 1a or 1b therapy: predictive factors of thyroid disease development and duration. J Clin Endocrinol Metab, Vol. 90, No. 7 (Jul 2005), pp. 4133-4137, issn 0021-972X (Print) 0021-972X (Linking).

Caraccio, N., Ferrannini, E., Monzani, F. (2002). Lipoprotein profile in subclinical hypothyroidism: response to levothyroxine replacement, a randomized placebo-controlled study. J Clin Endocrinol Metab, Vol. 87, No. 4 (Apr 2002), pp. 1533-1538, issn 0021-972X (Print) 0021-972X (Linking).

Carle, A., Laurberg, P., Pedersen, I.B., Perrild, H., Ovesen, L., Rasmussen, L.B., Jorgensen, T., Knudsen, N. (2007). Age modifies the pituitary TSH response to thyroid failure. Thyroid, Vol. 17, No. 2 (Feb 2007), pp. 139-144, issn 1050-7256 (Print) 1050-7256 (Linking).

Ceresini, G., Lauretani, F., Maggio, M., Ceda, G.P., Morganti, S., Usberti, E., Chezzi, C., Valcavi, R., Bandinelli, S., Guralnik, J.M., Cappola, A.R., Valenti, G., Ferrucci, L. (2009). Thyroid function abnormalities and cognitive impairment in elderly people: results of the Invecchiare in Chianti study. J Am Geriatr Soc, Vol. 57, No. 1 (Jan 2009), pp. 89-93, issn 1532-5415 (Electronic) 0002-8614 (Linking).

Ceresini, G., Morganti, S., Maggio, M., Usberti, E., Fiorino, I., Artoni, A., Teresi, G., Belli, S., Ridolfi, V., Valenti, G., Ceda, G.P. (2010). Subclinical thyroid disease in elderly subjects. Acta Biomed, Vol. 81 Suppl 1, No. 2010), pp. 31-36, issn 0392-4203 (Print) 0392-4203 (Linking).

Chadarevian, R., Bruckert, E., Leenhardt, L., Giral, P., Ankri, A., Turpin, G. (2001). Components of the fibrinolytic system are differently altered in moderate and severe hypothyroidism. J Clin Endocrinol Metab, Vol. 86, No. 2 (Feb 2001), pp. 732-737, issn 0021-972X (Print) 0021-972X (Linking).

Chait, A., Bierman, E.L., Albers, J.J. (1979). Regulatory role of triiodothyronine in the degradation of low density lipoprotein by cultured human skin fibroblasts. J Clin Endocrinol Metab, Vol. 48, No. 5 (May 1979), pp. 887-889, issn 0021-972X (Print) 0021-972X (Linking).

Chavanne, D., Constans, T., Petit, A., Mondon, K., Hommet, C. (2011). Hypothyroidism and cognition in the elderly. Geriatr Psychol Neuropsychiatr Vieil, Vol. 9, No. 4 (Dec 1 2011), pp. 477-489, issn 2115-8789 (Print) 2115-7863 (Linking).

Christ-Crain, M., Meier, C., Guglielmetti, M., Huber, P.R., Riesen, W., Staub, J.J., Muller, B. (2003). Elevated C-reactive protein and homocysteine values: cardiovascular risk factors in hypothyroidism? A cross-sectional and a double-blind, placebo-controlled trial. Atherosclerosis, Vol. 166, No. 2 (Feb 2003), pp. 379-386, issn 0021-9150 (Print) 0021-9150 (Linking).

Colantuoni, A., Marchiafava, P.L., Lapi, D., Forini, F.S., Iervasi, G. (2005). Effects of tetraiodothyronine and triiodothyronine on hamster cheek pouch microcirculation. Am J Physiol Heart Circ Physiol, Vol. 288, No. 4 (Apr 2005), pp. H1931-1936, issn 0363-6135 (Print) 0363-6135 (Linking).

Cooper, D.S. (2001). Clinical practice. Subclinical hypothyroidism. N Engl J Med, Vol. 345, No. 4 (Jul 26 2001), pp. 260-265, issn 0028-4793 (Print) 0028-4793 (Linking).

Cooper, D.S., Halpern, R., Wood, L.C., Levin, A.A., Ridgway, E.C. (1984). L-Thyroxine therapy in subclinical hypothyroidism. A double-blind, placebo-controlled trial. Ann Intern Med, Vol. 101, No. 1 (Jul 1984), pp. 18-24, issn 0003-4819 (Print) 0003-4819 (Linking).

Correia, N., Mullally, S., Cooke, G., Tun, T.K., Phelan, N., Feeney, J., Fitzgibbon, M., Boran, G., O'Mara, S., Gibney, J. (2009). Evidence for a specific defect in hippocampal memory in overt and subclinical hypothyroidism. J Clin Endocrinol Metab, Vol. 94, No. 10 (Oct 2009), pp. 3789-3797, issn 1945-7197 (Electronic) 0021-972X (Linking).

Corsonello, A., Montesanto, A., Berardelli, M., De Rango, F., Dato, S., Mari, V., Mazzei, B., Lattanzio, F., Passarino, G. (2010). A cross-section analysis of FT3 age-related changes in a group of old and oldest-old subjects, including centenarians' relatives, shows that a down-regulated thyroid function has a familial component and is related to longevity. Age Ageing, Vol. 39, No. 6 (Nov 2010), pp. 723-727, issn 1468-2834 (Electronic) 0002-0729 (Linking).

Dardano, A.M., Monzani F. (2008). Hypothyroidism and endothelial function: a markers of early atherosclerosis? . Recent Patents on Endocrine, Metabolic & Immune Drug Discovery, Vol. 2, No. 2 (May 2008 2008), pp. 79-96, issn 1872-2148.

Davis, J.D., Podolanczuk, A., Donahue, J.E., Stopa, E., Hennessey, J.V., Luo, L.G., Lim, Y.P., Stern, R.A. (2008). Thyroid hormone levels in the prefrontal cortex of post-mortem brains of Alzheimer's disease patients. Curr Aging Sci, Vol. 1, No. 3 (Dec 2008), pp. 175-181, issn 1874-6128 (Electronic).

Dayan, C.M. (2001). Interpretation of thyroid function tests. Lancet, Vol. 357, No. 9256 (Feb 24 2001), pp. 619-624, issn 0140-6736 (Print) 0140-6736 (Linking).

Dernellis, J., Panaretou, M. (2002). Effects of thyroid replacement therapy on arterial blood pressure in patients with hypertension and hypothyroidism. Am Heart J, Vol. 143, No. 4 (Apr 2002), pp. 718-724, issn 1097-6744 (Electronic) 0002-8703 (Linking).

Diez, J.J., Iglesias, P. (2004). Spontaneous subclinical hypothyroidism in patients older than 55 years: an analysis of natural course and risk factors for the development of overt thyroid failure. J Clin Endocrinol Metab, Vol. 89, No. 10 (Oct 2004), pp. 4890-4897, issn 0021-972X (Print) 0021-972X (Linking).

Dillmann, W.H. (2002). Cellular action of thyroid hormone on the heart. Thyroid, Vol. 12, No. 6 (Jun 2002), pp. 447-452, issn 1050-7256 (Print) 1050-7256 (Linking).

Duntas, L.H., Mantzou, E., Koutras, D.A. (2002). Circulating levels of oxidized low-density lipoprotein in overt and mild hypothyroidism. Thyroid, Vol. 12, No. 11 (Nov 2002), pp. 1003-1007, issn 1050-7256 (Print) 1050-7256 (Linking).

Egger, M., Smith, G.D., Sterne, J.A. (2001). Uses and abuses of meta-analysis. Clin Med, Vol. 1, No. 6 (Nov-Dec 2001), pp. 478-484, issn 1470-2118 (Print) 1470-2118 (Linking).

Etgen, T., Sander, D., Bickel, H., Forstl, H. (2011). Mild cognitive impairment and dementia: the importance of modifiable risk factors. Dtsch Arztebl Int, Vol. 108, No. 44 (Nov 2011), pp. 743-750, issn 1866-0452 (Electronic) 1866-0452 (Linking).

Faber, J., Petersen, L., Wiinberg, N., Schifter, S., Mehlsen, J. (2002). Hemodynamic changes after levothyroxine treatment in subclinical hypothyroidism. Thyroid, Vol. 12, No. 4 (Apr 2002), pp. 319-324, issn 1050-7256 (Print) 1050-7256 (Linking).

Fatourechi, V. (2009). Subclinical hypothyroidism: an update for primary care physicians. Mayo Clin Proc, Vol. 84, No. 1 2009), pp. 65-71, issn 1942-5546 (Electronic) 0025-6196 (Linking).

Fommei, E., Iervasi, G. (2002). The role of thyroid hormone in blood pressure homeostasis: evidence from short-term hypothyroidism in humans. J Clin Endocrinol Metab, Vol. 87, No. 5 (May 2002), pp. 1996-2000, issn 0021-972X (Print) 0021-972X (Linking).

Fu, A.L., Zhou, C.Y., Chen, X. (2010). Thyroid hormone prevents cognitive deficit in a mouse model of Alzheimer's disease. Neuropharmacology, Vol. 58, No. 4-5 (Mar-Apr 2010), pp. 722-729, issn 1873-7064 (Electronic) 0028-3908 (Linking).

Fukuyama, K., Ichiki, T., Takeda, K., Tokunou, T., Iino, N., Masuda, S., Ishibashi, M., Egashira, K., Shimokawa, H., Hirano, K., Kanaide, H., Takeshita, A. (2003). Downregulation of vascular angiotensin II type 1 receptor by thyroid hormone. Hypertension, Vol. 41, No. 3 (Mar 2003), pp. 598-603, issn 1524-4563 (Electronic) 0194-911X (Linking).

Galli, E., Pingitore, A., Iervasi, G. (2010). The role of thyroid hormone in the pathophysiology of heart failure: clinical evidence. Heart Fail Rev, Vol. 15, No. 2 (Mar 2010), pp. 155-169, issn 1573-7322 (Electronic) 1382-4147 (Linking).

Gardner, D.F. (2004). The neuromuscular system and brain in hypothyroidism, In: The Thyroid, A Fundamental and Clinical Text, Bravermann, L.E., Utiger, R.D. pp. 837841, Ninth Edition, Lippincott Williams and Wilkins, ISBN 0-7817-5047-4(HC), Philadelphia, USA

Geul, K.W., van Sluisveld, I.L., Grobbee, D.E., Docter, R., de Bruyn, A.M., Hooykaas, H., van der Merwe, J.P., van Hemert, A.M., Krenning, E.P., Hennemann, G., et al. (1993). The importance of thyroid microsomal antibodies in the development of elevated serum TSH in middle-aged women: associations with serum lipids. Clin Endocrinol (Oxf), Vol. 39, No. 3 (Sep 1993), pp. 275-280, issn 0300-0664 (Print) 0300-0664 (Linking).

Gharib, H., Tuttle, R.M., Baskin, H.J., Fish, L.H., Singer, P.A., McDermott, M.T. (2005a). Consensus Statement #1: Subclinical thyroid dysfunction: a joint statement on management from the American Association of Clinical Endocrinologists, the American Thyroid Association, and The Endocrine Society. Thyroid, Vol. 15, No. 1 (Jan 2005a), pp. 24-28; response 32-23, issn 1050-7256 (Print) 1050-7256 (Linking).

Gharib, H., Tuttle, R.M., Baskin, H.J., Fish, L.H., Singer, P.A., McDermott, M.T. (2005b). Subclinical thyroid dysfunction: a joint statement on management from the American Association of Clinical Endocrinologists, the American Thyroid Association, and the Endocrine Society. J Clin Endocrinol Metab, Vol. 90, No. 1 (Jan 2005b), pp. 581-585; discussion 586-587, issn 0021-972X (Print) 0021-972X (Linking).

Graham, J.E., Rockwood, K., Beattie, B.L., Eastwood, R., Gauthier, S., Tuokko, H., McDowell, I. (1997). Prevalence and severity of cognitive impairment with and without dementia in an elderly population. Lancet, Vol. 349, No. 9068 (Jun 21 1997), pp. 1793-1796, issn 0140-6736 (Print) 0140-6736 (Linking).

Gussekloo, J., van Exel, E., de Craen, A.J., Meinders, A.E., Frolich, M., Westendorp, R.G. (2004). Thyroid status, disability and cognitive function, and survival in old age. JAMA, Vol. 292, No. 21 (Dec 1 2004), pp. 2591-2599, issn 1538-3598 (Electronic) 0098-7484 (Linking).

Gussekloo, J., van Exel, E., de Craen, A.J., Meinders, A.E., Frolich, M., Westendorp, R.G. (2006). [Thyroid function, activities of daily living and survival in extreme old age: the 'Leiden 85-plus Study']. Ned Tijdschr Geneeskd, Vol. 150, No. 2 (Jan 14 2006), pp. 90-96, issn 0028-2162 (Print) 0028-2162 (Linking).

Hak, A.E., Pols, H.A., Visser, T.J., Drexhage, H.A., Hofman, A., Witteman, J.C. (2000). Subclinical hypothyroidism is an independent risk factor for atherosclerosis and myocardial infarction in elderly women: the Rotterdam Study. Ann Intern Med, Vol. 132, No. 4 (Feb 15 2000), pp. 270-278, issn 0003-4819 (Print) 0003-4819 (Linking).

Hancock, S.L., Cox, R.S., McDougall, I.R. (1991). Thyroid diseases after treatment of Hodgkin's disease. N Engl J Med, Vol. 325, No. 9 (Aug 29 1991), pp. 599-605, issn 0028-4793 (Print) 0028-4793 (Linking).

Helfand, M. (2004). Screening for subclinical thyroid dysfunction in nonpregnant adults: a summary of the evidence for the U.S. Preventive Services Task Force. Ann Intern Med, Vol. 140, No. 2 (Jan 20 2004), pp. 128-141, issn 1539-3704 (Electronic) 0003-4819 (Linking).

Herholz, K. (2010). Cerebral glucose metabolism in preclinical and prodromal Alzheimer's disease. Expert Rev Neurother, Vol. 10, No. 11 (Nov 2010), pp. 1667-1673, issn 1744-8360 (Electronic) 1473-7175 (Linking).

Hogervorst, E., Huppert, F., Matthews, F.E., Brayne, C. (2008). Thyroid function and cognitive decline in the MRC Cognitive Function and Ageing Study. Psychoneuroendocrinology, Vol. 33, No. 7 (Aug 2008), pp. 1013-1022, issn 0306-4530 (Print) 0306-4530 (Linking).

Hollowell, J.G., Staehling, N.W., Flanders, W.D., Hannon, W.H., Gunter, E.W., Spencer, C.A., Braverman, L.E. (2002). Serum TSH, T(4), and thyroid antibodies in the United States population (1988 to 1994): National Health and Nutrition Examination Survey (NHANES III). J Clin Endocrinol Metab, Vol. 87, No. 2 (Feb 2002), pp. 489-499, issn 0021-972X (Print) 0021-972X (Linking).

Imaizumi, M., Akahoshi, M., Ichimaru, S., Nakashima, E., Hida, A., Soda, M., Usa, T., Ashizawa, K., Yokoyama, N., Maeda, R., Nagataki, S., Eguchi, K. (2004). Risk for ischemic heart disease and all-cause mortality in subclinical hypothyroidism. J Clin Endocrinol Metab, Vol. 89, No. 7 (Jul 2004), pp. 3365-3370, issn 0021-972X (Print) 0021-972X (Linking).

Jaeschke, R., Guyatt, G., Gerstein, H., Patterson, C., Molloy, W., Cook, D., Harper, S., Griffith, L., Carbotte, R. (1996). Does treatment with L-thyroxine influence health status in middle-aged and older adults with subclinical hypothyroidism? J Gen Intern Med, Vol. 11, No. 12 (Dec 1996), pp. 744-749, issn 0884-8734 (Print) 0884-8734 (Linking).

Kahaly, G.J. (2000). Cardiovascular and atherogenic aspects of subclinical hypothyroidism. Thyroid, Vol. 10, No. 8 (Aug 2000), pp. 665-679, issn 1050-7256 (Print) 1050-7256 (Linking).

Kahaly, G.J., Dillmann, W.H. (2005). Thyroid hormone action in the heart. Endocr Rev, Vol. 26, No. 5 (Aug 2005), pp. 704-728, issn 0163-769X (Print) 0163-769X (Linking).

Kalmijn, S., Foley, D., White, L., Burchfiel, C.M., Curb, J.D., Petrovitch, H., Ross, G.W., Havlik, R.J., Launer, L.J. (2000). Metabolic cardiovascular syndrome and risk of dementia in Japanese-American elderly men. The Honolulu-Asia aging study. Arterioscler Thromb Vasc Biol, Vol. 20, No. 10 (Oct 2000), pp. 2255-2260, issn 1524-4636 (Electronic) 1079-5642 (Linking).

Kanaya, A.M., Harris, F., Volpato, S., Perez-Stable, E.J., Harris, T., Bauer, D.C. (2002). Association between thyroid dysfunction and total cholesterol level in an older biracial population: the health, aging and body composition study. Arch Intern Med, Vol. 162, No. 7 (Apr 8 2002), pp. 773-779, issn 0003-9926 (Print) 0003-9926 (Linking).

Karmisholt, J., Andersen, S., Laurberg, P. (2011). Variation in thyroid function in subclinical hypothyroidism: importance of clinical follow-up and therapy. Eur J Endocrinol, Vol. 164, No. 3 (Mar 2011), pp. 317-323, issn 1479-683X (Electronic) 0804-4643 (Linking).

Klein, I. (2004). The cardiovascular system in hypothyroidism, In: The Thyroid, A Fundamental and Clinical Text, Bravermann, L.E., Utiger, R.D. pp. 774-80, Ninth Edition, Lippincott Williams and Wilkins, ISBN 0-7817-5047-4(HC), Philadelphia, USA

Klein, I., Danzi, S. (2007). Thyroid disease and the heart. Circulation, Vol. 116, No. 15 (Oct 9 2007), pp. 1725-1735, issn 1524-4539 (Electronic) 0009-7322 (Linking).

Klein, I., Ojamaa, K. (2001). Thyroid hormone and the cardiovascular system. N Engl J Med, Vol. 344, No. 7 (Feb 15 2001), pp. 501-509, issn 0028-4793 (Print) 0028-4793 (Linking).

Kong, W.M., Sheikh, M.H., Lumb, P.J., Naoumova, R.P., Freedman, D.B., Crook, M., Dore, C.J., Finer, N. (2002). A 6-month randomized trial of thyroxine treatment in women with mild subclinical hypothyroidism. Am J Med, Vol. 112, No. 5 (Apr 1 2002), pp. 348-354, issn 0002-9343 (Print) 0002-9343 (Linking).

Kumar, N., Allen, K.A., Riccardi, D., Bercu, B.B., Cantor, A., Minton, S., Balducci, L., Jacobsen, P.B. (2004). Fatigue, weight gain, lethargy and amenorrhea in breast cancer patients on chemotherapy: is subclinical hypothyroidism the culprit? Breast Cancer Res Treat, Vol. 83, No. 2 (Jan 2004), pp. 149-159, issn 0167-6806 (Print) 0167-6806 (Linking).

Kvetny, J., Heldgaard, P.E., Bladbjerg, E.M., Gram, J. (2004). Subclinical hypothyroidism is associated with a low-grade inflammation, increased triglyceride levels and predicts cardiovascular disease in males below 50 years. Clin Endocrinol (Oxf), Vol. 61, No. 2 (Aug 2004), pp. 232-238, issn 0300-0664 (Print) 0300-0664 (Linking).

Ladenson, P.W., Singer, P.A., Ain, K.B., Bagchi, N., Bigos, S.T., Levy, E.G., Smith, S.A., Daniels, G.H., Cohen, H.D. (2000). American Thyroid Association guidelines for detection of thyroid dysfunction. Arch Intern Med, Vol. 160, No. 11 (Jun 12 2000), pp. 1573-1575, issn 0003-9926 (Print) 0003-9926 (Linking).

Laurberg, P., Andersen, S., Carle, A., Karmisholt, J., Knudsen, N., Pedersen, I.B. (2011). The TSH upper reference limit: where are we at? Nat Rev Endocrinol, Vol. 7, No. 4 (Apr 2011), pp. 232-239, issn 1759-5037 (Electronic) 1759-5029 (Linking).

Lee, W.Y., Suh, J.Y., Rhee, E.J., Park, J.S., Sung, K.C., Kim, S.W. (2004). Plasma CRP, apolipoprotein A-1, apolipoprotein B and Lpa levels according to thyroid function status. Arch Med Res, Vol. 35, No. 6 (Nov-Dec 2004), pp. 540-545, issn 0188-4409 (Print) 0188-4409 (Linking).

Lekakis, J., Papamichael, C., Alevizaki, M., Piperingos, G., Marafelia, P., Mantzos, J., Stamatelopoulos, S., Koutras, D.A. (1997). Flow-mediated, endothelium-dependent vasodilation is impaired in subjects with hypothyroidism, borderline hypothyroidism, and high-normal serum thyrotropin (TSH) values. Thyroid, Vol. 7, No. 3 (Jun 1997), pp. 411-414, issn 1050-7256 (Print) 1050-7256 (Linking).

Luboshitzky, R., Aviv, A., Herer, P., Lavie, L. (2002). Risk factors for cardiovascular disease in women with subclinical hypothyroidism. Thyroid, Vol. 12, No. 5 (May 2002), pp. 421-425, issn 1050-7256 (Print) 1050-7256 (Linking).

Luboshitzky, R., Herer, P. (2004). Cardiovascular risk factors in middle-aged women with subclinical hypothyroidism. Neuro Endocrinol Lett, Vol. 25, No. 4 (Aug 2004), pp. 262-266, issn 0172-780X (Print) 0172-780X (Linking).

Mariotti, S. (2005). Thyroid function and aging: do serum 3,5,3'-triiodothyronine and thyroid-stimulating hormone concentrations give the Janus response? J Clin Endocrinol Metab, Vol. 90, No. 12 (Dec 2005), pp. 6735-6737, issn 0021-972X (Print) 0021-972X (Linking).

Mariotti, S., Barbesino, G., Caturegli, P., Bartalena, L., Sansoni, P., Fagnoni, F., Monti, D., Fagiolo, U., Franceschi, C., Pinchera, A. (1993). Complex alteration of thyroid function in healthy centenarians. J Clin Endocrinol Metab, Vol. 77, No. 5 (Nov 1993), pp. 1130-1134, issn 0021-972X (Print) 0021-972X (Linking).

Mariotti, S., Franceschi, C., Cossarizza, A., Pinchera, A. (1995). The aging thyroid. Endocr Rev, Vol. 16, No. 6 (Dec 1995), pp. 686-715, issn 0163-769X (Print) 0163-769X (Linking).

Meier, C., Staub, J.J., Roth, C.B., Guglielmetti, M., Kunz, M., Miserez, A.R., Drewe, J., Huber, P., Herzog, R., Muller, B. (2001). TSH-controlled L-thyroxine therapy reduces cholesterol levels and clinical symptoms in subclinical hypothyroidism: a double blind, placebo-controlled trial (Basel Thyroid Study). J Clin Endocrinol Metab, Vol. 86, No. 10 (Oct 2001), pp. 4860-4866, issn 0021-972X (Print) 0021-972X (Linking).

Mitrou, P., Raptis, S.A., Dimitriadis, G. (2011). Thyroid disease in older people. Maturitas, Vol., No. (Jun 28 2011), pp. issn 1873-4111 (Electronic) 0378-5122 (Linking).

Mohandas, R., Gupta, K.L. (2003). Managing thyroid dysfunction in the elderly. Answers to seven common questions. Postgrad Med, Vol. 113, No. 5 (May 2003), pp. 54-56, 65-58, 100, issn 0032-5481 (Print) 0032-5481 (Linking).

Monzani, F., Caraccio, N., Kozakowa, M., Dardano, A., Vittone, F., Virdis, A., Taddei, S., Palombo, C., Ferrannini, E. (2004). Effect of levothyroxine replacement on lipid profile and intima-media thickness in subclinical hypothyroidism: a double-blind, placebo-controlled study. J Clin Endocrinol Metab, Vol. 89, No. 5 (May 2004), pp. 2099-2106, issn 0021-972X (Print) 0021-972X (Linking).

Monzani, F., Dardano, A., Caraccio, N. (2006). Does treating subclinical hypothyroidism improve markers of cardiovascular risk? Treat Endocrinol, Vol. 5, No. 2 2006), pp. 65-81, issn 1175-6349 (Print) 1175-6349 (Linking).

Monzani, F., Del Guerra, P., Caraccio, N., Pruneti, C.A., Pucci, E., Luisi, M., Baschieri, L. (1993). Subclinical hypothyroidism: neurobehavioral features and beneficial effect of L-thyroxine treatment. Clin Investig, Vol. 71, No. 5 (May 1993), pp. 367-371, issn 0941-0198 (Print) 0941-0198 (Linking).

Muller, B., Tsakiris, D.A., Roth, C.B., Guglielmetti, M., Staub, J.J., Marbet, G.A. (2001). Haemostatic profile in hypothyroidism as potential risk factor for vascular or thrombotic disease. Eur J Clin Invest, Vol. 31, No. 2 (Feb 2001), pp. 131-137, issn 0014-2972 (Print) 0014-2972 (Linking).

Nystrom, E., Caidahl, K., Fager, G., Wikkelso, C., Lundberg, P.A., Lindstedt, G. (1988). A double-blind cross-over 12-month study of L-thyroxine treatment of women with 'subclinical' hypothyroidism. Clin Endocrinol (Oxf), Vol. 29, No. 1 (Jul 1988), pp. 63-75, issn 0300-0664 (Print) 0300-0664 (Linking).

Ochs, N., Auer, R., Bauer, D.C., Nanchen, D., Gussekloo, J., Cornuz, J., Rodondi, N. (2008). Meta-analysis: subclinical thyroid dysfunction and the risk for coronary heart disease and mortality. Ann Intern Med, Vol. 148, No. 11 (Jun 3 2008), pp. 832-845, issn 1539-3704 (Electronic) 0003-4819 (Linking).

Ojamaa, K., Klemperer, J.D., Klein, I. (1996). Acute effects of thyroid hormone on vascular smooth muscle. Thyroid, Vol. 6, No. 5 (Oct 1996), pp. 505-512, issn 1050-7256 (Print) 1050-7256 (Linking).

Olsen, K.J. (1978). Scintigraphic estimation of thyroid volume and dose distribution at treatment with 131I. Acta Radiol Oncol Radiat Phys Biol, Vol. 17, No. 1 1978), pp. 74-80, issn 0348-5196 (Print) 0348-5196 (Linking).

Ooka, H., Fujita, S., Yoshimoto, E. (1983). Pituitary-thyroid activity and longevity in neonatally thyroxine-treated rats. Mech Ageing Dev, Vol. 22, No. 2 (Jun 1983), pp. 113-120, issn 0047-6374 (Print) 0047-6374 (Linking).

Osterweil, D., Syndulko, K., Cohen, S.N., Pettler-Jennings, P.D., Hershman, J.M., Cummings, J.L., Tourtellotte, W.W., Solomon, D.H. (1992). Cognitive function in non-demented older adults with hypothyroidism. J Am Geriatr Soc, Vol. 40, No. 4 (Apr 1992), pp. 325-335, issn 0002-8614 (Print) 0002-8614 (Linking).

Palmieri, E.A., Fazio, S., Lombardi, G., Biondi, B. (2004). Subclinical hypothyroidism and cardiovascular risk: a reason to treat? Treat Endocrinol, Vol. 3, No. 4 2004), pp. 233-244, issn 1175-6349 (Print) 1175-6349 (Linking).

Patel, J., Landers, K., Li, H., Mortimer, R.H., Richard, K. (2011). Thyroid hormones and fetal neurological development. J Endocrinol, Vol. 209, No. 1 (Apr 2011), pp. 1-8, issn 1479-6805 (Electronic) 0022-0795 (Linking).

Prinz, P.N., Scanlan, J.M., Vitaliano, P.P., Moe, K.E., Borson, S., Toivola, B., Merriam, G.R., Larsen, L.H., Reed, H.L. (1999). Thyroid hormones: positive relationships with cognition in healthy, euthyroid older men. J Gerontol A Biol Sci Med Sci, Vol. 54, No. 3 (Mar 1999), pp. M111-116, issn 1079-5006 (Print) 1079-5006 (Linking).

Razvi, S., Ingoe, L., Keeka, G., Oates, C., McMillan, C., Weaver, J.U. (2007). The beneficial effect of L-thyroxine on cardiovascular risk factors, endothelial function, and quality of life in subclinical hypothyroidism: randomized, crossover trial. J Clin Endocrinol Metab, Vol. 92, No. 5 (May 2007), pp. 1715-1723, issn 0021-972X (Print) 0021-972X (Linking).

Razvi, S., Shakoor, A., Vanderpump, M., Weaver, J.U., Pearce, S.H. (2008). The influence of age on the relationship between subclinical hypothyroidism and ischemic heart disease: a metaanalysis. J Clin Endocrinol Metab, Vol. 93, No. 8 (Aug 2008), pp. 2998-3007, issn 0021-972X (Print) 0021-972X (Linking).

Razvi, S., Weaver, J.U., Vanderpump, M.P., Pearce, S.H. (2010). The incidence of ischemic heart disease and mortality in people with subclinical hypothyroidism: reanalysis of the Whickham Survey cohort. J Clin Endocrinol Metab, Vol. 95, No. 4 (Apr 2010), pp. 1734-1740, issn 1945-7197 (Electronic) 0021-972X (Linking).

Rivolta, G., Cerutti, R., Colombo, R., Miano, G., Dionisio, P., Grossi, E. (1999). Prevalence of subclinical hypothyroidism in a population living in the Milan metropolitan area. J Endocrinol Invest, Vol. 22, No. 9 (Oct 1999), pp. 693-697, issn 0391-4097 (Print) 0391-4097 (Linking).

Roberts, L.M., Pattison, H., Roalfe, A., Franklyn, J., Wilson, S., Hobbs, F.D., Parle, J.V. (2006). Is subclinical thyroid dysfunction in the elderly associated with depression or cognitive dysfunction? Ann Intern Med, Vol. 145, No. 8 (Oct 17 2006), pp. 573-581, issn 1539-3704 (Electronic) 0003-4819 (Linking).

Rodondi, N., Aujesky, D., Vittinghoff, E., Cornuz, J., Bauer, D.C. (2006). Subclinical hypothyroidism and the risk of coronary heart disease: a meta-analysis. Am J Med, Vol. 119, No. 7 (Jul 2006), pp. 541-551, issn 1555-7162 (Electronic) 0002-9343 (Linking).

Rodondi, N., den Elzen, W.P., Bauer, D.C., Cappola, A.R., Razvi, S., Walsh, J.P., Asvold, B.O., Iervasi, G., Imaizumi, M., Collet, T.H., Bremner, A., Maisonneuve, P., Sgarbi, J.A., Khaw, K.T., Vanderpump, M.P., Newman, A.B., Cornuz, J., Franklyn, J.A., Westendorp, R.G., Vittinghoff, E., Gussekloo, J. (2010). Subclinical hypothyroidism and the risk of coronary heart disease and mortality. JAMA, Vol. 304, No. 12 (Sep 22 2010), pp. 1365-1374, issn 1538-3598 (Electronic) 0098-7484 (Linking).

Ross, D.S., (2004). subclinical hypothyroidism, in: The thyroid, A Fundamental and Clinical Text. Lippincott Williams and Wilkins, isbn 0-7817-5047-4 (HC), Philadelphia.

Rozing, M.P., Houwing-Duistermaat, J.J., Slagboom, P.E., Beekman, M., Frolich, M., de Craen, A.J., Westendorp, R.G., van Heemst, D. (2010). Familial longevity is associated with decreased thyroid function. J Clin Endocrinol Metab, Vol. 95, No. 11 (Nov 2010), pp. 4979-4984, issn 1945-7197 (Electronic) 0021-972X (Linking).

Samuels, M.H. (1998). Subclinical thyroid disease in the elderly. Thyroid, Vol. 8, No. 9 (Sep 1998), pp. 803-813, issn 1050-7256 (Print) 1050-7256 (Linking).

Sawin, C.T., Castelli, W.P., Hershman, J.M., McNamara, P., Bacharach, P. (1985). The aging thyroid. Thyroid deficiency in the Framingham Study. Arch Intern Med, Vol. 145, No. 8 (Aug 1985), pp. 1386-1388, issn 0003-9926 (Print) 0003-9926 (Linking).

Sawin, C.T., Chopra, D., Azizi, F., Mannix, J.E., Bacharach, P. (1979). The aging thyroid. Increased prevalence of elevated serum thyrotropin levels in the elderly. JAMA, Vol. 242, No. 3 (Jul 20 1979), pp. 247-250, issn 0098-7484 (Print) 0098-7484 (Linking).

Shih, C.H., Chen, S.L., Yen, C.C., Huang, Y.H., Chen, C.D., Lee, Y.S., Lin, K.H. (2004). Thyroid hormone receptor-dependent transcriptional regulation of fibrinogen and coagulation proteins. Endocrinology, Vol. 145, No. 6 (Jun 2004), pp. 2804-2814, issn 0013-7227 (Print) 0013-7227 (Linking).

Singh, S., Duggal, J., Molnar, J., Maldonado, F., Barsano, C.P., Arora, R. (2008). Impact of subclinical thyroid disorders on coronary heart disease, cardiovascular and all-cause mortality: a meta-analysis. Int J Cardiol, Vol. 125, No. 1 (Mar 28 2008), pp. 41-48, issn 1874-1754 (Electronic) 0167-5273 (Linking).

Spencer, C.A., Schwarzbein, D., Guttler, R.B., LoPresti, J.S., Nicoloff, J.T. (1993). Thyrotropin (TSH)-releasing hormone stimulation test responses employing third and fourth generation TSH assays. J Clin Endocrinol Metab, Vol. 76, No. 2 (Feb 1993), pp. 494-498, issn 0021-972X (Print) 0021-972X (Linking).

Squizzato, A., Romualdi, E., Piantanida, E., Gerdes, V.E., Buller, H.R., Tanda, M., Bartalena, L., Venco, A., Ageno, W. (2007). Subclinical hypothyroidism and deep venous thrombosis. A pilot cross-sectional study. Thromb Haemost, Vol. 97, No. 5 (May 2007), pp. 803-806, issn 0340-6245 (Print) 0340-6245 (Linking).

St John, J.A., Henderson, V.W., Gatto, N.M., McCleary, C.A., Spencer, C.A., Hodis, H.N., Mack, W.J. (2009). Mildly elevated TSH and cognition in middle-aged and older adults. Thyroid, Vol. 19, No. 2 (Feb 2009), pp. 111-117, issn 1557-9077 (Electronic) 1050-7256 (Linking).

Staub, J.J., Althaus, B.U., Engler, H., Ryff, A.S., Trabucco, P., Marquardt, K., Burckhardt, D., Girard, J., Weintraub, B.D. (1992). Spectrum of subclinical and overt hypothyroidism:

effect on thyrotropin, prolactin, and thyroid reserve, and metabolic impact on peripheral target tissues. Am J Med, Vol. 92, No. 6 (Jun 1992), pp. 631-642, issn 0002-9343 (Print) 0002-9343 (Linking).

Surks, M.I., Hollowell, J.G. (2007). Age-specific distribution of serum thyrotropin and antithyroid antibodies in the US population: implications for the prevalence of subclinical hypothyroidism. J Clin Endocrinol Metab, Vol. 92, No. 12 (Dec 2007), pp. 4575-4582, issn 0021-972X (Print) 0021-972X (Linking).

Surks, M.I., Ocampo, E. (1996). Subclinical thyroid disease. Am J Med, Vol. 100, No. 2 (Feb 1996), pp. 217-223, issn 0002-9343 (Print) 0002-9343 (Linking).

Surks, M.I., Ortiz, E., Daniels, G.H., Sawin, C.T., Col, N.F., Cobin, R.H., Franklyn, J.A., Hershman, J.M., Burman, K.D., Denke, M.A., Gorman, C., Cooper, R.S., Weissman, N.J. (2004). Subclinical thyroid disease: scientific review and guidelines for diagnosis and management. JAMA, Vol. 291, No. 2 (Jan 14 2004), pp. 228-238, issn 1538-3598 (Electronic) 0098-7484 (Linking).

Szabolcs, I., Podoba, J., Feldkamp, J., Dohan, O., Farkas, I., Sajgo, M., Takats, K.I., Goth, M., Kovacs, L., Kressinszky, K., Hnilica, P., Szilagyi, G. (1997). Comparative screening for thyroid disorders in old age in areas of iodine deficiency, long-term iodine prophylaxis and abundant iodine intake. Clin Endocrinol (Oxf), Vol. 47, No. 1 (Jul 1997), pp. 87-92, issn 0300-0664 (Print) 0300-0664 (Linking).

Taddei, S., Caraccio, N., Virdis, A., Dardano, A., Versari, D., Ghiadoni, L., Ferrannini, E., Salvetti, A., Monzani, F. (2006). Low-grade systemic inflammation causes endothelial dysfunction in patients with Hashimoto's thyroiditis. J Clin Endocrinol Metab, Vol. 91, No. 12 (Dec 2006), pp. 5076-5082, issn 0021-972X (Print) 0021-972X (Linking).

Taddei, S., Caraccio, N., Virdis, A., Dardano, A., Versari, D., Ghiadoni, L., Salvetti, A., Ferrannini, E., Monzani, F. (2003). Impaired endothelium-dependent vasodilatation in subclinical hypothyroidism: beneficial effect of levothyroxine therapy. J Clin Endocrinol Metab, Vol. 88, No. 8 (Aug 2003), pp. 3731-3737, issn 0021-972X (Print) 0021-972X (Linking).

Tan, Z.S., Beiser, A., Vasan, R.S., Au, R., Auerbach, S., Kiel, D.P., Wolf, P.A., Seshadri, S. (2008). Thyroid function and the risk of Alzheimer disease: the Framingham Study. Arch Intern Med, Vol. 168, No. 14 (Jul 28 2008), pp. 1514-1520, issn 1538-3679 (Electronic) 0003-9926 (Linking).

Tappy, L., Randin, J.P., Schwed, P., Wertheimer, J., Lemarchand-Beraud, T. (1987). Prevalence of thyroid disorders in psychogeriatric inpatients. A possible relationship of hypothyroidism with neurotic depression but not with dementia. J Am Geriatr Soc, Vol. 35, No. 6 (Jun 1987), pp. 526-531, issn 0002-8614 (Print) 0002-8614 (Linking).

Tunbridge, W.M., Evered, D.C., Hall, R., Appleton, D., Brewis, M., Clark, F., Evans, J.G., Young, E., Bird, T., Smith, P.A. (1977). The spectrum of thyroid disease in a community: the Whickham survey. Clin Endocrinol (Oxf), Vol. 7, No. 6 (Dec 1977), pp. 481-493, issn 0300-0664 (Print) 0300-0664 (Linking).

Turemen, E.E., Cetinarslan, B., Sahin, T., Canturk, Z., Tarkun, I. (2011). Endothelial dysfunction and low grade chronic inflammation in subclinical hypothyroidism due to autoimmune thyroiditis. Endocr J, Vol. 58, No. 5 2011), pp. 349-354, issn 1348-4540 (Electronic) 0918-8959 (Linking).

van den Beld, A.W., Visser, T.J., Feelders, R.A., Grobbee, D.E., Lamberts, S.W. (2005). Thyroid hormone concentrations, disease, physical function, and mortality in elderly men. J Clin Endocrinol Metab, Vol. 90, No. 12 (Dec 2005), pp. 6403-6409, issn 0021-972X (Print) 0021-972X (Linking).

Vanderpump, M.P., Tunbridge, W.M., French, J.M., Appleton, D., Bates, D., Clark, F., Grimley Evans, J., Hasan, D.M., Rodgers, H., Tunbridge, F., et al. (1995). The incidence of thyroid disorders in the community: a twenty-year follow-up of the Whickham Survey. Clin Endocrinol (Oxf), Vol. 43, No. 1 (Jul 1995), pp. 55-68, issn 0300-0664 (Print) 0300-0664 (Linking).

Villar, H.C., Saconato, H., Valente, O., Atallah, A.N. (2007). Thyroid hormone replacement for subclinical hypothyroidism. Cochrane Database Syst Rev, Vol., No. 3 2007), pp. CD003419, issn 1469-493X (Electronic) 1361-6137 (Linking).

Volpato, S., Guralnik, J.M., Fried, L.P., Remaley, A.T., Cappola, A.R., Launer, L.J. (2002). Serum thyroxine level and cognitive decline in euthyroid older women. Neurology, Vol. 58, No. 7 (Apr 9 2002), pp. 1055-1061, issn 0028-3878 (Print) 0028-3878 (Linking).

Walsh, J.P., Bremner, A.P., Bulsara, M.K., O'Leary, P., Leedman, P.J., Feddema, P., Michelangeli, V. (2005). Thyroid dysfunction and serum lipids: a community-based study. Clin Endocrinol (Oxf), Vol. 63, No. 6 (Dec 2005), pp. 670-675, issn 0300-0664 (Print) 0300-0664 (Linking).

Walton, K.W., Campbell, D.A., Tonks, E.L. (1965). The significance of alterations in serum lipids in thyroid dysfunction. I. The relation between serum lipoproteins, carotenoids and vitamin A in hypothyroidism and thyrotoxicosis. Clin Sci, Vol. 29, No. 2 (Oct 1965), pp. 199-215, issn 0009-9287 (Print) 0009-9287 (Linking).

Wang, C., Crapo, L.M. (1997). The epidemiology of thyroid disease and implications for screening. Endocrinol Metab Clin North Am, Vol. 26, No. 1 (Mar 1997), pp. 189-218, issn 0889-8529 (Print) 0889-8529 (Linking).

Yamamoto, N., Ishizawa, K., Ishikawa, M., Yamanaka, G., Yamanaka, T., Murakami, S., Hiraiwa, T., Okumiya, K., Ishine, M., Matsubayashi, K., Otsuka, K. (2012). Cognitive function with subclinical hypothyroidism in elderly people without dementia: One year follow up. Geriatr Gerontol Int, Vol. 12, No. 1 (Jan 2012), pp. 164-165, issn 1447-0594 (Electronic) 1447-0594 (Linking).

Zoeller, R.T., Rovet, J. (2004). Timing of thyroid hormone action in the developing brain: clinical observations and experimental findings. J Neuroendocrinol, Vol. 16, No. 10 (Oct 2004), pp. 809-818, issn 0953-8194 (Print) 0953-8194 (Linking).

Zulewski, H., Muller, B., Exer, P., Miserez, A.R., Staub, J.J. (1997). Estimation of tissue hypothyroidism by a new clinical score: evaluation of patients with various grades of hypothyroidism and controls. J Clin Endocrinol Metab, Vol. 82, No. 3 (Mar 1997), pp. 771-776, issn 0021-972X (Print) 0021-972X (Linking).

Section 5

Thyroid Hormone in Special Situations

Chapter 8

Obesity and Weight Loss: The Influence of Thyroid Hormone on Adipokines

Renata de Azevedo Melo Luvizotto, Sandro José Conde, Miriane de Oliveira, Maria Teresa De Sibio, Keize Nagamati Jr and Célia Regina Nogueira

Additional information is available at the end of the chapter

1. Introduction

The primary function of adipose tissue is storing energy in triacylglycerol (TG) form, neutralizing the excess of circulating lipids and saving non-adipose tissues of a fat overload. Under normal conditions, in the postprandial state, there is lipogenic endocrine system stimulation, allowing that positive energy balance can be stored as TG in adipose tissue, a process called lipogenesis. In contrast, the mobilization of fat in adipocytes occurs through the hydrolysis of TG by hormone sensitive lipase (HSL), a phenomenon called lipolysis. At the center of this interface - lipolysis and lipogenesis - is the insulin hormone, which exerts a potent inhibitory role on the HSL, allowing lower rates of lipolysis and hence, highest fat mass [1]. However, adipose tissue is not only a passive stock organ of triacylglycerol, being currently recognized as an endocrine organ with multiple functions [1, 2]. Produces several biologically active substances called adipokines, among them tumor necrosis factor-α (TNF-α), monocyte chemoattractant protein 1 (MCP-1), interleukin-6 (IL-6), leptin, resistin and adiponectin. These substances actively participate in, among others, body energy regulation, mainly, by endocrine, paracrine and autocrine signals, which allow the adipocyte play a metabolic role in other tissues [3-5].

However, in obesity there is an imbalance in adipokines production, a fact which, together with the inability to store fat in the adipocytes, results in a process of adipose tissue dysfunction [6], a known risk factor for developing obesity-associated metabolic disorders [1, 2, 6]. This fact occurs because the adipocytes (hypertrophic and hyperactive) initiates the production of adipokines and chemotactic factors (such as MCP-1), which attract macrophages into the adipose tissue [7]. Consequently there is a synergistic interaction on proinflammatory adipokines production - mainly TNF-α - and antagonistic on adiponectin. These substances lead to insulin resistance, reducing the lipogenic action of insulin in adipocytes, which results in higher rates of lipolysis in the adipose tissue [8, 9]. On the other hand, calorie restriction affects the regulation of adipose tissue gene expression, normalizing the adipokines changes observed in obesity [10].

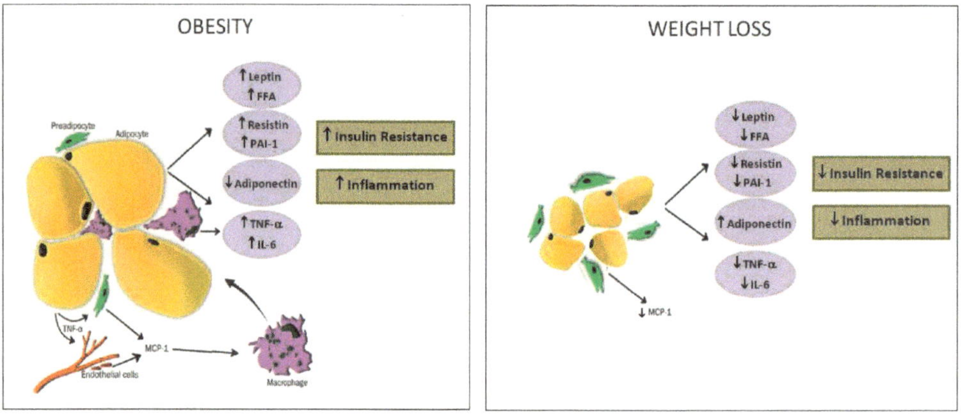

Figure 1. Adapted from van Kruijsdijk et al, 2009 [6]. In obesity the hypertrophic and hyperactive adipocytes initiate the production of MCP-1, which attract macrophages into the adipose tissue, increasing proinflammatory adipokines production (mainly TNF-α) and decreasing adiponectin production, leading to insulin resistance and inflammation. The weight loss process revert this alterations, improving insulin resistance and inflammation. FFA: fatty free acids; PAI1: Plasminogen activator inhibitor 1; TNFα: tumor necrosis factor-α; MCP1: monocyte chemoattractant protein 1; IL6: interleukin 6.

In this chapter will be revised about the influence of thyroid hormones on adipokines in obesity and weight loss. Also will be discussed the physiological role of adipokines as well as the effect of obesity and weight loss on the adipokines.

2. Adipokines physiological role

The adipose tissue is considered an endocrine organ and shows great dynamism. Since 1940 there is a hypothesis that adipose tissue has signals to communicate with other tissues [11], but only later was shown that this tissue is able to synthesize and secrete a large number of protein factors (which also act as cytokines) collectively called adipokines. These adipokines, in most part, are related, directly or indirectly, in processes involving atherosclerosis, hypertension, insulin resistance (IR) and type 2 diabetes (DM2), dyslipidemia, ie, represent the link between adiposity, metabolic syndrome and cardiovascular diseases [12-15]. Among these is Leptin, Resistin, Adiponectin, and others such as tumor necrosis factor-alpha (TNF-alpha), interleukin-6 (IL-6), plasminogen activator inhibitor-1 (PAI-1), acylation stimulating protein (ASP) and factors involved in the renin-angiotensin system (RAS).

2.1. Leptin

With its gene identified in 1994 [16] leptin is the adipokine most studied and thenceforth it has been identified more than 30 biochemical products secreted by adipocytes. Leptin is a peptidic hormone with 167 amino acids and 16kDa of molecular weight and synthesized from the "ob" gene in adipocytes, being more common in subcutaneous adipose tissue than in visceral fat [17]. Besides to be considered an important lipostate, or energy balance regulator according to body fat mass in long-term [18, 19] has been implicated in the regulation of immune, respiratory and reproductive systems [20]. The term Leptin comes from Greek "leptos" which means "thin" due to the fact that this protein lead to increased energy expenditure and act on satiety signals in hypothalamus, reducing caloric intake [21].

The expression and circulating leptin levels are controlled by a number of factors that may increase its secretion (insulin, glucocorticoids, TNF-α, estrogens, thyroid hormone and CCAAT/enhancer-binding protein-alpha) or decrease (Beta3-adrenergic activity, androgens , free fatty acids, GH, and peroxisome proliferator-activated receptor-gamma agonists) depending on the physiological assembly expressed by the body, especially on satiety and energy intake [22].

When circulating this adipokine reaches various body tissues as pancreas, increasing insulin secretion; liver, causing a satiety sensation by the increase in glucose production and increasing energy expenditure; hypothalamus, increasing stimulation of hypothalamic-pituitary-adrenal axis, and decreasing the stimulus of hypothalamic-pituitary-thyroid and hypothalamic-pituitary-gonadal axis; muscle tissue, increasing glucose uptake and metabolism [23].

Many of the effects of leptin result from their actions on the central nervous system, particularly in the hypothalamus, which acts in satiety and appetite regulation. Reaching these tissues after crossing the blood-brain barrier, leptin acts in the arcuate nucleus where there is a large concentration of leptin receptors, when binding to reduce the action of neurons that use neuropeptide Y (NPY) signaling and agouti-related protein (ARGP). NPY is a peptide of 36 amino acids, synthesized mainly in the arcuate nucleus, which projects to the paraventricular nucleus, ventromedial, perifornical and lateral, also involved in energy balance regulation. It is the most potent orexigenic. The ARGP also synthesized in the arcuate nucleus, also is projected to paratentricular nucleus, ventromedial and lateral, acting as a melanocortin system analogue on receptors MC-3 and MC-4, stimulating food intake. Leptin acts by decreasing the activity of these orexigenics signals, inhibiting food intake and increasing energy expenditure by activating the sympathetic nervous system [24, 25]. Also in the hypothalamus, leptin activates neurons pro-opiomelanocortin (POMC) producing alpha-melanocyte stimulating hormone (alpha-MHS). All substances expressed in this system are anorexigenics, ie, act on reducing food intake [14]. This product acts on malanocortin-4 receptors and also on neurons that express cocaine and amphetamine-regulated transcript (CART). POMC/CART neurones also have projections to the lateral hypothalamus and paraventricular nucleus, with a reciprocal innervation of these nuclei to the arcuate nucleus. Both alpha-MSH and CART are potent anorexigenic agents. The nucleus tractus solitarius (NTS) participates in the satiety control, involved in the end of food intake process. Afferent inputs related satiety signals include neurological vagus nerve and sympathetic system associated with chemical signals such as endocrine factors of gut cholecystokinin. There are many interconnections between hypothalamic nuclei including the paraventricular nucleus and the NTS (Figure 2).

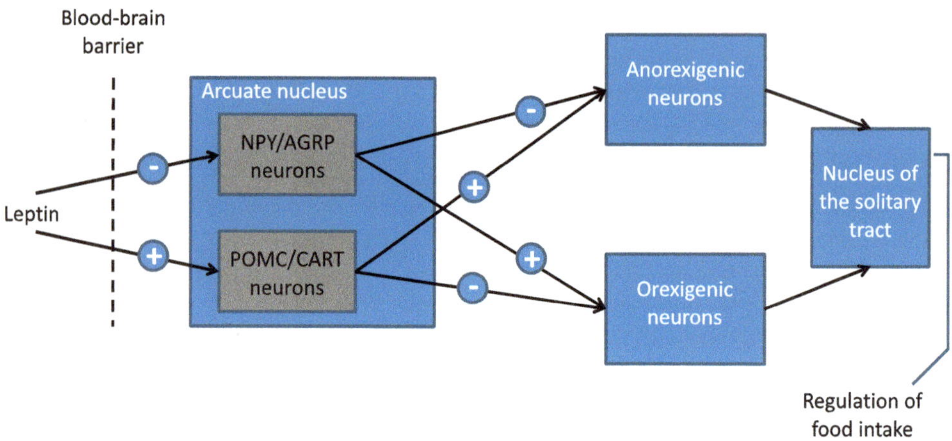

Figure 2. Food intake regulation by leptin at arcuate nucleus level. NPY: Neuropeptide Y; AGRP: Agouti-related protein; POMC: Pro-opiomelanocortin; CART: Cocaine and amphetamine-regulated transcript.

Among the actions taken by other hypothalamic nuclei in relation to energy homeostasis, can be highlight the ventromedial nucleus as a satiety center, lateral hypothalamus as the center of hunger and paraventricular nucleus on increased energy expenditure effects, as production of corticotropin releasing hormone and thyrotropin releasing hormone, activators the sympathetic nervous system. In perifornical nucleus, there is production of peptides termed orexins A and B, which act in the ventromedial nucleus and inhibits satiety and increase food intake. These areas receive nucleus axons of neurons in the arcuate nucleus, POMC/CART and NPY/ARGP, being considered as secondary action areas of leptin (downstream) [14, 26]. The leptin role in the CNS as a regulator is thus triggering mechanism (cascading effect), in order to stimulate or inhibit substances that act directly or indirectly in the hypothalamic areas involved in energy balance control.

In addition to their central effects, leptin also interacts with numerous peripheral tissues. Essentially, there are two major isoforms of leptin receptor, a long isoform which is required for full stimulation of the janus kinase-signal transducers and activators of transcription (JAK-STAT) pathway, and the short isoforms which result in the activation of JAK2 but not STAT. In skeletal muscle, for example, there are the two isoforms but the expression of short isoform is greater than the long one, making the leptin signalization in skeletal muscle activate various kinases including PI3-kinase, Akt (or PKB), PKC, MAP kinase kinase and Jun ERK [27, 28].

In the immune system the leptin receptor are expressed in hematopoietic cells, where leptin produced by adipocytes stimulates the normal growth of myeloid and erythroid [14]. In addition, leptin synergistically acts with other cytokines by increasing the proliferation of leukocytes, specifically T4 cells.

Leptin effects on reproduction are varied and the target organs range of hypothalamus, ovary and endometrial. In the hypothalamic-pituitary axis there is a stimulatory effect [29]. Its levels have a circadian and ultradian cycle, and these variations are associated with varying levels of luteinizing hormone (LH) and estradiol, informing to the brain about the critical fat stores necessary for secretion of luteinizing releasing hormone and activation of hypothalamic-pituitary-gonadal axis [30]. The amount of leptin released in the brain is greater in women than in men, suggesting that women may be more resistant to the leptin action and require higher levels to achieve an appropriate response [31]. It is known that leptin, in ovaries, may affect the menstrual cycle by a direct inhibitory effect on the follicles development [29]. Leptin may still have an important role in the early stages of cleavage and embryonic development [32], in the fetal growth regulation and development, hematopoiesis and angiogenesis, as leptin receptors were found in syncytiotrophoblast, suggesting that leptin may play an important role in fetal endocrine function of feto-placental unit [33]. In addition, leptin may play a central role in other target organs for reproduction, such as endometrial and mammary gland, influencing important functions including lactation and prevention of misbirth [34].

In the respiratory system leptin acts as a growth factor in the lung and as a modulator in the mechanisms of breathing central control. Leptin levels are elevated in patients with sleep apnea, independent of body fat, being associated with leptin resistance [14].

For hypothalamic-pituitary-thyroid axis leptin acts on the expression of thyrotropin-releasing hormone (TRH). Mice *in vitro* and *in vivo* study has demonstrated that leptin stimulates neurons directly in the paraventricular nucleus, which express TRH, increasing proTRH expression [35]. During fasting, the prohormone convertases 1 and 2 (PC1 and PC2) are decreased and leptin showed to restore PC1 and PC2 to pre-fasting levels [36]. Studies in rodents have shown that calorie restriction rapidly suppresses TRH expression in the paraventricular nucleus, leading to decreased thyroxine (T_4) and triiodothyronine (T_3) levels [37], and leptin can reverse these changes [38].

Both partial and complete deficiency of leptin is associated with hypothyroidism. Ob/ob mice exhibit hypothyroidism at birth [39] and normal mice have decreased T_4 levels during fasting [38]. Individuals with congenital leptin deficiency have a disorganized TSH secretion, suggesting that leptin may regulate the pulsatile characteristics of TSH and the circadian cycle [40]. In women with hypothalamic amenorrhea leptin treatment significantly increased free T_3 and free T_4, however did not affect TSH levels [41]. The lack of significant changes in TSH levels in many studies may be due to pulsatile nature of this hormone, but leptin can directly stimulate the T_4 release from the thyroid gland and/or increase TSH bioactivity [42, 43].

2.2. Resistin

Resistin is a polypeptide at approximately 12kDa and belongs to proteins family with cysteine-rich C-terminal domain call resistin-like molecules, which are identical to those found in inflammatory zone family, giving to resistin the alias FIZZ3 [44]. Its expression is 15 fold higher in visceral adipose tissue when compared to subcutaneous adipose tissue, in rodents [44], but it is also expressed in human macrophages [45]. Its name is due to the resistin presents a significant role in obesity-associated insulin resistance [46] and its molecular structure is very similar to adiponectin. Resistin production increases with food intake and obesity, and decreases in the presence of PPAR-gamma ligands [47].

Resistin promotes insulin resistance by increasing hepatic gluconeogenesis, and presenting rapid effect on this tissue [47]. Other *in vivo* study also found effects of administration and neutralization of resistin on glucose tolerance in skeletal muscle and adipose tissue, indicating resistin action also in these tissues by negative modulation of insulin signaling on glucose uptake [46].

Regarding the specific body fat deposits, resistin expressions 2-3 fold higher is found in visceral adipose tissue, followed by subcutaneous, abdominal and gluteal-femoral subcutaneous. Its expression is 3 fold higher in preadipocytes compared with mature adipocytes, also functioning as a potential regulator of adipogenesis [48].

Resistin deficient mice have weight and fat mass similar to wild-type mice, even when high-fat fed. However, resistin deficient mice significantly improved fasting glucose levels in control diet and improved glucose tolerance in high-fat diet. Insulin sensitivity is unaffected. The improvement in glucose homeostasis in resistin deficient mice is associated with decreased hepatic gluconeogenesis. Whereas these data support a resistin role in glucose homeostasis during fasting in rodents, a similar role in humans remains to be determined [3].

2.3. Adiponectin

Adiponectin, also known as ACRP 30 (adipocyte complement related protein of 30kDa), apM1 (adipose most abundant gene transcript 1), AdipQ or GBP28 (gelatin binding protein of 28 kDa) [49-52], is a protein exclusively expressed in differentiated adipocytes and circulates in high levels in the blood [53], presenting greater expression in subcutaneous adipose tissue than in visceral adipose tissue [54]. Unlike other factors secreted by adipose tissue, adiponectin acts as a protective factor for cardiovascular disease and increases insulin sensitivity. It is an approximately 30 kDa polypeptide that shows high homology with collagen VIII and X, and complement component C1q. A proteolytic cleavage product containing the globular domain of adiponectin circulate in physiologically significant levels and has biological activity [53].

Except for cases of severe malnutrition [55] and in neonates [56], there is a strong negative correlation between plasma adiponectin and fat mass [52].

Were identified two adiponectin receptors isoforms (Adipo-R1 and -R2) [57]. This receptors present seven transmembrane domains but are functionally different of receptors coupled to G protein. AdipoR1 is expressed mainly in muscle tissue and has high affinity for globular adiponectin, and low affinity for full-length adiponectin. AdipoR2 has high expression in liver and has intermediate affinity for both isoforms of circulating adiponectin. Thus, it is noted that the biological effects of adiponectin depends not only on circulating levels or the properties of each isoform but also receptor subtype and its expression in each tissue [3].

Adiponectin anti-inflammatory and anti-atherogenic actions occurs through decreased expression of adhesion molecule-1 (via reduced expression of TNF-alpha activity and resistin); decreased macrophage chemotaxis to fat cells formation; and inhibition of inflammatory signaling in endothelial tissue [58]. It increases insulin sensitivity via increased fatty acid oxidation and glucose uptake and utilization in skeletal muscle and adipose tissue; reduction of hepatic glucose release, leading to better control of glucose serum levels, free fatty acids and triglycerides [59]. In rat adipocytes, *in vitro,* the 60% reduction in adiponectin expression increased significantly insulin resistance. The presence of nucleotide polymorphisms in adiponectin caused by genetic or environmental factors (diet rich in fat, for example), can be a determining factor in reducing their insulin sensitizing action [60].

In the liver, adiponectin increases insulin sensitivity by reducing nonesterified fatty acids uptake, increasing fatty acid oxidation and decreasing glucose output. In muscle, adiponectin stimulates glucose metabolism and fatty acid oxidation. In the endothelium, it inhibits monocyte adherence by reducing adhesion molecules; inhibits macrophages transformation and reduces migrating smooth muscle cells proliferation in response to growth factors. Adiponectin also increases nitric oxide production by endothelial cells and stimulates angiogenesis. Taken together, these effects suggest that adiponectin is the only adipokine that present antidiabetic, anti-inflammatory and anti-atherogenic effects [3].

2.4. Others adipokines

Tumor Necrose Factor - alpha (TNF-α) – TNF-α is a cytokine expressed by adipocytes and stromovascular cells, with higher expression in subcutaneous adipose tissue compared to visceral adipose tissue, acting directly on adipocytes, promoting apoptosis induction, lipogenesis inhibition, by inhibiting lipoprotein lipase (LLP), GLUT-4 and the acetyl CoA synthetase expressions, as well as increased lipolysis, therefore exerting an important regulatory role in fat accumulation in adipose tissue [61, 62]. TNF-α is a transmembrane protein of 26 kDa, which, after being cleaved generates a portion of 17-kDa, which is biologically active and exerts its effects through TNF-α receptor type I and II. It is a cytokine initially described as an endotoxin-induced factor causing necrosis in tumors. The ability of TNF to induce cachexia *in vivo* led to an extensive evaluation of its role in energy homeostasis [3]. TNF-α alters gene expression of metabolically important tissues such as adipose tissue and liver [63] and impairs the insulin signaling by activation of serine kinases that increase the insulin receptor substrate-1 and -2 phosphorylation, increasing its degradation [64]. Both TNF-α and triiodothyronine are involved in the tissue homeostasis maintenance of the anterior pituitary gland, however, triiodothyronine inhibit the signaling cascade that TNF-α promotes on this tissue in signaling pathways affecting MAPK p38 and nuclear factor kappaB [65].

Interleukin-6 (IL-6) – IL-6 is also a cytokine with pro-inflammatory effect in acute responses and action on carbohydrates and lipids metabolism [66, 67]. IL-6 circulates in glycosylated form ranging from 22 to 27 kDa. Its receptor (IL-6R) is homologous to the leptin receptor and exists in two isoforms, a membrane-bound and soluble. The infusion of IL-6 near physiological doses, in healthy humans, increase lipolysis independently of catecholamines, glucagon and insulin modulation [68], indicating IL-6 as an important factor in lipid metabolism. As TNF-α, it inhibits the LLP and increases free fatty acids and glycerol release. Furthermore, the increased expression may be related to leptin suppression and stimulation of C-reactive protein production, as well as in reducing IRS-1 and GLUT-4 expression in the liver and muscle [66]. IL-6 is secreted by adipocytes and macrophages, which are responsible for 30% of its secretion [67]. Catecholamines can stimulate IL-6 expression via β2-and β3-adrenoceptors in adipose tissue, when in high concentrations [69]. The IL-6 central administration increases energy expenditure and decreases body fat in rodents. Also, transgenic mice with IL-6 overexpressed showed generalized growth deficiency and reduced body mass, however, IL-6 deficient mice develop obesity and metabolic abnormalities, suggesting that IL-6 may prevent, rather than cause these conditions [70].

Monocyte chemotactic protein-1 (MCP-1) – MCP-1 is a chemokine and a member of the small inducible cytokine family, which plays a role in the recruitment of monocytes and T lymphocytes to sites of injury and infection. Its main receptor is the chemokine CC motif receptor (CCR) 2 that is expressed in various cell types including adipocytes, skeletal muscle cells and macrophages. MCP-1 was first described as a secretory product of monocytes and endothelial cells with a role in atherosclerosis. MCP-1, acting through its receptor CCR2, is now thought to play a central role in the recruitment of monocytes to atherosclerotic lesions and in the development of intimal hyperplasia after arterial injury. Owing to their crucial roles in monocyte recruitment in vascular and nonvascular diseases, MCP-1 and CCR2 have become important therapeutic targets in cardiovascular research. Furthermore, MCP-1 plays a role in inflammation in insulin-responsive tissues. As for skeletal muscle, MCP-1 is increased during myopathies and can be induced by interferon-gamma. Recently, MCP-1 has been attributed an additional role in the pathophysiology of obesity [71].

Plasminogen activator inhibitor (PAI)-1 – Adipocytes can secrete many proteins in hemostasis and fibrinolytic system as PAI-1 [72]. PAI-1 is a member of the serine protease inhibitor family and is the primary inhibitor of fibrinolysis by inactivating urokinase-type and tissue-type plasminogen activator. PAI-1 has also been implicated in a variety of other biological processes including angiogenesis and atherogenesis. PAI-1 is expressed by many cell types within adipose tissue including adipocytes [3]. PAI-1 expression and secretion are greater in visceral adipose tissue relative to subcutaneous adipose tissue [54]. PAI-1 promotes thrombi formation and unstable atherogenic plaque rupture, and change the fibrinolytic balance by inhibition of plasmin production, contributing to vascular architecture remodeling and atherosclerotic process [66, 73].

Adipsin and acylation stimulating protein (ASP) – Also secreted by adipose tissue it has an important effect on lipogenesis [59]. APS inhibits the lipolysis by inhibition of hormone sensitive lipase (HSL), and stimulating lipogenesis by increasing GLUT4 translocation from cytosol to membrane; increases glycerol-3-phosphate production and increases diacylglycerol acyltransferase activity, an catalyst enzyme in triglycerides synthesis [74]. Thus affects both the glucose and the lipid metabolism.

Proteins of the renin angiotensin system (RAS) – Pathogenic models have been proposed to explain the association between adiposity and the renin angiotensin system [75]. This seems to be related to fat accumulation in adipose tissue, as well as its involvement in inflammatory and atherogenic process. Adipose tissue secretes many proteins related to the RAS as renin, angiotensinogen (AGT), angiotensin I, angiotensin II, angiotensin type I receptors (AT1) and type 2 (AT2) angiotensin-converting enzyme (ACE), and other proteases capable of producing angiotensin II (chymase, cathepsins D and G) [76, 77]. The angiotensin I receptor is secretion inductor of series 2 prostaglandins which participates in preadipocytes cell differentiation, and the angiotensin II stimulates adipocytes differentiation and lipogenesis in time of angiotensin I to II conversion, indicating their involvement in the accumulation of fat mass process [78].

3. Adipokines and thyroid hormones

The thyroid gland mainly produces the thyroid hormones T_3 and T_4. However, also produces small amounts of other iodothyronines as reverse T_3 and 3,5-diiodo-L-thyronine. This gland is part of hypothalamic-pituitary-thyroid axis. Thyroid hormones secretion is regulated by the classical mechanism of negative feedback; briefly, thyroid releasing hormone (TRH), produced predominantly by neurons of the paraventricular nucleus in the hypothalamus, stimulates the release of thyroid stimulating hormone (TSH) in pituitary and this in turn, stimulates the synthesis and release of thyroid hormones. The increase in thyroid hormones serum concentrations inhibit the production of both TRH and TSH, leading to decreased thyroid function. The subsequent decrease in thyroid hormones serum levels, in turn, stimulates TRH and TSH, again increasing the concentration of hormones [79]. Thyroid hormones act in the body through the coupling to its receptor α (TRα) and β (TRβ). The thyroid hormone receptors (TRs), members of the superfamily of nuclear receptors interact with a specific DNA sequence, called responsive element in the promoter region of target gene and regulates gene transcription [80]. Generally, TRs are repressors in the absence of binding T_3 and transcriptional activators in its presence [81].

Although the thyroid hormones are essential for the survival [37], thyroid function disorder leads to changes in metabolic parameters, for example, thyroid hormone excess is associated with weight loss and reduced muscle and fat mass [82] , showing that thyroid hormones play a central role in regulating the adipose tissue metabolism [83]. Furthermore, Viguerie et al. [84] showed by microarray that 19 genes of human white adipose tissue are regulated by thyroid hormone. These modulated genes give rise to proteins involved in transduction signal, lipid metabolism, apoptosis and inflammatory responses. The thyroid hormones inhibit proliferation and stimulate differentiation of adipocytes [85], regulate lipid metabolism by upregulation lipolytic enzymes expression, increase oxygen consumption and modulate tissue sensitivity to other hormones [84].

Since thyroid hormones affect adipose tissue metabolism, it is interesting to evaluate the relationship between thyroid hormones and adipokines in obese and weight loss, the focus of discussion in next sections.

4. Thyroid hormone effect on adipokines in obesity

4.1. Leptin

A potential interaction between leptin and thyroid hormones has been suggested since both hormones are associated with body weight and energy expenditure regulation.

Leptin deficiency leads to severe obesity, however, in humans it's usually find high levels of leptin associated with leptin-resistance state [86-91]. Although thyroid function is usually normal in obese subjects, many studies have demonstrated that TSH levels are slightly increased in obese subjects [92-94]. Several studies have suggested that leptin influences TSH release, suggesting a regulatory role by leptin on thyroid axis at least in some conditions [35, 40, 95-101]. Thyroid hormones regulate the expression of several genes in human adipocyte [84], however, the role of thyroid hormones in leptin modulation remains controversial (Figure 3).

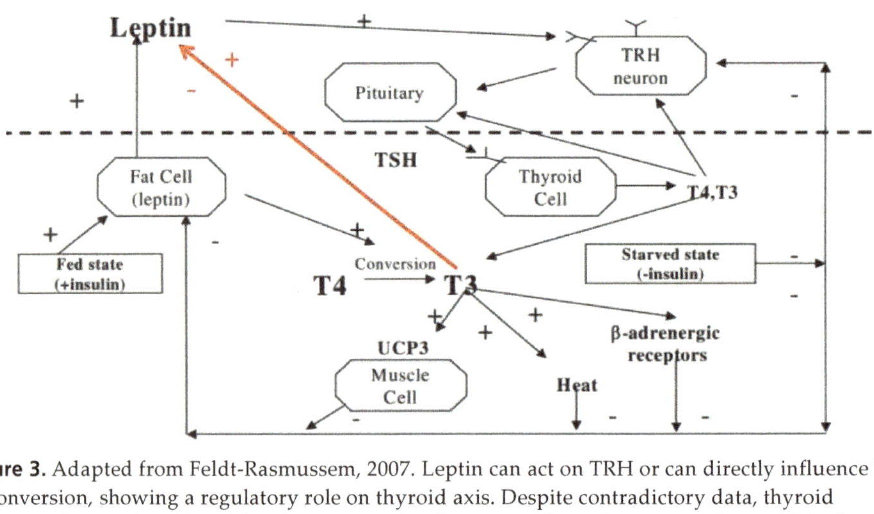

Figure 3. Adapted from Feldt-Rasmussem, 2007. Leptin can act on TRH or can directly influence T_4 – T_3 conversion, showing a regulatory role on thyroid axis. Despite contradictory data, thyroid hormone also regulates leptin levels increasing or decreasing depending on condition. TRH: thyroid release hormone; TSH: thyroid stimulating hormone; UCP3: uncoupling protein 3; T_4: thyroxine; T_3: triiodothyronine.

Studies with rodents indicate that thyroid hormones exert a negative influence on serum leptin concentrations [102-105]. Syed et al. [106] also found similar results, but report that thyroid hormones influence leptin levels indirectly through the regulation of fat mass. Wang et al. [107] reported that although leptin and thyroid hormones might affect the same pathways to regulate energy metabolism, the leptin effects on metabolism are not dependent upon the presence of thyroid hormones. In agreement, Luvizotto et al. [108] reported that T_3 administration in obese rats promotes weight loss and diminishes serum levels and gene expression of leptin and other adipokines. Contrary to these results, Yoshida et al. [109] founds increased leptin mRNA levels in 3T3-L1 cell cultures treated with T_3 at physiological and supraphysiological doses.

Obese human subjects have high serum leptin levels as leptin concentrations are directly proportional to body fat mass, more specifically to adipocyte volume [110, 111]. Regarding to thyroid hormones, there is indications that human obesity is usually associated with increased TSH and T_3 levels [92, 112]. As in rats, studies with humans reached to controversial results about the effect of thyroid hormones over leptin concentrations. In fact, human studies present more difficulties in terms of controlling variables as patient characteristics, treatments and method for measuring leptin levels and body composition. In hypothyroid subjects serum leptin was found to be increased [83, 113], decreased [114, 115] or unchanged [116, 117] when compared with euthyroid subjects. The same controversial results are found in studies with hyperthyroid subjects [83, 113, 115-118].

These conflicting results might be explained by the existence of many factors influencing leptin levels and thyroid hormones, and more studies are needed to fully understand the relationship between leptin and thyroid hormones.

4.2. Resistin

Resistin is strongly related to insulin resistance, showing increased resistin concentrations in obese and diabetic animals [46], and additionally it has been associated with inflammatory condition [119]. There is evidence that the hyperlipidic diet-induced obesity as well as leptin gene mutations are associated with high resistin circulating levels [120]. Resistin administered intraperitoneally increases plasma glucose and induces a hepatic insulin resistance. Other studies involving administration of resistin-recombinant promoted insulin resistance and reduced glucose transport stimulated by insulin, whereas administration of anti-resistin antibodies produced the opposite effect in rats [46]. Moreover, anti-resistin antibodies decrease blood glucose levels and improve the insulin sensitivity in obese rats [121, 122]. In mice with diet-induced obesity, immunoneutralization of resistin resulted in a 20% drop in blood glucose and improved insulin sensitivity as measured by insulin tolerance testing [46].

Resistin in humans is primarily produced in peripheral blood monocytes and its levels correlate with IL-6 concentrations [120], the question of its inflammatory role has been raised [123, 124], however the physiological role of resistin is far from clear and its role in obesity and insulin resistance and/or diabetes is controversial. Janke et al. [121] describes in adipose tissue of obese individuals, although this adipokine has been identified, there was no correlation between resistin gene expression and their body weight, adiposity and insulin resistance. In contrast, high resistin levels are related to obesity and insulin resistance [46], and since body mass index has a possible association with thyroid hormones during periods of weight gain [125], could be establish a relationship between thyroid hormones and resistin in obesity.

Thyroid hormones appear to regulate resistin, at least in rats, however, in humans, studies on resistin levels and thyroid status have produced conflicting results. Some studies report that patients with hyperthyroidism have elevated resistin concentrations when compared with euthyroid control subjects [126]. Normalization of circulating thyroid hormones was accompanied by a significant decrease in resistin concentrations [126]. Others showed that hyperthyroid patients exhibit a significant decrease in resistin levels compared with euthyroid individuals. Normalization of circulating thyroid hormones levels was not accompanied by any significant change in resistin levels [127]. After adjusting the weight by the body mass index, the resistin levels of hyperthyroid patients were similar to euthyroid individuals [128].

Azza et al. [129] in their study with hypothyroid rats found an increase in body mass index without changes in resistin levels. On the other hand, Nogueiras et al. [130], found that adipose tissue resistin mRNA levels were increased in hypothyroid rats and decreased, to almost undetectable levels, in hyperthyroid rats. These data may help to explain previous findings showing a marked improvement in insulin resistance observed in obese rats after treatment with exogenous thyroid hormones [106]. Luvizotto et al. [108] reported that administration of T_3 supraphysiological doses decreased resistin serum levels and ressitin mRNA gene expression in adipose tissue in obese rats.

Data on the effect of thyroid hormones on resistin are scarce and controversial, so more studies are needed to elucidate the exact mechanism by which thyroid hormones may influence resistin levels.

4.3. Adiponectin

The main target tissue and the precise mechanism of adiponectin action are not fully understood. The adiponectin activity is probably regulated at several levels, including gene expression, post-transcriptional modifications, oligomeric complexes formation, and proteolytic cleavage into smaller and perhaps more active fragments [131]. Some experimental models suggest that reduced adiponectin expression is associated with obesity and insulin resistance. Adiponectin expression may be activated during adipogenesis, but the feedback inhibition on its production may be involved in obesity development. It has been shown that adipogenic genes expression was suppressed during obesity and diabetes development in mice [132]. A negative correlation between obesity and circulating adiponectin has been well accepted.

Studies of a possible relationship between adiponectin and lipid metabolism changes associated with thyroid dysfunction are scarce. Hyperthyroid patients showed an increase in body weight, body mass index and cholesterol serum levels after controlling for thyrotoxicosis. The lack of correlation between these parameters and serum adiponectin suggests that changes in body composition and lipid profile observed in hyperthyroidism are independent of adiponectin. In contrast, patients with hypothyroidism showed elevated cholesterol and triglycerides levels when compared to normal subjects. Thyroid function control was followed by a significant decrease in serum cholesterol and triglyceride concentrations. However no relationship between adiponectin and lipid profile before and after therapy was evidenced. Furthermore, after adjusting adiponectin levels for body mass index, no significant change was observed in patients with hyper- and hypothyroidism, suggesting that thyroid hormones play a small role in adiponectin levels modulation [128].

An experimental study of rats with hyperthyroidism showed an important rise in serum adiponectin [133]. However, in contrast, Cabanelas et al. [134] show reduced adiponectin gene expression in inguinal explants of normal rats. Confirming this data Luvizotto et. al. [108] demonstrate that obese animals had decreased adiponectin serum levels when compared to control animals; and the administration of T_3, interestingly, even diminishing the body fat mass, presented lower levels of adiponectin; showing that supraphysiological T_3 doses alter adiponectin expression in obesity, suggesting that T_3 may cause undesirable effects on adipose tissue.

4.4. Others adipokines

TNF-α - Fruhbeck et al. [135] in their investigations revealed a narrow molecular link between TNF-α and obesity, verifying that TNF-α expression is increased in obesity, which in turn decreased insulin sensitivity, the same way of resistin. High-fat fed rodents showed significantly increased TNF-α expression and alteration in insulin signaling pathway *in vivo* [136]. Anti-TNF-α antibodies improves insulin sensitivity in obese rats, whereas TNF-α deficient animals, even when subjected to high-fat diet, present themselves "protected" from obesity development and insulin resistance. TNF-α is a cytokine that may be involved in autoimmune thyroid disease development [137, 138]. Jiskra & Telicka [138] examined the relationship between thyroid function and cytokines, using patients with Graves' disease (characterized by hyperthyroidism), and patients with Hashimoto thyroiditis (disease characterized by hypothyroidism). The cytokine profile was assessed and patients with Hashimoto's thyroiditis present body mass index above the ideal level and TNF-α serum levels smaller than in patients with Graves' disease, who had body mass index within normal limits. Díez et al. [139] show that patients with hyperthyroidism before treatment present TNF-α serum levels higher than in control group, but hyperthyroidism treatment was accompanied by normalization of TNF-α levels. However TNF-α reduction was not observed in patients with hypothyroidism who have had the thyroid function normalized, despite a positive correlation between the TNF-α post-treatment levels and weight loss.

IL-6 - IL-6 levels are increased in obesity [140], and is also a marker of insulin resistance [141, 142]. According Nonogaki et al [143], metabolic impact produced by increased expression of

IL-6 in the body fat deposits can be very importante in the obesity pathogenesis. The increase in IL-6 plasmatic could stimulate the hepatic synthesis of triacylglycerol, contributing to hypertriglyceridemia associated with visceral obesity. Data on relationship of thyroid hormones and IL-6 in obesity are scarce, but the association between reduction of T_3 circulating levels and increasing pro-inflammatory cytokines, particularly IL-6, is described in the literature in both animals' models and human studies - septic patients and in patients with systemic inflammatory response [144, 145]. The acute subcutaneous administration of IL-6 (5 mg) in rats was associated with decrease in T_4,T_3 and TSH serum concentrations, while the T_4/T_3 ratio decreased, suggesting that T_4 deiodination was not affected [144]. Changes in serum thyroid hormone concentrations could effectively be ascribed to IL-6, since they could be prevented by IL-6 preincubation with its neutralizing antibody [144]. The continuous IL-6 intraperitoneal infusion (15 mg/day for 7 consecutive days) in rats was associated with a transient decrease in serum T_4 and TSH, although less than that caused by IL-1 [145]. In latter study, pro-TRH mRNA hypothalamic and pituitary TSH-b mRNA were unaffected by IL-6, suggesting that the effects of IL-6 on TSH might not necessarily be associated with a decreased synthesis of thyrotropin [145]. On the other hand, the observation that the intracerebroventricular IL-6 administration to rats was followed by a decrease in serum TSH and an increase in serum adrenocorticotropin (ACTH) concentrations, while these changes could be reproduced in hemipituitaries only for ACTH, but not for TSH, suggested that the action of IL-6 on TSH might be exerted predominantly at the hypothalamic levels [146]. Increased concentrations of cytokines, especially IL-6, are often found in nonthyroidal illness patients and correlate with changes in thyroid hormone concentrations [144].

MCP-1 - Expression in adipose tissue and plasma MCP-1 levels have been found to correlate positively with the degree of obesity [7, 147-149]. Elevated circulating levels of MCP-1 as well as MCP-1 mRNA have been reported in obese mice [149, 150]. The possibility that MCP-1 formation in adipose tissue is due to macrophage infiltration must be considered since obesity is associated with various degrees of macrophage accumulation in adipose tissue [7, 147]. No data on this adipokines and thyroid hormone have been published.

PAI-1 - Adipose tissue PAI-1 gene expression and serum concentration have been reported in several pathological conditions, such as obesity, hyperinsulinemia, and hyperglycemia [151, 152]. The thyroid hormones T_4 and T_3 also have cardiovascular effects, probably through the regulation of circulating clotting proteins and fibrinolytic activity [153]; however, the mechanisms leading to cardiovascular and thromboembolytic diseases in thyroid dysfunction are controversial. Some reports have described an increase in serum PAI-1 concentration in hyperthyroidism, whereas others did not detect any differences [154, 155]. Biz, et al. [158] determined the effects of *in vivo* treatment of rats with the thyroid hormone T_4 on gene expression and the serum concentration of PAI-1. Additionally, the effects of T_3 and T_4 on PAI-1 gene expression in 3T3-L1 adipocytes were also evaluated. The results demonstrated that adipocytes present different responses to thyroid hormones when considering *in vivo* and *in vitro* experiments. Other investigations have also demonstrated different *in vivo* and *in vitro* responses. The diverse *in vivo* and *in vitro* effects of thyroid hormones on PAI-1 gene expression regulation are not related to the inhibitory effect of T_4 on thyroid-stimulating hormone (TSH) secretion, since the literature has not shown any relationship between TSH and PAI-1 serum concentration [157]. However, it could be suggested that the lower amount of thyroid hormone receptors and deiodinase present in white adipose tissue than in brain, liver, brown adipose tissue, and kidney may be involved in this process. In addition, the low blood flow in white adipose tissue in comparison to other tissue types [158] could contribute to hormone distribution *in vivo*, suggesting that lower amounts of T_4 and T_3 were achieved in adipocytes *in vivo* in comparison to the *in vitro* study. Thyroid hormones have different effects in relation to PAI-1 gene expression in adipocytes in the intact rat (*in vivo* study) and in cultured adipocytes (*in vitro* study). Further studies are required to better elucidate the diverse *in vivo* and *in vitro* effects of thyroid hormone on adipocytes PAI-1 gene expression [156].

ASP - In a number of studies, ASP has been demonstrated to be increased in obesity, diabetes and cardiovascular disease [159-161]. Plasma ASP levels correlate positively with body mass index, as well as with plasma lipids. Study using culture of human adipocytes revealed increased secretion of chylomicrons induced by ASP [162]. There is evidence that circulating lipids also stimulate the expression of ASP after drinking large quantities of these nutrients [163]. There is no data available regarding the effect of thyroid hormones on ASP levels in obesity.

RAS- Adipose tissue synthesizes and secretes the major components of RAS [164]. There is evidence for overactivation of adipose tissue RAS in obesity in rodents [165], and for a positive correlation between adipose tissue angiotensinogen levels and BMI in humans [166]. Also Ang II secretion from adipose tissue is increased in obese, but not lean, individuals [167]. Increased production of angiotensinogen with excess gain in white adipose tissue contributes to glucose intolerance development, insulin resistance, cardiovascular and renal diseases [76, 168, 169]. In addition, increased RAS activity contributes to inflammation in fat tissue [170]. The interaction of RAS with other adipokines also contributes to the development of metabolic syndrome. Ang II appears to stimulate leptin production by adipocytes [76]; which in turn, hyperleptinemia may further hyperactivity of RAS by stimulating renin release by the kidney. Ang II may also regulate negatively adipocyte production of adiponectin in both rodents and humans [171, 172]. Thyroid hormones are important regulators of cardiac and renal functions while RAS components act systemically and locally in individual organs also to control cardiovascular and renal functions. Several studies have implicated the systemic and local RAS in the mediation of functional and structural changes in cardiovascular and renal tissues due to abnormal thyroid hormone levels [173, 174]. Thyroid hormones also appear to stimulate expression and synthesis of RAS components [175-177].

5. Thyroid hormone effects on adipokines in weight loss

5.1. Leptin

After weight loss, leptin levels decrease [178-180], as well TSH and T_3 reduces to normal levels [92, 93, 112]. In starvation conditions, serum leptin levels decrease and thyroid hormones levels are quickly supressed, leading to a consequent reduction in energy expenditure [83].

Varady et al. [181] studying severely obese women have suggested that a minimum weigh loss of 5% is required to improve adipokines profile, including the reduction of leptin levels. Not only a minimal weight loss is required but a maximal weigh loss beyond which further improvements in circulating adipokine levels are no longer observed has been suggested [179, 182]. The method or diet content by which weigh loss is achieved seems to be less important than the overall weight loss [179, 183].

As mentioned before, studies investigating the correlation between thyroid hormones and leptin levels present conflicting results. Luvizotto et al. showed that administration of physiologic levels of T_3 increases leptin mRNA expression with no influence on body weight in calorie-restricted obese rats [108], while administration of supraphysiological T_3 dose promotes weight loss and diminishes serum levels and gene expression of leptin [108] (Figure 3). Again, as Syed et al. [106] reported, the effects of thyroid hormones in leptin concentrations might be indirect trough the regulation of fat mass (Figure 4). The decline of TSH release and T_3 concentrations associated with decrease in leptin levels after weight loss may contribute to the compensatory reductions of energy expenditure and catabolism that typically accompany weight loss [184].

As both thyroid hormones and leptin have major roles in energy balance and regulation of body weight, an interaction between these hormones could not be discarded to achieve or maintain weight loss but further studies are necessary to elucidate the relationship between leptin and thyroid hormones.

5.2. Resistin

Since obesity is considered a global epidemic and one of majors public health problem, affecting developed and developing countries [185, 186], and obese subjects may presente increased resistin levels [46], which can worse insulin resistance and inflammation [119], one of the most used strategies is the weight loss by reduction of caloric intake [187]. Caloric restriction affects the regulation of adipose tissue gene expression, normalizing the adipokines changes caused by obesity [10], while thyroid hormones play a central role in regulating adipose tissue metabolism [83], being related to body weight changes, thyroid hormones may therefore play a key role in the normalization of resistin in weight loss.

Nogueiras et al. [130] show a decrease in resistin mRNA expression in epididymal adipose tissue of pregnant and nonpregnant rats that were subjected to food restriction. Kim et al. [188] showed that resistin mRNA levels were decreased during fasting, but increased considerably when the animals were refed or after insulin infusion. T_3 had no effect on resistin mRNA levels in adipose tissue of obese animals submitted to calorie restriction [189].

Normalization of circulating thyroid hormones was accompanied by a significant decrease in resistin concentrations [126]. Others showed that hyperthyroid patients exhibit a significant decrease in resistin levels compared with euthyroid individuals, and the normalization of circulating thyroid hormones was not accompanied by any significant change in resistin levels [127]. After adjusting the weight by the body mass index, the resistin levels in hyperthyroid patients were similar to euthyroid subjects [128] (Figure 4).

The association between thyroid hormone and resistin in weight loss present conflicting data, requiring further studies to evaluate this relation.

5.3. Adiponectin

Negative correlation between obesity and circulanting adiponectin has been well accept, and adiponectin concentration increases concomitantly to weight loss [190].

Experimental study on caloric restriction showed increased levels of circulating adiponectin [191]. Accordingly, Zhu et al. [194] showed that calorically restricted animals exhibited a significant increase in plasma adiponectin levels accompanied by significant decline in triglyceride levels, showing that adiponectin levels are inversely proportional to the degree of adiposity [192, 193].

Thyroid hormones perform a central role in adipose tissue metabolism regulation [83], which produces the biologically active substances adipocytokines, or adipokines, that include adiponectin [127, 194], indeed thyroid hormones share some physiological actions with adiponectin, such as reduction of body fat by increased thermogenesis and lipid oxidation [194].

The interaction between thyroid hormones and adiponectin concentration remains unclear. In humans, hyperthyroidism has been associated with both similar [128, 195] and elevated adiponectin concentrations [196], while experimental study with hyperthyroid rats found an increase in adiponectin serum concentration [133]. In agreement, some data shown that therapy to normalize hyperthyroidism significantly reduced circulating adiponectin levels [197]. In contrast Luvizotto et al. [189] show that thyroid hormone, at the doses of 5 and 25 μg T_3 / 100 g BW, diminishes adiponectin gene expression, suggesting that thyroid hormone modulates negatively adiponectin expression in calorie-restricted obese rats (Figure 4).

5.4. Others adipokines

TNF-α - The first information about the TNF-α biological effects indicated an involvement in insulin resistance, weight loss and anorexia. The increase in lipolysis result from TNF-α stimulus in hormone-sensitive lipase expression, leading to decreased activity of lipoprotein lipase. However, more recent investigations have revealed a molecular mechanism of weight loss on TNF-α levels, showing TNF-α expression is increased in obesity and decreases with weight loss, thereby improving insulin sensitivity [135, 198]. After weight loss there is a decrease of macrophages number in adipose tissue [199], this can lead to decreased TNF-α levels, since both adipose tissue and macrophages produce this cytokine. There are few studies correlating the thyroid status with TNF-α levels in weight loss. Patients with HIV tend to lose weight and in some cases it is observed a decrease in T_3 levels accompanied by increased TNF-α levels, when these individuals are compared to patients with HIV with normal T_3 levels. These results corroborate to other study linking the sick euthyroid syndrome to high TNF-α levels in cachectic patients with HIV [200].

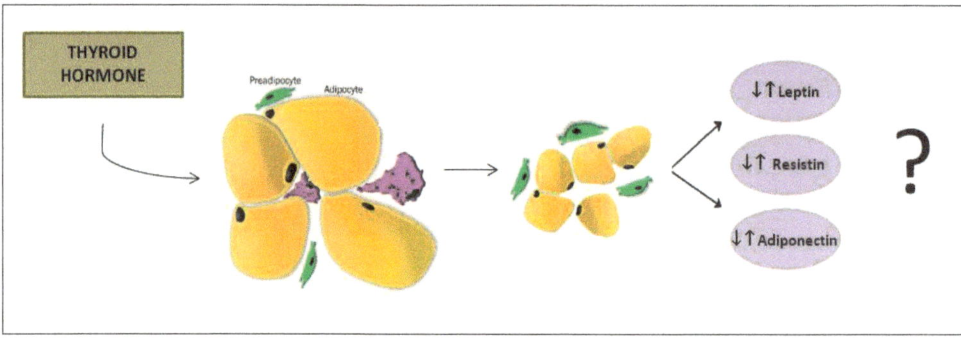

Figure 4. Thyroid hormone may modulate adipokines concentration by regulating adipose tissue metabolism by, *i.e.*, increasing lipid oxidation leading to body fat decreased. The exact influence of thyroid hormone on adipokines remains unclear.

IL-6 - IL-6 levels decrease with weight loss [140-142]. The intracerebroventricular administration of this cytokine can decrease body fat [201]. Association studies between thyroid hormones and IL-6 in weight loss are scarce, but studies in critically patients demonstrated a direct association between decreased T_3 levels and high IL-6 plasma levels, demonstrating that approximately 28% of T_3 fall could be directly related to increased IL-6 [202]. In another study, of 270 patients admitted to intensive care unit, serum T_3, T_4 and IL-6 were measured and again was observed a negative correlation between T_3 and T_4 levels and IL-6 levels, demonstrating that this cytokine could be an important factor associated with decreased circulating thyroid hormones levels [203].

MCP-1 - Chronic inflammation associated with obesity exists in dogs, and it is evident that weight loss decreases this inflammation as observed by decreasing MCP-1 after weight loss [204]. In agreement, Kanda et al. [205] demonstrated that MCP-1 deficient mice have reduced adipose tissue macrophage infiltration. Few studies correlate weight loss and MCP-1 levels, and no data was found regarding weight loss, MCP-1 and thyroid association.

PAI-1 - Weight loss secondary to calorie restriction is associated with reduced PAI-1 activity in adults [206, 207]. However, in children no significant change in PAI-1 levels was observed in 43 obese children after a physical training program [208]. This may be explain by the increase in fibrinolytic activity due to a decrease in PAI-1 antigen levels in obese children after weight loss, and a significant positive correlation was observed between variations in body mass index and variations in PAI-1 levels. Moreover, the largest decrease in PAI-1 levels was observed in the obese children with the highest previous PAI-1 levels [209]. Weight loss induced by a low calorie diet causes a decrease in plasma PAI-1 levels especially among obese individuals [210, 211], and these increase once again if weight is regained [212]. Surgically removing fat confers the same beneficial effect [212]. Antidiabetic drugs such as thiazolidinediones, metformin, and AT1-receptor antagonists reduce adipose PAI-1 expression [211]. Interestingly, waist-to-hip ratio, a reflection of central fat accumulation, has been found in women to be the only independent predictor of circulating PAI-1 activity [213]. In individuals subjected to a calorie restricted diet, PAI-1 levels were more closely related to changes in the central fat deposit than in the subcutaneous fat deposit [214]. Thus, the visceral fat deposit may be importante for the occurrence of increased plasma PAI-1 levels. There is few data available regarding the thyroid hormones and PAI-1. Studies have been focused on serum measurements, in severe hypothyroidism was found decreased PAI-1 levels [215], while in hyperthyroidism some studies show increased [113, 216, 217], other decreased [83, 218] as well as unaffected PAI-1 levels [219, 220].

RAS - Studies with RAS manipulation (deletion) showed that function loss in any single component of RAS tested so far, provides protection from diet-induced obesity and insulin resistance [221-224]. Therefore, RAS seems to play a role in obesity development; however systemic RAS overactivation via gene overexpression or chronic Ang II infusion also induces insulin resistance, but not necessarily obesity [225]. Weight loss in humans results in decreases in circulating components of the RAS [226]. In fact, Engeli et al. [226] suggest that a 5% reduction in body fat mass can reduce meaningfully the RAS in plasma and adipose tissue, which may contribute to reduce blood pressure. Genetic polymorphisms of RAS may also play a role in response to weight loss in obese individuals [227]. Decrease of RAS leads to improvement in insulin sensitivity, blood pressure, and renal function. As RAS interacts with others adipokines, reduction in RAS concentrations followed weight loss may also contributes to improvement of other adipokines levels and, consequently, improve other metabolic disorders [226, 228]. As mentioned, thyroid hormones appear to stimulate expression and synthesis of RAS components [175-177]. However, precise interaction between thyroid hormones and RAS components in weight loss process are scarce in the literature.

Literature on newer adipokines and thyroid disorders is scarce. No data on ASP and weight loss is available and no data on these adipokines and thyroid hormone have been published so far. Future research studying these associations is awaited.

6. The use of TRβ analogues

Thyroid hormone analogues, termed thyromimetics, are molecules with activate signaling pathway property similar to thyroid hormones, sometimes with tissue specificity or by activating a singular pathway stimulated by thyroid hormones, other with less effect, but even with a way close to thyroid hormones. The thyromimetics have a great pharmaceutical potential since they present certain specificity as intracellular signaling that stimulate and thus may have a tissue specific action. However, only the past 20 years, with increasing resolution of three-dimensional models, docking experiments and crystallography models the specificity of thyromimetics has been revealed.

Thyroid hormone is one of the most responsible for metabolism controlling and cell oxygen consumption, affecting growth, cell differentiation and homeostasis control [229]. The thyroid hormone also has specific functions depending on tissue: in liver, controlling lipid metabolism [230-232]; in heart, regulating the calcium handling and the heart rate [233]. As for lipid deposits, the thyroid hormone acts in brown adipose tissue by controlling heating and adaptive thermogenesis during rest [234]. Under high hormone levels conditions in the organism, such as hyperthyroidism, there is an increase in metabolic rate with consequent weight loss and decrease cholesterol serum levels, desirable conditions for metabolic diseases treatment such as obesity [235] and hyperlipidemia [230-232]. In this context, the possible specificity through thyroid homone analogues may lead to desirable effects on adipokines release control and obesity, without the undesirable symptoms on heart or on TSH release.

Thyromimetics can be seen as thyroid hormone derivative or its metabolites derivative. Studies on the direct influence of these analogues on adipokines levels are scarce, but the tissue selectivity shown may be interesting in the study of non thyroid diseases, mainly involving the lipid rate control in adipose tissue and decreased cholesterol by the liver. This selectivity in many cases is related to action pathway stimulate by thyromimetics. Some of them may have actions in liver and adipose tissue through its selective binding to TR-β1, while not lead to effects such as tachycardia since there is no selectivity for the TR-α1 (most expressed isoform in the heart). Thus we can highlight some known thyromimetics and some details of their actions.

The first developed analogue, in the mid-1980s, was 3,5-dibromo-3-pyridazinone-L-thyronine (L-94901) present 50% of binding T_3 to TRs in liver, and only 1.3% effective for cardiac TRs [236, 237]. L-94901 showed an increase of oxygen overall consumption and a reduction in cholesterol serum levels in animal models submitted to low dose, sufficient to prevent cardiotoxic effects, however, also led to lower TSH, T_4 and T_3 plasma levels [236].

An analogue selectivity-related to TR-β1 is 3,5-Dichloro-4-[(4-hydroxy-3-isopropylphenoxy)-phenyl] acetic acid (KB-141), with 10-fold greater ability to reduce the cholesterol rate than increase heart rate [238, 239], stimulating metabolic rate and oxygen consumption [240]. Eprotirome (KB2115) is a thyroid hormone analogue that has a low uptake by non-hepatic tissues. It has preferential selectivity for the TRβ, leading to decreased total cholesterol, LDL and apolipoprotein B levels without apparent side-effects. It showed good results in hypercholesterolemia treatment and associated with statin was effective in reducing atherogenic lipoproteins levels without extra-hepatics effects of thyroid hormone [241].

One of the most widely studied thyroid hormone analogues is 3,5-dimethyl-4-[(4'-hydroxy-3'-isopropylbenzyl)-phenoxy] acetic acid (CG-1), with selectivity for TRβ 10-fold greater than for TR-α. Hypercholesterolemic rats models treated with GC-1 showed decrease in cholesterol, LDL and triglyceride serum levels, without significantly altering heart function or regulated-thyroid hormone gene expression as MHC-HT and α, β-MHC and SERCA2

[242]. The same results were observed with KB-141 use, but with a subtle increase in heart rate. Contributing to cholesterol serum levels reduction by GC-1 is the increased SR-BI expression, a receptor that promotes cholesterol uptake in the liver, stimulating the bile acids production [243]. Deleterious effects absence of GC-1 on cardiac structure and function [244], skeletal muscle and bone mass [245] suggests that GC-1 has potential therapeutic use for metabolic disorders such as obesity and hyperlipidemia [246].

Started studies during the mid-1990s, N-[3,5-dimethyl-4-(4'-hydroxy-3'-isopropylphenoxy)-phenyl] oxamic acid (CGS-23425) was a potent ability to decrease cholesterol in rats and dogs at dose 25 times higher than the minimum for producing lipid lowering effects [247]. In hypercholesterolemic rats, CGS-23425 had the desired effects of decreasing serum LDL and increased apoA1, with a corresponding increase in apoA1 gene transcription by TR-β1 selectively [248].

A thyroid hormone analogue currently in phase II clinical trial is the 3.5-diiodothyropropionic acid (DITPA), with affinity equivalent between TR-α1 and β1 but with 100 times less affinity than T3 [249]. In hypothyroid rats, DITPA improved cardiac performance with half the chronotropic effect and less metabolic stimulation than levothyroxine [250]. In normal volunteers, DITPA does not affect the heart rate or blood pressure, while the serum cholesterol and triglycerides were significantly decreased [251]. Observations have shown that DIPTA exerts its action by stimulating nongenomic pathways stimulated by T3 as the αVβ3 integrin receptor, activating the MAPK cascade and causing similar effects to those seen with GC-1, leading to angiogenesis, indicating that some cardiac effects may be caused by nongenomic pathway activation [252].

Although there are few studies on thyromimetics and adipokines, studies on obesity and lipid lowering show interesting results. Other compounds have been studied as thyroid hormone natural metabolic intermediates: 3-iodothyronamine (T1AM) showed effects on cardiac output, heart hate and decreased body temperature with neuroprotective action; Diiodothyronine-3.5 (T2) with effects such as increased lipid peroxidation and fatty acids oxidation, among others; 3,3 ', 5'-triiodothyronine (rT3) able to initiate actin polymerization; triiodothyroacetic acid (Triac) that increases the metabolic rate and thermogenesis, and one of the few identified analogues able to increase leptin secretion [246]. Like thyromimetics, these natural metabolites, collectively, show body weight and fat mass reduction, while thyromimetics are more specific to reduce cholesterol serum levels, but both have effects saving cardiac activity. However, before they are used in large scale, attention should be paid to non-selectivity presented by natural metabolites, and for TSH suppression showed by thyromimetics, which may lead to undesirable tissue hypothyroidism. Thus, the tissue specificity and selectivity for TR brings a good perspective for thyromimetics, however there is still a long way from its use as therapeutic agent.

7. Final considerations

Adipose tissue produces a wide range of biological active substances, named adipokines, involved in glucose metabolism, lipid metabolism, inflammation, coagulation, blood pressure, and feeding behavior, thus affecting metabolism and function of many organs and tissues including muscle, liver, vasculature, and brain. Obesity cause imbalance in the adipokines production, while the weight loss are able to normalize these changes. In obese, the stabilization of weight loss even in calorie restricted diet has been attributed to the decrease in serum T_3 concentrations, leading to a reduction in metabolic rate. Because of this, and despite not being accepted as an obesity treatment, the administration of thyroid hormones, in isolation or in association with hypocaloric diets, is sometimes used illicitly. The thyroid hormones regulate the energetic balance and act on the adipokines, regulating several genes in adipose tissue. However, the available data on the effects of thyroid hormone on adipokines in obesity or weight loss are conflicting. A clear association has not yet been established between in obesity and calorie restriction in obesity and the effect of thyroid hormone on adipokines, requiring further studies. Despite studies of TRβ analogs show good results, the direct influence of these analogues on adipokines levels are scarce. More research is needed to fully elucidate the exact mechanism of thyroid hormone and its analogues on adipokines in obesity and weight loss.

Author details

Renata de Azevedo Melo Luvizotto*, Sandro José Conde, Miriane de Oliveira,
Maria Teresa De Sibio, Keize Nagamati Jr and Célia Regina Nogueira
Department of Internal Medicine, Botucatu School of Medicine, University of São Paulo State, Botucatu, SP, Brazil

8. References

[1] Hajer G R, van Haeften T W and Visseren F L 2008 Adipose tissue dysfunction in obesity, diabetes, and vascular diseases *Eur Heart J* 29 2959-71

[2] Torres-Leal F L, Fonseca-Alaniz M H, Rogero M M and Tirapegui J 2010 The role of inflamed adipose tissue in the insulin resistance *Cell Biochem Funct* 28 623-31

[3] Kershaw E E and Flier J S 2004 Adipose tissue as an endocrine organ *J Clin Endocrinol Metab* 89 2548-56

[4] Ahima R S, Qi Y, Singhal N S, Jackson M B and Scherer P E 2006 Brain adipocytokine action and metabolic regulation *Diabetes* 55 Suppl 2 S145-54

[5] Ahima R S 2006 Adipose tissue as an endocrine organ *Obesity (Silver Spring)* 14 Suppl 5 242S-9S

[6] van Kruijsdijk R C, van der Wall E and Visseren F L 2009 Obesity and cancer: the role of dysfunctional adipose tissue *Cancer Epidemiol Biomarkers Prev* 18 2569-78

[7] Xu H, Barnes G T, Yang Q, Tan G, Yang D, Chou C J, Sole J, Nichols A, Ross J S, Tartaglia L A and Chen H 2003 Chronic inflammation in fat plays a crucial role in the development of obesity-related insulin resistance *J Clin Invest* 112 1821-30

[8] Skurk T, Alberti-Huber C, Herder C and Hauner H 2007 Relationship between adipocyte size and adipokine expression and secretion *J Clin Endocrinol Metab* 92 1023-33

* Corresponding Authors

[9] Rasouli N and Kern P A 2008 Adipocytokines and the metabolic complications of obesity *J Clin Endocrinol Metab* 93 S64-73

[10] Fontana L 2009 Neuroendocrine factors in the regulation of inflammation: excessive adiposity and calorie restriction *Exp Gerontol* 44 41-5

[11] Miner J L 2004 The adipocyte as an endocrine cell *J Anim Sci* 82 935-41

[12] Kennedy G C 1953 The role of depot fat in the hypothalamic control of food intake in the rat *Proc R Soc Lond B Biol Sci* 140 578-96

[13] Zhang Y, Proenca R, Maffei M, Barone M, Leopold L and Friedman J M 1994 Positional cloning of the mouse obese gene and its human homologue *Nature* 372 425-32

[14] Janeckova R 2001 The role of leptin in human physiology and pathophysiology *Physiol Res* 50 443-59

[15] Havel P J 2001 Peripheral signals conveying metabolic information to the brain: short-term and long-term regulation of food intake and energy homeostasis *Exp Biol Med (Maywood)* 226 963-77

[16] Aronne L J and Thornton-Jones Z D 2007 New targets for obesity pharmacotherapy *Clin Pharmacol Ther* 81 748-52

[17] Klein I and Ojamaa K 2001 Thyroid hormone and the cardiovascular system *N Engl J Med* 344 501-9

[18] Baranowska B, Radzikowska M, Wasilewska-Dziubinska E, Roguski K and Borowiec M 2000 Disturbed release of gastrointestinal peptides in anorexia nervosa and in obesity *Diabetes Obes Metab* 2 99-103

[19] Ramacciotti C E, Coli E, Paoli R, Marazziti D and Dell'Osso L 2003 Serotonergic activity measured by platelet [3H]paroxetine binding in patients with eating disorders *Psychiatry Res* 118 33-8

[20] Kaye W H, Barbarich N C, Putnam K, Gendall K A, Fernstrom J, Fernstrom M, McConaha C W and Kishore A 2003 Anxiolytic effects of acute tryptophan depletion in anorexia nervosa *Int J Eat Disord* 33 257-67; discussion 68-70

[21] Metwally M, Ledger W L and Li T C 2008 Reproductive endocrinology and clinical aspects of obesity in women *Ann N Y Acad Sci* 1127 140-6

[22] Lopez D, Abisambra Socarras J F, Bedi M and Ness G C 2007 Activation of the hepatic LDL receptor promoter by thyroid hormone *Biochim Biophys Acta* 1771 1216-25

[23] Ladenson P W, McCarren M, Morkin E, Edson R G, Shih M C, Warren S R, Barnhill J G, Churby L, Thai H, O'Brien T, Anand I, Warner A, Hattler B, Dunlap M, Erikson J and Goldman S 2010 Effects of the thyromimetic agent diiodothyropropionic acid on body weight, body mass index, and serum lipoproteins: a pilot prospective, randomized, controlled study *J Clin Endocrinol Metab* 95 1349-54

[24] Banks W A and Lebel C R 2002 Strategies for the delivery of leptin to the CNS *J Drug Target* 10 297-308

[25] Niswender K D and Schwartz M W 2003 Insulin and leptin revisited: adiposity signals with overlapping physiological and intracellular signaling capabilities *Front Neuroendocrinol* 24 1-10

[26] Schwartz M W, Woods S C, Porte D, Jr., Seeley R J and Baskin D G 2000 Central nervous system control of food intake *Nature* 404 661-71

[27] Muoio D M and Lynis Dohm G 2002 Peripheral metabolic actions of leptin *Best Pract Res Clin Endocrinol Metab* 16 653-66
[28] Sweeney G 2002 Leptin signalling *Cell Signal* 14 655-63
[29] Moschos S, Chan J L and Mantzoros C S 2002 Leptin and reproduction: a review *Fertil Steril* 77 433-44
[30] Mantzoros C S 2000 Role of leptin in reproduction *Ann N Y Acad Sci* 900 174-83
[31] Schwartz M W, Peskind E, Raskind M, Boyko E J and Porte D, Jr. 1996 Cerebrospinal fluid leptin levels: relationship to plasma levels and to adiposity in humans *Nat Med* 2 589-93
[32] Brannian J D and Hansen K A 2002 Leptin and ovarian folliculogenesis: implications for ovulation induction and ART outcomes *Semin Reprod Med* 20 103-12
[33] Henson M C and Castracane V D 2000 Leptin in pregnancy *Biol Reprod* 63 1219-28
[34] Laird S M, Quinton N D, Anstie B, Li T C and Blakemore A I 2001 Leptin and leptin-binding activity in women with recurrent miscarriage: correlation with pregnancy outcome *Hum Reprod* 16 2008-13
[35] Legradi G, Emerson C H, Ahima R S, Flier J S and Lechan R M 1997 Leptin prevents fasting-induced suppression of prothyrotropin-releasing hormone messenger ribonucleic acid in neurons of the hypothalamic paraventricular nucleus *Endocrinology* 138 2569-76
[36] Sanchez V C, Goldstein J, Stuart R C, Hovanesian V, Huo L, Munzberg H, Friedman T C, Bjorbaek C and Nillni E A 2004 Regulation of hypothalamic prohormone convertases 1 and 2 and effects on processing of prothyrotropin-releasing hormone *J Clin Invest* 114 357-69
[37] Flier J S, Harris M and Hollenberg A N 2000 Leptin, nutrition, and the thyroid: the why, the wherefore, and the wiring *J Clin Invest* 105 859-61
[38] Ahima R S, Prabakaran D, Mantzoros C, Qu D, Lowell B, Maratos-Flier E and Flier J S 1996 Role of leptin in the neuroendocrine response to fasting *Nature* 382 250-2
[39] van der Kroon P H, Boldewijn H and Langeveld-Soeter N 1982 Congenital hypothyroidism in latent obese (ob/ob) mice *Int J Obes* 6 83-90
[40] Mantzoros C S, Ozata M, Negrao A B, Suchard M A, Ziotopoulou M, Caglayan S, Elashoff R M, Cogswell R J, Negro P, Liberty V, Wong M L, Veldhuis J, Ozdemir I C, Gold P W, Flier J S and Licinio J 2001 Synchronicity of frequently sampled thyrotropin (TSH) and leptin concentrations in healthy adults and leptin-deficient subjects: evidence for possible partial TSH regulation by leptin in humans *J Clin Endocrinol Metab* 86 3284-91
[41] Welt C K, Chan J L, Bullen J, Murphy R, Smith P, DePaoli A M, Karalis A and Mantzoros C S 2004 Recombinant human leptin in women with hypothalamic amenorrhea *N Engl J Med* 351 987-97
[42] Rosenbaum M, Goldsmith R, Bloomfield D, Magnano A, Weimer L, Heymsfield S, Gallagher D, Mayer L, Murphy E and Leibel R L 2005 Low-dose leptin reverses skeletal muscle, autonomic, and neuroendocrine adaptations to maintenance of reduced weight *J Clin Invest* 115 3579-86
[43] Dardeno T A, Chou S H, Moon H S, Chamberland J P, Fiorenza C G and Mantzoros C S 2010 Leptin in human physiology and therapeutics *Front Neuroendocrinol* 31 377-93

[44] Banerjee R R and Lazar M A 2003 Resistin: molecular history and prognosis *J Mol Med (Berl)* 81 218-26

[45] Patel L, Buckels A C, Kinghorn I J, Murdock P R, Holbrook J D, Plumpton C, Macphee C H and Smith S A 2003 Resistin is expressed in human macrophages and directly regulated by PPAR gamma activators *Biochem Biophys Res Commun* 300 472-6

[46] Steppan C M, Bailey S T, Bhat S, Brown E J, Banerjee R R, Wright C M, Patel H R, Ahima R S and Lazar M A 2001 The hormone resistin links obesity to diabetes *Nature* 409 307-12

[47] Rajala M W, Qi Y, Patel H R, Takahashi N, Banerjee R, Pajvani U B, Sinha M K, Gingerich R L, Scherer P E and Ahima R S 2004 Regulation of resistin expression and circulating levels in obesity, diabetes, and fasting *Diabetes* 53 1671-9

[48] McTernan P G, McTernan C L, Chetty R, Jenner K, Fisher F M, Lauer M N, Crocker J, Barnett A H and Kumar S 2002 Increased resistin gene and protein expression in human abdominal adipose tissue *J Clin Endocrinol Metab* 87 2407

[49] Maeda K, Okubo K, Shimomura I, Funahashi T, Matsuzawa Y and Matsubara K 1996 cDNA cloning and expression of a novel adipose specific collagen-like factor, apM1 (AdiPose Most abundant Gene transcript 1) *Biochem Biophys Res Commun* 221 286-9

[50] Scherer P E, Williams S, Fogliano M, Baldini G and Lodish H F 1995 A novel serum protein similar to C1q, produced exclusively in adipocytes *J Biol Chem* 270 26746-9

[51] Nakano Y, Tobe T, Choi-Miura N H, Mazda T and Tomita M 1996 Isolation and characterization of GBP28, a novel gelatin-binding protein purified from human plasma *J Biochem* 120 803-12

[52] Hu E, Liang P and Spiegelman B M 1996 AdipoQ is a novel adipose-specific gene dysregulated in obesity *J Biol Chem* 271 10697-703

[53] Chandran M, Phillips S A, Ciaraldi T and Henry R R 2003 Adiponectin: more than just another fat cell hormone? *Diabetes Care* 26 2442-50

[54] Fain J N, Madan A K, Hiler M L, Cheema P and Bahouth S W 2004 Comparison of the release of adipokines by adipose tissue, adipose tissue matrix, and adipocytes from visceral and subcutaneous abdominal adipose tissues of obese humans *Endocrinology* 145 2273-82

[55] Iwahashi H, Funahashi T, Kurokawa N, Sayama K, Fukuda E, Okita K, Imagawa A, Yamagata K, Shimomura I, Miyagawa J I and Matsuzawa Y 2003 Plasma adiponectin levels in women with anorexia nervosa *Horm Metab Res* 35 537-40

[56] Lindsay R S, Walker J D, Havel P J, Hamilton B A, Calder A A and Johnstone F D 2003 Adiponectin is present in cord blood but is unrelated to birth weight *Diabetes Care* 26 2244-9

[57] Yamauchi T, Kamon J, Ito Y, Tsuchida A, Yokomizo T, Kita S, Sugiyama T, Miyagishi M, Hara K, Tsunoda M, Murakami K, Ohteki T, Uchida S, Takekawa S, Waki H, Tsuno N H, Shibata Y, Terauchi Y, Froguel P, Tobe K, Koyasu S, Taira K, Kitamura T, Shimizu T, Nagai R and Kadowaki T 2003 Cloning of adiponectin receptors that mediate antidiabetic metabolic effects *Nature* 423 762-9

[58] Kawanami D, Maemura K, Takeda N, Harada T, Nojiri T, Imai Y, Manabe I, Utsunomiya K and Nagai R 2004 Direct reciprocal effects of resistin and adiponectin on

vascular endothelial cells: a new insight into adipocytokine-endothelial cell interactions *Biochem Biophys Res Commun* 314 415-9

[59] Rajala M W and Scherer P E 2003 Minireview: The adipocyte--at the crossroads of energy homeostasis, inflammation, and atherosclerosis *Endocrinology* 144 3765-73

[60] Kubota N, Terauchi Y, Yamauchi T, Kubota T, Moroi M, Matsui J, Eto K, Yamashita T, Kamon J, Satoh H, Yano W, Froguel P, Nagai R, Kimura S, Kadowaki T and Noda T 2002 Disruption of adiponectin causes insulin resistance and neointimal formation *J Biol Chem* 277 25863-6

[61] Arner P 1995 Differences in lipolysis between human subcutaneous and omental adipose tissues *Ann Med* 27 435-8

[62] Montague C T, Prins J B, Sanders L, Zhang J, Sewter C P, Digby J, Byrne C D and O'Rahilly S 1998 Depot-related gene expression in human subcutaneous and omental adipocytes *Diabetes* 47 1384-91

[63] Ruan H, Miles P D, Ladd C M, Ross K, Golub T R, Olefsky J M and Lodish H F 2002 Profiling gene transcription in vivo reveals adipose tissue as an immediate target of tumor necrosis factor-alpha: implications for insulin resistance *Diabetes* 51 3176-88

[64] Hotamisligil G S 2003 Inflammatory pathways and insulin action *Int J Obes Relat Metab Disord* 27 Suppl 3 S53-5

[65] Lasa M, Gil-Araujo B, Palafox M and Aranda A 2010 Thyroid hormone antagonizes tumor necrosis factor-alpha signaling in pituitary cells through the induction of dual specificity phosphatase 1 *Mol Endocrinol* 24 412-22

[66] Lyon C J, Law R E and Hsueh W A 2003 Minireview: adiposity, inflammation, and atherogenesis *Endocrinology* 144 2195-200

[67] Mohamed-Ali V, Flower L, Sethi J, Hotamisligil G, Gray R, Humphries S E, York D A and Pinkney J 2001 beta-Adrenergic regulation of IL-6 release from adipose tissue: in vivo and in vitro studies *J Clin Endocrinol Metab* 86 5864-9

[68] van Hall G, Steensberg A, Sacchetti M, Fischer C, Keller C, Schjerling P, Hiscock N, Moller K, Saltin B, Febbraio M A and Pedersen B K 2003 Interleukin-6 stimulates lipolysis and fat oxidation in humans *J Clin Endocrinol Metab* 88 3005-10

[69] Rexrode K M, Pradhan A, Manson J E, Buring J E and Ridker P M 2003 Relationship of total and abdominal adiposity with CRP and IL-6 in women *Ann Epidemiol* 13 674-82

[70] De Benedetti F, Alonzi T, Moretta A, Lazzaro D, Costa P, Poli V, Martini A, Ciliberto G and Fattori E 1997 Interleukin 6 causes growth impairment in transgenic mice through a decrease in insulin-like growth factor-I. A model for stunted growth in children with chronic inflammation *J Clin Invest* 99 643-50

[71] Sell H and Eckel J 2007 Monocyte chemotactic protein-1 and its role in insulin resistance *Curr Opin Lipidol* 18 258-62

[72] Mertens I and Van Gaal L F 2002 Obesity, haemostasis and the fibrinolytic system *Obes Rev* 3 85-101

[73] Hsueh W A and Law R 2003 The central role of fat and effect of peroxisome proliferator-activated receptor-gamma on progression of insulin resistance and cardiovascular disease *Am J Cardiol* 92 3J-9J

[74] Van Harmelen V, Reynisdottir S, Cianflone K, Degerman E, Hoffstedt J, Nilsell K, Sniderman A and Arner P 1999 Mechanisms involved in the regulation of free fatty acid

release from isolated human fat cells by acylation-stimulating protein and insulin *J Biol Chem* 274 18243-51
[75] Siani A, Cappuccio F P, Barba G, Trevisan M, Farinaro E, Lacone R, Russo O, Russo P, Mancini M and Strazzullo P 2002 The relationship of waist circumference to blood pressure: the Olivetti Heart Study *Am J Hypertens* 15 780-6
[76] Engeli S, Schling P, Gorzelniak K, Boschmann M, Janke J, Ailhaud G, Teboul M, Massiera F and Sharma A M 2003 The adipose-tissue renin-angiotensin-aldosterone system: role in the metabolic syndrome? *Int J Biochem Cell Biol* 35 807-25
[77] Goossens G H, Blaak E E and van Baak M A 2003 Possible involvement of the adipose tissue renin-angiotensin system in the pathophysiology of obesity and obesity-related disorders *Obes Rev* 4 43-55
[78] Giacchetti G, Faloia E, Mariniello B, Sardu C, Gatti C, Camilloni M A, Guerrieri M and Mantero F 2002 Overexpression of the renin-angiotensin system in human visceral adipose tissue in normal and overweight subjects *Am J Hypertens* 15 381-8
[79] Silvestri E, Schiavo L, Lombardi A and Goglia F 2005 Thyroid hormones as molecular determinants of thermogenesis *Acta Physiol Scand* 184 265-83
[80] Yen P M 2001 Physiological and molecular basis of thyroid hormone action *Physiol Rev* 81 1097-142
[81] Bassett J H, Harvey C B and Williams G R 2003 Mechanisms of thyroid hormone receptor-specific nuclear and extra nuclear actions *Mol Cell Endocrinol* 213 1-11
[82] Feldt-Rasmussen U 2007 Thyroid and leptin *Thyroid* 17 413-9
[83] Pinkney J H, Goodrick S J, Katz J, Johnson A B, Lightman S L, Coppack S W and Mohamed-Ali V 1998 Leptin and the pituitary-thyroid axis: a comparative study in lean, obese, hypothyroid and hyperthyroid subjects *Clin Endocrinol (Oxf)* 49 583-8
[84] Viguerie N, Millet L, Avizou S, Vidal H, Larrouy D and Langin D 2002 Regulation of human adipocyte gene expression by thyroid hormone *J Clin Endocrinol Metab* 87 630-4
[85] Darimont C, Gaillard D, Ailhaud G and Negrel R 1993 Terminal differentiation of mouse preadipocyte cells: adipogenic and antimitogenic role of triiodothyronine *Mol Cell Endocrinol* 98 67-73
[86] Ozata M, Ozdemir I C and Licinio J 1999 Human leptin deficiency caused by a missense mutation: multiple endocrine defects, decreased sympathetic tone, and immune system dysfunction indicate new targets for leptin action, greater central than peripheral resistance to the effects of leptin, and spontaneous correction of leptin-mediated defects *J Clin Endocrinol Metab* 84 3686-95
[87] Considine R V, Sinha M K, Heiman M L, Kriauciunas A, Stephens T W, Nyce M R, Ohannesian J P, Marco C C, McKee L J, Bauer T L and et al. 1996 Serum immunoreactive-leptin concentrations in normal-weight and obese humans *N Engl J Med* 334 292-5
[88] Friedman J M and Halaas J L 1998 Leptin and the regulation of body weight in mammals *Nature* 395 763-70
[89] Montague C T, Farooqi I S, Whitehead J P, Soos M A, Rau H, Wareham N J, Sewter C P, Digby J E, Mohammed S N, Hurst J A, Cheetham C H, Earley A R, Barnett A H, Prins J B and O'Rahilly S 1997 Congenital leptin deficiency is associated with severe early-onset obesity in humans *Nature* 387 903-8

[90] Carlsson B, Lindell K, Gabrielsson B, Karlsson C, Bjarnason R, Westphal O, Karlsson U, Sjostrom L and Carlsson L M 1997 Obese (ob) gene defects are rare in human obesity *Obes Res* 5 30-5
[91] Pelleymounter M A, Cullen M J, Baker M B, Hecht R, Winters D, Boone T and Collins F 1995 Effects of the obese gene product on body weight regulation in ob/ob mice *Science* 269 540-3
[92] Reinehr T, Isa A, de Sousa G, Dieffenbach R and Andler W 2008 Thyroid hormones and their relation to weight status *Horm Res* 70 51-7
[93] Reinehr T and Andler W 2002 Thyroid hormones before and after weight loss in obesity *Arch Dis Child* 87 320-3
[94] Reinehr T, de Sousa G and Andler W 2006 Hyperthyrotropinemia in obese children is reversible after weight loss and is not related to lipids *J Clin Endocrinol Metab* 91 3088-91
[95] Fekete C, Kelly J, Mihaly E, Sarkar S, Rand W M, Legradi G, Emerson C H and Lechan R M 2001 Neuropeptide Y has a central inhibitory action on the hypothalamic-pituitary-thyroid axis *Endocrinology* 142 2606-13
[96] Fekete C, Legradi G, Mihaly E, Tatro J B, Rand W M and Lechan R M 2000 alpha-Melanocyte stimulating hormone prevents fasting-induced suppression of corticotropin-releasing hormone gene expression in the rat hypothalamic paraventricular nucleus *Neurosci Lett* 289 152-6
[97] Legradi G, Emerson C H, Ahima R S, Rand W M, Flier J S and Lechan R M 1998 Arcuate nucleus ablation prevents fasting-induced suppression of ProTRH mRNA in the hypothalamic paraventricular nucleus *Neuroendocrinology* 68 89-97
[98] Kim M S, Small C J, Stanley S A, Morgan D G, Seal L J, Kong W M, Edwards C M, Abusnana S, Sunter D, Ghatei M A and Bloom S R 2000 The central melanocortin system affects the hypothalamo-pituitary thyroid axis and may mediate the effect of leptin *J Clin Invest* 105 1005-11
[99] Seoane L M, Carro E, Tovar S, Casanueva F F and Dieguez C 2000 Regulation of in vivo TSH secretion by leptin *Regul Pept* 92 25-9
[100] Orban Z, Bornstein S R and Chrousos G P 1998 The interaction between leptin and the hypothalamic-pituitary-thyroid axis *Horm Metab Res* 30 231-5
[101] Gibson W T, Farooqi I S, Moreau M, DePaoli A M, Lawrence E, O'Rahilly S and Trussell R A 2004 Congenital leptin deficiency due to homozygosity for the Delta133G mutation: report of another case and evaluation of response to four years of leptin therapy *J Clin Endocrinol Metab* 89 4821-6
[102] Fain J N, Coronel E C, Beauchamp M J and Bahouth S W 1997 Expression of leptin and beta 3-adrenergic receptors in rat adipose tissue in altered thyroid states *Biochem J* 322 (Pt 1) 145-50
[103] Escobar-Morreale H F, Serrano-Gotarredona J, Varela C, Garcia-Robles R and Sancho J M 1997 Circulating leptin concentrations in women with hirsutism *Fertil Steril* 68 898-906
[104] Fain J N and Bahouth S W 1998 Effect of tri-iodothyronine on leptin release and leptin mRNA accumulation in rat adipose tissue *Biochem J* 332 (Pt 2) 361-6

[105] Iossa S, Lionetti L, Mollica M P, Crescenzo R, Barletta A and Liverini G 2001 Fat balance and serum leptin concentrations in normal, hypothyroid, and hyperthyroid rats *Int J Obes Relat Metab Disord* 25 417-25

[106] Syed M A, Thompson M P, Pachucki J and Burmeister L A 1999 The effect of thyroid hormone on size of fat depots accounts for most of the changes in leptin mRNA and serum levels in the rat *Thyroid* 9 503-12

[107] Wang J L, Chinookoswong N, Yin S and Shi Z Q 2000 Calorigenic actions of leptin are additive to, but not dependent on, those of thyroid hormones *Am J Physiol Endocrinol Metab* 279 E1278-85

[108] Luvizotto R A, Conde S J, Sibio M T, Nascimento A F, Lima-Leopoldo A P, Leopoldo A S, Padovani C R, Cicogna A C and Nogueira C R 2010 Administration of physiologic levels of triiodothyronine increases leptin expression in calorie-restricted obese rats, but does not influence weight loss *Metabolism* 59 1-6

[109] Yoshida T, Monkawa T, Hayashi M and Saruta T 1997 Regulation of expression of leptin mRNA and secretion of leptin by thyroid hormone in 3T3-L1 adipocytes *Biochem Biophys Res Commun* 232 822-6

[110] Couillard C, Mauriege P, Imbeault P, Prud'homme D, Nadeau A, Tremblay A, Bouchard C and Despres J P 2000 Hyperleptinemia is more closely associated with adipose cell hypertrophy than with adipose tissue hyperplasia *Int J Obes Relat Metab Disord* 24 782-8

[111] Hamilton B S, Paglia D, Kwan A Y and Deitel M 1995 Increased obese mRNA expression in omental fat cells from massively obese humans *Nat Med* 1 953-6

[112] Kok P, Roelfsema F, Langendonk J G, Frolich M, Burggraaf J, Meinders A E and Pijl H 2005 High circulating thyrotropin levels in obese women are reduced after body weight loss induced by caloric restriction *J Clin Endocrinol Metab* 90 4659-63

[113] Chen M D, Song Y M, Tsou C T, Lin W H and Sheu W H 2000 Leptin concentration and the Zn/Cu ratio in plasma in women with thyroid disorder *Biol Trace Elem Res* 75 99-105

[114] Valcavi R, Zini M, Peino R, Casanueva F F and Dieguez C 1997 Influence of thyroid status on serum immunoreactive leptin levels *J Clin Endocrinol Metab* 82 1632-4

[115] Diekman M J, Romijn J A, Endert E, Sauerwein H and Wiersinga W M 1998 Thyroid hormones modulate serum leptin levels: observations in thyrotoxic and hypothyroid women *Thyroid* 8 1081-6

[116] Sreenan S, Caro J F and Refetoff S 1997 Thyroid dysfunction is not associated with alterations in serum leptin levels *Thyroid* 7 407-9

[117] Matsubara M, Yoshizawa T, Morioka T and Katayose S 2000 Serum leptin and lipids in patients with thyroid dysfunction *J Atheroscler Thromb* 7 50-4

[118] Pinkney J H, Goodrick S J, Katz J R, Johnson A B, Lightman S L, Coppack S W, Medbak S and Mohamed-Ali V 2000 Thyroid and sympathetic influences on plasma leptin in hypothyroidism and hyperthyroidism *Int J Obes Relat Metab Disord* 24 Suppl 2 S165-6

[119] Janowska J, Zahorska-Markiewicz B and Olszanecka-Glinianowicz M 2006 Relationship between serum resistin concentration and proinflammatory cytokines in obese women with impaired and normal glucose tolerance *Metabolism* 55 1495-9

[120] Savage D B, Sewter C P, Klenk E S, Segal D G, Vidal-Puig A, Considine R V and O'Rahilly S 2001 Resistin / Fizz3 expression in relation to obesity and peroxisome proliferator-activated receptor-gamma action in humans *Diabetes* 50 2199-202

[121] Janke J, Engeli S, Gorzelniak K, Luft F C and Sharma A M 2002 Resistin gene expression in human adipocytes is not related to insulin resistance *Obes Res* 10 1-5

[122] Ukkola O 2002 Resistin - a mediator of obesity-associated insulin resistance or an innocent bystander? *Eur J Endocrinol* 147 571-4

[123] Steppan C M and Lazar M A 2004 The current biology of resistin *J Intern Med* 255 439-47

[124] Reilly M P, Lehrke M, Wolfe M L, Rohatgi A, Lazar M A and Rader D J 2005 Resistin is an inflammatory marker of atherosclerosis in humans *Circulation* 111 932-9

[125] Rosenbaum M, Hirsch J, Murphy E and Leibel R L 2000 Effects of changes in body weight on carbohydrate metabolism, catecholamine excretion, and thyroid function *Am J Clin Nutr* 71 1421-32

[126] Krassas G E, Pontikides N, Loustis K, Koliakos G, Constantinidis T and Panidis D 2005 Resistin levels in hyperthyroid patients before and after restoration of thyroid function: relationship with body weight and body composition *Eur J Endocrinol* 153 217-21

[127] Tilg H and Moschen A R 2006 Adipocytokines: mediators linking adipose tissue, inflammation and immunity *Nat Rev Immunol* 6 772-83

[128] Iglesias P, Alvarez Fidalgo P, Codoceo R and Diez J J 2003 Serum concentrations of adipocytokines in patients with hyperthyroidism and hypothyroidism before and after control of thyroid function *Clin Endocrinol (Oxf)* 59 621-9

[129] Nagwa M A, Elhussein A M, Azza M and Abdulhadi N H 2011 Alarming high prevalence of overweight/obesity among Sudanese children *Eur J Clin Nutr* 65 409-11

[130] Nogueiras R, Gualillo O, Caminos J E, Casanueva F F and Dieguez C 2003 Regulation of resistin by gonadal, thyroid hormone, and nutritional status *Obes Res* 11 408-14

[131] Shklyaev S, Aslanidi G, Tennant M, Prima V, Kohlbrenner E, Kroutov V, Campbell-Thompson M, Crawford J, Shek E W, Scarpace P J and Zolotukhin S 2003 Sustained peripheral expression of transgene adiponectin offsets the development of diet-induced obesity in rats *Proc Natl Acad Sci U S A* 100 14217-22

[132] Nedvidkova J, Smitka K, Kopsky V and Hainer V 2005 Adiponectin, an adipocyte-derived protein *Physiol Res* 54 133-40

[133] Aragao C N, Souza L L, Cabanelas A, Oliveira K J and Pazos-Moura C C 2007 Effect of experimental hypo- and hyperthyroidism on serum adiponectin *Metabolism* 56 6-11

[134] Cabanelas A, Cordeiro A, Santos Almeida N A, Monteiro de Paula G S, Coelho V M, Ortiga-Carvalho T M and Pazos-Moura C C 2010 Effect of triiodothyronine on adiponectin expression and leptin release by white adipose tissue of normal rats *Horm Metab Res* 42 254-60

[135] Fruhbeck G, Gomez-Ambrosi J, Muruzabal F J and Burrell M A 2001 The adipocyte: a model for integration of endocrine and metabolic signaling in energy metabolism regulation *Am J Physiol Endocrinol Metab* 280 E827-47

[136] Morin C L, Eckel R H, Marcel T and Pagliassotti M J 1997 High fat diets elevate adipose tissue-derived tumor necrosis factor-alpha activity *Endocrinology* 138 4665-71

[137] Wang S H and Baker J R 2007 The role of apoptosis in thyroid autoimmunity *Thyroid* 17 975-9
[138] Jiskra J, Antosova M, Limanova Z, Telicka Z and Lacinova Z 2009 The relationship between thyroid function, serum monokine induced by interferon gamma and soluble interleukin-2 receptor in thyroid autoimmune diseases *Clin Exp Immunol* 156 211-6
[139] Diez J J, Hernanz A, Medina S, Bayon C and Iglesias P 2002 Serum concentrations of tumour necrosis factor-alpha (TNF-alpha) and soluble TNF-alpha receptor p55 in patients with hypothyroidism and hyperthyroidism before and after normalization of thyroid function *Clin Endocrinol (Oxf)* 57 515-21
[140] Bastard J P, Lagathu C, Caron M and Capeau J 2007 Point-counterpoint: Interleukin-6 does/does not have a beneficial role in insulin sensitivity and glucose homeostasis *J Appl Physiol* 102 821-2; author reply 5
[141] Prins J B 2002 Adipose tissue as an endocrine organ *Best Pract Res Clin Endocrinol Metab* 16 639-51
[142] Berg A H and Scherer P E 2005 Adipose tissue, inflammation, and cardiovascular disease *Circ Res* 96 939-49
[143] Nonogaki K 1999 Obesity: autonomic circuits versus feeding *Nat Med* 5 742-3
[144] Bartalena L, Bogazzi F, Brogioni S, Grasso L and Martino E 1998 Role of cytokines in the pathogenesis of the euthyroid sick syndrome *Eur J Endocrinol* 138 603-14
[145] van Haasteren G A, van der Meer M J, Hermus A R, Linkels E, Klootwijk W, Kaptein E, van Toor H, Sweep C G, Visser T J and de Greef W J 1994 Different effects of continuous infusion of interleukin-1 and interleukin-6 on the hypothalamic-hypophysial-thyroid axis *Endocrinology* 135 1336-45
[146] Lyson K and McCann S M 1991 The effect of interleukin-6 on pituitary hormone release in vivo and in vitro *Neuroendocrinology* 54 262-6
[147] Weisberg S P, McCann D, Desai M, Rosenbaum M, Leibel R L and Ferrante A W, Jr. 2003 Obesity is associated with macrophage accumulation in adipose tissue *J Clin Invest* 112 1796-808
[148] Christiansen T, Richelsen B and Bruun J M 2005 Monocyte chemoattractant protein-1 is produced in isolated adipocytes, associated with adiposity and reduced after weight loss in morbid obese subjects *Int J Obes (Lond)* 29 146-50
[149] Sartipy P and Loskutoff D J 2003 Monocyte chemoattractant protein 1 in obesity and insulin resistance *Proc Natl Acad Sci U S A* 100 7265-70
[150] Takahashi K, Mizuarai S, Araki H, Mashiko S, Ishihara A, Kanatani A, Itadani H and Kotani H 2003 Adiposity elevates plasma MCP-1 levels leading to the increased CD11b-positive monocytes in mice *J Biol Chem* 278 46654-60
[151] Sudi K M, Gallistl S, Trobinger M, Payerl D, Weinhandl G, Muntean W, Aigner R and Borkenstein M H 2001 The influence of weight loss on fibrinolytic and metabolic parameters in obese children and adolescents *J Pediatr Endocrinol Metab* 14 85-94
[152] Alessi M C, Poggi M and Juhan-Vague I 2007 Plasminogen activator inhibitor-1, adipose tissue and insulin resistance *Curr Opin Lipidol* 18 240-5
[153] Horne M K, 3rd, Singh K K, Rosenfeld K G, Wesley R, Skarulis M C, Merryman P K, Cullinane A, Costello R, Patterson A, Eggerman T, Bernstein D M, Pucino F and Csako

G 2004 Is thyroid hormone suppression therapy prothrombotic? *J Clin Endocrinol Metab* 89 4469-73
[154] Erem C, Ersoz H O, Karti S S, Ukinc K, Hacihasanoglu A, Deger O and Telatar M 2002 Blood coagulation and fibrinolysis in patients with hyperthyroidism *J Endocrinol Invest* 25 345-50
[155] Wahrenberg H, Wennlund A and Hoffstedt J 2002 Increased adipose tissue secretion of interleukin-6, but not of leptin, plasminogen activator inhibitor-1 or tumour necrosis factor alpha, in Graves' hyperthyroidism *Eur J Endocrinol* 146 607-11
[156] Biz C, Oliveira C, Mattos A B, Oliveira J, Ribeiro E B, Oller do Nascimento C M and Oyama L M 2009 The effect of thyroid hormones on the white adipose tissue gene expression of PAI-1 and its serum concentration *Braz J Med Biol Res* 42 1163-6
[157] Donnini D, Ambesi-Impiombato F S and Curcio F 2003 Thyrotropin stimulates production of procoagulant and vasodilative factors in human aortic endothelial cells *Thyroid* 13 517-21
[158] Closa D, Gomez-Sierra J M, Latres E, Alemany M and Remesar X 1993 Short-term oscillations of aortic core temperature and thermogenic organ blood flow in the rat *Exp Physiol* 78 243-53
[159] Cianflone K, Xia Z and Chen L Y 2003 Critical review of acylation-stimulating protein physiology in humans and rodents *Biochim Biophys Acta* 1609 127-43
[160] Maslowska M, Vu H, Phelis S, Sniderman A D, Rhode B M, Blank D and Cianflone K 1999 Plasma acylation stimulating protein, adipsin and lipids in non-obese and obese populations *Eur J Clin Invest* 29 679-86
[161] Cianflone K and Maslowska M 1995 Differentiation-induced production of ASP in human adipocytes *Eur J Clin Invest* 25 817-25
[162] Scantlebury T, Maslowska M and Cianflone K 1998 Chylomicron-specific enhancement of acylation stimulating protein and precursor protein C3 production in differentiated human adipocytes *J Biol Chem* 273 20903-9
[163] Maslowska M, Scantlebury T, Germinario R and Cianflone K 1997 Acute in vitro production of acylation stimulating protein in differentiated human adipocytes *J Lipid Res* 38 1-11
[164] Engeli S, Negrel R and Sharma A M 2000 Physiology and pathophysiology of the adipose tissue renin-angiotensin system *Hypertension* 35 1270-7
[165] Rahmouni K, Mark A L, Haynes W G and Sigmund C D 2004 Adipose depot-specific modulation of angiotensinogen gene expression in diet-induced obesity *Am J Physiol Endocrinol Metab* 286 E891-5
[166] Van Harmelen V, Ariapart P, Hoffstedt J, Lundkvist I, Bringman S and Arner P 2000 Increased adipose angiotensinogen gene expression in human obesity *Obes Res* 8 337-41
[167] Goossens G H, Jocken J W, Blaak E E, Schiffers P M, Saris W H and van Baak M A 2007 Endocrine role of the renin-angiotensin system in human adipose tissue and muscle: effect of beta-adrenergic stimulation *Hypertension* 49 542-7
[168] Kalupahana N S, Massiera F, Quignard-Boulange A, Ailhaud G, Voy B H, Wasserman D H and Moustaid-Moussa N 2012 Overproduction of angiotensinogen from adipose tissue induces adipose inflammation, glucose intolerance, and insulin resistance *Obesity (Silver Spring)* 20 48-56

[169] Henegar J R, Bigler S A, Henegar L K, Tyagi S C and Hall J E 2001 Functional and structural changes in the kidney in the early stages of obesity *J Am Soc Nephrol* 12 1211-7
[170] Fischer-Posovszky P, Wabitsch M and Hochberg Z 2007 Endocrinology of adipose tissue - an update *Horm Metab Res* 39 314-21
[171] Hattori Y, Akimoto K, Gross S S, Hattori S and Kasai K 2005 Angiotensin-II-induced oxidative stress elicits hypoadiponectinaemia in rats *Diabetologia* 48 1066-74
[172] Yilmaz M I, Sonmez A, Caglar K, Celik T, Yenicesu M, Eyileten T, Acikel C, Oguz Y, Yavuz I and Vural A 2007 Effect of antihypertensive agents on plasma adiponectin levels in hypertensive patients with metabolic syndrome *Nephrology (Carlton)* 12 147-53
[173] Vargas F, Rodriguez-Gomez I, Vargas-Tendero P, Jimenez E and Montiel M 2012 The renin-angiotensin system in thyroid disorders and its role in cardiovascular and renal manifestations *J Endocrinol* 213 25-36
[174] Barreto-Chaves M L, Carrillo-Sepulveda M A, Carneiro-Ramos M S, Gomes D A and Diniz G P 2010 The crosstalk between thyroid hormones and the Renin-Angiotensin System *Vascul Pharmacol* 52 166-70
[175] Chen K, Carey L C, Valego N K and Rose J C 2007 Thyroid hormone replacement normalizes renal renin and angiotensin receptor expression in thyroidectomized fetal sheep *Am J Physiol Regul Integr Comp Physiol* 293 R701-6
[176] Kobori H, Hayashi M and Saruta T 2001 Thyroid Hormone Stimulates Renin Gene Expression Through the Thyroid Hormone Response Element *Hypertension* 37 99-104
[177] Chen K, Carey L C, Valego N K, Liu J and Rose J C 2005 Thyroid hormone modulates renin and ANG II receptor expression in fetal sheep *Am J Physiol Regul Integr Comp Physiol* 289 R1006-14
[178] Maffei M, Halaas J, Ravussin E, Pratley R E, Lee G H, Zhang Y, Fei H, Kim S, Lallone R, Ranganathan S and et al. 1995 Leptin levels in human and rodent: measurement of plasma leptin and ob RNA in obese and weight-reduced subjects *Nat Med* 1 1155-61
[179] Rolland C, Hession M and Broom I 2011 Effect of weight loss on adipokine levels in obese patients *Diabetes Metab Syndr Obes* 4 315-23
[180] Xenachis C, Samojlik E, Raghuwanshi M P and Kirschner M A 2001 Leptin, insulin and TNF-alpha in weight loss *J Endocrinol Invest* 24 865-70
[181] Varady K A, Tussing L, Bhutani S and Braunschweig C L 2009 Degree of weight loss required to improve adipokine concentrations and decrease fat cell size in severely obese women *Metabolism* 58 1096-101
[182] Mitterberger M C, Mattesich M, Klaver E, Lechner S, Engelhardt T, Larcher L, Pierer G, Piza-Katzer H and Zwerschke W 2010 Adipokine profile and insulin sensitivity in formerly obese women subjected to bariatric surgery or diet-induced long-term caloric restriction *J Gerontol A Biol Sci Med Sci* 65 915-23
[183] Havel P J, Kasim-Karakas S, Mueller W, Johnson P R, Gingerich R L and Stern J S 1996 Relationship of plasma leptin to plasma insulin and adiposity in normal weight and overweight women: effects of dietary fat content and sustained weight loss *J Clin Endocrinol Metab* 81 4406-13
[184] Webber J 2003 Energy balance in obesity *Proc Nutr Soc* 62 539-43
[185] O'Brien P E and Dixon J B 2002 The extent of the problem of obesity *Am J Surg* 184 4S-8S

[186] Aranceta J, Moreno B, Moya M and Anadon A 2009 Prevention of overweight and obesity from a public health perspective *Nutr Rev* 67 Suppl 1 S83-8
[187] Weiss E C, Galuska D A, Khan L K and Serdula M K 2006 Weight-control practices among U.S. adults, 2001-2002 *Am J Prev Med* 31 18-24
[188] Kim K H, Lee K, Moon Y S and Sul H S 2001 A cysteine-rich adipose tissue-specific secretory factor inhibits adipocyte differentiation *J Biol Chem* 276 11252-6
[189] Luvizotto R A, Sibio M T, Olimpio R M, Nascimento A F, Lima-Leopoldo A P, Leopoldo A S, Padovani C R, Cicogna A C and Nogueira C R 2011 Supraphysiological triiodothyronine doses diminish leptin and adiponectin gene expression, but do not alter resistin expression in calorie restricted obese rats *Horm Metab Res* 43 452-7
[190] Faraj M, Havel P J, Phelis S, Blank D, Sniderman A D and Cianflone K 2003 Plasma acylation-stimulating protein, adiponectin, leptin, and ghrelin before and after weight loss induced by gastric bypass surgery in morbidly obese subjects *J Clin Endocrinol Metab* 88 1594-602
[191] Wolfe B E, Jimerson D C, Orlova C and Mantzoros C S 2004 Effect of dieting on plasma leptin, soluble leptin receptor, adiponectin and resistin levels in healthy volunteers *Clin Endocrinol (Oxf)* 61 332-8
[192] Arita Y, Kihara S, Ouchi N, Takahashi M, Maeda K, Miyagawa J, Hotta K, Shimomura I, Nakamura T, Miyaoka K, Kuriyama H, Nishida M, Yamashita S, Okubo K, Matsubara K, Muraguchi M, Ohmoto Y, Funahashi T and Matsuzawa Y 1999 Paradoxical decrease of an adipose-specific protein, adiponectin, in obesity *Biochem Biophys Res Commun* 257 79-83
[193] Hotta K, Funahashi T, Arita Y, Takahashi M, Matsuda M, Okamoto Y, Iwahashi H, Kuriyama H, Ouchi N, Maeda K, Nishida M, Kihara S, Sakai N, Nakajima T, Hasegawa K, Muraguchi M, Ohmoto Y, Nakamura T, Yamashita S, Hanafusa T and Matsuzawa Y 2000 Plasma concentrations of a novel, adipose-specific protein, adiponectin, in type 2 diabetic patients *Arterioscler Thromb Vasc Biol* 20 1595-9
[194] Ahima R S and Flier J S 2000 Adipose tissue as an endocrine organ *Trends Endocrinol Metab* 11 327-32
[195] Santini F, Marsili A, Mammoli C, Valeriano R, Scartabelli G, Pelosini C, Giannetti M, Centoni R, Vitti P and Pinchera A 2004 Serum concentrations of adiponectin and leptin in patients with thyroid dysfunctions *J Endocrinol Invest* 27 RC5-7
[196] Yaturu S, Prado S and Grimes S R 2004 Changes in adipocyte hormones leptin, resistin, and adiponectin in thyroid dysfunction *J Cell Biochem* 93 491-6
[197] Saito T, Kawano T, Ikoma A, Namai K, Tamemoto H, Kawakami M and Ishikawa S E 2005 Elevation of serum adiponectin levels in Basedow disease *Metabolism* 54 1461-6
[198] Kern P A, Ranganathan S, Li C, Wood L and Ranganathan G 2001 Adipose tissue tumor necrosis factor and interleukin-6 expression in human obesity and insulin resistance *Am J Physiol Endocrinol Metab* 280 E745-51
[199] Cancello R, Henegar C, Viguerie N, Taleb S, Poitou C, Rouault C, Coupaye M, Pelloux V, Hugol D, Bouillot J L, Bouloumie A, Barbatelli G, Cinti S, Svensson P A, Barsh G S, Zucker J D, Basdevant A, Langin D and Clement K 2005 Reduction of macrophage infiltration and chemoattractant gene expression changes in white adipose tissue of morbidly obese subjects after surgery-induced weight loss *Diabetes* 54 2277-86

[200] Tevi-Benissan C, Di Costanzo B, Gresenguet G and Belec L 1997 [Overproduction of tumor necrosis factor-alpha in African patients with HIV-1 infection, cachexia and low tri-iodothyronine syndrome] *Med Trop (Mars)* 57 349-52
[201] Wallenius K, Wallenius V, Sunter D, Dickson S L and Jansson J O 2002 Intracerebroventricular interleukin-6 treatment decreases body fat in rats *Biochem Biophys Res Commun* 293 560-5
[202] Lado-Abeal J, Romero A, Castro-Piedras I, Rodriguez-Perez A and Alvarez-Escudero J 2010 Thyroid hormone receptors are down-regulated in skeletal muscle of patients with non-thyroidal illness syndrome secondary to non-septic shock *Eur J Endocrinol* 163 765-73
[203] Davies P H, Black E G, Sheppard M C and Franklyn J A 1996 Relation between serum interleukin-6 and thyroid hormone concentrations in 270 hospital in-patients with non-thyroidal illness *Clin Endocrinol (Oxf)* 44 199-205
[204] Wakshlag J J, Struble A M, Levine C B, Bushey J J, Laflamme D P and Long G M 2011 The effects of weight loss on adipokines and markers of inflammation in dogs *Br J Nutr* 106 Suppl 1 S11-4
[205] Kanda H, Tateya S, Tamori Y, Kotani K, Hiasa K, Kitazawa R, Kitazawa S, Miyachi H, Maeda S, Egashira K and Kasuga M 2006 MCP-1 contributes to macrophage infiltration into adipose tissue, insulin resistance, and hepatic steatosis in obesity *J Clin Invest* 116 1494-505
[206] Mavri A, Stegnar M, Krebs M, Sentocnik J T, Geiger M and Binder B R 1999 Impact of adipose tissue on plasma plasminogen activator inhibitor-1 in dieting obese women *Arterioscler Thromb Vasc Biol* 19 1582-7
[207] Primrose J N, Davies J A, Prentice C R, Hughes R and Johnston D 1992 Reduction in factor VII, fibrinogen and plasminogen activator inhibitor-1 activity after surgical treatment of morbid obesity *Thromb Haemost* 68 396-9
[208] Ferguson M A, White L J, McCoy S, Kim H W, Petty T and Wilsey J 2004 Plasma adiponectin response to acute exercise in healthy subjects *Eur J Appl Physiol* 91 324-9
[209] Estelles A, Dalmau J, Falco C, Berbel O, Castello R, Espana F and Aznar J 2001 Plasma PAI-1 levels in obese children--effect of weight loss and influence of PAI-1 promoter 4G/5G genotype *Thromb Haemost* 86 647-52
[210] Mertens I and Van Gaal L F 2005 Visceral fat as a determinant of fibrinolysis and hemostasis *Semin Vasc Med* 5 48-55
[211] Skurk T and Hauner H 2004 Obesity and impaired fibrinolysis: role of adipose production of plasminogen activator inhibitor-1 *Int J Obes Relat Metab Disord* 28 1357-64
[212] Mutch N J, Wilson H M and Booth N A 2001 Plasminogen activator inhibitor-1 and haemostasis in obesity *Proc Nutr Soc* 60 341-7
[213] Toft I, Bonaa K H, Ingebretsen O C, Nordoy A, Birkeland K I and Jenssen T 1997 Gender differences in the relationships between plasma plasminogen activator inhibitor-1 activity and factors linked to the insulin resistance syndrome in essential hypertension *Arterioscler Thromb Vasc Biol* 17 553-9
[214] Svendsen O L, Hassager C, Christiansen C, Nielsen J D and Winther K 1996 Plasminogen activator inhibitor-1, tissue-type plasminogen activator, and fibrinogen: Effect of dieting with or without exercise in overweight postmenopausal women *Arterioscler Thromb Vasc Biol* 16 381-5

[215] Chadarevian R, Bruckert E, Leenhardt L, Giral P, Ankri A and Turpin G 2001 Components of the fibrinolytic system are differently altered in moderate and severe hypothyroidism *J Clin Endocrinol Metab* 86 732-7

[216] Li Y, Chen H, Tan J, Wang X, Liang H and Sun X 1998 Impaired release of tissue plasminogen activator from the endothelium in Graves' disease - indicator of endothelial dysfunction and reduced fibrinolytic capacity *Eur J Clin Invest* 28 1050-4

[217] Nakamura T, Nagasaka S, Ishikawa S, Hayashi H, Saito T, Kusaka I and Higashiyama M 2000 Association of hyperthyroidism with serum leptin levels *Metabolism* 49 1285-8

[218] Obermayer-Pietsch B M, Fruhauf G E, Lipp R W, Sendlhofer G and Pieber T R 2001 Dissociation of leptin and body weight in hyperthyroid patients after radioiodine treatment *Int J Obes Relat Metab Disord* 25 115-20

[219] Corbetta S, Englaro P, Giambona S, Persani L, Blum W F and Beck-Peccoz P 1997 Lack of effects of circulating thyroid hormone levels on serum leptin concentrations *Eur J Endocrinol* 137 659-63

[220] Leonhardt U, Ritzel U, Schafer G, Becker W and Ramadori G 1998 Serum leptin levels in hypo- and hyperthyroidism *J Endocrinol* 157 75-9

[221] Jayasooriya A P, Mathai M L, Walker L L, Begg D P, Denton D A, Cameron-Smith D, Egan G F, McKinley M J, Rodger P D, Sinclair A J, Wark J D, Weisinger H S, Jois M and Weisinger R S 2008 Mice lacking angiotensin-converting enzyme have increased energy expenditure, with reduced fat mass and improved glucose clearance *Proc Natl Acad Sci U S A* 105 6531-6

[222] Takahashi N, Li F, Hua K, Deng J, Wang C H, Bowers R R, Bartness T J, Kim H S and Harp J B 2007 Increased energy expenditure, dietary fat wasting, and resistance to diet-induced obesity in mice lacking renin *Cell Metab* 6 506-12

[223] Yvan-Charvet L, Even P, Bloch-Faure M, Guerre-Millo M, Moustaid-Moussa N, Ferre P and Quignard-Boulange A 2005 Deletion of the angiotensin type 2 receptor (AT2R) reduces adipose cell size and protects from diet-induced obesity and insulin resistance *Diabetes* 54 991-9

[224] Massiera F, Seydoux J, Geloen A, Quignard-Boulange A, Turban S, Saint-Marc P, Fukamizu A, Negrel R, Ailhaud G and Teboul M 2001 Angiotensinogen-deficient mice exhibit impairment of diet-induced weight gain with alteration in adipose tissue development and increased locomotor activity *Endocrinology* 142 5220-5

[225] Brink M, Wellen J and Delafontaine P 1996 Angiotensin II causes weight loss and decreases circulating insulin-like growth factor I in rats through a pressor-independent mechanism *J Clin Invest* 97 2509-16

[226] Engeli S, Bohnke J, Gorzelniak K, Janke J, Schling P, Bader M, Luft F C and Sharma A M 2005 Weight loss and the renin-angiotensin-aldosterone system *Hypertension* 45 356-62

[227] Hamada T, Kotani K, Nagai N, Tsuzaki K, Sano Y, Matsuoka Y, Fujibayashi M, Kiyohara N, Tanaka S, Yoshimura M, Egawa K, Kitagawa Y, Kiso Y, Moritani T and Sakane N 2011 Genetic polymorphisms of the renin-angiotensin system and obesity-related metabolic changes in response to low-energy diets in obese women *Nutrition* 27 34-9

[228] Masuo K, Mikami H, Ogihara T and Tuck M L 2001 Weight reduction and pharmacologic treatment in obese hypertensives *Am J Hypertens* 14 530-8

[229] Silva J E 1995 Thyroid hormone control of thermogenesis and energy balance *Thyroid* 5 481-92

[230] Engelken S F and Eaton R P 1981 The effects of altered thyroid status on lipid metabolism in the genetic hyperlipemic Zucker rat *Atherosclerosis* 38 177-88

[231] Hansson P, Valdemarsson S and Nilsson-Ehle P 1983 Experimental hyperthyroidism in man: effects on plasma lipoproteins, lipoprotein lipase and hepatic lipase *Horm Metab Res* 15 449-52

[232] Scarabottolo L, Trezzi E, Roma P and Catapano A L 1986 Experimental hypothyroidism modulates the expression of the low density lipoprotein receptor by the liver *Atherosclerosis* 59 329-33

[233] Klein I 1990 Thyroid hormone and the cardiovascular system *Am J Med* 88 631-7

[234] Lowell B B and Spiegelman B M 2000 Towards a molecular understanding of adaptive thermogenesis *Nature* 404 652-60

[235] Loireau A, Autissier N, Dumas P, Michel O, Jorgensen E C and Michel R 1986 Comparative effects of 3,5-dimethyl-3'-isopropyl-L-thyronine (DIMIT) and 3,5-diiodo-3'-isopropylthyroacetic acid (IpTA2) on body weight gain and lipid metabolism in genetically obese Zucker rats *Biochem Pharmacol* 35 1691-6

[236] Underwood A H, Emmett J C, Ellis D, Flynn S B, Leeson P D, Benson G M, Novelli R, Pearce N J and Shah V P 1986 A thyromimetic that decreases plasma cholesterol levels without increasing cardiac activity *Nature* 324 425-9

[237] Leeson P D, Ellis D, Emmett J C, Shah V P, Showell G A and Underwood A H 1988 Thyroid hormone analogues. Synthesis of 3'-substituted 3,5-diiodo-L-thyronines and quantitative structure-activity studies of in vitro and in vivo thyromimetic activities in rat liver and heart *J Med Chem* 31 37-54

[238] Ye L, Li Y L, Mellstrom K, Mellin C, Bladh L G, Koehler K, Garg N, Garcia Collazo A M, Litten C, Husman B, Persson K, Ljunggren J, Grover G, Sleph P G, George R and Malm J 2003 Thyroid receptor ligands. 1. Agonist ligands selective for the thyroid receptor beta1 *J Med Chem* 46 1580-8

[239] Yokoyama N, Walker G N, Main A J, Stanton J L, Morrissey M M, Boehm C, Engle A, Neubert A D, Wasvary J M, Stephan Z F and et al. 1995 Synthesis and structure-activity relationships of oxamic acid and acetic acid derivatives related to L-thyronine *J Med Chem* 38 695-707

[240] Grover G J, Mellstrom K, Ye L, Malm J, Li Y L, Bladh L G, Sleph P G, Smith M A, George R, Vennstrom B, Mookhtiar K, Horvath R, Speelman J, Egan D and Baxter J D 2003 Selective thyroid hormone receptor-beta activation: a strategy for reduction of weight, cholesterol, and lipoprotein (a) with reduced cardiovascular liability *Proc Natl Acad Sci U S A* 100 10067-72

[241] Ladenson P W, Kristensen J D, Ridgway E C, Olsson A G, Carlsson B, Klein I, Baxter J D and Angelin B 2010 Use of the thyroid hormone analogue eprotirome in statin-treated dyslipidemia *N Engl J Med* 362 906-16

[242] Brenta G, Danzi S and Klein I 2007 Potential therapeutic applications of thyroid hormone analogs *Nat Clin Pract Endocrinol Metab* 3 632-40

[243] Johansson L, Rudling M, Scanlan T S, Lundasen T, Webb P, Baxter J, Angelin B and Parini P 2005 Selective thyroid receptor modulation by GC-1 reduces serum lipids and

stimulates steps of reverse cholesterol transport in euthyroid mice *Proc Natl Acad Sci U S A* 102 10297-302

[244] Trost S U, Swanson E, Gloss B, Wang-Iverson D B, Zhang H, Volodarsky T, Grover G J, Baxter J D, Chiellini G, Scanlan T S and Dillmann W H 2000 The thyroid hormone receptor-beta-selective agonist GC-1 differentially affects plasma lipids and cardiac activity *Endocrinology* 141 3057-64

[245] Freitas F R, Moriscot A S, Jorgetti V, Soares A G, Passarelli M, Scanlan T S, Brent G A, Bianco A C and Gouveia C H 2003 Spared bone mass in rats treated with thyroid hormone receptor TR beta-selective compound GC-1 *Am J Physiol Endocrinol Metab* 285 E1135-41

[246] Moreno M, de Lange P, Lombardi A, Silvestri E, Lanni A and Goglia F 2008 Metabolic effects of thyroid hormone derivatives *Thyroid* 18 239-53

[247] Stephan Z F, Yurachek E C, Sharif R, Wasvary J M, Leonards K S, Hu C W, Hintze T H and Steele R E 1996 Demonstration of potent lipid-lowering activity by a thyromimetic agent devoid of cardiovascular and thermogenic effects *Atherosclerosis* 126 53-63

[248] Taylor A H, Stephan Z F, Steele R E and Wong N C 1997 Beneficial effects of a novel thyromimetic on lipoprotein metabolism *Mol Pharmacol* 52 542-7

[249] Pennock G D, Raya T E, Bahl J J, Goldman S and Morkin E 1992 Cardiac effects of 3,5-diiodothyropropionic acid, a thyroid hormone analog with inotropic selectivity *J Pharmacol Exp Ther* 263 163-9

[250] Mahaffey K W, Raya T E, Pennock G D, Morkin E and Goldman S 1995 Left ventricular performance and remodeling in rabbits after myocardial infarction. Effects of a thyroid hormone analogue *Circulation* 91 794-801

[251] Morkin E, Pennock G, Spooner P H, Bahl J J, Underhill Fox K and Goldman S 2002 Pilot studies on the use of 3,5-diiodothyropropionic acid, a thyroid hormone analog, in the treatment of congestive heart failure *Cardiology* 97 218-25

[252] Mousa S A, O'Connor L J, Bergh J J, Davis F B, Scanlan T S and Davis P J 2005 The proangiogenic action of thyroid hormone analogue GC-1 is initiated at an integrin *J Cardiovasc Pharmacol* 46 356-60

Chapter 9

Thyroid Hormone and Energy Expenditure

Einav Yehuda-Shnaidman, Bella Kalderon and Jacob Bar-Tana

Additional information is available at the end of the chapter

1. Introduction

One of the most pronounced effects of Thyroid Hormone (TH, Triiodothyronine (T3), Tetraiodothyronine (T4)) is modulation of metabolic efficiency, energy expenditure and calorigenesis. Thus, hypothyroidism results in decreased energy expenditure and basal metabolic rate accompanied by weight gain and cold intolerance, while hyperthyroidism results in hypermetabolism, weight loss despite increased energy intake, intolerance to heat, loss of lean mass, bone resorption and tachycardia. TH role in modulating metabolic efficiency has been realized for over a century but its cellular mode-of-action remained to be resolved.

2. Mode-of-action of TH in modulating metabolic efficiency

The first description of TH-induced calorigenesis dates to 1895 (1). That initial report has been followed by exhaustive data focusing on the phenomenology of TH action as reflected by hyper- and hypothyroidsm. Thus, high levels of TH in mammals increase oxygen consumption and heat production, resulting in pronounced body weight loss, while low levels of TH are associated with a decrease in metabolic rate and the oxidation of energy substrates (glucose, fatty acids and amino acids), resulting in pronounced increase in body weight (2-6). Although it was widely accepted that TH stimulates calorigenesis by affecting respiration, its cellular mode-of-action remained to be resolved. Hence, exhaustive attempts were made by the scientific community throughout the twentieth century to verify the mechanism(s) involved in modulating metabolic efficiency by TH. Studies by Lardy and Feldott (7) and Hess and Martius (8) have pointed out during the 1950s, that the respiratory control ratio of isolated mitochondria was robustly decreased in the presence of added T4. TH was thus claimed to have direct action at the mitochondrial level by inducing 'mitochondrial uncoupling', namely, dissociating mitochondrial phosphorylation from its substrate oxidation driver. However, the high T4 doses used in those studies implied possible non-physiological activity rather than authentic TH-induced calorigenesis. Later evidence in support of 'mitochondrial uncoupling' has however indicated increase in oxygen consumption and mitochondrial proton permeability of isolated liver mitochondria derived from hyperthyroid rats, with concomitant decrease in mitochondrial phosphate potential and inner mitochondrial membrane (IMM) potential (9, 10). These observations were further corroborated by increase in liver oxidizing capacity of hyperthyroid rats accompanied by decrease in phosphate and cytosolic redox potential (11), while opposite effects were reported in livers of hypothyroid rats (12). Similarly, hepatocytes isolated from T3-treated rats show higher oxygen consumption and lower IMM potential as compared with non-treated control (13-16). Also, a decrease in IMM potential has been reported in TH-treated human lymphocytes or those derived from hyperthyroid patients (17). Overall, these findings suggested that TH indeed induces mitochondrial uncoupling, and that mitochondrial uncoupling may account for the cellular mode-of-action of TH in modulating metabolic efficiency *in vivo*.

Concomitantly with the proposed mitochondrial paradigm of TH, others have proposed non-mitochondrial activity of TH in modulating metabolic efficiency. Thus, TH was claimed to induce "futile substrate cycles", namely, opposing energy-requiring metabolic pathways that proceed simultaneously without generating net products, e.g. glycolysis accompanied by gluconeogenesis, lipolysis with lipogenesis (18, 19), Na+/K+ ATPase with concomitant Na+/K+ leakage (13), or glycerol-3- phosphate/NADH mitochondrial shuttling (20). However, these proposed mechanisms could account for only a small fraction (about 15%) of the total increase in oxygen consumption induced by TH (13, 21), resulting in a mitochondrial paradigm consensus for TH-induced calorigenesis. Yet, the concerned mitochondrial targets still remained enigmatic.

3. Nuclear / mitochondrial targets of TH

TH effects in the mitochondrial context may consist of long-term effects that are dependent upon gene expression, and short-term effects that are refractory to inhibitors of protein synthesis. An important finding reported by Tata et al (2), indicated that the calorigenic activity of TH was abrogated by actinomycin D, implying that TH-induced mitochondrial uncoupling is mediated by modulating nuclear gene expression of respective mitochondrial and/or extra-mitochondrial proteins. These results were followed by extensive studies ((22, 23) and others) that resulted in discovering the nuclear TH receptors (THR) of the superfamily of nuclear receptors, acting as target for TH in modulating nuclear gene expression. THR are encoded by two distinct tissue-dependent genes coding for splice variants of the THRα (brain, bone, heart) and THRβ (liver, brain, heart) isoforms. THR homodimers or heterodimers with other members of the superfamily of nuclear receptors (e.g., retinoic X receptor (RXR)) may interact with TH-response elements (TRE) in the promoters of TH-responsive genes, resulting in transcriptional activation or suppression as function of transcriptional co-activators or co-suppressors recruited by TH/THR to the transcriptional complex of respective promoters. Indeed, TH binding to nuclear THR results in direct transcriptional activation of the expression of genes coding for components of mitochondrial oxidative phosphorylation (i.e. βF1-adenosine triphosphatase, adenine nucleotide translocase (ANT), cytochrome c1) (24, 25), or genes coding for intermediate factors that are indirectly involved in promoting the nuclear expression of mitochondrial components (i.e. nuclear respiratory factors 1 and -2, peroxisome proliferator-activated receptor-γ coactivator-1) (26), or in stimulating mitochondrial DNA replication (27). Hence, TH-induced mitochondrial uncoupling was believed to be accounted for by TH-induced gene expression of respective protein targets that modulate mitochondrial oxidative phosphorylation. In pursuing putative proteins involved in TH-induced mitochondrial uncoupling, a number of candidates have been suggested. These included the adenine nucleotide translocase, proteins that are involved in phosphatidylglycerol and cardiolipin synthesis (28), and in particular the mitochondrial uncoupling proteins (UCPs).

4. Mitochondrial uncoupling proteins (UCPs)

With the discovery of UCPs, extensive efforts were invested in verifying their putative role in mediating the calorigenic effect of TH. In fact, the UCP-coding genes have TREs in their promoters and their expression level is increased by TH treatment, implying their putative role in mediating TH-induced calorigenesis (40). UCP1 (29) mediates proton leak in brown adipose tissue IMM (30), resulting in uncoupling fuel oxidation from ATP synthesis and in dissipating IMM potential as heat. The adaptive thermogenic response of UCP1 is driven by the sympathetic nervous system in response to cold temperature or high-energy cafeteria diet, and could apparently serve as target for TH in modulating total body energy expenditure. Indeed, recent findings by Lopez et al (31) have indicated that TH treatment results in suppressing hypothalamic AMP-activated protein kinase (AMPK) activity, resulting in SNS-induced thermogenic response of brown adipose fat. However, UCP1 is specifically expressed in brown adipose tissue, which is sparse in adult humans. While recent findings point to some brown adipose islets in adult humans (32-37), their putative impact on total body energy expenditure still remains to be resolved. Hence, other proteins that share sequence homology with UCP1(38), including the ubiquitously expressed UCP2, and in particular the UCP3 that is expressed in skeletal muscle, were pursued for their role in mediating TH-induced calorigenesis (39). However, the following observations may indicate that UCP2 and UCP3 may not account for TH-induced mitochondrial uncoupling (41). Thus, findings suggest that UCP2/3 do not contribute to adaptive thermogenesis (42), but may have a role in ROS signaling (43) and/or in exporting fatty acid anions from the mitochondrial matrix (44). Also, the expression of liver UCP2/3 proteins is restricted to Kupffer cells, implying that the uncoupling effect of TH in liver parenchymal cells is not due to UCPs. Most importantly, UCP3 knock-out mice are lean and show normal response to TH (45), leaving unresolved the specific proteins that may mediate TH metabolic effects in the mitochondrial context.

5. Mitochondrial permeability transition pore (PTP)

In analogy to UCPs, mitochondria consist of Permeability Transition Pores (PTP) (46-50) located at the contact sites of the inner (IMM) and outer (OMM) mitochondrial membranes. The molecular composition and structure of mitochondrial PTP still remains to be resolved. The current model of PTP consists of the integral proteins ANT (in the IMM), the voltage-dependent anion channel (VDAC, in the OMM), cyclophylin D (CypD, in the mitochondrial matrix) and the Bcl2 family of proteins (in the OMM). PTP gating may present itself in definitive or transient modes, differing in reversibility and synchronization (51, 52). Definitive synchronized PTP gating is induced by intramitochondrial Ca^{+2} load (53), and is enhanced by oxidative stress, depletion of adenine nucleotides, increased inorganic phosphate, increased matrix pH, and depolarization of the IMM (54-56). This opening/gating mode results in high-conductance PTP (HC-PTP), extensive depolarization of the IMM (~70% decrease in IMM potential), rapid passage of ions and solutes of less than 1500 Da across the IMM, and mitochondrial swelling. These may lead to rupture of the OMM, release of mitochondrial proapoptotic proteins (such as cytochrome c, apoptotic intrinsic factor), followed by programmed cell death/apoptosis (57). Alternatively, spontaneous, non-synchronized, transient/flickering PTP gating due to cyclic opening and closure of individual PTP channels may result in reversible and limited depolarization of the IMM (~30% decrease in IMM potential), moderate decrease in proton motive force, and passage of solutes of less than 300 Da, accompanied by mitochondrial contraction rather than swelling (58-63). Most importantly, in contrast to the irreversible proapoptotic depolarization inflicted by definitive PTP gating, transient low conductance PTP (LC-PTP) gating is innocuous and reversible, leading to mild mitochondrial uncoupling. These findings may indicate that LC-PTP may serve as mitochondrial target of TH in inducing physiological mitochondrial uncoupling and calorigenesis.

6. Mitochondrial PTP gating by TH

In testing the role played by PTP gating in TH action, a straightforward approach would be to examine whether TH-induced uncoupling is inhibited by the PTP specific inhibitor, cyclosporin A (CSA). CSA acts as a potent inhibitor of PTP gating due to its binding to CypD, resulting in interfering with CypD interaction with PTP-ANT (64, 65). Indeed, TH-induced lowering of mitochondrial membrane potential and proton gradient followed by mitochondrial swelling are all eliminated by added CSA, pointing to PTP involvement in TH mitochondrial activity (66, 67). In addition, liver mitochondria of hypothyroid rats show decrease in mitochondrial Ca^{+2} efflux, swelling and protein release, being restored by TH treatment (68-70). Furthermore, TH treatment of Jurkat cells induces induce LC-PTP gating (71), implying that mitochondrial PTP may serve as target for TH in inducing mitochondrial uncoupling. However, as described below, TH activity in gating PTP is not accounted for by modulating gene expression of structural components of mitochondrial PTP.

Adenine Nucleotide Translocase (ANT): ANT is a central player in oxidative phosphorylation due to its primary function in translocating adenine-nucleotides via the IMM. ANT function in the PTP context has been verified by its direct association with CypD and VDAC (72), as well as by PTP gating being activated and inhibited by the ANT ligands Atractylate and Bongrekic acid, respectively (73). Moreover, ANT/CypD/VDAC- reconstituted liposomes show PTP characteristics in terms of sensitivity to Ca^{+2}, CSA and ANT ligands ((74, 75) but see also (76)). Also, over-expression of ANT isoforms (ANT1, ANT3) promotes apoptosis, being inhibited by CSA (77, 78). Moreover, ANT expression levels affect mitochondrial IMM potential, with high ANT levels resulting in IMM depolarization and mitochondrial proton leak (71, 77, 79). Hence, in light of ANT structural and regulatory functions in the PTP context, and since the expression level of ANT2, the only ANT isoform expressed in liver, is increased in hyperthyroidism and decreased by hypothyroidism (80), TH-induced ANT expression could apparently account for liver TH-induced LC-PTP gating. However, over-expression of ANT2 in HeLa cell line or in rat primary hepatocytes resulted in extensive mitochondrial depolarization that was not inhibited by CSA (71), implying the formation of PTP-nonrelated ANT channels (81), or of CSA-insensitive PTP (82). Lack of an obligatory linkage between PTP and ANT conforms to other findings pointing to PTP gating by proapoptotic ligands in liver cells or isolated mitochondria that lack ANT (76).

Cyclophilin D (CypD): CypD is a member of the family of peptidyl-prolyl cis-trans isomerases (PPIase) (83). The CypD protein contains a mitochondrial-targeting sequence that directs it specifically to the mitochondrial matrix. The link between CypD and PTP has been verified by CypD direct association with ANT (72) as well as by CSA inhibition of PTP gating due to its interaction and inhibition of CypD activity (64, 65, 84). Moreover, PTP opening by Ca^{+2} and oxidative stress was enhanced in isolated mitochondria of neurons over-expressing CypD (85), while CSA-sensitive PTP opening was abrogated in isolated mitochondria of CypD knock-out mice (86). These CypD characteristics may indicate that CypD could apparently serve as protein target of TH in inducing PTP opening and mitochondrial uncoupling. Indeed, liver mitochondria of hyperthyroid rats show increased expression of CypD as well as its PPIase enzymatic activity (71), while opposite effects prevailed in liver mitochondria isolated from hypothyroid rats. However, over-expression of CypD in HeLa cell line, or in rat primary hepatocytes, resulted in mitochondrial hyperpolarization rather than PTP opening (71, 87). Moreover, over-expressed CypD was found to desensitize cells to apoptotic stimuli or to protect cells from mitochondrial depolarization and apoptosis induced by over-expression of ANT1 (77, 78). Hence, TH-induced CypD expression may not account for TH-induced PTP gating and calorigenesis. CypD induction by TH may reflect TH activity in inducing peptidyl-prolyl cis-trans isomerase activity and protein folding rather than PTP opening (88).

Voltage Dependent Anion Channel (VDAC): VDAC is a highly abundant protein of the OMM. Its primary function consists of exchanging anions between the cytosol and the inter-membrane mitochondrial space (89). Previous findings have indicated its putative role in gating mitochondrial PTP (90-94). However, its expression level is not changed by *in vivo* TH treatment (71), excluding VDAC from being a molecular target of TH in inducing mitochondrial uncoupling.

7. Modulation of Bcl2-family proteins by TH

The family of Bcl2 proteins consists of more than 20 proteins that were extensively studied in terms of their role in cell death (95). The Bcl2 family is grouped into two main subfamilies: proapoptotic proteins (e.g. Bax, Bak, and others) and anti-apoptotic proteins (e.g. Bcl2), which promote or inhibit PTP gating, respectively (95-97). Bcl2-family proteins may directly interact with PTP components such as ANT (98-100) or VDAC (101), and when over-expressed or added to isolated mitochondria may specifically induce (e.g. Bax and Bak) (102-104) or antagonize (e.g. Bcl2) (105) PTP gating. Similarly, depletion of proapoptotic Bax or Bak results in failure of PTP gating (98, 105, 106), whereas Bcl2 inactivation results in definitive PTP gating triggered by oxidative stress (107). Thus, mitochondrial Bcl2-family proteins and their respective heterodimers (e.g., Bax/Bcl2, Bad/Bcl2) may apparently serve as candidate targets of TH in inducing mitochondrial uncoupling (108-110). Indeed, TH-induced PTP gating is accompanied by increase in mitochondrial Bax and Bak, together with decrease in mitochondrial Bcl2 content, whereas hypothyroidism results in opposite effects that are reversed by TH (71). Modulation of the mitochondrial content of Bcl2 proteins by TH is due to their specific translocation in/out of mitochondria, rather than reflecting modulation of their expression and total cellular content. Amplifying the ratio of mitochondrial pro- vs. anti-apoptotic proteins, results in robust decrease in mitochondrial Bax/Bcl2 heterodimer with concomitant increase in free Bax, leading to PTP gating by free mitochondrial Bax (111). Indeed, over-expression of Bcl2 protects against TH-induced mitochondrial PTP gating (71), implying that depletion of mitochondrial Bcl2 by TH may account for TH-induced mitochondrial uncoupling.

8. Extra-mitochondrial upstream signals that induce TH-induced PTP gating mediated by Bcl2-family proteins

Since Bcl2-Bax hetrodimerization may depend on Bcl2(S70) phosphorylation state (112), mitochondrial Bcl2 depletion by T3 was further verified in terms of Bcl2(S70) phosphorylation profile. Indeed, concomitantly with decrease in mitochondrial Bcl2, T3 treatment results in decreased phosphorylation of monomeric mitochondrial Bcl2(S70) as well as of Bcl2(S70)-Bax heterodimer (113), indicating that mitochondrial Bcl2 depletion may reflect Bcl2(S70) dephosphorylation by TH. In pursuing kinases (e.g. PKA, PKC) or phosphatases (e.g. PP2A, PP2B/Calcineurin) reported to be involved in Bcl2(S70) phosphorylation (112, 114), neither PKA, PKC nor PP2A were found to mediate phosphorylation/dephosphorylation of Bcl2(S70) by TH (113). In contrast, dephosphorylation of Bcl2(S70) and the depletion of mitochondrial Bcl2 protein by T3 are both reversed by the FK506 inhibitor of PP2B, indicating that the TH effect may be mediated by activation of PP2B (113). Furthermore, added FK506 blocksT3-induced opening of PTP, indicating that dephosphorylation of Bcl2(S70) and its mitochondrial depletion by T3-activated PP2B may account for mitochondrial PTP opening by TH. Since TH-induced PP2B activation was not accompanied by increase in PP2B expression, PP2B activation was further pursued by searching for TH-induced increase in cytosolic Ca^{+2} (113). Indeed, Ca^{+2} -activated PP2B has previously been reported to bind and dephosphorylate Bcl2(S70) (115, 116). Most importantly, T3 treatment resulted in pronounced increase in Ca^{+2}, while Ca^{+2} chelation by BAPTA resulted in abrogating LC-PTP gating by TH, indicating that TH-induced PP2B activity involved mobilization of intracellular Ca^{+2} (113). Indeed, T3-induced mobilization of intracellular Ca^{+2} has recently been reported to mediate a variety of non-genomic effects of TH (117, 118).

The dynamic equilibrium between cytosolic Ca^{+2} ($[Ca^{+2}]c$) and endoplasmic reticulum (ER) Ca^{+2} ($[Ca^{+2}]ER$) is maintained by an interplay between the inositol 1,4,5-trisphosphate receptor (IP3R1) and the sarcoplasmic Ca^{+2} ATPase (SERCA) that catalyzes ER Ca^{+2} efflux and influx, respectively (119). IP3R1 is activated by binding of the IP3 ligand and may further be modulated by its phosphorylation by PKA, PKC or CaMKII, its dephosphorylation by PP2B, or by its association with one or more of about 50 proteins, including FKBP12 or Bcl2 (120, 121). The putative role played by IP3R1 in TH-induced PTP gating was evaluated by verifying the effect of TH in cells lacking IP3R1 (113). Thus, PTP opening, dephosphorylation of mitochondrial Bcl2(S70) and depletion of mitochondrial Bcl2 are all abrogated in cells lacking IP3R1, indicating that IP3R1 is indeed required for TH-induced mitochondrial uncoupling. Similarly, T3 is ineffective in increasing $[Ca^{+2}]c$ upon inhibition of IP3R1 by 2APB, indicating a specific requirement for IP3R1 activity in modulating $[Ca^{+2}]c$ by TH. Furthermore, T3-induced gating of IP3R1 is accounted for by both, increase in IP3R1 expression and protein levels, complemented by IP3R1 truncation into channel-only isoforms. Truncated IP3R1 isoforms have been reported to serve as channel-only peptides capable of carrying out $[Ca^{+2}]ER$ efflux in the absence of added IP3 (122-126). IP3R1 truncation by TH may reflect TH activation of IP3R1 proteases that remain to be further verified. The IP3R1 / PP2B crosstalk in mediating TH-induced PTP gating is supported by constitutive PP2B-induced PTP gating under conditions of suppressing IP3R1 expression by siRNA (127). Hence, PP2B is acting downstream to TH-induced IP3R1, and is obligatory as well as sufficient in mediating PTP by $[Ca^{+2}]c$.

Over all, TH-induced expression of the IP3R1 channel accompanied by its truncation is proposed to result in $[Ca^{+2}]ER$ efflux, increase in $[Ca^{+2}]c$ and $[Ca^{+2}]c$-activated PP2B, followed by dephosphorylation of mitochondrial Bcl2(S70) with concomitant decrease in mitochondrial Bcl2 protein levels and increase in mitochondrial free Bax (Scheme 1). The decrease in mitochondrial Bcl2 and/or the respective increase in mitochondrial free Bax may initiate and promote variable PTP gating, resulting in physiological LC-PTP–induced calorigenesis. LC-PTP gating may drift to HC-PTP–induced apoptosis as function of additional prevailing conditions that may affect mitochondrial permeability transition.

9. Thyromimetic agents and energy expenditure

Increase in energy expenditure by TH has long been considered for treating obesity. Indeed, treating obesity by thyroid extracts was quite popular throughout the 20th century and well into the 1970s, being later abandoned due to severe side effects consisting of cardiac dysrhythmias, bone resorption / osteoporosis, electrolyte disturbances, and loss of lean body mass (128). Thus, a final ruling warning against the use of thyroid preparations for the treatment of obesity of euthyroid subjects has been issued by the FDA on 1978. Similarly to TH, treating obesity by uncoupling of mitochondrial oxidative phosphorylation by 2,4-dinitrophenol (DNP) has been introduced on 1933, but abandoned on 1938 due to fatal hyperthermia (129).

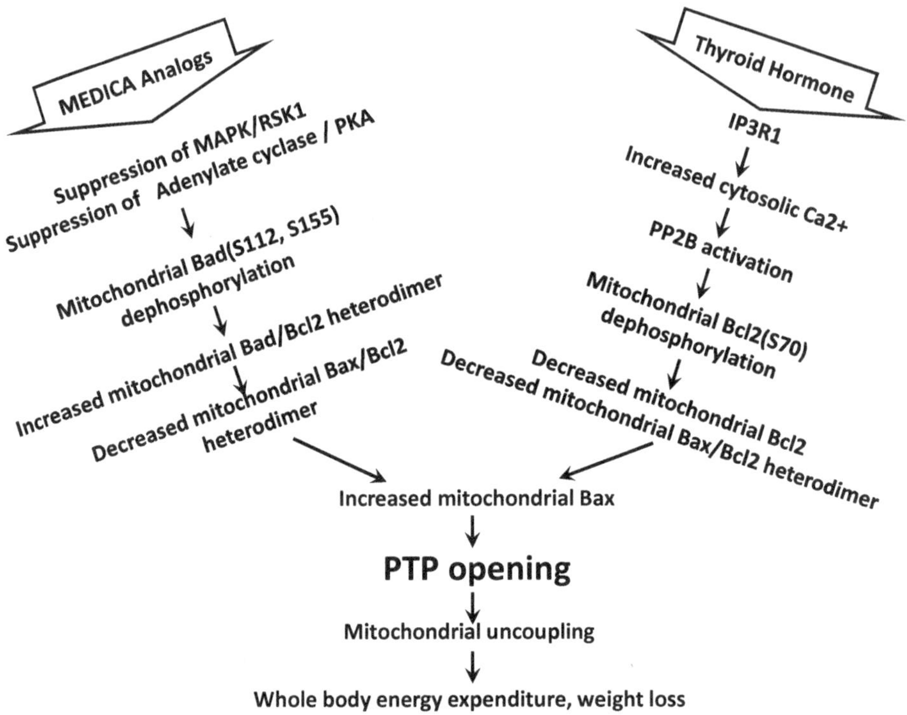

Scheme 1. PTP-induced calorigenesis by Thyroid Hormone and MEDICA Analogs

These early attempts were followed by rational drug design of synthetic structural analogs of TH that may avoid the lethal chronotropic cardiac effects of TH, while maintaining the beneficial effects of TH in the context of diseases of the Metabolic Syndrome (130, 131). Most efforts in that direction were invested in designing thyromimetics that selectively target the liver TH-receptor isoforms (THRβ) while avoiding the heart isoforms (THRα). Tissue selectivity has been further pursued by designing thyromimetics that undergo selective hepatic uptake. These efforts have mainly resulted in thyromimetics effective in treating dyslipidemia, due to increased expression of hepatic LDL-receptors together with CYP7A1 / 7-alpha-cholesterol hydroxylase, resulting in enhancing hepatic uptake of LDL-cholesterol and its conversion into bile. Liver-specific thyromimetics were further found to induce the expression of the hepatic scavenger receptor SR-B1 that mediates reverse cholesterol transport. However, in contrast to the advances made in designing hypolipidemic thyromimetics, the efficacy of thyromimetics in treating obesity and obesity-induced diabetes type 2 still remains to be verified. Moreover, the use of thyromimetics for treating diseases of the Metabolic Syndrome involves potential harmful risks due to: a. The partial selectivity of thyromimetics for hepatic THRβ, resulting in positive chronotropic effects as well as enhanced bone and muscle catabolism induced by high-dose. Hence, the safety of hypolipidemic thyromimetics still remains to be verified in subjects suffering from congestive heart failure or coronary heart disease. b. Since THRβ regulates the feedback loop of hypothalamic TSH, thyromimetics may suppress the production of endogenous TH, resulting in combined hypo- and hyperthyroidsm. These limitations, combined with our present view of the mode-of-action of TH in the mitochondrial context, may however point to an alternative strategy, namely synthesizing thyromimetics that may directly target mitochondrial PTP while avoiding the TH/THR transduction pathway altogether.

Long chain fatty acids (LCFA) have long been shown to induce mitochondrial uncoupling due to their protonophoric activity (81, 132) and/or PTP gating ((51, 133), and ref therein), implying a potential mitochondrial thyromimetic activity. However, the uncoupling activity of LCFA is confounded by their dual role as putative uncouplers of oxidative phosphorylation and as substrates for oxidation or esterification. MEDICA analogs consist of long chain dioic acids (HOOC-C(α')-C(β')-(CH2)n-C(β)-C(α)-COOH (n=10-14)) that are substituted in the $\alpha\alpha'$ or $\beta\beta'$ carbons (134). MEDICA analogs may be thioesterified endogenously into their respective mono acyl-CoA thioesters (135), however, they are not esterified into lipids nor β-oxidized, thus dissociating between the substrate role and the putative uncoupling activity of natural LCFA.

Similarly to TH, MEDICA analogs induce calorigenesis in animal models *in vivo*. Thus, treatment of rats with MEDICA analogs results in an increase in oxygen consumption accompanied by a decrease in liver mitochondrial phosphate potential and cytosolic redox potential, reflecting mitochondrial uncoupling *in vivo* (136). Furthermore, treatment of obese leptin receptor-deficient rats (*e.g.* Zucker, cp/cp) with MEDICA analogs results in increased oxygen consumption and food consumption together with weight loss, implying increased total body energy expenditure (137, 138). Also, the non-protonophoric mitochondrial activity of MEDICA analogs is similar to that of TH (71), in terms of promoting CSA-sensitive decrease in phosphate and redox potentials with concomitant increase in oxygen consumption in cultured cells as well as *in vivo* (11, 16, 67, 139, 140), indicating that both MEDICA analogs and TH do converge onto LC/HC-PTP gating (11, 71). Indeed, similarly to TH, PTP gating by MEDICA analogs is mediated by modulating the profile of mitochondrial Bcl2-family proteins, resulting in decrease in mitochondrial Bcl2-Bax heterodimer with concomitant increase in mitochondrial free Bax (71, 113). However, different transduction pathways are involved in modulating the mitochondrial content of free Bax by TH or MEDICA analogs. Thus, dissociation of the Bcl2-Bax heterodimer by TH is driven by dephosphorylation of Bcl2(Ser-70) by T3-activated PP2B (113), whereas dissociation of the Bcl2/Bax heterodimer by MEDICA analogs is driven by dephosphorylation of Bad(Ser-112, Ser-155) (141). The decrease in phosphorylated Bad(Ser-112, Ser-155) results in its decreased binding to14-3-3 followed by its increased binding to mitochondrial Bcl2, resulting in Bax displacement and PTP gating (142, 143). Decrease in phosphorylated Bad by MEDICA analogs is due to suppression of the Raf1/MAPK/RSK1 and the adenylate cyclase/PKA transduction pathways, and their respective downstream targets Bad(Ser-112) and Bad(Ser-155) (141). Hence, the TH and MEDICA transduction pathways converge at their downstream Bax target but diverge upstream of the Bcl2/Bax heterodimer (Scheme 1). LC-PTP gating by MEDICA analogs may account for their thyromimetic calorigenic activity in *vivo*.

10. Conclusion

Energy expenditure by TH has long been realized to be accounted for by uncoupling of mitochondrial oxidative phosphorylation. However, the mode-of-action of TH in promoting mitochondrial uncoupling remained elusive. Mitochondrial uncoupling by TH is transduced by TH-induced gating of mitochondrial PTP due to modulating its Bcl2-family proteins. This mode-of-action underscores the physiological aspects of mitochondrial PTP in modulating metabolic rate, in contrast to most previous studies that analyzed mitochondrial PTP in its apoptotic context. TH-induced gating of mitochondrial PTP may offer a whole new dimension of developing novel anti-obesity drugs that promote weight loss by targeting mitochondrial PTP.

Author details

Einav Yehuda-Shnaidman, Bella Kalderon and Jacob Bar-Tana
Human Nutrition and Metabolism, Hebrew University Medical School, Jerusalem, Israel

11. References

[1] 1. Mittheilung K M-LS. Uiiber den respiratorischen Gaswechsel unter dem Einfluss der Thvreoidea so wie unter verschiedenen pathologische Zustandem. Berlin Klin Wochenschr. 1895;32:650-6.

[2] Tata JR, Ernster L, Lindberg O. Control of basal metabolic rate by thyroid hormones and cellular function. Nature. 1962 Mar 17;193:1058-60.

[3] Tata JR, Ernster L, Lindberg O, Arrhenius E, Pedersen S, Hedman R. The action of thyroid hormones at the cell level. Biochem J. 1963 Mar;86:408-28.

[4] Krotkiewski M. Thyroid hormones in the pathogenesis and treatment of obesity. Eur J Pharmacol. 2002 Apr 12;440(2-3):85-98.

[5] Brunova J, Bruna J, Joubert G, Koning M. Weight gain in patients after therapy for hyperthyroidism. S Afr Med J. 2003 Jul;93(7):529-31.

[6] Tata JR. The road to nuclear receptors of thyroid hormone. Biochim Biophys Acta. 2012 Mar 17.

[7] Lardy HA, Feldott G. Metabolic effects of thyroxine in vitro. Ann N Y Acad Sci. 1951 Dec;54(4):636-48.

[8] Hess B, Martius C. The mode of action of thyroxin. Arch Biochem Biophys. 1951 Oct;33(3):486-7.

[9] Hafner RP, Nobes CD, McGown AD, Brand MD. Altered relationship between protonmotive force and respiration rate in non-phosphorylating liver mitochondria isolated from rats of different thyroid hormone status. Eur J Biochem. 1988 Dec 15;178(2):511-8.

[10] Brand MD, Steverding D, Kadenbach B, Stevenson PM, Hafner RP. The mechanism of the increase in mitochondrial proton permeability induced by thyroid hormones. Eur J Biochem. 1992 Jun 15;206(3):775-81.

[11] Kalderon B, Hertz R, Bar-Tana J. Effect of thyroid hormone treatment on redox and phosphate potentials in rat liver. Endocrinology. 1992 Jul;131(1):400-7.

[12] Pehowich DJ. Thyroid hormone status and membrane n-3 fatty acid content influence mitochondrial proton leak. Biochim Biophys Acta. 1999 Apr 21;1411(1):192-200.

[13] Nobes CD, Lakin-Thomas PL, Brand MD. The contribution of ATP turnover by the Na+/K+-ATPase to the rate of respiration of hepatocytes. Effects of thyroid status and fatty acids. Biochim Biophys Acta. 1989 Sep 28;976(2-3):241-5.

[14] Shears SB, Bronk JR. The influence of thyroxine administered in vivo on the transmembrane protonic electrochemical potential difference in rat liver mitochondria. Biochem J. 1979 Feb 15;178(2):505-7.

[15] Gregory RB, Berry MN. The administration of triiodothyronine to rats results in a lowering of the mitochondrial membrane potential in isolated hepatocytes. Biochim Biophys Acta. 1991 Dec 3;1133(1):89-94.

[16] Harper ME, Brand MD. The quantitative contributions of mitochondrial proton leak and ATP turnover reactions to the changed respiration rates of hepatocytes from rats of different thyroid status. J Biol Chem. 1993 Jul 15;268(20):14850-60.

[17] Mihara S, Suzuki N, Wakisaka S, Suzuki S, Sekita N, Yamamoto S, et al. Effects of thyroid hormones on apoptotic cell death of human lymphocytes. J Clin Endocrinol Metab. 1999 Apr;84(4):1378-85.

[18] Shulman GI, Ladenson PW, Wolfe MH, Ridgway EC, Wolfe RR. Substrate cycling between gluconeogenesis and glycolysis in euthyroid, hypothyroid, and hyperthyroid man. J Clin Invest. 1985 Aug;76(2):757-64.

[19] Freake HC, Oppenheimer JH. Thermogenesis and thyroid function. Annu Rev Nutr. 1995;15:263-91.

[20] Muller MJ, Seitz HJ. Rapid and direct stimulation of hepatic gluconeogenesis by L-triiodothyronine (T3) in the isolated-perfused rat liver. Life Sci. 1980 Sep 8;27(10):827-35.

[21] Sestoft L. Metabolic aspects of the calorigenic effect of thyroid hormone in mammals. Clin Endocrinol (Oxf). 1980 Nov;13(5):489-506.

[22] Oppenheimer JH, Koerner D, Schwartz HL, Surks MI. Specific nuclear triiodothyronine binding sites in rat liver and kidney. J Clin Endocrinol Metab. 1972 Aug;35(2):330-3.

[23] Samuels HH, Tsai JS. Thyroid hormone action in cell culture: domonstration of nuclear receptors in intact cells and isolated nuclei. Proc Natl Acad Sci U S A. 1973 Dec;70(12):3488-92.

[24] Li R, Luciakova K, Zaid A, Betina S, Fridell E, Nelson BD. Thyroid hormone activates transcription from the promoter regions of some human nuclear-encoded genes of the oxidative phosphorylation system. Mol Cell Endocrinol. 1997 Apr 4;128(1-2):69-75.

[25] Goglia F, Silvestri E, Lanni A. Thyroid hormones and mitochondria. Biosci Rep. 2002 Feb;22(1):17-32.

[26] Weitzel JM, Iwen KA, Seitz HJ. Regulation of mitochondrial biogenesis by thyroid hormone. Exp Physiol. 2003 Jan;88(1):121-8.
[27] Wrutniak-Cabello C, Casas F, Cabello G. Thyroid hormone action in mitochondria. J Mol Endocrinol. 2001 Feb;26(1):67-77.
[28] Schlame M, Hostetler KY. Cardiolipin synthase from mammalian mitochondria. Biochim Biophys Acta. 1997 Sep 4;1348(1-2):207-13.
[29] Nicholls DG, Bernson VS, Heaton GM. The identification of the component in the inner membrane of brown adipose tissue mitochondria responsible for regulating energy dissipation. Experientia Suppl. 1978;32:89-93.
[30] Cannon B, Nedergaard J. Brown adipose tissue: function and physiological significance. Physiol Rev. 2004 Jan;84(1):277-359.
[31] Lopez M, Varela L, Vazquez MJ, Rodriguez-Cuenca S, Gonzalez CR, Velagapudi VR, et al. Hypothalamic AMPK and fatty acid metabolism mediate thyroid regulation of energy balance. Nat Med. 2010 Sep;16(9):1001-8.
[32] Nedergaard J, Bengtsson T, Cannon B. Unexpected evidence for active brown adipose tissue in adult humans. Am J Physiol Endocrinol Metab. 2007 Aug;293(2):E444-52.
[33] van Marken Lichtenbelt WD, Vanhommerig JW, Smulders NM, Drossaerts JM, Kemerink GJ, Bouvy ND, et al. Cold-activated brown adipose tissue in healthy men. N Engl J Med. 2009 Apr 9;360(15):1500-8.
[34] Cypess AM, Lehman S, Williams G, Tal I, Rodman D, Goldfine AB, et al. Identification and importance of brown adipose tissue in adult humans. N Engl J Med. 2009 Apr 9;360(15):1509-17.
[35] Virtanen KA, Lidell ME, Orava J, Heglind M, Westergren R, Niemi T, et al. Functional brown adipose tissue in healthy adults. N Engl J Med. 2009 Apr 9;360(15):1518-25.
[36] Zingaretti MC, Crosta F, Vitali A, Guerrieri M, Frontini A, Cannon B, et al. The presence of UCP1 demonstrates that metabolically active adipose tissue in the neck of adult humans truly represents brown adipose tissue. Faseb J. 2009 Sep;23(9):3113-20.
[37] Saito M, Okamatsu-Ogura Y, Matsushita M, Watanabe K, Yoneshiro T, Nio-Kobayashi J, et al. High incidence of metabolically active brown adipose tissue in healthy adult humans: effects of cold exposure and adiposity. Diabetes. 2009 Jul;58(7):1526-31.
[38] Ricquier D, Bouillaud F. The uncoupling protein homologues: UCP1, UCP2, UCP3, StUCP and AtUCP. Biochem J. 2000 Jan 15;345 Pt 2:161-79.
[39] Lanni A, Moreno M, Lombardi A, Goglia F. Thyroid hormone and uncoupling proteins. FEBS Lett. 2003 May 22;543(1-3):5-10.
[40] Barbe P, Larrouy D, Boulanger C, Chevillotte E, Viguerie N, Thalamas C, et al. Triiodothyronine-mediated up-regulation of UCP2 and UCP3 mRNA expression in human skeletal muscle without coordinated induction of mitochondrial respiratory chain genes. FASEB J. 2001 Jan;15(1):13-5.
[41] Harper ME, Seifert EL. Thyroid hormone effects on mitochondrial energetics. Thyroid. 2008 Feb;18(2):145-56.

[42] Brand MD, Esteves TC. Physiological functions of the mitochondrial uncoupling proteins UCP2 and UCP3. Cell Metab. 2005 Aug;2(2):85-93.

[43] Pi J, Collins S. Reactive oxygen species and uncoupling protein 2 in pancreatic beta-cell function. Diabetes Obes Metab. 2010 Oct;12 Suppl 2:141-8.

[44] Seifert EL, Bezaire V, Estey C, Harper ME. Essential role for uncoupling protein-3 in mitochondrial adaptation to fasting but not in fatty acid oxidation or fatty acid anion export. J Biol Chem. 2008 Sep 12;283(37):25124-31.

[45] Gong DW, Monemdjou S, Gavrilova O, Leon LR, Marcus-Samuels B, Chou CJ, et al. Lack of obesity and normal response to fasting and thyroid hormone in mice lacking uncoupling protein-3. J Biol Chem. 2000 May 26;275(21):16251-7.

[46] Halestrap AP, McStay GP, Clarke SJ. The permeability transition pore complex: another view. Biochimie. 2002 Feb-Mar;84(2-3):153-66.

[47] Kinnally KW, Peixoto PM, Ryu SY, Dejean LM. Is mPTP the gatekeeper for necrosis, apoptosis, or both? Biochim Biophys Acta. 2011 Apr;1813(4):616-22.

[48] Miura T, Tanno M. The mPTP and its regulatory proteins: final common targets of signalling pathways for protection against necrosis. Cardiovasc Res. 2011 Dec 7.

[49] Azzolin L, von Stockum S, Basso E, Petronilli V, Forte MA, Bernardi P. The mitochondrial permeability transition from yeast to mammals. FEBS Lett. 2010 Jun 18;584(12):2504-9.

[50] Zorov DB, Juhaszova M, Yaniv Y, Nuss HB, Wang S, Sollott SJ. Regulation and pharmacology of the mitochondrial permeability transition pore. Cardiovasc Res. 2009 Jul 15;83(2):213-25.

[51] Koshkin V, Dai FF, Robson-Doucette CA, Chan CB, Wheeler MB. Limited mitochondrial permeabilization is an early manifestation of palmitate-induced lipotoxicity in pancreatic beta-cells. J Biol Chem. 2008 Mar 21;283(12):7936-48.

[52] Ichas F, Mazat JP. From calcium signaling to cell death: two conformations for the mitochondrial permeability transition pore. Switching from low- to high-conductance state. Biochim Biophys Acta. 1998 Aug 10;1366(1-2):33-50.

[53] Bernardi P. Mitochondrial transport of cations: channels, exchangers, and permeability transition. Physiol Rev. 1999 Oct;79(4):1127-55.

[54] Zoratti M, Szabo I. The mitochondrial permeability transition. Biochim Biophys Acta. 1995 Jul 17;1241(2):139-76.

[55] Penzo D, Tagliapietra C, Colonna R, Petronilli V, Bernardi P. Effects of fatty acids on mitochondria: implications for cell death. Biochim Biophys Acta. 2002 Sep 10;1555(1-3):160-5.

[56] Wieckowski MR, Brdiczka D, Wojtczak L. Long-chain fatty acids promote opening of the reconstituted mitochondrial permeability transition pore. FEBS Lett. 2000 Nov 3;484(2):61-4.

[57] Crompton M. The mitochondrial permeability transition pore and its role in cell death. Biochem J. 1999 Jul 15;341 (Pt 2):233-49.

[58] Zorov DB, Kinnally KW, Perini S, Tedeschi H. Multiple conductance levels in rat heart inner mitochondrial membranes studied by patch clamping. Biochim Biophys Acta. 1992 Apr 13;1105(2):263-70.
[59] Ichas F, Jouaville LS, Mazat JP. Mitochondria are excitable organelles capable of generating and conveying electrical and calcium signals. Cell. 1997 Jun 27;89(7):1145-53.
[60] Jacobson J, Duchen MR. Mitochondrial oxidative stress and cell death in astrocytes--requirement for stored Ca2+ and sustained opening of the permeability transition pore. J Cell Sci. 2002 Mar 15;115(Pt 6):1175-88.
[61] Novgorodov SA, Gudz TI. Permeability transition pore of the inner mitochondrial membrane can operate in two open states with different selectivities. J Bioenerg Biomembr. 1996 Apr;28(2):139-46.
[62] Brustovetsky N, Dubinsky JM. Dual responses of CNS mitochondria to elevated calcium. J Neurosci. 2000 Jan 1;20(1):103-13.
[63] Hausenloy D, Wynne A, Duchen M, Yellon D. Transient mitochondrial permeability transition pore opening mediates preconditioning-induced protection. Circulation. 2004 Apr 13;109(14):1714-7.
[64] Nicolli A, Basso E, Petronilli V, Wenger RM, Bernardi P. Interactions of cyclophilin with the mitochondrial inner membrane and regulation of the permeability transition pore, and cyclosporin A-sensitive channel. J Biol Chem. 1996 Jan 26;271(4):2185-92.
[65] Griffiths EJ, Halestrap AP. Further evidence that cyclosporin A protects mitochondria from calcium overload by inhibiting a matrix peptidyl-prolyl cis-trans isomerase. Implications for the immunosuppressive and toxic effects of cyclosporin. Biochem J. 1991 Mar 1;274 (Pt 2):611-4.
[66] Kalderon B, Hermesh O, Bar-Tana J. Mitochondrial permeability transition is induced by in vivo thyroid hormone treatment. Endocrinology. 1995 Aug;136(8):3552-6.
[67] Hermesh O, Kalderon B, Berman B, Bar-Tana J. Mitochondrial protonophoric activity induced by a thyromimetic fatty acid analogue. Biochim Biophys Acta. 2000 Apr 21;1457(3):166-74.
[68] Vacca RA, Moro L, Caraccio G, Guerrieri F, Marra E, Greco M. Thyroid hormone administration to hypothyroid rats restores the mitochondrial membrane permeability properties. Endocrinology. 2003 Sep;144(9):3783-8.
[69] Chavez E, Franco M, Reyes-Vivas H, Zazueta C, Ramirez J, Carrillo R. Hypothyroidism renders liver mitochondria resistant to the opening of membrane permeability transition pore. Biochim Biophys Acta. 1998 Sep 30;1407(3):243-8.
[70] Venditti P, De Rosa R, Di Meo S. Effect of thyroid state on susceptibility to oxidants and swelling of mitochondria from rat tissues. Free Radic Biol Med. 2003 Sep 1;35(5):485-94.
[71] Yehuda-Shnaidman E, Kalderon B, Bar-Tana J. Modulation of mitochondrial transition pore components by thyroid hormone. Endocrinology. 2005 May;146(5):2462-72.
[72] Woodfield K, Ruck A, Brdiczka D, Halestrap AP. Direct demonstration of a specific interaction between cyclophilin-D and the adenine nucleotide translocase confirms their

role in the mitochondrial permeability transition. Biochem J. 1998 Dec 1;336 (Pt 2):287-90.

[73] Belzacq AS, Brenner C. The adenine nucleotide translocator: a new potential chemotherapeutic target. Curr Drug Targets. 2003 Oct;4(7):517-24.

[74] Brustovetsky N, Tropschug M, Heimpel S, Heidkamper D, Klingenberg M. A large Ca2+-dependent channel formed by recombinant ADP/ATP carrier from Neurospora crassa resembles the mitochondrial permeability transition pore. Biochemistry. 2002 Oct 1;41(39):11804-11.

[75] Haworth RA, Hunter DR. Control of the mitochondrial permeability transition pore by high-affinity ADP binding at the ADP/ATP translocase in permeabilized mitochondria. J Bioenerg Biomembr. 2000 Feb;32(1):91-6.

[76] Kokoszka JE, Waymire KG, Levy SE, Sligh JE, Cai J, Jones DP, et al. The ADP/ATP translocator is not essential for the mitochondrial permeability transition pore. Nature. 2004 Jan 29;427(6973):461-5.

[77] Bauer MK, Schubert A, Rocks O, Grimm S. Adenine nucleotide translocase-1, a component of the permeability transition pore, can dominantly induce apoptosis. J Cell Biol. 1999 Dec 27;147(7):1493-502.

[78] Schubert A, Grimm S. Cyclophilin D, a component of the permeability transition-pore, is an apoptosis repressor. Cancer Res. 2004 Jan 1;64(1):85-93.

[79] Brand MD, Pakay JL, Ocloo A, Kokoszka J, Wallace DC, Brookes PS, et al. The basal proton conductance of mitochondria depends on adenine nucleotide translocase content. Biochem J. 2005 Dec 1;392(Pt 2):353-62.

[80] Dummler K, Muller S, Seitz HJ. Regulation of adenine nucleotide translocase and glycerol 3-phosphate dehydrogenase expression by thyroid hormones in different rat tissues. Biochem J. 1996 Aug 1;317 (Pt 3):913-8.

[81] Skulachev VP. Fatty acid circuit as a physiological mechanism of uncoupling of oxidative phosphorylation. FEBS Lett. 1991 Dec 9;294(3):158-62.

[82] He L, Lemasters JJ. Regulated and unregulated mitochondrial permeability transition pores: a new paradigm of pore structure and function? FEBS Lett. 2002 Feb 13;512(1-3):1-7.

[83] Fischer G, Wittmann-Liebold B, Lang K, Kiefhaber T, Schmid FX. Cyclophilin and peptidyl-prolyl cis-trans isomerase are probably identical proteins. Nature. 1989 Feb 2;337(6206):476-8.

[84] McGee AM, Baines CP. Phosphate is not an absolute requirement for the inhibitory effects of cyclosporin A or cyclophilin D deletion on mitochondrial permeability transition. Biochem J. 2012 Apr 1;443(1):185-91.

[85] Li Y, Johnson N, Capano M, Edwards M, Crompton M. Cyclophilin-D promotes the mitochondrial permeability transition but has opposite effects on apoptosis and necrosis. Biochem J. 2004 Oct 1;383(Pt 1):101-9.

[86] Basso E, Fante L, Fowlkes J, Petronilli V, Forte MA, Bernardi P. Properties of the permeability transition pore in mitochondria devoid of Cyclophilin D. J Biol Chem. 2005 May 13;280(19):18558-61.
[87] Lin DT, Lechleiter JD. Mitochondrial targeted cyclophilin D protects cells from cell death by peptidyl prolyl isomerization. J Biol Chem. 2002 Aug 23;277(34):31134-41.
[88] Andreeva L, Heads R, Green CJ. Cyclophilins and their possible role in the stress response. Int J Exp Pathol. 1999 Dec;80(6):305-15.
[89] Pavlov E, Grigoriev SM, Dejean LM, Zweihorn CL, Mannella CA, Kinnally KW. The mitochondrial channel VDAC has a cation-selective open state. Biochim Biophys Acta. 2005 Dec 20;1710(2-3):96-102.
[90] Crompton M, Virji S, Doyle V, Johnson N, Ward JM. The mitochondrial permeability transition pore. Biochem Soc Symp. 1999;66:167-79.
[91] Narita M, Shimizu S, Ito T, Chittenden T, Lutz RJ, Matsuda H, et al. Bax interacts with the permeability transition pore to induce permeability transition and cytochrome c release in isolated mitochondria. Proc Natl Acad Sci U S A. 1998 Dec 8;95(25):14681-6.
[92] Shi Y, Chen J, Weng C, Chen R, Zheng Y, Chen Q, et al. Identification of the protein-protein contact site and interaction mode of human VDAC1 with Bcl-2 family proteins. Biochem Biophys Res Commun. 2003 Jun 13;305(4):989-96.
[93] Rapizzi E, Pinton P, Szabadkai G, Wieckowski MR, Vandecasteele G, Baird G, et al. Recombinant expression of the voltage-dependent anion channel enhances the transfer of Ca2+ microdomains to mitochondria. J Cell Biol. 2002 Nov 25;159(4):613-24.
[94] Abu-Hamad S, Sivan S, Shoshan-Barmatz V. The expression level of the voltage-dependent anion channel controls life and death of the cell. Proc Natl Acad Sci U S A. 2006 Apr 11;103(15):5787-92.
[95] Gross A, McDonnell JM, Korsmeyer SJ. BCL-2 family members and the mitochondria in apoptosis. Genes Dev. 1999 Aug 1;13(15):1899-911.
[96] Jacotot E, Costantini P, Laboureau E, Zamzami N, Susin SA, Kroemer G. Mitochondrial membrane permeabilization during the apoptotic process. Ann N Y Acad Sci. 1999;887:18-30.
[97] Renault TT, Manon S. Bax: Addressed to kill. Biochimie. 2011 Sep;93(9):1379-91.
[98] Marzo I, Brenner C, Zamzami N, Jurgensmeier JM, Susin SA, Vieira HL, et al. Bax and adenine nucleotide translocator cooperate in the mitochondrial control of apoptosis. Science. 1998 Sep 25;281(5385):2027-31.
[99] Belzacq AS, Vieira HL, Verrier F, Vandecasteele G, Cohen I, Prevost MC, et al. Bcl-2 and Bax modulate adenine nucleotide translocase activity. Cancer Res. 2003 Jan 15;63(2):541-6.
[100] Zhivotovsky B, Galluzzi L, Kepp O, Kroemer G. Adenine nucleotide translocase: a component of the phylogenetically conserved cell death machinery. Cell Death Differ. 2009 Nov;16(11):1419-25.
[101] Shimizu S, Tsujimoto Y. Proapoptotic BH3-only Bcl-2 family members induce cytochrome c release, but not mitochondrial membrane potential loss, and do not

directly modulate voltage-dependent anion channel activity. Proc Natl Acad Sci U S A. 2000 Jan 18;97(2):577-82.
[102] Pastorino JG, Tafani M, Rothman RJ, Marcinkeviciute A, Hoek JB, Farber JL. Functional consequences of the sustained or transient activation by Bax of the mitochondrial permeability transition pore. J Biol Chem. 1999 Oct 29;274(44):31734-9.
[103] Shimizu S, Eguchi Y, Kamiike W, Funahashi Y, Mignon A, Lacronique V, et al. Bcl-2 prevents apoptotic mitochondrial dysfunction by regulating proton flux. Proc Natl Acad Sci U S A. 1998 Feb 17;95(4):1455-9.
[104] Pastorino JG, Chen ST, Tafani M, Snyder JW, Farber JL. The overexpression of Bax produces cell death upon induction of the mitochondrial permeability transition. J Biol Chem. 1998 Mar 27;273(13):7770-5.
[105] Boya P, Morales MC, Gonzalez-Polo RA, Andreau K, Gourdier I, Perfettini JL, et al. The chemopreventive agent N-(4-hydroxyphenyl)retinamide induces apoptosis through a mitochondrial pathway regulated by proteins from the Bcl-2 family. Oncogene. 2003 Sep 18;22(40):6220-30.
[106] Kandasamy K, Srinivasula SM, Alnemri ES, Thompson CB, Korsmeyer SJ, Bryant JL, et al. Involvement of proapoptotic molecules Bax and Bak in tumor necrosis factor-related apoptosis-inducing ligand (TRAIL)-induced mitochondrial disruption and apoptosis: differential regulation of cytochrome c and Smac/DIABLO release. Cancer Res. 2003 Apr 1;63(7):1712-21.
[107] Ravagnan L, Marzo I, Costantini P, Susin SA, Zamzami N, Petit PX, et al. Lonidamine triggers apoptosis via a direct, Bcl-2-inhibited effect on the mitochondrial permeability transition pore. Oncogene. 1999 Apr 22;18(16):2537-46.
[108] Zhang L, Yu J, Park BH, Kinzler KW, Vogelstein B. Role of BAX in the apoptotic response to anticancer agents. Science. 2000 Nov 3;290(5493):989-92.
[109] Raisova M, Hossini AM, Eberle J, Riebeling C, Wieder T, Sturm I, et al. The Bax/Bcl-2 ratio determines the susceptibility of human melanoma cells to CD95/Fas-mediated apoptosis. J Invest Dermatol. 2001 Aug;117(2):333-40.
[110] Perez-Navarro E, Gavalda N, Gratacos E, Alberch J. Brain-derived neurotrophic factor prevents changes in Bcl-2 family members and caspase-3 activation induced by excitotoxicity in the striatum. J Neurochem. 2005 Feb;92(3):678-91.
[111] Guan QH, Pei DS, Xu TL, Zhang GY. Brain ischemia/reperfusion-induced expression of DP5 and its interaction with Bcl-2, thus freeing Bax from Bcl-2/Bax dimmers are mediated by c-Jun N-terminal kinase (JNK) pathway. Neurosci Lett. 2006 Jan 30;393(2-3):226-30.
[112] Deng X, Kornblau SM, Ruvolo PP, May WS, Jr. Regulation of Bcl2 phosphorylation and potential significance for leukemic cell chemoresistance. J Natl Cancer Inst Monogr. 2001(28):30-7.
[113] Yehuda-Shnaidman E, Kalderon B, Azazmeh N, Bar-Tana J. Gating of the mitochondrial permeability transition pore by thyroid hormone. FASEB J. 2010 Jan;24(1):93-104.

[114] Ruvolo PP, Deng X, May WS. Phosphorylation of Bcl2 and regulation of apoptosis. Leukemia. 2001 Apr;15(4):515-22.
[115] Shibasaki F, Kondo E, Akagi T, McKeon F. Suppression of signalling through transcription factor NF-AT by interactions between calcineurin and Bcl-2. Nature. 1997 Apr 17;386(6626):728-31.
[116] Erin N, Bronson SK, Billingsley ML. Calcium-dependent interaction of calcineurin with Bcl-2 in neuronal tissue. Neuroscience. 2003;117(3):541-55.
[117] D'Arezzo S, Incerpi S, Davis FB, Acconcia F, Marino M, Farias RN, et al. Rapid nongenomic effects of 3,5,3'-triiodo-L-thyronine on the intracellular pH of L-6 myoblasts are mediated by intracellular calcium mobilization and kinase pathways. Endocrinology. 2004 Dec;145(12):5694-703.
[118] Yamauchi M, Kambe F, Cao X, Lu X, Kozaki Y, Oiso Y, et al. Thyroid hormone activates adenosine 5'-monophosphate-activated protein kinase via intracellular calcium mobilization and activation of calcium/calmodulin-dependent protein kinase kinase-beta. Mol Endocrinol. 2008 Apr;22(4):893-903.
[119] Gorlach A, Klappa P, Kietzmann T. The endoplasmic reticulum: folding, calcium homeostasis, signaling, and redox control. Antioxid Redox Signal. 2006 Sep-Oct;8(9-10):1391-418.
[120] Patterson RL, Boehning D, Snyder SH. Inositol 1,4,5-trisphosphate receptors as signal integrators. Annu Rev Biochem. 2004;73:437-65.
[121] Joseph SK, Hajnoczky G. IP3 receptors in cell survival and apoptosis: Ca2+ release and beyond. Apoptosis. 2007 May;12(5):951-68.
[122] Assefa Z, Bultynck G, Szlufcik K, Nadif Kasri N, Vermassen E, Goris J, et al. Caspase-3-induced truncation of type 1 inositol trisphosphate receptor accelerates apoptotic cell death and induces inositol trisphosphate-independent calcium release during apoptosis. J Biol Chem. 2004 Oct 8;279(41):43227-36.
[123] Verbert L, Lee B, Kocks SL, Assefa Z, Parys JB, Missiaen L, et al. Caspase-3-truncated type 1 inositol 1,4,5-trisphosphate receptor enhances intracellular Ca2+ leak and disturbs Ca2+ signalling. Biol Cell. 2008 Jan;100(1):39-49.
[124] Wojcikiewicz RJ, Oberdorf JA. Degradation of inositol 1,4,5-trisphosphate receptors during cell stimulation is a specific process mediated by cysteine protease activity. J Biol Chem. 1996 Jul 12;271(28):16652-5.
[125] Nakayama T, Hattori M, Uchida K, Nakamura T, Tateishi Y, Bannai H, et al. The regulatory domain of the inositol 1,4,5-trisphosphate receptor is necessary to keep the channel domain closed: possible physiological significance of specific cleavage by caspase 3. Biochem J. 2004 Jan 15;377(Pt 2):299-307.
[126] Szlufcik K, Missiaen L, Parys JB, Callewaert G, De Smedt H. Uncoupled IP3 receptor can function as a Ca2+-leak channel: cell biological and pathological consequences. Biol Cell. 2006 Jan;98(1):1-14.

[127] Jayaraman T, Marks AR. Calcineurin is downstream of the inositol 1,4,5-trisphosphate receptor in the apoptotic and cell growth pathways. J Biol Chem. 2000 Mar 3;275(9):6417-20.

[128] Bray GA. Use and abuse of appetite-suppressant drugs in the treatment of obesity. Ann Intern Med. 1993 Oct 1;119(7 Pt 2):707-13.

[129] Parascandola J. Dinitrophenol and bioenergetics: an historical perspective. Mol Cell Biochem. 1974 Nov 15;5(1-2):69-77.

[130] Baxter JD, Webb P. Thyroid hormone mimetics: potential applications in atherosclerosis, obesity and type 2 diabetes. Nat Rev Drug Discov. 2009 Apr;8(4):308-20.

[131] Tancevski I, Rudling M, Eller P. Thyromimetics: a journey from bench to bed-side. Pharmacol Ther. 2011 Jul;131(1):33-9.

[132] Wojtczak L, Wieckowski MR, Schonfeld P. Protonophoric activity of fatty acid analogs and derivatives in the inner mitochondrial membrane: a further argument for the fatty acid cycling model. Arch Biochem Biophys. 1998 Sep 1;357(1):76-84.

[133] Bernardi P, Penzo D, Wojtczak L. Mitochondrial energy dissipation by fatty acids. Mechanisms and implications for cell death. Vitam Horm. 2002;65:97-126.

[134] Bar-Tana J, Ben-Shoshan S, Blum J, Migron Y, Hertz R, Pill J, et al. Synthesis and hypolipidemic and antidiabetogenic activities of beta,beta,beta',beta'-tetrasubstituted, long-chain dioic acids. J Med Chem. 1989 Sep;32(9):2072-84.

[135] Kalderon B, Sheena V, Shachrur S, Hertz R, Bar-Tana J. Modulation by nutrients and drugs of liver acyl-CoAs analyzed by mass spectrometry. J Lipid Res. 2002 Jul;43(7):1125-32.

[136] Kalderon B, Hertz R, Bar-Tana J. Tissue selective modulation of redox and phosphate potentials by beta,beta'-methyl-substituted hexadecanedioic acid. Endocrinology. 1992 Oct;131(4):1629-35.

[137] Russell JC, Shillabeer G, Bar-Tana J, Lau DC, Richardson M, Wenzel LM, et al. Development of insulin resistance in the JCR:LA-cp rat: role of triacylglycerols and effects of MEDICA 16. Diabetes. 1998 May;47(5):770-8.

[138] Mayorek N, Kalderon B, Itach E, Bar-Tana J. Sensitization to insulin induced by beta,beta'-methyl-substituted hexadecanedioic acid (MEDICA 16) in obese Zucker rats in vivo. Diabetes. 1997 Dec;46(12):1958-64.

[139] Soboll S. Thyroid hormone action on mitochondrial energy transfer. Biochim Biophys Acta. 1993 Aug 16;1144(1):1-16.

[140] Bobyleva V, Pazienza TL, Maseroli R, Tomasi A, Salvioli S, Cossarizza A, et al. Decrease in mitochondrial energy coupling by thyroid hormones: a physiological effect rather than a pathological hyperthyroidism consequence. FEBS Lett. 1998 Jul 3;430(3):409-13.

[141] Samovski D, Kalderon B, Yehuda-Shnaidman E, Bar-Tana J. Gating of the mitochondrial permeability transition pore by long chain fatty acyl analogs in vivo. J Biol Chem. 2010 Mar 5;285(10):6879-90.

[142] Yang E, Zha J, Jockel J, Boise LH, Thompson CB, Korsmeyer SJ. Bad, a heterodimeric partner for Bcl-XL and Bcl-2, displaces Bax and promotes cell death. Cell. 1995 Jan 27;80(2):285-91.

[143] Zha J, Harada H, Yang E, Jockel J, Korsmeyer SJ. Serine phosphorylation of death agonist BAD in response to survival factor results in binding to 14-3-3 not BCL-X(L). Cell. 1996 Nov 15;87(4):619-28.

Chapter 10

Thyroid Disorders and Bone Mineral Homeostasis

Eva Feigerlova, Marc Klein, Anna Angelousi, Lelia Groza, Bruno Leheup and Georges Weryha

Additional information is available at the end of the chapter

1. Introduction

Thyroid hormones play a crucial role in the skeletal growth, peak bone mass acquisition and maintenance of bone mass. Abnormalities in hypothalamic–pituitary–thyroid axis in infancy and childhood have been shown to interfere with a normal linear growth and skeletal maturation. Hypothyroidism compromises normal bone formation and results in slowing of linear growth. Thyrotoxicosis leads to growth acceleration, diminution of bone mass and advance in bone age. Studies in animal models have demonstrated the importance of thyroid hormone signaling in the maintenance of bone mass in adulthood. Increased risk of fracture has been demonstrated in both hypothyroidism and hyperthyroidism. The thyroid hormone, 3,5,3′-triiodothyronine (T3), has long been considered to play a primordial role in the skeletal homeostasis. However, recent studies have shown that TSH acts as a direct regulator of bone remodeling, highlighting the importance of integrity of the hypothalamo-pituitary-thyroid axis.

This chapter will review our current understanding regarding the action of thyroid hormones on the bone development and maintenance of bone mass, under normal conditions and as a result of thyroid gland dysfunction. Mechanism of thyroid hormone action will be illustrated in relation to bone with the focus on the genetic regulation and the molecular interactions between thyroid hormones and skeletal cells. Clinical consequences of thyroid dysfunction on the growth and skeletal maturation will be detailed. We will review the published literature regarding BMD in hyperthyroid and hypothyroid patients including patients on medical therapy, as well as the influence of sex and menopause on the maintenance of bone mass. The impact of treatments for thyroid dysfunction on the bone mineral metabolism will be discussed.

2. Role of thyroid hormones in bone growth and metabolism

Thyroid hormones are critical for the skeletal development and the bone maintenance. The thyroid hormone, 3,5,3'-triiodothyronine (T3), is responsible for major actions of thyroid hormones. T3 binds to nuclear receptors that regulate gene transcription via interaction with thyroid hormone response elements of specific genes (Sap et al., 1986; Weinberger et al., 1986; Thompson et al., 1987). Recently, non-genomic actions of T3 and T4 have been described (Cheng et al., 2010). Local tissue availability of T3 seems to be regulated by type 2 and 3 deiodinase (St Germain et al, 2009). The nuclear thyroid hormone receptors (TRs) are derived from the THRA and THRB genes coding for the TRα1 and β1-2 T3-binding isoforms, truncated isoforms Δα1, Δα2 and Δβ3, and a TRa2 non-T3-binding isoform of unknown function (Lazar et Chin et al, 1990; Lazar, 1993; Chassande et al, 1997; Williams, 2000; Cheng et al, 2010). Expression of TRα1 and TRβ1 was described in growth plate chondrocytes, osteoblasts, and stromal cells of bone marrow (Williams et al, 1994; Abu et al, 1997; Ballock et al, 1999; Bradley et al, 1992; Bassett et Williams, 2003; Siddiqi et al, 2002). Expression of TRα in the skeleton is higher than that of TRβ (Bookout et al, 2006; O'Shea et al, 2003).

2.1. Thyroid hormone and bone development

Studies on animal models have brought valuable insights into role of TRs in bone development and growth. Mice lacking TRβ or TRα1 did not display abnormalities in skeletal development (Forrest et al, 1996; Wikstrom et al, 1998). On the other hand, genetic disruption of both receptors (TRα1 and TRβ) led to delayed ossification and disorders in development of epiphyseal growth plates (EGPs; Gothe et al, 1999). Pax-8$^{-/-}$ mice, expressing all TR isoforms, but lacking the follicular cells producing T4 and T3 in the thyroid gland, displayed more severe abnormalities in bone development than mice KO for all TRs (TR$\alpha^{0/0}$, TR$\beta^{-/-}$) (Flamant et al, 2002). The authors concluded that the unliganded TRs (aporeceptors) on thyroid hormone responsive genes have repressor effects during bone development. In support of this, Pax-8$^{-/-}$TR$\alpha^{0/0}$, but not Pax-8$^{-/-}$TR$\beta^{-/-}$, compound mutants presented a partial rescue of the bone phenotype (O'Shea et Williams, 2002; Flamant et al, 2002). Another study was realized employing mice invalidated for TRα. These animals were euthyroid, but displayed a growth delay with abnormal bone development and ossification (Bassett et al 2007a, 2007b; Gauthier et al, 1999, 2001; O'Shea 2003, 2005). Mice lacking all TRα isoforms presented a less severe impairment of bone development than TRα-/- mice, pointing to the role of non-T3 binding TRα isoforms (Δα1 and Δα2) (Gauthier et al, 2001). On the other hand, mice with nonfunctional TRβ displayed augmentation in circulating thyroid hormone levels associated with dysregulation of hypothalamo-pituitary-thyroid axis. These animals had skeletal signs of hyperthyroidism, increased bone mineral deposition and acceleration of growth-plate maturation, resulting in a short adult body size (Bassett et al, 2007a; O'Shea et al, 2003). These findings suggested an increased skeletal response to T3 via TRα, which was consistent with the hypothesis that elevated circulating thyroid hormone levels in TRβ mutant mice result in an increased skeletal response to T3 via TRα (O'Shea et al, 2006). Recently, GC-1, thyroid hormone analogue targeting preferentially TRβ1 over TRα1, has partially reverted skeletal development and maturation defects in hypothyroid rats (Freitas et al, 2005). This finding is suggestive of TRβ1 involvement in bone growth.

Thyroid hormones regulate bone development also indirectly through the growth hormone (GH) and insulin-like growth factor-I (IGF-I) axis. Previously, it was demonstrated that T4 enhanced the growth promoting effect of GH/IGF-I (Thorngren et Hansson, 1974) and could stimulate longitudinal bone growth in hypophysectomized rats (Thorngren et Hansson, 1973; Ray et al, 1954). T3 was shown to interact with the thyroid hormone receptor - thyroid hormone responsive element complex (TR-TRE) in the GH promoter to regulate GH gene transcription (Glass et al, 1987; Koenig et al, 1987). However, GH without T3 did not promote the maturation (Ballock et Reddi, 1994) and organization (Lewinson et al, 1989) of growth plate chondrocytes and GH replacement could not rescue the impaired ossification in TRα and TRβ-null mice (Kindblom et al, 2001). In $TR\alpha1^{-/-}\beta^{-/-}$ mice, GH substitution reversed the growth phenotype, but not the defective ossification (Kindblom et al, 2001). On the other hand, inactivation of GH or IGF-I receptors in mice was associated with delayed ossification (Liu et al, 1993; Sjogren et al, 2000).

Overall, the literature data indicate importance of both TRs and GH-IGF-I axis in skeletal development. Other factors, such as the Indian Hedgehog (Ihh), parathyroid hormone-related peptide (PTHrP), fibroblast growth factor receptor and Wnt-β-catenin signaling pathways, are implicated in this process (Barnard et al, 2005; O'Shea et al, 2005; Stevens et al, 2000, 2003; Wang et al, 2007). Further studies are warranted to clarify the exact mechanisms underlying the physiological regulation of bone development.

2.2. Thyroid hormone and bone remodeling

Literature evidence points to the critical importance of thyroid hormones in bone remodeling and maintenance. Adult euthyroid mice invalidated for TRα have reduced osteoclastic bone resorption and increased trabecular bone volume and mineralization (Bassett et al, 2007a, 2007b), indicating a critical role of TRα in T3 action in bone cells. On the other hand, increased osteoclastic bone resorption and severe osteoporosis were demonstrated in adult TRβ mutant mice, suggestive of thyroid hormone excess in TRα-expressing skeletal cells (Bassett et al, 2007a, 2007b; Gauthier et al, 2001; O'Shea et al, 2006).

The bone architecture and strength are maintained by a balanced process of remodeling, which involves recruitment of osteoclast and osteoblasts. T3 can induce differentiation and inhibits proliferation of osteoblastic cells. T3 was shown to promote production of IL-6, IL-8, IGF-I and its binding proteins IGFBP2-4 in bone marrow stromal cells and osteoblasts (Milne et al, 2001; Siddiqi et al, 1998), and to increase the expression of several bone-related genes, including osteocalcin, collagen type I, gelatinase B and collagenase 3 (Gouveia et al 2001; Milne et al 1998; Pereira 1999; Varga et al 1997; Williams et al 1994). T3 is implicated in chondrogenesis, angiogenesis, bone matrix formation and mineralization (Himeno et al, 2002; Makihira et al, 2003; Pereira et al, 1999). In primary cultures of growth plate chondrocytes, T3 inhibits chondrocyte clonal expansion and cell proliferation, induces hypertrophic chondrocyte differentiation and promotes cartilage matrix mineralization (Robson et al, 2000).

Furthermore, T3 is involved in local signaling pathways by stimulating osteoblast responses to IGF1-I, PTH and fibroblast growth factors. T3 is a critical regulator of the Ihh - bone morphogenetic protein (BMP) – PTHrP feedback loop (Stevens et al, 2000). Hypothyroidism is marked by increased PTHrP expression and impaired hypertrophic chondrocyte differentiation (Stevens et al, 2000). In hyperthyroidism, reduced expression of PTHrP associated with augmentation of BMP enhances hypertrophic chondrocyte differentiation (Lassova et al, 2009; Stevens et al, 2000). It has also been shown that T3 regulates terminal differentiation of growth plate chondrocytes in part through controlling cell cycle progression at the G1/S restriction point (Ballock et al, 2000). T3 mediates osteoclastic bone resorption through activation of osteoblasts, which then release receptor activator for NF-κB ligand (RANKL), a member of the TNF cytokine family. RANKL is a ligand for osteoprotegerin, a cytokine that regulates osteoclastic differentiation, and functions as a key factor for osteoclast differentiation and activation by inhibiting osteoclasts apoptosis (Allain et al, 1992; Britto et al, 1994).

Overall, T3 seems to enhance activity of osteoblasts by various mechanisms and signaling loops. Although the effects of thyrotoxicosis in adult bone are characterized by increased bone resorption, it is not known whether T3 acts directly in osteoclasts or whether effects on osteoclasts are secondary to the actions of T3 in osteoblasts.

2.3. Role of TSH on bone

Thyroid stimulating hormone (TSH) is a ligand hormone between hypothalamic-pituitary axis and the thyroid gland. TSH has long been recognized to act on the thyroid gland to control follicle development and thyroid hormone production and secretion. Beyond thyroid, TSH has also been shown to have additional effects on other tissues. TSH can exert a direct effect on bone metabolism independently of the peripheral thyroid hormone (thyroxine, T4, and triiodothyronine, T3) levels. This effect is mediated through the receptor for binding the thyroid-stimulating hormone (TSH-R), which is a pituitary G protein-coupled transmembrane receptor. Its expression has been demonstrated on osteoblast and osteoclast precursors. The TSH-R haploinsufficient mice display osteoporosis and focal osteosclerosis and thyroid hormone replacement did not restore bone mass but corrected growth deficiency in these animals (Abe et al, 2003). It has been suggested that the effects of TSH on the skeleton are independent of thyroid hormone levels.

In vitro and *in vivo* studies have provided evidence that TSH has negative effects on both osteoclasts and osteoblasts (Abe et al, 2003; Hase et al, 2006; Sun et al, 2006; Ma et al, 2011). TSH inhibits osteoclastogenesis by attenuating Janus N-terminal kinase (JNK) and NF-KB signaling. The osteoclast-inhibitory actions of TSH are partially mediated also through effects on tumor necrosis factor (TNF)-alpha production as it has been demonstrated in murine models (Abe et al, 2003). Mice lacking the TSHR present osteoporosis, early in embryogenesis, due to increased osteoclast formation (Abe et al, 2003; Hase et al 2006; Ma et al, 2009). These observations have not been confirmed in double-null mice of TSHR and TNF-alpha supporting thus the role of TNF-alpha in increased osteoclastogenesis (Abe et al,

2003; Hase et al 2006; Ma et al, 2009). Yamoah et al (2008) have recently described RANKL-responsive elements on the TNF alpha gene providing new insights into regulation of TNF transcription in osteoclast formation. The role of TSH on RANKL remains controversial since the administration of the exogenous recombinant TSH in animal models and humans has been shown to increase and in other series to decrease RANKL serum levels (Martini et al, 2008; Sampath et al, 2007; Abe et al, 2003). Role of TSH in osteoblastogenesis seems to be mediated through attenuation of Wnt and VEGF signaling (Abe et al, 2003). Enhanced osteoblastogenesis in TSHR deficiency was found to be associated with increased expression of low-density lipoprotein receptor–like protein-5 and Flk-1 proteins (Abe et al, 2003). Expression of these receptors, but not that of osteoblastic transcription factors, was inhibited by rhTSH. Altogether, these observations suggest that TSH negatively modulates bone turnover, however, further research is warranted to explain in detail the regulatory pathways.

3. Thyroid hormones and skeletal growth in infancy and adolescence

In prepubertal children, the linear growth is controlled mainly by GH-IGF-I axis, with influence from glucocorticoids and thyroid hormones. Thyroid hormones were shown to play an essential role for normal onset of the childhood component of growth (Heyerdahl, 1997). Role of the GH/IGF-I axis in the regulation of thyroid gland growth has recently been demonstrated (Boas et al, 2009). During pubertal period, sex steroids are important co-regulators of skeletal growth. Age related consequences of thyroid dysfunction on bone development have largely been described. Nevertheless, the exact role of thyroid hormone in the peak bone mass acquisition during childhood and early adulthood is not well understood. The same is for the gender specific action of T3 in the developing skeleton (Gauthier et al, 1999).

Euthyroid status is essential for normal skeletal development and linear growth. Generalized retardation in endochondral and intramembranous ossification associated with alterations in the EGPs, such as reduced thickness, disorganized columns of chondrocytes, and impaired differentiation of hypertrophic chondrocytes, have been reported in hypothyroid status during development (Lewinson et al, 1989; Stevens et al, 2000). The clinical consequences are reduced growth and skeletal abnormalities (Allain & McGregor, 1993). Theodore Kocher was awarded the Nobel Prize in Medicine in 1909 for his description of consequences of thyroidectomy. He showed the impact of hypothyroidism on the child growth (Kocher, 1883). Hypothyroid children present with the growth retardation and disproportionately short limbs in relation to the trunk. Radiographic skeletal examination may reveal, depending on the age and onset of hypothyroidism, a delayed closure of the fontanelles, enlargement of pituitary fossa and epiphyseal dysgenesis. Reilly & Smyth have described in 1937 stippled appearance of epiphyses on X-ray films in hypothyroid children. The pathognomonic nature of these changes was later confirmed by Wilkis (Wilkis, 1941). Epiphyseal dysgenesis has been demonstrated in the ossification centers that normally ossify after the onset of the hypothyroid status. Delayed appearance of ossification centers and delayed bone age are also noted in hypothyroid children. BMD seems to be also affected by a hypothyroid status during childhood. In one cross-sectional study, BMD was reported to be lower in prepubertal children with congenital hypothyroidism than in controls (Demartini et al, 2007).

Treatment with thyroxine results in a period of rapid catch-up growth, although predicted final height based on midparental height calculations may not be achieved, particularly when hypothyroidism is prolonged (Rivkees et al, 1988). The LT4 replacement for 8 years in children with congenital hypothyroidism did not have a negative effect on BMD for the lumbar spine and the femoral site and on biochemical markers of bone turnover (Leger et al, 1997). The results showed normal serum levels of calcium, phosphate, alkaline phosphatase, parathyroid hormone and 25-hydroxyvitamin D and did not demonstrate any relationship between BMD and L-T4 dosage or biochemical markers of bone formation. These findings were confirmed by other studies reporting no alterations of bone mass in adolescents and young adults with congenital hypothyroidism, treated from the neonatal period (Salerno et al, 2004, Demeester-Mirkine et al, 1990).

On the other hand, thyroid hormone excess results in accelerated skeletal maturation, premature closure of the EGPs and subsequent decrease in longitudinal bone growth with a compromised final adult height (Allain & McGregor, 1993; O'Shea et al, 1993; Harvey et al, 2002). In severe cases, hyperthyroidism during early childhood may also cause craniosynostosis due to premature fusion of the sutures of the skull (Segni et al 1999). Low bone density values and high bone resorption rates were demonstrated at diagnosis of hyperthyroidism in children and adolescents (Mora et al, 1999). Successful treatment of hyperthyroidism was shown to increase BMD in children and improve the conditions for the best obtainable peak bone mass (Mora et al, 1999).

Consequences of syndrome of resistance to thyroid hormone (RTH) on the skeletal development have been described in literature. RTH results from dominant negative mutations in the carboxyl terminus of the thyroid hormone receptor β gene. The mutant receptors are transcriptionally impaired and inhibit thyroid hormone receptor action. RTH is characterized by phenotypic variability including skeletal manifestations (Weiss et Refetoff, 2000). Our current understanding is based mainly on the published case reports. Involvement of the skeleton can cause a short stature, advanced or delayed bone age, increased bone turnover, osteoporosis, fractures, craniofacial abnormalities and craniosynostosis. The clinical variability might be secondary to functional properties of mutant proteins and heterogeneity of cofactors mediating action of TR (Kvistad et al, 2004).

4. Effects of thyroid dysfunction on bone turnover in adult bone

4.1. Hypothyroidism

Reduced bone turnover in hypothyroidism impairs bone formation and mineralization (Eriksen et al, 1986). Results of population studies indicate an increased fracture risk in hypothyroid individuals (Ahmed et al, 2006; Vestegaard et al 2002, 2005). The association between subclinical hypothyroidism and decreased BMD with increased fracture risk has also been reported, but has not been confirmed by others (Lee et al, 2006, 2010; Bertoli et al, 2002). Overall, the literature data have so far presented conflicting results. We will review the current literature and discuss changes in the bone metabolism, BMD and fracture risk in adult men and women with overt and subclinical hypothyroidism.

4.1.1. Mineral metabolism in hypothyroidism

Slight perturbations in some parameters of bone and mineral metabolism have been reported in hypothyroid patients. Minor abnormalities of calcium metabolism may exist with slightly elevated serum calcium, PTH and 1,25(OH)$_2$ vitamin D, decreased level of alkaline phosphatase, decreased urinary calcium excretion and glomerular filtration rate. The exchangeable pool of calcium and its rate of turnover may be reduced, reflecting decreased bone formation and resorption. However, these changes seem not to be different, even during the treatment, in hypothyroid patients compared to euthyroid controls (Sabuncu et al, 2001).

4.1.2. Overt hypothyroidism and skeletal changes

Large population based studies identified an increased fracture risk in individuals with hypothyroidism (Vestegaard et al 2000; 2002). The first of these studies (Vestegaard et al, 2000) analyzed 408 patients with primary hypothyroidism and found a temporary increase in fracture risk within the first 2 years after diagnosis, mainly in the age group $\geq$50 years, and was limited to the forearms. In the following study (Vestegaard, 2002), 4473 patients with autoimmune hypothyroidism (mean age, 66.1 +/- 17.3) were shown to present a significantly increased fracture risk up to 8 years prior to diagnosis with a peak around the time of diagnosis. The fracture risk was found to return to normal more than 5 years after its diagnosis.

An increased fracture risk in hypothyroid patients is not probably due to modifications of bone density. There are no convincing literature data as to changes in bone architecture during hypothyroidism. Neuromuscular symptoms and impaired muscle energy metabolism could be responsible for bone changes in this population. Hypothyroid patients have been shown to display impaired neuromuscular response to exercise persisting even after restoration of euthyroid status (Caraccio et al, 2005).

4.1.3. Subclinical hypothyroidism and skeletal changes

Subclinical hypothyroidism is a relatively frequent clinical condition, particularly among aged population, characterized by a low-normal free T4 level and a slightly elevated TSH level. The prevalence of subclinical hypothyroidism has been reported between 3.9 and 6.5% (Hollowell et al, 2002; Huber et al, 2002)

In Trosmo study, Grimnes et al. (2008) have demonstrated that, after multivariate adjustment, 25 out of 950 postmenopausal women with serum TSH above the 97.5 percentile had significantly higher BMD at the femoral neck than women with serum TSH in the normal range. However, there was no association between TSH and BMD, and serum TSH as a continuous variable had no effect on BMD.

Bone quality was studied by Nagata et al. using quantitative ultrasound in postmenopausal women with subclinical hypothyroidism. The results demonstrated that calcaneo osteo sono assessment indices of right feet measured by ultrasound bone densitometer decreased according to the increase in TSH concentration. The authors have suggested that hypothyroidism affects bone structure (Nagata et al, 2007).

4.2. Hyperthyroidism

Hyperthyroid patients present with an increased bone turnover and a risk for osteoporosis. The activity of osteoblasts and osteoclasts are increased, the latter predominates favoring resorption, negative balance of calcium, and bone loss (Melsen & Mosekilde, 1977; Mosekilde et al, 1990). Thyrotoxicosis in adults is a recognized cause of high-bone-turnover osteoporosis. Reduced bone mineral density was noted in hyperthyroid patients with an increased susceptibility to fragility fracture (Mosekilde et al, 1990; Vestergaard et al, 2002, 2005).

In both, clinical and subclinical hyperthyroidism, elevation of markers of bone turnover and decreased BMD have been reported (Kumeda et al, 2000; Heemstra et al, 2006; Lee et al, 2006). Previous studies that investigated impact of thyroid dysfunction on BMD and fracture risk did not provide conclusive results. Recently published population studies indicate association of endogenous subclinical hyperthyroidism with an increased fracture risk (Bauer et al, 2001; Jamal et al, 2005; Vadiveloo et al, 2011). Consequences of the hyperthyroid status (overt and subclinical) on bone turnover, BMD and fracture risk will be discussed and compared with the data in healthy population.

4.2.1. Mineral metabolism in hyperthyroidism

Hyperthyroidism is associated with impaired mineral metabolism. Increased serum calcium levels have been reported in up to 27% of hyperthyroid patients (Begic-Karup et al, 2001), but severe and symptomatic hypercalcemia is rare. Concentrations of serum alkaline phosphatase and osteocalcin are also frequently elevated. These findings are reminiscent of those in primary hyperparathyroidism, however, serum parathyroid hormone is mostly low-normal (Iqbal et al, 2003). True primary hyperparathyroidism and thyrotoxicosis may coexist (Beus & Stack, 2004; Wagner et al, 1999). Decreased plasma 25-hydroxycholecalciferol levels observed in hyperthyroidism could participate to the lower intestinal absorption of calcium and osteopenia in these patients (Mohan et al, 2004). Bone resorption markers, urinary pyridinoline and deoxypyridinoline, are increased 7-8 times more than in age and sex matched controls (Kraenzlin et al, 2008). Furthermore, hyperthyroid patients display a greater increase in urinary pyridinoline cross-links than that in serum markers of bone formation (osteocalcin, bone-specific alkaline phosphatase) (Akalin et al, 2002; Kisakol et al, 2003). Altogether, an increased bone turnover in these patients is in favor of osteoclastic bone resorption.

After initiation of anti-thyroid treatment, biochemical markers of bone resorption, such as urinary hydroxyproline, serum pyridinoline, serum deoxypiridinoline cross-links, have been found to fall, with a subsequent rise of the bone formation markers (Mosekilde et al 1990; Siddiqi et al, 1997; Garnero et al, 1994). Elevation of serum PTH has been reported in some patients with severe thyrotoxicosis under anti-thyroid treatment (Pantazi et al, 2000). This rise in PTH was suggested to play a role in inducing some temporal changes in mineral metabolism and participate to the reversal of the catabolic bone status of hyperthyroidism to anabolic. Furthermore, another study found that in hyperthyroidism, despite normal or high IGF-I levels, IGF-I bioactivity is reduced, probably because of high levels of IGF-binding protein-1 (Miell et al, 1993). Treatment of thyrotoxicosis reverses this abnormality. The rise in IGF-I bioactivity may therefore have a positive effect on the bone metabolism.

4.2.2. Overt hyperthyroidism and skeletal changes

Pathological skeletal changes, including osteopenia and osteoporosis, with higher incidence of fracture rates have been reported in hyperthyroid patients. Accordingly, hyperthyroidism was found 2.5-fold more often in postmenopausal women presenting with hip fracture than in controls. Among postmenopausal women, risk of hip fracture was significantly higher in patients with overt untreated hyperthyroidism and a history of past hyperthyroidism (Wejda et al, 1995). These findings were confirmed by a prospective follow-up study realized in 9516 Caucasian women, 65 years of age or older (Cummings et al, 1995). The authors demonstrated a higher risk of hip fracture among women who had previous hyperthyroidism. Another study reported that the prevalence of all types of fractures in patients with a history of thyroid disease was not different from that of control subjects.

However, women with a history of hyperthyroidism or thyroid cancer appeared to have their first fracture earlier than women without thyroid disease (Solomon et al, 1993). Median lumbar BMD in patients with thyrotoxicosis was shown to be 12.6% lower than that of normal individuals before the initiation of treatment (Krolner et al, 1983). Decreased BMD in hyperthyroid patients was demonstrated particularly in areas consisting of cortical bone. The risk of hip fracture increased significantly with age at diagnosis of hyperthyroidism (Campos-Pastor et al, 1993; Udayakmar et al, 2006; Vestergaard et al, 2002, 2005). The etiology of hyperthyroidism is not believed to play a role in the severity of hyperthyroid bone disease (Jodar et al, 1997).

A recent meta-analysis (Vestergaard et al, 2005) evaluated data regarding BMD and fracture risk in 20 (962 patients) and 5 publications, respectively (62 830 patients and controls). The results showed that patients with hyperthyroidism have a significantly decreased BMD. These values were lower in untreated patients compared to those under treatment, particularly for the lumbar spine (-0.83 vs. -0.27 Z-score) and the femoral site (-0.75 vs. -0.15 Z-score). The risk of hip fracture at the moment of diagnosis of hyperthyroidism was 1.6 (95% CI 0.7 to 3.4), and the value of BMD alone was associated with a risk of hip fracture corresponding to 1.2 (95% CI 0.9-1.5).

Decreased bone density in hyperthyroid patients tended to normalize under treatment (Wejda et al, 1995, Jodar et al, 1997). The improvement of BMD was noted even though no other specific anti-osteoporotic measures were introduced. The type of treatment of hyperthyroidism, iodine 131 or anti-thyroid drugs was not shown to alter the fracture risk (Vestergaard et al, 2005).

4.2.3. Subclinical hyperthyroidism and skeletal changes

Subclinical hyperthyroidism is defined as subnormal serum TSH with normal serum free thyroid hormones without signs or symptoms of thyrotoxicosis. Its prevalence in the U.S. population has been reported 0.7% (Hollowell et al, 2002). By definition, such patients should not have any clinical abnormalities associated with thyrotoxicosis (Biondi et al, 2005). However, a reduced bone mass was reported among postmenopausal patients (Bauer et al 2001). These observations could thus have a broader impact on the healthcare systems, as the subclinical hyperthyroidism is more frequent than overt thyrotoxicosis (Hollowell et al, 2002). Improvement of bone mineral density was shown in postmenopausal women with subclinical hyperthyroidism after normalization of their thyroid function (Faber et al, 1998). These data would justify indications of treatment in the older population. However, the risk/benefit ratio needs to be demonstrated by long-term, randomized studies.

On the other hand, the bone mineral density of the lumbar spine, femoral neck and the midshaft of the radius were not significantly decreased in premenopausal women (Foldes et al, 1993). The impact of subclinical hyperthyroidism in men is less known. A recent work suggests that a serum TSH concentration at the lower end of the reference range may be associated with low BMD in men (Kim et al, 2010).

5. Impact of thyroid hormone treatment on bone metabolism

Effects of thyroid replacement therapy or thyroid suppressive therapy on bone mineral density (BMD) are controversial. Results of previous studies are confounded by differences in study design, insufficient prospective data and small numbers of subjects. In the population study by Vestergaard et al (2005), the use of anti-thyroid drugs was associated with a significantly reduced fracture risk, no effect of levothyroxine on fracture risk was observed. No influence of L-thyroxine therapy on BMD was reported in young adults with congenital hypothyroidism (Salerno et al, 2004). Recently published population based case-control study has demonstrated a significantly increased fracture risk in adults over 70 years treated by levothyroxine (Turner et al, 2011). Publications on the association between the thyroid replacement and suppressive treatments and the bone mineral metabolism will be discussed.

5.1. Thyroid hormone replacement therapy

The objective of thyroid hormone replacement therapy is to normalize TSH levels. Some authors have suggested that treatment with levothyroxine may cause long-term osteoporosis, but there is no evidence to support this theory, and studies have shown no difference in bone density or fracture risk in patients undergoing treatment.

Previously, the effects of thyroid hormone treatment upon lumbar spine BMD were studied in a consecutive series of patients with myxedema. Patients with myxoedema did not differ from normal individuals as regards initial lumbar BMD, but levothyroxine-treatment caused a significant reduction in this variable. The median decrease in lumbar BMC after 1 year was 8.9% (95% confidence limits 1.5-15.4%, P less than 0.05). This loss of bone might be attributed to an inappropriate increase in bone turnover in the euthyroid status (Krolner et al, 1983). Accelerated bone turnover was shown to occur in women with subclinical hypothyroidism during replacement L-T4 treatment and normal TSH levels (Meier et al, 2004; Tarraga Lopez et al, 2011). In these women, bone loss was attributed to an adaptive mechanism on decreased bone turnover in pre-existent hypothyroidism. Finally, a long-term L-T4 treatment in children and adolescents with congenital hypothyroidism, diffuse goiter or with chronic lymphocytic thyroiditis did not affect BMD nor had a negative effect on the attainment of peak bone mass (Kooh et al, 1996; Saggese et al, 1996; Tumer et al, 1999). These results suggest that careful regulation of thyroid replacement is critical. Significant effects of prolonged L-T4-replacement therapy on bone tissue in patients with congenital hypothyroidism can be avoided by careful monitoring of serum TSH and adjustment of doses of L-T4 (Salerno et al, 2004).

5.2. Thyroid hormone suppressive therapy

Treatment with thyroid hormones with the objective to suppress TSH levels is used for example after surgery and radioiodine in differentiated thyroid carcinomas. The patients are maintained in subclinical hyperthyroidism, a condition associated with increased bone turnover.

Previous studies indicated that adults receiving high doses of L-T4-replacement therapy may be at risk of excessive bone loss. Reduction in BMD was observed after exogenous administration of high L-T4 doses used to fully suppress TSH in cases of thyroid cancer, goiters or nodules. Further, a review of cross-sectional and prospective studies examining the effect of thyroid hormone suppression on skeletal integrity in adults showed neither significant negative effect nor a decrease in BMD (Greenspan et al, 1990). Conflicting results were reported also in children. A significant reduction in peripheral BMD was found in children and adolescents receiving suppressive doses of L-T4 treatment for endemic goiter, Hashimoto's thyroiditis or thyroid cancer (Radetti et al, 1993).

More recently, suppression of TSH in hyperthyroidism or after thyroid hormone treatment has been shown to result in decrease in BMD and increase in fracture risk in postmenopausal women (Vestergaard et al, 2000; Bauer et al, 2001; Jamal et al, 2005; Kim et al, 2006). Similar results have been demonstrated in premenopausal women and men by Karner et al (2005). Recently realized systematic reviews analyzing effects of subclinical hyperthyroidism showed that postmenopausal women with subclinical hyperthyroidism may present an increased risk, whereas no increased risk has been demonstrated in men and premenopausal women (Quan et al, 2002; Heemstra et al, 2006). However, both reviews found methodological differences between different studies, making a structured meta-analysis impossible. Lately, a randomized prospective controlled trial has shown significant adverse effects of TSH suppressive therapy on BMD in women ≥ 50 years of age (Sugitani et Fujimoto, 2011). However, the results have not been adjusted for confounding factors, such as menopause status, dietary calcium, vitamin D intake, and smoking.

Overall, literature data enhance the hypothesis that low TSH levels may have a deleterious effect on bone homeostasis. Nevertheless, the exact relationship between subclinical hyperthyroidism and osteoporosis remains to be explained.

6. TSH as a metabolic regulator

We previously discussed (see paragraph 1.2) the role of TSH in the control of bone remodeling in animal models (Abe E, Marians RC et al, 2003). Systemic administration of TSH to ovariectomised rats has been shown to prevent bone loss and restore bone mass (Sampath et al, 2007; Sun et al, 2008) have demonstrated that intermittent administration of exogenous TSH in ovariectomised rats and mice have anti-resorptive effects. Recent findings indicate that TSH might play a crucial role in bone turnover in humans. Bone loss has been shown in women with polymorphism in the TSHR gene (Onigata et al, 2005).

There is a growing body of evidence that variations of TSH even in its reference range may influence BMD. A higher BMD has been reported in postmenopausal women with TSH within the physiological range comparing to these with the low level of TSH (Baqi et al, 2010). Clinical observations show that patients with subclinical hyperthyroidism and normal circulating thyroid hormone levels display osteoporotic changes (De Menis et al, 1992; Kisakol et al, 2003). Strong correlation between serum TSH and bone status has been demonstrated in postmenopausal women (Bauer et al, 2001; Morris et al, 2007). Based on these findings it has been suggested that it is the suppressed TSH rather than the elevated thyroid hormones that exert a deleterious effect on bone density. In a recent observational study, low-normal TSH values were shown to be associated with high prevalence of vertebral fractures in women with post-menopausal osteoporosis or osteopenia, even after correction for age, BMD, BMI and serum free-thyroxine values (Mazziotti et al, 2010). Svare et al, 2009, in a cross-sectional, population-based study, analyzed 5778 women without and 944 with self-reported thyroid disease aged ≥40 years. Women with the TSH level <0.50 mU/l had lower forearm BMD than the reference group and the prevalence of osteoporosis was higher in women who reported hyperthyroidism than in women without self-reported thyroid disease. Finally, Kim et al, 2010 investigated the association between serum thyrotropin (TSH) concentration and bone mineral density (BMD) in 1478 healthy euthyroid men in a cross-sectional community based survey. Lumbar spine BMD and femoral neck BMD were shown to increase with TSH level after adjustment for age, weight and height. The odds of lower BMD were significantly increased in subjects with low-normal TSH, when compared to high-normal TSH after adjustment for confounding factors. These results suggested that a serum TSH concentration at the lower end of the reference range may be associated with low BMD in men.

The role of TSH on bone metabolism has also been analyzed through markers of bone metabolism after administration of recombinant TSH (rhTSH). TSH has been demonstrated to activate directly osteoblasts according to the increased levels of N-terminal propeptide of type I procollagen (PINP) (Martini et al, 2008). Others showed that TSH promotes the production and activity of alkaline phosphatase and of osteocalcin (Sampath et al, 2007; Abe et al, 2003), while some studies found inhibition of osteoblast differentiation induced by the administration of TSH (Abe et al, 2003). These finding suggested that TSH may enhance the differentiation of osteoblasts precursors.

Clinically, it has been found that the administration of exogenous TSH may have antiresorptive effects of TSH on bone turnover. In women monitored for thyroid carcinoma, a short-term stimulation with rhTSH had inhibitory effect on bone resorption. Acute administration of rhTSH in thyroidectomised postmenopausal women with suppressed endogenous serum TSH resulted in diminution in serum C-telopeptides of type-1 collagen and increase in bone alkaline phosphatase (Mazziotti et al., 2005). A transient inhibition of bone resorption and increase in osteoblastic activity, measured by markers of bone metabolism, after acute TSH administration was demonstrated also by other studies (Karga et al, 2010; Iakovou et al, 2010; Martini et al, 2008).

Overall, these data constitute the evidence for relationship between TSH and a change in bone mass in humans.

7. Bone effects of thyroid hormone analogues

Synthetic analogues of thyroid hormones display tissue-specific actions (Baxter and Webb 2009). They have been developed for their lipid lowering activity by preferential activation of the TRβ1 isoform in the liver while sparing the TRα1 mediated cardiac effects (Angelin & Rudling, 2010; Pramfalk et al., 2010; Webb, 2010). Previous animal and human studies have demonstrated that thyromimetics can influence bone metabolism. Skeletal effects of thyroid hormone analogues recently reported in literature on cell lines, animal models and humans are summarized in Table 1.

Previously studied selective thyromimetic, tiratricol (3,5,3′-triiodothyroacetic acid; Triac) was shown to enhance skeletal metabolic activity (Sherman, et al 1997) and to produce adverse effects on bone metabolism (Alvarez et al 2004; Brenta et al 2003; Kawaguchi et al 1994a, 1994b). DITPA, 3,5-diiodothyropropionic acid, has a higher affinity for the TRβ compared to the TRα. Administration of DITPA to humans for 24 weeks was associated with a significant rise in serum osteocalcin, N-telopeptide, and deoxypyridinoline levels, indicating an increased bone turnover (Ladenson el al 2010b). GC-1, [3,5-dimethyl-4-(4′-hydroxy-3′isopropylbenzyl)-phenoxy acetic acid], binds TRβ1 with the same affinity as T3, but TRα1 with a 10-fold lower affinity (Scanlan, 2010). Bone sparing effects in adult female rats have been observed after treatment by GC-1 for 64 days (Freitas et al, 2003). In another

Thyromimetic	Study Design	Skeletal effects	Reference
Tiratricol (Triac)	Cultured neonatal mouse calvariae: Triac vs. T3	More potent stimulation of resorption and less potent stimulation of formation vs. T3	Kawaguchi 1994a
Tiratricol (Triac)	Cultured fetal rat long bones and neonatal mouse calvariae; Triac vs. T3	Equal or greater stimulation of bone resorption by Triac than T3	Kawaguchi 1994b
Tiratricol (Triac)	Rats; Triac vs. T3	Greater increase in beta-CTX levels, no alteration of BMD	Alvarez 2004
Tiratricol (Triac)	Randomized clinical trial (2 months); athyreotic patients: Triac vs. L-T4	Increased serum osteocalcin and urinary excretion of calcium and pyridinium cross-links	Sherman 1997
Tiratricol (Triac)	Randomized clinical trial (11 months); euthyroid goitrous women: Triac vs. L-T4	Significant increase in serum deoxypyridinoline and significant decrease in hip bone density, but ns compared to L-T4;	Brenta 2003
DITPA	Prospective, controlled, double-blind clinical trial (24 weeks): DITPA vs. placebo	Increase in serum osteocalcin, N-telopeptide and deoxypyridinoline	Ladenson 2010b
Sobetirome (GC-1)	Rat and mouse osteoblast-like cells	Induction of differentiation and activity of osteoblasts	Beber 2009
Sobetirome (GC-1)	Female adult Wistar rats; study groups (64 days): GC-1; T3 ; control	No effects on BMD in L2-L5, femur, and tibia; no changes in histomorphometric parameters of the femur	Freitas 2003
Sobetirome (GC-1)	21-day old female hypothyroid rats, treatment for 5 weeks: GC-1 vs. placebo	Induction of ossification, HC differentiation, expression of collagen II and X mRNA, increase in EGP thickness	Freitas 2005
Eprotirome (KB2115)	Randomized, double-blind, multicenter 12-week clinical trial: Eprotirome vs. placebo	No changes in b-ALP and type I collagen breakdown product; ns increase in PINP	Ladenson 2010a

Table 1. Skeletal effects of thyroid hormone analogues: b-ALP – bone alcalic phosphatase; BMD - bone mineral density; EGP - epiphyseal growth plate; HC – hypertrophic chondrocytes; ns – non significant; PINP - procollagen type I N-terminal propeptide

study, partial reversion of the skeletal development and maturation defects has been shown in hypothyroid rats after 5 week therapy by GC-1 (Freitas et al 2005). Eprotirome, (KB2115), 3-[[3,5-dibromo-4-[4-hydroxy-3-(1-methylethyl)-phenoxy]-phenyl]-amino]-3-oxopropanoic acid, displays a higher affinity for TRβ1 isoform with hepatic uptake (Berkenstam 2008). Administration of eprotirome to humans for 12 weeks has not been associated with unfavorable bone effects (Ladenson et al 2010a).

Altogether the data are consistent with potentially adverse skeletal effects of thyroid hormone analogues. However, no conclusive evidence can be drawn and further investigations would be justified to establish an accurate benefice/risk ratio before their clinical use.

8. Conclusion

The last decades have seen an increasing interest in the action of thyroid hormones in bone mineral homeostasis. *In vivo* and *in vitro* studies in cell lines as well as animal models have demonstrated a critical role of thyroid hormones, TSH and their receptors in the skeletal growth and its maintenance. However, many of the molecular mechanisms of thyroid hormone action remain still poorly defined.

Clinical studies, consistently with animal data, indicate a close association between thyroid status and bone metabolism. Thyrotoxicosis results in an increased bone turnover, osteoporosis and a risk of fragility fracture. Thyroid hormone deficiency decreases bone turnover with a subsequent risk of bone fragility. Exogenous administration of suppressive doses of thyroxine was shown to negatively influences BMD and bone turnover. In future, prospective studies a prolonged time of observation will be necessary, as well as to increase the number of studied patients, in order to better assess the relative risk of osteoporosis in patients undergoing TSH-suppressive treatment. Another question that remains to be answered is if there is a benefit from treatment of subclinical thyroid disease on skeletal health.

Finally, thyroid hormone analogues represent a promising therapeutic option for their lipid lowering activity. Nevertheless, literature data suggest their potentially adverse skeletal effects. No conclusive evidence can be drawn and further investigations would be justified to establish an accurate benefice/risk ratio before their clinical use.

Author details

Eva Feigerlova, Marc Klein, Anna Angelousi, Lelia Groza and Georges Weryha*
Department of Endocrinology, CHU Nancy, Vandoeuvre, France

Bruno Leheup
Department of Pediatric Endocrinology, CHU Nancy, Vandoeuvre, France

* Corresponding Author

9. References

[1] Abe E, Marians RC, Yu W, Wu XB, Ando T, Li Y, Iqbal J, Eldeiry L, Rajendren G, Blair HC, Davies TF, Zaidi M. (2003) TSH is a negative regulator of skeletal remodeling. Cell 115: 151–162.

[2] Abu EO, Bord S, Horner A, Chatterjee VKK, and Compston JE (1997) The expression of thyroid hormone receptors in human bone. Bone 21: 137–142.

[3] Ahmed LA, Schirmer H, Berntsen GK et al (2006) Self-reported diseases and the risk of non-vertebral fractures: the Tromso study. Osteoporos Int 17: 46–53.

[4] Akalin A, Colak O, Alatas O, Efe B (2002) Bone remodeling markers and serum cytokines in patients with hyperthyroidism. Clin Endocrinol 57:125-129

[5] Allain TJ, Chambers TJ, Flanagan AM, McGregor AM (1992) Tri-iodothyronine stimulates rat osteoclastic bone resorption by an indirect effect. J Endocrinol 133:327–331.

[6] Allain TJ, McGregor AM (1993) Thyroid hormones and bone. J Endocrinol 139:9–18.

[7] Alvarez L, Burgueño A, Zeni S, Randi AS, Hernández S, Hockl P, et al (2004) Comparison of the effects of 3,5,3′-triiodothyroacetic Acid and triiodothyronine on goiter prevention and involution and on hepatic and skeletal parameters in rats. Horm. Metab. Res. 36:291–7.

[8] Angelin, B., & Rudling, M. (2010). Lipid lowering with thyroid hormone and thyromimetics. Curr Opin Lipidol 21(6), 499–506.

[9] Ballock R, Mita BC, Zhou X, Chen DH, and Mink LM (1999) Expression of thyroid hormone receptor isoforms in rat growth plate cartilage in vivo. J Bone Miner Res 14: 1550–1556, 1999.

[10] Ballock RT, Reddi AH (1994) Thyroxine is the serum factor that regulates morphogenesis of columnar cartilage from isolated chondrocytes in chemically defined medium. J Cell Biol 126:1311–1318.

[11] Ballock RT, Zhou X, Mink LM, Chen DH, Mita BC, Stewart MC (2000) Expression of cyclin-dependent kinase inhibitors in epiphyseal chondrocytes induced to terminally differentiate with thyroid hormone. Endocrinology. 141:4552-7.

[12] Baqi L, Payer J, Killinger Z, Susienkova K et al (2010) The level of TSH appeared favourable in maintaining bone mineral density in postmenopausal women. Endocr Regul. 44: 9-15.

[13] Barnard, J.C. et al. (2005) Thyroid hormones regulate fibroblast growth factor receptor signaling during chondrogenesis. Endocrinology 146: 5568–5580

[14] Bassett JH, Williams GR (2003) The molecular actions of thyroid hormone in bone. Trends Endocrinol Metab 14: 356–364.

[15] Bassett, J.H. et al. (2007a) Thyroid hormone excess rather than thyrotropin deficiency induces osteoporosis in hyperthyroidism. Mol. Endocrinol. 21: 1095–1107

[16] Bassett, J.H. et al. (2007b) Thyroid status during skeletal development determines adult bone structure and mineralization. Mol. Endocrinol. 21: 1893–1904

[17] Bauer DC, Ettinger B, Nevitt MC et al (2001) Risk for fracture in women with low serum levels of thyroid-stimulating hormone. Ann Intern Med134: 561–568.

[18] Baxter, J. D., & Webb, P. (2009). Thyroid hormone mimetics: Potential applications in atherosclerosis, obesity and type 2 diabetes. Nat Rev Drug Discov 8(4), 308–320.

[19] Beber EH, Capelo LP, Fonseca TL, Costa CC, Lotfi CF, Scanlan TS, et al (2009) The thyroid hormone receptor (TR) beta-selective agonist GC-1 inhibits proliferation but induces differentiation and TR beta mRNA expression in mouse and rat osteoblast-like cells. Calcif. Tissue Int. 84:324–33

[20] Begic-Karup S, Wagner B, Raber W, Schneider B, Hamwi A, Waldhäusl W, Vierhapper H (2001) Serum calcium in thyroid disease. Wien Klin Wochenschr. 113(1-2):65-8.

[21] Berkenstam, A., Kristensen, J., Mellstrom, K., Carlsson, B., Malm, J., Rehnmark, S., et al. (2008). The thyroid hormone mimetic compound KB2115 lowers plasma LDL cholesterol and stimulates bile acid synthesis without cardiac effects in humans. Proc Natl Acad Sci U S A 105(2), 663–667.

[22] Bertoli A, Fusco A, Andreoli A, Magnani A et al (2002) Effect of subclinical hypothyroidism and obesity on whole-body and regional bone mineral content. Horm Res. 57:79-84.

[23] Beus KS, Stack BC Jr (2004) Synchronous thyroid pathology in patients presenting with primary hyperparathyroidism. Am J Otolaryngol. 25:308-12.

[24] Biondi B, Palmieri EA, Klain M, Schlumberger M, Filetti S, Lombardi G (2005) Subclinical hyperthyroidism: clinical features and treatment options. Eur J Endocrinol 152:1-9.

[25] Boas M et al (2009) Association of Thyroid Gland Volume, Serum Insulin-Like Growth Factor-I, and Anthropometric Variables in Euthyroid Prepubertal Children. J Clin Endocrinol Metab 94: 4031–4035.

[26] Bookout, A.L. et al. (2006) Anatomical profiling of nuclear receptor expression reveals a hierarchical transcriptional network. Cell 126: 789–799

[27] Bradley DJ, Towle HC, & Young WS 3rd (1992) Spatial and temporal expression of alpha- and beta-thyroid hormone receptor mRNAs, including the beta 2-subtype, in the developing mammalian nervous system. J Neurosci 12: 2288–2302

[28] Brenta G, Schnitman M, Fretes O, Facco E, Gurfinkel M, Damilano S, et al (2003) Comparative efficacy and side effects of the treatment of euthyroid goiter with levo-thyroxine or triiodothyroacetic acid. J. Clin. Endocrinol. Metab. 88:5287–92.

[29] Britto JM, Fenton AJ, Holloway WR, Nicholson GC (1994) Osteoblasts mediate thyroid hormone stimulation of osteoclastic bone resorption. Endocrinology 134:169–176.

[30] Campos-Pastor MM, Munoz-Torres M, Escobar-Jimenez F, et al (1993) Bone mass in females with different thyroid disorders: influence of menopausal status. Bone and Mineral 21:1-8.

[31] Caraccio N, Natali A, Sironi A, et al (2005) Muscle metabolism and exercise tolerance in subclinical hypothyroidism: a controlled trial of levothyroxine. J Clin Endocrinol Metab 90:4057–62

[32] Chassande O, Fraichard A, Gauthier K, Flamant F, Legrand C, Savatier P, Laudet V, Samarut J (1997) Identification of transcripts initiated from an internal promoter in the c-erbA alpha locus that encode inhibitors of retinoic acid receptor-alpha and triiodothyronine receptor activities. Mol Endocrinol 11:1278–1290.

[33] Cheng SY, Leonard JL, & Davis PJ (2010) Molecular aspects of thyroid hormone actions. Endocr Rev 31: 139–170

[34] Cummings SR, Nevitt MC, Browner WS, et al (1995) Risk factors for hip fracture in white women. Study of Osteoporotic Fractures Research Group. N Engl J Med 332:767–73.

[35] Demartini Ade A, Kulak CA, Borba VC, Cat MN, Dondoni RS, Sandrini R, et al (2007) Bone mineral density of children and adolescents with congenital hypothyroidism. Arq Bras Endocrinol Metabol. 51:1084–92.

[36] De Menis E, Da Rin G, Roiter I, et al. (1992) Bone turnover in overt and subclinical hyperthyroidism due to autonomous thyroid adenoma. Horm Res 37:217–220.

[37] Demeester-Mirkine N, Bergmann P, Body JJ, et al (1990) Calcitonin and bone mass status in congenital hypothyroidism. Calcif Tissue Int 46:222–6

[38] Eriksen EF, Mosekilde L, Melsen F (1986) Kinetics of trabecular bone resorption and formation in hypothyroidism: evidence for a positive balance per remodeling cycle. Bone 7: 101–108.

[39] Faber J, Jensen IW, Petersen L, Nygaard B, Hegedüs L, Siersbaek-Nielsen K (1998) Normalization of serum thyrotrophin by means of radioiodine treatment in subclinical hyperthyroidism: effect on bone loss in postmenopausal women. Clin Endocrinol (Oxf). 1998 48:285-90.

[40] Flamant F, Poguet AL, Plateroti M, Chassande O, Gauthier K, Streichenberger N, Mansouri A, Samarut J (2002) Congenital hypothyroid Pax8(–/–) mutant mice can be rescued by inactivating the TRalpha gene. Mol Endocrinol 16:24–32.

[41] Foldes J, Tarjan G, Szathmari M, et al (1993) Bone mineral density in patients with endogenous subclinical hyperthyroidism: is this thyroid status a risk factor for osteoporosis? Clin Endocrinol (Oxf) 39:521–7.

[42] Forrest D, Erway LC, Ng L, Altschuler R, Curran T (1996) Thyroid hormone receptor beta is essential for development of auditory function. Nat Genet 13:354–357.

[43] Freitas FRS, Capelo LP, O'Shea PJ, Jorgetti V, Moriscot AS, Scanlan TS, et al. (2005) The thyroid hormone receptor beta-specific agonist GC-1 selectively affects the bone development of hypothyroid rats. J. Bone Miner. Res. 20:294–304.

[44] Freitas FRS, Moriscot AS, Jorgetti V, Soares AG, Passarelli M, Scanlan TS, et al (2003) Spared bone mass in rats treated with thyroid hormone receptor TR beta-selective compound GC-1. Am. J. Physiol. Endocrinol. Metab.285:E1135–1141.

[45] Glass CK, Franco R, Weinberger C, Albert VR, Evans RM, Rosenfeld MG (1987) A c-erb-A binding site in rat growth hormone gene mediates trans-activation by thyroid hormone. Nature 329:738–741.

[46] Garnero P, Vassy V, Bertholin A, Riou JP, Delmas PD (1994) Markers of bone turnover in hyperthyroidism an the effects of treatment. J Clin Endocrinol Metab. 78:955–959.

[47] Gauthier, K. et al. (1999) Different functions for the thyroid hormone receptors TRalpha and TRbeta in the control of thyroid hormone production and post-natal development. EMBO J. 18, 623–631

[48] Gauthier K, Plateroti M, Harvey CB, Williams GR, Weiss RE, Refetoff S, Willott JF, Sundin V, Roux JP, Malaval L, Hara M, Samarut J, Chassande O (2001) Genetic analysis

reveals different functions for the products of the thyroid hormone receptor alpha locus. Mol Cell Biol 21:4748–4760.

[49] Gothe S, Wang Z, Ng L, Kindblom JM, Barros AC, Ohlsson C, Vennstrom B, Forrest D (1999) Mice devoid of all known thyroid hormone receptors are viable but exhibit disorders of the pituitary-thyroid axis, growth, and bone maturation. Genes Dev 13:1329–1341.

[50] Gouveia CH, Schultz JJ, Bianco AC, Brent GA (2001) Thyroid hormone stimulation of osteocalcin gene expression in ROS17/2.8 cells is mediated by transcriptional and post-transcriptional mechanisms. J Endocrinol 170:667–675

[51] Greenspan SL & Greenspan FS (1999) The effect of thyroid hormone on skeletal integrity. Annals of Internal Medicine 130:750–758.

[52] Grimnes G, Emaus N, Joakimsen RM, Figenschau Y, Jorde R (2008) The relationship between serum TSH and bone mineral density in men and postmenopausal women: The Tromsø study. Thyroid. 18:1147–55.

[53] Harvey CB, O'Shea PJ, Scott AJ, Robson H, Siebler T, Shalet SM, Samarut J, Chassande O, Williams GR (2002) Molecular mechanisms of thyroid hormone effects on bone growth and function. Mol Genet Metab 75:17–30.

[54] Hase H, Ando T, Eldeiry L, Brebene A, Peng Y, Liu L, Amano H, Davies TF, Sun L, Zaidi M, Abe E (2006) TNF mediates the skeletal effects of thyroid-stimulating hormone. Proc Natl Acad Sci USA 103:12849–12854.

[55] Heemstra KA, Hamdy NA, Romijn JA & Smit JW (2006) The effects of thyrotropin-suppressive therapy on bone metabolism in patients with well-differentiated thyroid carcinoma. Thyroid 16:583–591.

[56] Heyerdahl S (1997) Linear growth in early treated children with congenital hypothyroidism. Acta Paediatr. 86:479-83.

[57] Himeno, M. et al. (2002) Impaired vascular invasion of Cbfa1-deficient cartilage engrafted in the spleen. J. Bone Miner. Res. 17, 1297–1305

[58] Hollowell JG, Staehling NW, Flanders WD, Hannon WH, Gunter EW, Spencer CA, Braverman LE (2002) Serum TSH, T(4), and thyroid antibodies in the United Statuss population (1988 to 1994): National Health and Nutrition Examination Survey (NHANES III). J Clin Endocrinol Metab.87:489-99.

[59] Huber G, Staub JJ, Meier C, Mitrache C, Guglielmetti M, Huber P, Braverman LE (2002) Prospective study of the spontaneous course of subclinical hypothyroidism: prognostic value of thyrotropin, thyroid reserve, and thyroid antibodies. J Clin Endocrinol Metab 87:3221-6.

[60] Iakovou I, Chrisoulidou A, Balaris V, Balaris C, Doumas A, Karatzas N (2010) Acute effects of recombinant human TSH on bone markers in differentiated thyroid cancer. Hell J Nucl Med 13:208-12.

[61] Iqbal AA, Burgess EH, Gallina DL, Nanes MS, Cook CB (2003) Hypercalcemia in hyperthyroidism: patterns of serum calcium, parathyroid hormone, and 1,25-dihydroxyvitamin D3 levels during management of thyrotoxicosis. Endocr Pract 9:517-21.

[62] Jamal SA, Leiter RE, Bayoumi AM et al (2005) Clinical utility of laboratory testing in women with osteoporosis. Osteoporos Int 16: 534–540.
[63] Jodar E, Munoz-Torres M, Escobar-Jimenez F, et al (1997) Bone loss in hyperthyroid patients and in former hyperthyroid patients controlled on medical therapy: influence of aetiology and menopause. Clin Endocrinol (Oxf) 47: 279–85.
[64] Karga H, Papaioannou G, Polymeris A, Papamichael K, Karpouza A, Samouilidou E, Papaioannou P (2010) The effects of recombinant human TSH on bone turnover in patients after thyroidectomy. J Bone Miner Metab 28:35-41.
[65] Karner I, Hrgović Z, Sijanović S, Buković D, Klobucar A, Usadel KH, Fassbender WJ (2005) Bone mineral density changes and bone turnover in thyroid carcinoma patients treated with supraphysiologic doses of thyroxine. Eur J Med Res. 10:480-8.
[66] Kawaguchi H, Pilbeam CC, Raisz LG (1994a) Anabolic effects of 3,3′,5-triiodothyronine and triiodothyroacetic acid in cultured neonatal mouse parietal bones. Endocrinology 135: 971–6.
[67] Kawaguchi H, Pilbeam CC, Woodiel FN, Raisz LG (1994b) Comparison of the effects of 3,5,3′-triiodothyroacetic acid and triiodothyronine on bone resorption in cultured fetal rat long bones and neonatal mouse calvariae. J. Bone Miner. Res. 9:247–53.
[68] Kim DJ, Khang YH, Koh JM, Shong YK, Kim GS (2006) Low normal TSH levels are associated with low bone mineral density in healthy postmenopausal women. Clin Endocrinol (Oxf) 64:86–90
[69] Kim BJ, Lee SH, Bae SJ, Kim HK, Choe JW, Kim HY, Koh JM, Kim GS (2010) The association between serum thyrotropin (TSH) levels and bone mineral density in healthy euthyroid men. Clin Endocrinol (Oxf). 73:396-403.
[70] Kindblom JM, Gothe S, Forrest D, Tornell J, Vennstrom B, Ohlsson C (2001) GH substitution reverses the growth phenotype but not the defective ossification in thyroid hormone receptor alpha $1^{-/-}$beta$^{-/-}$ mice. J Endocrinol 171:15–22.
[71] Kisakol G, Kaya A, Gonen S, Tunc R (2003) Bone and calcium metabolism in subclinical autoimmune hyperthyroidism and hypothyroidism. Endocr J 50:657–661.
[72] Kocher T (1883) Ueber Kropfexstirpation und ihre Folgen. Arch Klin Chir 29:254.
[73] Koenig RJ, Brent GA, Warne RL, Larsen PR, Moore DD (1987) Thyroid hormone receptor binds to a site in the rat growth hormone promoter required for induction by thyroid hormone. Proc Natl Acad Sci USA 84:5670–5674
[74] Kooh SW, Brnjac L, Ehlrich RM, Qureshi R & Krishnan S (1996) Bone mass in children with congenital hypothyroidism treated with thyroxine since birth. Journal of Pediatric Endocrinology and Metabolism 9:59–62.
[75] Kraenzlin ME, Kraenzlin CA, Meier C, Giunta C, Steinmann B (2008) Automated HPLC assay for urinary collagen cross-links: effect of age, menopause, and metabolic bone diseases. Clin Chem 54:1546-1553.
[76] Krolner B, Jorgensen JV, Nielsen SP (1983) Spinal bone mineral content in myxedema and thyrotoxicosis. Effects of thyroid hormone(s) and anti-thyroid treatment. Clin Endocrinol (Oxf) 18:439–46.
[77] Kumeda Y, Inaba M, Tahara H et al (2000) Persistent increase in bone turnover in Graves' patients with subclinical hyperthyroidism. J Clin Endocrinol Metab 85:4157-61.

[78] Kvistad PH, Lovas K, Boman H et al (2004) Retarded bone growth in thyroid hormone resistance. A clinical study of a large family with a novel thyroid hormone receptor mutation. Eur J Endocrinol 150: 425-430.

[79] Ladenson PW, Kristensen JD, Ridgway EC, Olsson AG, Carlsson B, Klein I, et al (2010a) Use of the thyroid hormone analogue eprotirome in statin-treated dyslipidemia. N. Engl. J. Med 362: 906–16.

[80] Ladenson PW, McCarren M, Morkin E, Edson RG, Shih M-C, Warren SR, et al (2010b) Effects of the thyromimetic agent diiodothyropropionic acid on body weight, body mass index, and serum lipoproteins: a pilot prospective, randomized, controlled study. J Clin Endocrinol Metab. 95:1349–54.

[81] Lassova, L. et al. (2009) Thyroid hormone treatment of cultured chondrocytes mimics in vivo stimulation of collagen X mRNA by increasing BMP 4 expression. J. Cell. Physiol. 219, 595–605

[82] Lazar MA (1993) Thyroid hormone receptors: Multiple forms, multiple possibilities. Endocr Rev 14: 184–193.

[83] Lazar MA, & Chin WW (1990) Nuclear thyroid hormone receptors. J Clin Invest 86: 1777–1782.

[84] Lee JS, Buzková P, Fink HA, Vu J, Carbone L, Chen Z et al (2010) Subclinical thyroid dysfunction and incident hip fracture in older adults. Arch Intern Med. 170:1876-83.

[85] Lee WY, Oh KW, Rhee EJ, Jung CH, Kim SW et al (2006) Relationship between subclinical thyroid dysfunction and femoral neck bone mineral density in women. Archives of Medical Research 37:511–516.

[86] Leger J, Ruiz JC, Guibourdenche J, Kindermans C, Garabedian M, Czernichow P (1997) Bone mineral density and metabolism in children with congenital hypothyroidism after prolonged L-thyroxine therapy. Acta Paediatr. 86:704-10.

[87] Lewinson D, Harel Z, Shenzer P, Silbermann M, Hochberg Z (1989) Effect of thyroid hormone and growth hormone on recovery from hypothyroidism of epiphyseal growth plate cartilage and its adjacent bone. Endocrinology 124:937–945.

[88] Liu JP, Baker J, Perkins AS, Robertson EJ, Efstratiadis A (1993) Mice carrying null mutations of the genes encoding insulin-like growth factor I (Igf-1) and type 1 IGF receptor (Igf1r). Cell 75:59–72.

[89] Ma R, Latif R, Zaidi M, Davies T (2009) Thyroid and bone: TSH inhibits osteoclastogenesis from embryonic stem cells. Presented at the 91st Annual Meeting of the Endocrine Society. Washington DC; June 10–13, 2009.

[90] Ma R, Morshed S, Latif R, Zaidi M, Davies TF (2011) The influence of thyroid-stimulating hormone and thyroid-stimulating hormone receptor antibodies on osteoclastogenesis. Thyroid 21:897-906.

[91] Makihira, S. et al. (2003) Thyroid hormone enhances aggrecanase-2/ADAM-TS5 expression and proteoglycan degradation in growth plate cartilage. Endocrinology 144, 2480–2488

[92] Martini G, Gennari L, De Paola V, Pilli T, Salvadori S, Merlotti D, Valleggi F, Campagna S, Franci B, Avanzati A, Nuti R, Pacini F (2008) The effects of recombinant TSH on bone turnover markers and serum osteoprotegerin and RANKL levels. Thyroid. 18:455-60.

[93] Mazziotti G, Sorvillo F, Piscopo M, Cioffi M, Pilla P, Biondi B, Iorio S, Giustina A, Amato G, Carella C (2005) Recombinant human TSH modulates in vivo C-telopeptides of type-1 collagen and bone alkaline phosphatase, but not osteoprotegerin production in postmenopausal women monitored for differentiated thyroid carcinoma. J Bone and Min Res 20:480-486.

[94] Mazziotti G, Porcelli T, Patelli I, Vescovi PP, Giustina A (2010) Serum TSH values and risk of vertebral fractures in euthyroid post-menopausal women with low bone mineral density. Bone. 46:747-51.

[95] Meier C, Beat M, Guglielmetti M, Christ-Crain M, Staub JJ, Kraenzlin M. (2004) Restoration of euthyroidism accelerates bone turnover in patients with subclinical hypothyroidism: a randomized controlled trial. Osteoporosis International 15:209–216.

[96] Melsen F, Mosekilde L (1977) Morphometric and dynamic studies of bone changes in hyperthyroidism. Acta Pathol Microbiol Scand A. 85A:141-50.

[97] Miell JP, Taylor AM, Zini M, Maheshwari G, Ross RJM, Valcani R (1993) Effects of hypothyroidism and hyperthyroidism on insulin-like growth factors (IGFs) and growth hormone- and IGF-binding proteins. J Clin Endocrinol Metab. 76:950 –955.

[98] Milne M, Kang MI, Quail JM, Baran DT (1998) Thyroid hormone excess increases insulin-like growth factor I transcripts in bone marrow cell cultures: divergent effects on vertebral and femoral cell cultures. Endocrinology 139:2527–2534

[99] Milne M, Quail JM, Rosen CJ, Baran DT (2001) Insulin-like growth factor binding proteins in femoral and vertebral bone marrow stromal cells: expression and regulation by thyroid hormone and dexamethasone. J Cell Biochem. 81:229-40.

[100] Mohan HK, Groves AM, Fogelman I, Clarke SE (2004) Thyroid hormone and parathyroid hormone competing to maintain calcium levels in the presence of vitamin D deficiency. Thyroid 14:789-91.

[101] Mora S, Weber G, Marenzi K, Signorini E, Rovelli R, Proverbio MC & Chiumello G (1999) Longitudinal changes of bone density and bone resorption in hyperthyroid girls during treatment. Journal of Bone and Mineral Research 14: 1971–1977.

[102] Morris MS (2007) The association between serum thyroid stimulating hormone in its reference range and bone status in postmenopausal American women. Bone 40:1128-1134.

[103] Mosekilde L, Eriksen EF, Charles P. Effects of thyroid hormones on bone and mineral metabolism. Endocrinol Metab Clin North Am 1990; 19: 35–63.

[104] Murphy E, Williams GR. The thyroid and the skeleton. Clin Endocrinol (Oxf) 2004; 61: 285–298.

[105] Nagata M, Suzuki A, Sekiguchi S, Ono Y, Nishiwaki-Yasuda K, Itoi T, et al (2007) Subclinical hypothyroidism is related to lower heel QUS in postmenopausal women. Endocr J 54:625–30.

[106] Onigata K, Kowasi T, Nishiyama S, Micuno H, Morikawa A. Bone mineral density in human cases with TSH receptor gene mutations. Proceedings of the New York Academy of Sciences 1rst Conference on Skeletal Development and Remodeling in Health, Disease, and Aging, May 18–21, 2005, New York, NY, USA.

[107] O'Shea PJ, Harvey CB, Suzuki H, Kaneshige M, Kaneshige K, Cheng SY, Williams GR (2003) A thyrotoxic skeletal phenotype of advanced bone formation in mice with resistance to thyroid hormone. Mol Endocrinol 17:1410–1424.

[108] O'Shea PJ, Williams GR (2002) Insight into the physiological actions of thyroid hormone receptors from genetically modified mice. J Endocrinol 175:553–570.

[109] O'Shea, P.J. et al. (2005) Contrasting skeletal phenotypes in mice with an identical mutation targeted to thyroid hormone receptor alpha1 or beta. Mol. Endocrinol. 19, 3045–3059

[110] O'Shea, P.J. et al. (2006) Characterization of skeletal phenotypes of TRalpha1 and TRbeta mutant mice: implications for tissue thyroid status and T3 target gene expression. Nucl. Receptor Signal. 4, e011

[111] Pantazi H, Papapetrou PD (2000) Changes in parameters of bone and mineral metabolism during therapy for hyperthyroidism. J Clin Endocrinol Metab. 85:1099-106.

[112] Pereira RC, Jorgetti V, Canalis E (1999) Triiodothyronine induces collagenase-3 and gelatinase B expression in murine osteoblasts. Am J Physiol 277:E496–E504

[113] Pramfalk C, Pedrelli M, & Parini P (2011) Role of thyroid receptor beta in lipid metabolism. Biochim Biophys Acta 1812:929-37

[114] Radetti G, Castellan C, Tato` L, Platter K, Gentili L & Adami S (1993) Bone mineral density in children and adolescent females treated with high doses of L-thyroxine. Hormon Research 39:127–131.

[115] Ray RD, Asling CW, Walker DG, Simpson ME, Li CH, Evans HM (1954) Growth and differentiation of the skeleton in thyroidectomized-hypophysectomized rats treated with thyroxin, growth hormone, and combination. J Bone Joint Surg Am 36:94–103

[116] Rivkees SA, Bode HH, Crawford JD (1988) Long-term growth in juvenile acquired hypothyroidism: the failure to achieve normal adult stature. N Engl J med 3:599-602.

[117] Robson H, Siebler T, Stevens DA et al (2000) Thyroid hormone acts directly on growth plate chondrocytes to promote hypertrophic differentiation and inhibit clonal expansion and cell proliferation. Endocrinology 141:3887–3897.

[118] Sabuncu T, Aksoy N, Arikan E, Ugur B, Tasan E, Hatemi H (2001) Early changes in parameters of bone and mineral metabolism during therapy for hyper- and hypothyroidism. Endocr Res. 27:203-13.

[119] Saggese G, Bertelloni S, Baroncelli GI, Costa S & Ceccarelli C (1996) Bone mineral denisty in adolescent females treated with L-thyroxine: a longitudinal study. European Journal of Pediatrics 155: 452–457.

[120] Salerno M, Lettiero T, Esposito-del Puente A et al. (2004) Effect of long-term L-thyroxine treatment on bone mineral density in young adults with congenital hypothyroidism. European Journal of Endocrinology 151:689–694.

[121] Sampath TK, Simic P, Sendak R, Draca N, Bowe AE, O'Brien S, Schiavi SC, McPherson JM, Vukicevic S (2007) Thyroid-stimulating hormone restores bone volume, microarchitecture, and strength in aged ovariectomized rats. J Bone Miner Res. 22:849-59.

[122] Sap J, Munoz A, Damm K, Goldberg Y, Ghysdael J, Leutz A, et al. (1986) The c-erb-A protein is a high-affinity receptor for thyroid hormone. Nature 324: 635–640.

[123] Scanlan TS (2010). Sobetirome: A case history of bench-to-clinic drug discovery and development. Heart Fail Rev 15(2), 177–182.

[124] Segni M et al. (1999) Special features of Graves' disease in early childhood. Thyroid 9: 871–877

[125] Sherman SI, Ringel MD, Smith MJ, Kopelen HA, Zoghbi WA, Ladenson PW (1997) Augmented hepatic and skeletal thyromimetic effects of tiratricol in comparison with levothyroxine. J. Clin. Endocrinol. Metab. 82:2153–8.

[126] Siddiqi A, Burrin JM, Noonan K, James I, Wood DF, Price CP, Monson JP (1997) A longitudinal study of markers of bone turnover in Graves' disease and their value in predicting bone mineral density. J Clin Endocrinol Metab. 82:753–759.

[127] Siddiqi A, Burrin JM, Wood DF, Monson JP (1998) Tri-iodothyronine regulates the production of interleukin-6 and interleukin-8 in human bone marrow stromal and osteoblast-like cells. J Endocrinol. 157:453-61.

[128] Siddiqi A, Parsons MP, Lewis JL et al. (2002) TR expression and function in human bone marrow stromal and osteoblast- like cells. J Clin Endocrinol Metab 87: 906–914.

[129] Sjogren K, Bohlooly YM, Olsson B, Coschigano K, Tornell J, Mohan S, Isaksson OG, Baumann G, Kopchick J, Ohlsson C (2000) Disproportional skeletal growth and markedly decreased bone mineral content in growth hormone receptor–/– mice. Biochem Biophys Res Commun 267:603–608.

[130] Solomon BL, Wartofsky L, Burman KD (1993) Prevalence of fractures in postmenopausal women with thyroid disease. Thyroid. 3:17-23.

[131] Stevens DA, Hasserjian RP, Robson H, Siebler T, Shalet SM, Williams GR (2000) Thyroid hormones regulate hypertrophic chondrocyte differentiation and expression of parathyroid hormone-related peptide and its receptor during endochondral bone formation. J Bone Miner Res 15:2431–2442.

[132] Stevens, D.A. et al. (2003) Thyroid hormone activates fibroblast growth factor receptor-1 in bone. Mol. Endocrinol. 17, 1751–1766

[133] St Germain, D.L. et al. (2009) Defining the roles of the iodothyronine deiodinases: current concepts and challenges. Endocrinology 150: 1097–1107

[134] Sugitani I, Fujimoto Y (2008) Effect of postoperative thyrotropin suppressive therapy on bone mineral density in patients with papillary thyroid carcinoma: a prospective controlled study. Surgery. 150:1250-7.

[135] Sun L et al. (2008) Intermittent recombinant TSH injections prevent ovariectomy-induced bone loss. PNAS. 105:4289-4294.

[136] Svare A, Nilsen TI, Bjøro T, Forsmo S, Schei B, Langhammer A (2009) Hyperthyroid levels of TSH correlate with low bone mineral density: the HUNT 2 study. Eur J Endocrinol. 161:779-86.

[137] Tárraga López PJ, López CF, de Mora FN, Montes JA, Albero JS, Mañez AN, Casas AG (2011) Osteoporosis in patients with subclinical hypothyroidism treated with thyroid hormone. Clin Cases Miner Bone Metab. 8:44-8.

[138] Thorngren KG, Hansson LI 1973 Effect of thyroxine and growth hormone on longitudinal bone growth in the hypophysectomized rat. Acta Endocrinol (Copenh) 74:24–40.

[139] Thorngren KG, Hansson LI 1974 Bioassay of growth hormone II. Determination of longitudinal bone growth with tetracycline in thyroxine-treated hypophysectomized rats. Acta Endocrinol (Copenh) 75:669–682.

[140] Thompson CC, Weinberger C, Lebo R, & Evans RM (1987) Identification of a novel thyroid hormone receptor expressed in the mammalian central nervous system. Science 237:1610–1614.

[141] Tumer L, Hasanoglu A, Cinaz P & Bideci A (1999) Bone mineral density and metabolism in children treated with L-thyroxine. Journal of Pediatric Endocrinology and Metabolism 12:519–523.

[142] Turner MR et al. (2011) Levothyroxine dose and risk of fractures in older adults: nested case-control study. BMJ. 342:d2238

[143] Udayakumar N, Chandrasekaran M, Rasheed MH, Suresh RV, Sivaprakash S (2006) Evaluation of bone mineral density in thyrotoxicosis. Singapore Med J 47:947-950.

[144] Varga F, Rumpler M, Luegmayr E, Fratzl-Zelman N, Glantschnig H, Klaushofer K (1997) Triiodothyronine, a regulator of osteoblastic differentiation: depression of histone H4, attenuation of c-fos/c-jun, and induction of osteocalcin expression. Calcif Tissue Int 61:404–411

[145] Vadiveloo T, Donnan PT, Cochrane L, Leese GP (2011) The Thyroid Epidemiology, Audit, and Research Study (TEARS): morbidity in patients with endogenous subclinical hyperthyroidism. J Clin Endocrinol Metab 96:1344-51.

[146] Vestergaard P, Mosekilde L (2002) Fractures in patients with hyperthyroidism and hypothyroidism: a nationwide follow-up study in 16,249 patients. Thyroid 12: 411–419.

[147] Vestergaard P, Rejnmark L, Mosekilde L (2005) Influence of hyper- and hypothyroidism, and the effects of treatment with anti-thyroid drugs and levothyroxine on fracture risk. Calcif Tissue Int 77: 139–144.

[148] Vestergaard P, Rejnmark L, Weeke J, Mosekilde L (2000) Fracture risk in patients treated for hyperthyroidism. Thyroid 10:341–348.

[149] Wagner B, Begic-Karup S, Raber W, Schneider B, Waldhäusl W, Vierhapper H (1999) Prevalence of primary hyperparathyroidism in 13387 patients with thyroid diseases, newly diagnosed by screening of serum calcium. Exp Clin Endocrinol Diabetes. 107:457-61.

[150] Wang, L. et al. (2007) Thyroid hormone interacts with the Wnt/betacatenin signaling pathway in the terminal differentiation of growth plate chondrocytes. J. Bone Miner. Res. 22, 1988–1995

[151] Webb P (2010). Thyroid hormone receptor and lipid regulation. Curr Opin Investig Drugs 11(10), 1135–1142.

[152] Weinberger C, Thompson CC, Ong, ES, Lebo R, Gruol DJ, & Evans RM (1986) The c-erb-A gene encodes a thyroid hormone receptor. Nature 324: 641–646.

[153] Weiss RE, Refetoff S (2000) Resistance to thyroid hormone. Rev Endocr Metab Disord 1:97–108.

[154] Wejda B, Hintze G, Katschinski B, Olbricht T, Benker G (1995) Hip fractures and the thyroid: A case study. J Intern Med 237:241–247

[155] Williams GR, Bland R, and Sheppard MC (1994) Characterization of thyroid hormone (T3) receptors in three osteosarcoma cell lines of distinct osteoblast phenotype: interactions among T3, vitamin D3, and retinoid signaling. Endocrinology 135: 2375–2385, 1994.

[156] Williams GR (2000) Cloning and characterization of two novel thyroid hormone receptor beta isoforms. Mol Cell Biol 20:8329–8342

[157] Wilkis L (1941) Epiphysial dysgenesis associated with hypothyroidism. Am J Dis Child. 61:13-34.

[158] Wikstrom L, Johansson C, Salto C, Barlow C, Campos Barros A, Baas F, Forrest D, Thoren P, Vennstrom B (1998) Abnormal heart rate and body temperature in mice lacking thyroid hormone receptor alpha 1. EMBO J 17:455–461.

[159] Yamoah K, Brebene A, Baliram R, et al (2008) High-mobility group box proteins modulate tumor necrosis factor-alpha expression in osteoclastogenesis via a novel deoxyribonucleic acid sequence. Mol Endocrinol 22:1141–1153.

Chapter 11

Thyroid Autoimmunity in Patients with Skin Disorders

Emina Kasumagic-Halilovic and Begler Begovic

Additional information is available at the end of the chapter

1. Introduction

Thyroid disorders are known to involve all the organ systems of the body and the skin is no exception. Some dermatological skin findings and diseases may be the first symptoms of thyroid disease [1]. Available data suggest that thyroid hormone plays a pivotal role in embryonic development of mammalian skin as well as in maintenance of normal cutaneous function an adult skin. Thyroid hormone stimulates epidermal oxygen consumption, protein synthesis, mitosis, and determination of epidermal thickness [2]. Thyroid hormone is an important regulator of epidermal homeostasis. In tissue culture studies using surrogates for DNA expression, T_3 has been shown to stimulate growth of both epidermal keratinocytes and dermal fibroblastes [3, 4]. In addition, thyroid hormone appears to be necessary for both the initiation and maintenance of hair growth and normal secretion of sebum.

Both hypothyroidism and hyperthyroidism are known to cause skin change. Hypothyroidism may result from either inadequate circulating levels of thyroid hormone or target cell resistance to hormonal action. Primary hypothyroidism is as a result of glandular failure is the most common cause and most frequently result from autoimmune disease [5]. In hypothyroidism, the skin is cold, xerotic and pale. The coldness is due to reduced core temperature and cutaneous vasoconstriction. The decreased skin perfusion has been documented with nail fold capillaroscopy [6]. It has been suggested that the diminished skin perfusion is reflex vasoconstriction compensatory to diminished core temperature. The diminished core temperature itself may be secondary to reduced thermogenesis [7]. Occasionally, purpura may be noted in hypothyroid patients as a result of diminished levels of clothing factors and the loss of vascular support secondary to the dermal mucin [8]. The dryness of hypothyroid skin results from decreased eccrine gland secretion. The mechanism for decreased sweating is not clear although the hypothyroid glands are atrophic on histologic examination [9]. Hypohidrosis, possibly accompanied by diminished epidermal sterol biosynthesis, may lead to acquired palmoplantar keratoderma. Xerosis is due to a change in skin texture and poor hydratation of the stratum corneum. The skin is rough and covered with fine scales. Palms and soles may be quite dry. The epidermis is thin and hyperkeratotic, and there is follicular plugging. Because the changes are generalized, they can be differentiated from similar alterations in the skin of atopic individuals and keratosis pilaris, where the findings are more prominent on the extremities [10]. Hypothyroidism also may affect the development of the lamellar granules (Odland bodies), which are vital in the establishment of a normal stratum corneum [11]. In hypothyroidism, the skin tends to be pale both because of the dermal mucopolysaccharides and dermal water content which alter the refraction of light. The name myxedema refers to the associated skin condition caused by increased glycosaminoglycan deposition in the skin. Generalized myxedema is still the classic cutaneous sign of hypothyroidism. The mucopolysaccharides that accumulate in the dermis are hyaluronic acid and chondriotin sulfate. They appear first in the papillary dermis and are most prominent around hair follicles and vassels. They separate the collagen bundles and there may be some secondary degeneration of collagen [10]. Generally, myxedema is diffuse, but focal mucinous papules have been describes. Skin may appear swollen, dry, pale, waxy, and firm to the touch. In addition, increased dermal carotene may appear as a prominent yellowish discoloration on the palms, soles and nasolabial folds. Hypothyroid patients may sometimes suffer *Candida* folliculitis. It has been theorized that because the sebaceous glands of hypothyroid patients secrete decreased sebum relative to those of euthyroid persons, the hair follicles may develop a flora with lipophilic organisms, which are replaced by *Candida albicans* (12). The hypothyroid skin heals slowly, and this tendency is proportional to the degree of hormone deficiency. In hypothyroidism, hair can be dry, coarse, brittle and slow growing. There is both patchy and diffuse loss of scalp hair, a very characteristic loss of the outer third of the eyebrow (madarosis), and diminished body hair. Pubic and axillary hair may be sparse. The alopecia connected to hypothyroidism may be mediated by hormone effects on the initiation as well as the duration of hair growth. Massive telogen effluvium may occur when there is abrupt onset of hypothyroidism, and the percentage of scalp hairs in telogen is generally increased in hypothyroid states [10]. Using DNA flow cytometry, Schell *et al.* observed that cell proliferation indices were reduced in hair bulbs of hypothyroid subjects and increased in hyperthyroidism compared with normal values [13]. Hypothyroid patients, especially children, frequently develop long, lanugo-type hair on the back, shoulders, and extremities [10]. Diminished sebum secretion contributes to the coarse appearance of the hair. Sometimes, hair loss is the only apparent symptom of hypothyroidism and the dermatologist is the first to diagnose and treat the condition. Nails grow slowly and tend to be thickened, striated and brittle. Onycholysis is also associated with hypothyroidism [1].

The specific pathophysiology linking hyperthyroidism to classic cutaneous findings remains to be well explained (5). In hyperthyroidism, the skin is warm, soft, moist and smooth. The epidermis is thin but not atrophic, and the stratum corneum is well hydrated. While the smooth skin is an epidermal finding, the warmth is caused by increased cutaneous blood flow and the moisture is a reflection of the underlying metabolic state [10]. The warmth is often accompanied by a persistent flush of the face, redness of the elbows, and palmar erythema. Hyperhydrosis, especially on palms and soles may be observed. Scalp hair may be fine and soft, and may be accompanied by a diffuse nonscarring alopecia. *In vitro* studies suggest increased hair growth rate in thyrotoxicosis. L-Triiodothyronine was shown to stimulate proliferation of outer root sheath keratinocytes and dermal papilla cells [14]. Hypertrichosis is can be observed in cases of thyroid dermatopathy and may be related to alterations in the proteoglycans associated with dermal papilla [15]. Sometimes an early symptom of hyperthyroidism is loss of pigment and early gray hair development. Nail changes may also occur, characterized by a concave contour accompanied by distal onycholysis (Plummer's nails). Hyperpigmentation has been described in thyrotoxic patients in both localized and generalized distribution. There is speculation that the hyperpigmentation is due to increased release of pituitary adrenocorticotropic hormone compensating for accelerated cortisol degradation [16]. Hyperthyroidism may also induce pruritus with or without urticaria [17]. Patients with autoimmune mediated thyrotoxicosis may also have distinct cutaneous manifestations such as pretibial myxedema and acropachy. Pretibial myxedema is the localized thickening of the pretibial skin due to accumulation of acid mukopolysaccharides. It usually present with firm nodules and plaques varying in colour from pink to purple-brown, and sometimes accompanied by woody induration on extensor surfaces. A diffuse brawny edema may be present without nodules. Localized hyperhydrosis has been reported in cases of pretibial myxedema. Less common is an elephantiasis nostras variant in which the extremity becomes enlarged and covered with verrucous nodules [10]. Thickening of the skin of the extensor surface of the forearm (preradial myxedema) has been reported [18]. Excessive amounts of hyaluronic acid and chondriotin are present in lesions as well as in clinically normal skin [19]. The precise pathogenesis of pretibial myxedema remains to be defined. One leading theory is that pretibial fibroblasts are the target for antithyroid antibodies. After stimulation by thyroid autoantibodies, fibroblasts may produce excess glukosaminglycans [5]. Other theories have implicated T cells as the primary effector of dermopathy. T-cells may interact with an autoantigen that is either identical or cross-reactive with a thyroid autoantigen in the dermis. In turn, this may induce secretion of cytokines such as glycosaminoglycan-stimulatory lymphokine, interleukin1, tumor necrosis factor, and gamma interferon, which activate fibroblasts to secrete hyaluronic acid and chondriotin sulfate [20]. Thyroid acropachy consist of the triad of digital clubbing, soft-tissue swelling of the hands and feet, and characteristic periostal reactions. The vast majority of cases are associated with Graves' disease, although it has been reported to occur in Hashimoto's thyroiditis. Scleromyxedema has been reported in the setting of hyperthyroidism. This rare entity is comprised of numerous firm, white, yellow, or pink papules scattered on the face, trunk, and extremitates. Cutaneous lesions are the result of accumulation of acid mucopolysaccharides, mostly hyaluronic acid, in the dermis, accompanied by large fibrocytes [5].

Skin manifestations of thyroid dysfunction may be divided into two main categories: (I) direct action of thyroid hormone on skin tissues, and (II) autoimmune skin disease associated with thyroid dysfunction of autoimmune etiology. Direct thyroid hormone action on skin is mediated through thyroid hormone receptor (TR). All three widely recognized thyroid hormone binding isoforms of TR have been identified in skin tissues [14, 21]. TRs have been detected in epidermal keratinocytes, skin fibroblasts, hair arrector pili muscle cells, sebaceous gland cells, vascular endothelial cells, and a number of cells types that make up the hair follicle [9]. The demonstration of TR expression in hair follicle cells indicates that thyroid hormone can affect hair growth directly, rather than through an intermediate mechanism such as a general metabolic status [22]. In addition, several thyroid hormone responsive genes have been identified in skin.

When thyroid disease is of autoimmune etiology, additional skin findings may be evident which reflect associated autoimmune disease [9]. Patients with autoimmune thyroid disease are at increased risk for other autoimmune diseases, both tissue-specific and generalized. In autoimmune disease such as Graves' disease and Hashimoto's thyroiditis the skin manifestations may be related to either thyroid hormone levels themselves or to associated T and/or B cell abnormalities [23]. A list of autoimmune conditions apparent when examining the skin includes alopecia areata, vitiligo, chronic urticaria, bullous disorders, connective tissue diseases and palmoplantar pustulosis.

There is convincing evidence of a significant association between thyroid autoimmunity and skin disorders. Most commonly reported cutaneous disorder related with thyroid diseases is alopecia areata, which have especially autoimmune etiology.

2. Thyroid autoimmunity in patients with alopecia areata

2.1. Introduction

Alopecia areata (AA) is a clinical condition characterized by well circumscribed, round, or oval patches of hair loss on the scalp or other parts of the body. Sometimes, alopecia totalis (AT), loss of all scalp hair, or alopacia universalis (AU), loss of all body hair, may develop. This disorder affects both sexes equally and occurs at all ages, although children and young adults are affected most often. The etiopathogenesis of AA is still unclear, but there is evidence that autoimmunity and endocrine dysfunction may be involved [24-26]. The autoimmune etiology has been proposed on the basis of its association with various autoimmune diseases, the presence of autoantibodies and various underlying immune abnormalities in the affected sites of these patients [27, 28]. One of the main associations is with thyroid abnormalities. This association was further supported by an increased incidence of abnormal thyroid structure, function tests and/or presence of thyroid autoantibodies found in many studies [29-32].

The aim of this study was to determine the prevalence of thyroid autoimmunity in patients with AA.

2.2. Patients and methods

The study included 70 patients with AA (40 female and 30 male). A detailed history and examination were taken in all study subjects, including patients age, age at onset, duration of disease, associated diseases, history of thyroid disorders and the extent and severity of disease. The diagnosis of AA was made on clinical grounds. Skin biopsy was performed in selected cases. No patient was diagnosed before this study as having any type of thyroid dysfunction. The control group consisted of 70 volunteers (40 female and 30 male) who had skin diseases other then AA or autoimmune disorders. Blood samples were taken and a physical examination and thyroid sonography was performed. All subjects gave their informed consent in accordance with the requirements of the institutional Ethichs Committee. Thyroid autoantibodies (thyroglobulin antibody, anti-Tg, and thyroid peroxidase antibody, anti-TPO) and thyroid hormones (thyroxine (T4), triiodthyronine (T3) and thyroid stimulating hormone (TSH) were measured in all subjects. Total T4 (normal range: 70-180 nmol/L) and total T3 (normal range: 1.3-3.3 nmol/L) were measured by use of radioimmunoassay (RIA); TSH (normal range: 0.3-4.2 mlU/L) was determined by use of immunoradiometric assay (IRMA) (BRAHMS Aktiengesellshaft, Hennigsdorf, Germany). Serum levels of anti-Tg (threshold value: 115 IU/mL) and anti-TPO (borderline value: 34 IU/mL) were measured by use of electrochemiluminiscence immunoassay (ECLIA) according to standard protocols (COBAS, Roche Diagnostics GmbH, Mannheim, Germany).

Baseline clinical characteristics for the two groups were compared with the use of Student's t-test for continuous variables, the chi-square test or Fisher' s exact test (two-sided) for categorical variables, as appropriate. Data were considered statistically significant at $P < 0.05$.

Statistical analyses were performed using MedCale for Windows, version 11.4.1.0 (MedCale Software, Mariakerke, Belgium).

2.3. Results

We performed a cross-sectional study in 70 consecutive patients with alopecia areata and 70 age- and sex-matched controls. Demographic data of patients and controls are shown in Table 1. The mean (SD) age of the patient and control groups was 40.39 (±14.39) and 40.71 (±15.30), respectively ($P = 0.896$). The onset of AA occurred in 14 (20%) of the patients before 16 years of age, 3 (4.28%) patients had AA more than 10 years. The duration of alopecia areata ranged from 1 to 150 months. A family history of the same disease was present in 7 (10%) patients. According to the clinical type of AA, 13 patients had unilocular lesion, 37 patients had multilocular lesions, 12 alopecia totalis and 8 alopecia universalis (Table 2).

Thyroid functional abnormalities were found in 8 (11,43%) patients. In the control group only one patient had abnormalities in hormonal status.

Hypoechogenic thyroid tissue was seen in 7 (10%) patients who all had elevated levels of thyroid autoatibodies. The thyroid gland was enlarged in 5 (7.14%) patients. Goitre was diagnosed in 4 (5.71%) cases. The ultrasound examination of the thyroid gland in control group was interpreted as normal in 64 (91.42%), and 6 (5.45%) volunteers had small simple goiter. Thyroid volume did not differ significantly between the study patients and the controls ($p>0.05$).

In patients with alopecia areata anti-Tg titers were ranging from 11.10 to 915.30 IU/mL and anti-TPO antibody titers from 5.10 to 714.40 IU/mL. In control group anti-Tg titers were ranging from 10.00 to 153.00 IU/mL, and anti-TPO antibody titers from 4.40 to 129.00 IU/mL. Anti-Tg antibody in 16 (23%) patients, anti-TPO antibody in 21 (30%) and both anti-Tg and anti-TPO antibodies in 13 (19%) were higher than the normal antibody titres. In the control group, one subject (1%) had positive anti-Tg and one volunteer (1%) had positive anti-TPO. The frequency of thyroid autoantibodies was significantly higher in alopecia areata patients than in control group (Table 3).

A Chi-square test for independence (with Yates Continuity Correction) indicated significant association between higher values of anti-Tg (values more than 115 IU/ml) and alopecia areata, χ^2 (1, n=140)= 13.123, P=0.0003.

A Chi-square test for independence (with Yates Continuity Correction) indicated significant association between higher values of anti-TPO (values more than 34 IU/ml) and alopecia areata, χ^2 (1, n=140)=19.468, P<0.0001.

	Alopecia areata group n (%)	Control group n (%)	P
Men, n (%)	30 (43)	30 (43)	
Women, n (%)	40 (57)	40 (57)	
Age range, years	17-66	16-66	
Age, mean years (SD)	40.39 (14.39)	40.71 (15.30)	0.896

Table 1. Demographic data of patients (Alopecia areata group) and volunteers (Control group)

Mean age of onset (SD) (year)	38.14 (14.61)
Age of onset range (year)	14-65
Mean duration (SD) (month)	21.93 (30.69)
Duration Range (month)	1-150
Type of alopecia areata n, (%)	
Unilocularis 13 (19)	
Multiloculares 37 (53)	
Universalis 8 (11)	
Totalis 12 (17)	

Table 2. Clinical characteristics of alopecia areata patients

	anti-Tg (threshold value115 IU/ml)		anti-TPO (threshold value 34 IU/ml)	
Group	Negative n(%)	Positive n(%)	Negative n(%)	Positive n(%)
Alopecia areata	54 (77)	16 (23)	49 (70)	21(30)
Control	69 (99)	1 (1)	69 (99)	1 (1)
Total	123 (88)	17 (12)	118 (84)	22 (16)
Difference n (%)	15 (22)		20 (29)	
χ^2, P	χ^2=13.123, P=0.0003		χ^2=19.468, P<0.0001	

Table 3. The frequencies of positive detectable thyroid autoantibody (anti-Tg and anti-TPO)

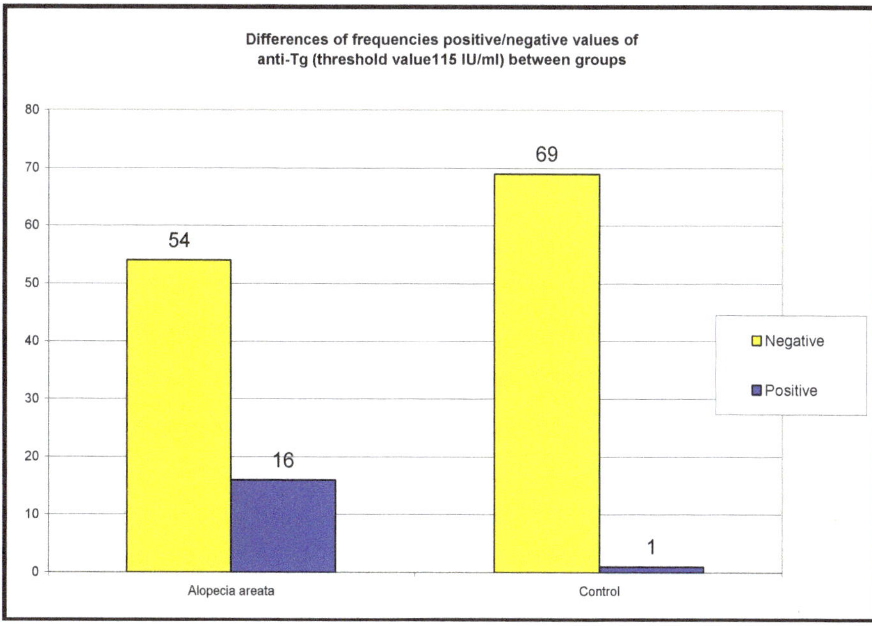

Scheme 1. Differences of frequencies positive/negative values of anti-Tg (threshold value115 IU/ml) between groups

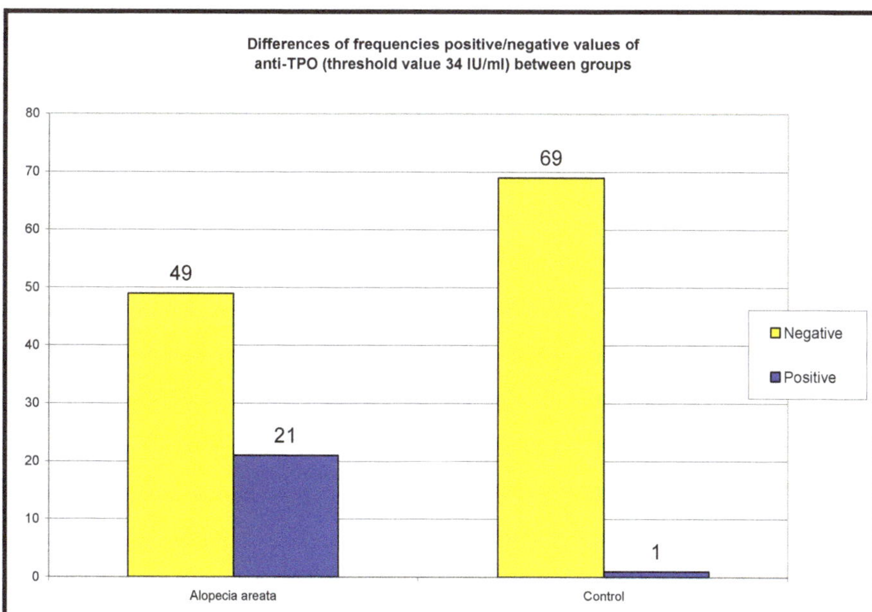

Scheme 2. Differences of frequencies positive/negative values of anti-TPO (threshold value 34 IU/ml) between groups

	anti-Tg (threshold value115 IU/ml)			Types of alopecia areata (P)		
Type of alopecia areata	Negative n	Positive n	Total	Multiloculares	Totalis	Universalis
Unilocularis	12	1	13	0.662246	0.160248	0.047472*
Multiloculares	30	7	37	N/A	0.426673	0.085080
Totalis	8	4	12	N/A	N/A	0.647916
Universalis	4	4	8	N/A	N/A	N/A
Total	54	16	70			

Table 4. The frequencies of positive detectable thyroid autoantibody (anti-Tg) and differences between types of alopecia areata

A Fisher's exact indicated significant association between higher values of anti-Tg (values more than 115 IU/ml) and some types of alopecia areata, Universalis vs Unilocularis (P=0.047472) (Table 4.)

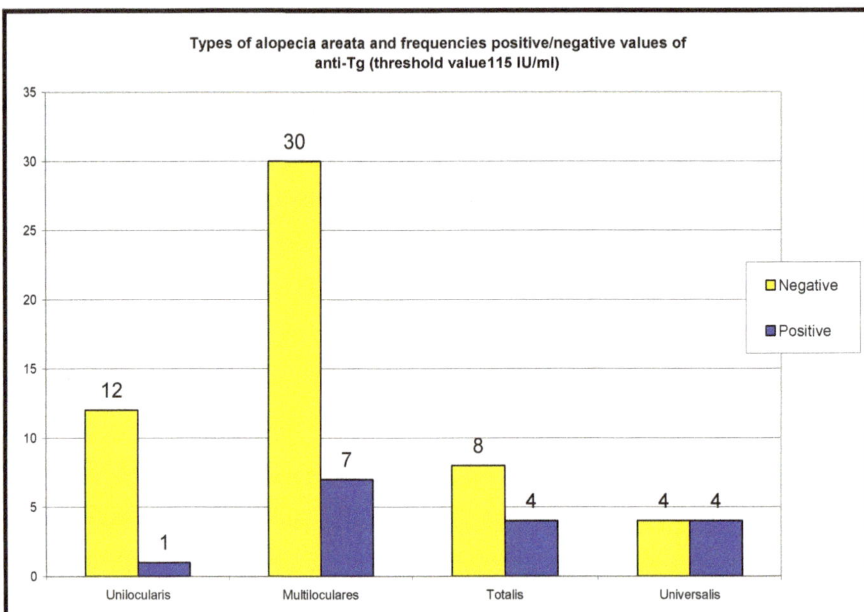

Scheme 3. Types of alopecia areata and frequencies positive/negative values of anti-Tg (threshold value115 IU/ml)

A Fisher's exact indicated significant association between higher values of anti-TPO (values more than 34 IU/ml) and some types of alopecia areata: Unilocularis vs Totalis (P=0.005217), Unilocularis vs Universalis (P=0.000069) and Multiloculares vs Universalis (P=0.000925) (Table 5).

	anti-TPO (threshold value 34 IU/ml)			Types of alopecia areata (P)		
Type of alopecia areata	Negative n	Positive n	Total	Multiloculares	Totalis	Universalis
Unilocularis	13	0	13	0.092788	0.005217*	0.000069*
Multiloculares	29	8	37	N/A	0.075803	0.000925*
Totalis	6	6	12	N/A	N/A	0.157688
Universalis	1	7	8	N/A	N/A	N/A
Total	49	21	70			

Table 5. The frequencies of positive detectable thyroid autoantibody (anti-TPO) and differences between types of alopecia areata

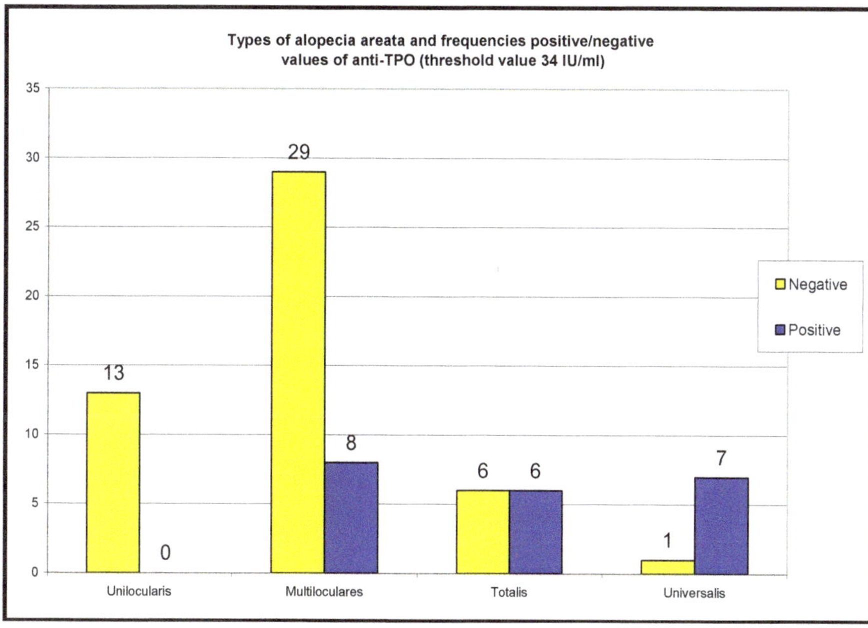

Scheme 4. Types of alopecia areata and frequencies positive/negative values of anti-TPO (threshold value 34 IU/ml)

2.4. Discusion

Alopecia areata is an ancient disease that was known to Egyptians even in the pre-Christian time [33]. Despite its long history, our knowledge is actually limited. Today, AA is hypothezed to be an autoimmune, organ specific T-cell mediated reaction directed against an unknown autoantigen of the hair follicle. T lymphocytes that have been shown to be oligoclonal and autoreactive are predominantly present in the peribulbous inflammatory infiltrate [34]. Although the skin is the primary location of the clinical phenotype, the determination of disease expression involves a complex interplay between different inflammatory cell subsets in the skin, skin draining lymphonodes, and spleen of the affected individuals [35].

Clinical association with AA has known for many years. AA frequently occurs in association with other autoimmune disorders such as vitiligo, lupus erythematosus, pernicious anemia and others [34, 36-38]. Among endocrine disorders, thyroid diseases are the commonest that has been described as associated with AA, but the issued values were different. In the greatest study reported till now, Muller and Winkelmann have found the evidences of different types of thyroid disease in 8% of 736 patients in compare to less than 2% of the control population in North America [39]. Broniarczyk-Dyla *et al.* observed abnormalities of thyroid structure and function in even 78% of AA patients [40]. Conversely, Puavilai *et al.* estimated that the prevalence of thyroid disease is relatively low (7.2%) and was not statistically different from the control group [41].

In accordance to previous studies, current study reported a high frequency of thyroid diseases in AA patients. We detected elevated anti-Tg in 16 (23%) and elevated anti-TPO in 21 (30%) of patients with AA. Compared with the control group, the frequency of the both anti-Tg and anti-TPO antibodies was significantly higher in those with AA. Statistically significant difference was also found in values of anti-Tg and anti-TPO between patients with different clinical type of the disease. The highest anti-Tg concentrations were observed in patients with alopecia universalis. Patients with thyroid diseases were on an average older and reported longer duration, but the results were not statistically significant. These results are consistent with a clinical study performed by Seyrafi *et al.* [32]. They analyzed serum TgAb level in 123 Iranian patients with AA and found it to be elevated in 29.3% of study patients. Grandolfo *et al.* observed the presence of thyroid autoantibodies in even 44% of AA patients [42]. Goh *et al.* also confirmed the frequent coexistence of AA and thyroid abnormalities [43]. They found 19% of probands with thyroid disease including simple goitre, Grave's disease and Hashomoto's thyroiditis. Our findings showed that the frequency of anti-TPO was more significant than anti-Tg. This antibody, historically referred to as the antimicrosomal antibody, is established as a sensitive tool for the detection of early subclinical autoimmune thyroid diseases and identification of at-risk cases for autoimmune thyroid diseases [44]. Nordyke *et al.* reported that anti-TPO antibody tends to have more correlation than does the anti-Tg antibody [45].

Alopecia areata offers many benefits as a model for the study of autoimmunity, in that it can be used to identify the contributing roles of immunogenetics and neuroendocrine factors in the initiation and propagation of autoimmune disease [24].

The study revealed a significant association between AA and thyroid disease and showed the tests used to detected thyroid autoantibodies to be relevant in patients with AA. Further exploration of this relationship in clinical setting and at a molecular level may help in the understanding of the pathogenesis of both diseases.

3. Conclusions

Thyroid autoimmunity is the most prevalent autoimmune condition in the general population, and is also associated with various skin diseases. The evidence is strong for the association with alopecia areata. Although their etiology is still unclear, the autoimmune hypothesis is most commonly accepted.

The nature of the relationship between anti-thyroid autoimmunity and the pathogenesis of autoimmune diseases is presently unknown. Some authors have shown that anti-Tg antibodies can form immune complexes [46], and anti-microsomal antibodies not only bind to thyroid peroxidase but also modulate natural killer cell activity in autoimmune thyroiditis [47]. Possible explanations for the relationship of these autoimmune diseases include: (1) immunomodulatory effects of antithyroid antibodies, (2) molecular mimicry between thyroid and disease-specific epitopes, and (3) genetic link between anti-thyroid autoimmunity and the susceptibility to autoimmune disease [48]. It is a multidisciplinary problem requiring cooperation of specialists in different fields of medicine. Both dermatologists and endocrinologists have to inquire their patients about the family history of autoimmune diseases and to look for associated autoimmune disorders.

This chapter is an attempt to update the current knowledge about the relationship between the thyroid and the skin diseases. Although cutaneous manifestations of autoimmune thyroid diseases are well described and thyroid hormone is known to regulate the development and function of skin, a better understanding of these processes is needed.

Author details

Emina Kasumagic-Halilovic*
Department of Dermatovenerology, Sarajevo University Clinical Center, Sarajevo, Bosnia and Herzegovina

Begler Begovic
Department of Clinical Pharmacology, Sarajevo University Clinical Center, Sarajevo, Bosnia and Herzegovina

4. References

[1] Mullin GE, Eastern JS (1986) Cutaneous signs of thyroid disease. Am Fam Physican. 34: 93-98.
[2] Mullin GE, Eastern JS (1986) Cutaneous consequences of accelerated thyroid function. Cutis. 37: 109-114.
[3] Safer JD, Crawford TM, Fraser LM, Hoa M, Ray S, Chen TC at al. (2003) Thyroid hormone action on skin: Diverging effects of topical varsus intraperitoneal administration. Thyroid. 13: 159-165.
[4] Holt PJA (1978) In vivo responses of the epidermis to triiodthyronine. J Invest Derm. 71: 202-204.
[5] Leonhardt JM, Heyman WR (2002) Thyroid disease and the skin. Dermatol Clin. 20:473-481.

* Corresponding Author

[6] Pazos-Moura CC, Moura EG, Breitenbach MMD et al. (1998) Nailfold capillaroscopy in hypothyroidism: blood flow velocity during rest and postocclusive reactive hyperemia. Angiology. 49: 471
[7] Silva JE (2003) The termogenic effect of thyroid hormone and its clinical implications. Anals of Internal Medicine. 139. 205-213.
[8] Christianson HB (1976) Cutaneous manifestations of hypothyroidism including purpura and ecchymoses. Cutis. 17: 45.
[9] Safer JD (2011) Thyroid hormone action on skin. Dermato Endocrinology 3: 211-215.
[10] Freinkel RK (1993) Cutaneous manifestations of endocrine disease. In: Fitzpatrick TB, Eisen AZ, Wolff K, Freedberg IM, Austen KF, editors. Dermatology in general medicine. McGraw-Hill, Inc. pp 2113-2131.
[11] Hanley K, Devaskar UP, Hicks SJ et al. (1997) Hypothyroidism delays fetal stratum corneum development in mice. Pediatr Res. 42: 610.
[12] Dekio S, Imaoka C, Jidoi J (1987) Candida folliculitis associated with hypothyroidism. Br J Dermatol. 117: 663.
[13] Schell H, Kiesewetter F, Seidel C et al. (1991) Cell cycle kinetiks of human anagen scalp hair bulbs in thyroid disorders determined byDNA flow cytometry. Dermatologica. 182: 23-26.
[14] Ahsan MK, Urano J, Kato S, Oura H, Arase S (1998) Immunohistochemical localization of thyroid hormone nuclear receptors in human hair follicles and in vitro effect of L-triiodothyronine on cultured cells of hair follicles and skin. J Med Invest. 44: 179-184.
[15] Westgate GE, Messenger AG, Watson LP, et al. (1991) Distribution of proteoglycans during the hair growth cycle in human skin. J Invest Dermatol. 96: 191.
[16] Diven DG, Gwinup G, Newton RC (1989) The thyroid. Dermatol Clin. 7: 547-557.
[17] Ai J, Leonhardt JM, Heymann WR (2003) Autoimmune thyroid diseases: etiology, pathogenesis, and dermatologic manifestations. J Am Acad Dermatol. 48: 641-659.
[18] Wortsman J, Dietrich J, Traycoff RB, Stone S (1981) Preradial myxedema in thyroid disease. Arch Dermatol. 117: 635-638.
[19] Bierewaltes WH, Bollet AJ (1959) Mucopolysaccharide content of skin in patients with pretibial myxedema. J Clin Invest. 38: 945
[20] Weetman AP (2001) Determinants of autoimmune thyroid disease. Nat Immunol. 2: 769-770.
[21] Billoni N, Buan B, Gautier B, Gaillard O, Mahe YF, Bernhard BA (2000) Thyroid hormone receptor beta-1 is expressed in the human hair follicle. Br J Dermatol. 142: 645-652.
[22] Messenger AG (2000) Thyroid hormone and hair growth. Br J Dermatol. 142: 631-635.
[23] Burman KD, McKinley-Grant L (2006) Dermatologic aspects of thyroid disease. Clin Dermatol. 24: 247-255.
[24] Gilhar A, Paus R, Kalish R (2007) Lymphocytes, neuropeptides, and genes involved in alopecia areata. J Clin Invest. 117: 2019-27.
[25] Alexis AF, Dudda-Subramanya R, Sinha AA (2004) Alopecia areata: autoimmune basis of hair loss. Eur J Dermatol. 14(6): 364-70.

[26] Milgraum SS, Mitchell AJ, Bacon GE, Rasmusen JE (1987) Alopecia areata, endocrine function, and antibodies in patients 16 years of age or younger. J Am Acad Dermatol. 17: 57-61.
[27] McDonagh AJG, Messenger AG (1996) The pathogenesis of alopecia areata. Dermatol Clin. 14: 661-70.
[28] Tobin DJ, Orentreich N, Fenton DA, Bystrin JC (1994) Antibodies to hair follicles in alopecia areata. J Invest Dermatol. 102: 721-4.
[29] Lewinski A, Broniarczyk-Dyla G, Sewerynek E. Zerek-Melen G, Szkudlinski M (1990) Abnormlities in structure and function of thyroid gland in patients with alopecia areata. J Am Acad Dermatol. 23: 768-9.
[30] Kasumagic-Halilovic E (2008) Thyroid autoimmunity in alopecia areata. Acta dermatovenerol Croat. 16(3): 123-25.
[31] Kurtev A, Ilev E (2005) Thyroid autoimmunity in children and adolescents with alopecia areata. Int J Dermatol. 44: 457-61.
[32] Seyrafi H, Akhiani M, Abbasi H, Mirpour S, Gholamrezanezahad A (2005) Evaluation of the profile of alopecia areata and the prevalence of thyroid function test abnormalities and serum autoantibodies in Iranien patients. BMC Dermatol. 5: 11-6.
[33] Ebel B (1937) The papyrus Ebers: The greatest Egyptian document. Copenhagen: Leivin and Munksgaard.
[34] Hordinsky M, Ericson M (2004) Autoimmunity: Alopecia areata. J Invest Dermatol Symp Proc. 9: 73-8.
[35] McElwee KJ, Hoffman R, Freyschmidt-Paul P, Wenzel E, Kissling S, Sundberg JP (2002) Resistence to alopecia areata in C3H/HeJ mice is associated with increased expression of regulatory cytokines and failure recruit CD4+ and CD8+ cells. J Invest Dermatol. 119: 1426-33.
[36] Gopal KV, Rama Rao GR, Kumar YH, Appa Rao MV, Vasudev P, Strikant (2007) Vitiligo: A part of a systemic autoimmune process. Indian J Dermatol Venereol Leprol. 73(3): 162-65.
[37] Werth VP, White WL, Sauchez MR, Franks AG (1992) Incidence of alopecia areata in lupus erythematosus. Arch Dermatol. 128(3): 368-71.
[38] Madani S, Shapiro J (2000) Alopecia areata update. J Am Acad Dermatol. 549-66.
[39] Muller SA, Winkelmann RK (1963) Alopecia areata. Arch Dermatol. 88: 290-97.
[40] Broniarczyk-Dyla G, Lewinski A, Zerek-Melen G, Sewerynek E, Wozniacka A (1989) Abnormalities of structure and function of the thyroid in patients with alopecia areata Przegl Dermatol. 76: 416-21.
[41] Puavilai S, Puavilai G, Charuwichitratana S, Sakuntabhai A, Sriprachya-Anunt S. Prevalence of thyroid diseases in patients with alopecia areata. Int J Dermatol 1994; 33(9): 632-3.
[42] Gandoldolfo M, Biscazzi AM, Pipoli M (2008) Alopecia areata and autoimmunity. G Ital Dermatol Venereol. 143(5): 277-81.
[43] Goh C, Finkel M, Christos PJ, Sinha AA (2006) Profile of 513 patients with alopecia areata: association of disease subtypes with atopy, autoimmune disease and positive family history. J Eur Acad Dermatol Venereol. 20: 1055-60.

[44] Kemp EH (2004) Autoantibodies as diagnostic and predictive markers of vitiligo. Autoimmunity. 37:287-90.

[45] Nordyke RA, Gilbert FI Jr, Miyamoto LA, Fleury KA (1993) The superiority of antimicrosomal over antithyreoglobulin antibodies for detecting Hashimoto's thyroiditis. Arch Intern Med. 153(7): 862-65.

[46] Dawe K, Hutchings P, Champion B, Cook A, Roitt I (1993) Autoantigens in thyroid diseases. Springer Semin Immunopathol. 14: 285-307.

[47] Robert DU (1991) The pathogenesis of autoimmune thyroiditis. N Engl J Med. 324: 278-279.

[48] Szyper-Kravitz M, Marai I, Shoenfeld Y (2005) Coexistence of thyroid autoimmunity with other autoimmune diseases: friend or foe? Additional aspects on the mosaic of autoimmunity. Autoimmunity. 38: 247-255.

Chapter 12

Thyroid Function Abnormalities in Patients Receiving Anticancer Agents

Francesco Torino, Agnese Barnabei,
Roberto Baldelli and Marialuisa Appetecchia

Additional information is available at the end of the chapter

1. Introduction

Advances in systemic chemotherapy and radiotherapy have had a profound effect on the prognosis of patients affected by many cancer histotypes. Nonetheless, one of the main challenges for modern oncology is in improving the tolerability of these treatments. The frequency and pathophysiology of the most common side effects induced by cytotoxic agents are well known. They may be immediate or delayed in onset and prevalently involve bone marrow, gastrointestinal system, liver, and cutaneous annexes.

Abnormalities in thyroid function and thyroid disease are variably associated with cancer or cancer therapy [1]. These disorders encompass a broad variety of pathophysiological mechanisms, may be subtle in presentation, sometimes difficult to be identified, and even more difficult to relate to a particular chemotherapeutic regimen due to the lack of specific wide clinical trials [2]. The alteration of thyroid hormone metabolism, more commonly known as "euthyroid sick syndrome", may occur in patients with advanced cancers. Thyroid dysfunction, such as the altered synthesis or clearance of thyroid hormone-binding proteins are observed in certain malignancies, or may be caused by treatments that modify total but not free concentration of thyroid hormones. However, the clinical influence of this abnormalities is marginal, if any.

Endocrine disorders are among the most commonly reported long-term complications of cancer treatment by adult survivors of childhood cancers [3]. In adults, cytotoxic drugs are infrequently associated to overt endocrine toxicity. However, excluding gonadotoxic consequence [4], only few studies thoroughly evaluated the endocrine dysfunction induced by cytotoxic anticancer therapy in this population [2]. Similarly, hormonal therapies, widely used as effective treatment of patients affected by endocrine responsive breast cancer and prostate cancer, have shown only marginally influence on thyroid function and thyroid toxicities attributed to these drugs are anecdotic.

In contrast to cytotoxics and hormonal therapies, several novel antineoplastic agents, including targeted therapies and immunotherapies, are unexpectedly associated with thyroid dysfunction and thyroid disease, despite their high selectivity of action [5].

Even diagnostic procedures using iodinated contrast agents can be associated with acute effects on the thyroid, including hyperthyroidism (i.e. in patients with thyroid autonomous nodules or mild Graves disease), or transient hypothyroidism (i.e. in patients with Hashimoto thyroiditis) [6,7]. Radiation therapy can be responsible for hypothyroidism from direct damage on the thyroid or secondary to hypopituitarism from brain irradiation. Irradiation received during childhood has been associated with thyroid nodules and thyroid cancer [8].

In this chapter, available data on thyroid abnormalities induced by anticancer drugs only are discussed.

2. Cytotoxic agents

Cytotoxic chemotherapy seems to alter endocrine functions in a relatively small proportion of patients and is infrequently associated with thyroid abnormalities in the absence of irradiation. Cytotoxics may sensitize the thyroid gland to the effects of concomitant radiation therapy, increasing the risk of radiation-induced primary hypothyroidism [9].

In a small published series, some agents such as 5-fluorouracil, glucocorticoids, estrogens, tamoxifen, podophyllin and L-asparaginase alter levels of thyroid hormone–binding proteins without any clinical consequence [10-15]. L-asparaginase can also be responsible for transient hypothalamic or pituitary hypothyroidism [16]. Other agents such as lomustine, vincristine, and cisplatin have *in vitro* effects on thyroid cells, but clinically relevant consequences have not been reported [17]. Mitotane is the only active agent against advanced adrenocortical cancer (ACC) and is under evaluation in patients who underwent radical resection of this rare disease. Mitotane showed a complex interference on the endocrine system that may require multiple hormone replacement therapy. In a prospective trial [18] on 17 patients who underwent radical resection for ACC, a marked reduction in free-T4 (FT4) levels was found, without any significant changes in serum thyroid stimulating hormone (TSH) and free-T3 (FT3) concentration. FT4 reduction was inversely correlated with mitotane concentrations and dropped in the hypothyroid range in most evaluable patients. These findings mimic central hypothyroidism and are consistent with data from clinical experiments which showed that mitotane directly reduces both secretory activity and cell viability on pituitary TSH-secreting mouse cells [19]. Alternatively, it has been suggested that mitotane may affect deiodase activity, thus changing the FT4 to FT3 ratio. However, despite limited information on free thyroid hormone concentrations during mitotane treatment has been reported, for some patients thyroxine replacement may be necessary [20].

An increased incidence of primary hypothyroidism has been documented in patients treated with multiple drug regimens, with or without radiotherapy [2]. In patients with testicular cancer who received combinations of cisplatin, bleomycin, vinblastine, etoposide, and dactinomycin, 4 out of 27 individuals (15%) developed primary hypothyroidism. In particular, the cumulative doses of cisplatin and vincristine seem to exacerbate these symptoms [21]. In another trial evaluating the combination of mechlorethamine, vinblastine, procarbazine and prednisolone (MOPP regimen) as treatment of Hodgkin's disease, 44% of patients developed elevated serum TSH concentrations, even though a causative role of iodine load during lymphangiograpy cannot be excluded [22]. Children with brain tumors (not involving the hypothalamic-pituitary axis) who receive vincristine, carmustine or lomustine, and procarbazine in combination and brain irradiation have a 35% incidence of hypothyroidism, compared with a 10% incidence in the group with brain irradiation alone [23]. Young age and use of chemotherapy have been associated with a higher incidence of hypothyroidism in patients receiving radiotherapy for medulloblastoma [24]. Again, the highest incidence occurred when the thyroid gland was included in the radiation field. Finally, there is no evidence that cytotoxic agents by itself may represent a risk factor for developing thyroid tumors, compared to radiotherapy [2].

3. Immunoregulatory agents

3.1. Cytokines

3.1.1. Interferon-α

Interferon-α is a human recombinant cytokine that increases the expression of major histocompatibility complex (MHC) class I and tumor-specific antigens on the tumor cell surface, stimulating immune-mediated destruction of these cells, as well as possibly exerting direct antitumor effects [25]. Interferon-α demonstrated variable efficacy in patients affected by melanoma, renal cell carcinoma (RCC), AIDS-related Kaposi's sarcoma, follicular lymphoma, hairy cell leukemia, and chronic myelogenous leukemia [25]. Reduction in viral load is another relevant activity of interferons. In combination with ribavidin, interferon-α prolongs survival in patients with hepatitis C [26,27]. Flu-like syndrome, malaise, neuropsychiatric disorders, hematologic and liver toxicity are the most common dose-limiting side-effects.

Thyroid diseases secondary to treatment with Interferon-α are common and may become clinically evident as destructive thyroiditis, autoimmune hypothyroidism or Graves-like hyperthyroidism. Patients receiving the drug for hepatitis appear more prone to present thyroid dysfunction than patients with malignant disease [28]. However, the infection from the hepatitis C virus itself has been demonstrated to increase the risk of thyroid damage [28]. The pegylated form of interferon-α is more effective than interferon-α in triggering antiviral response, but showed a similar rate of thyroid dysfunction [29].

Destructive or autoimmune thyroiditis is the most common thyroid abnormality following treatment with interferon-α. This condition may lead to hypothyroidism after a brief thyrotoxic phase and usually occurs in the first few weeks of interferon treatment and is in close temporal relationship with the appearance of thyroid autoantibodies, especially anti-thyroglobulin (anti-TG) antibodies. Another form of autoimmune thyroid toxicity associated to interferon-α is characterized by the development of thyroid antibodies without hypothyroidism. In the setting of interferon therapy, the risk of hypothyroidism is 2.4%–10% [30-35], with a risk of thyroid autoimmunity onset (including development of thyroid autoantibodies) approaching 20% [36,37]. Hypothyroidism is persistent in the majority of patients [33,38], even though although transient hypothyroidism has also been described [39]. The presence of anti-thyroperoxidase (anti-TPO) antibodies before treatment considerably increases the risk of hypothyroidism [40-42]. Thyroid abnormalities can occur as early as 4 weeks and as late as 23 months after initiating treatment, with a median of 4 months [30,34].

Interferon-α has also been associated with classical Graves disease and sometimes Graves' ophthalmopathy also develops, however the latter is less common [30]. This condition does not generally remit on withdrawal of the drug [35].

Several evidence supports the hypothesis that thyroid toxicity may likely be related to an autoimmune response to interferon-α. Overexpression of MHC class I antigens are associated with activation of cytotoxic T-cells resulting in cellular destruction [43]. It has been reported that interferon-α increases MHC class I expression on thyroid tissue from Graves patients, provided that lymphocytes are present in the thyroid tissue [44]. Hence, interferon-α might worsen local immune response in subjects who have preexisting subclinical thyroiditis with intrathyroidal lymphocytes [44]. In addition, interferon-α can shift the immune response to a Th1-mediated immune response, with increased production of the proinflammatory cytokines interferon-γ and interleukin-2, which may in turn amplify an autoimmune response. Interferon-α has been demonstrated to elicit a direct damage on thyroid cells, which may be responsible for the onset of destructive thyroiditis [28,35,42,45]. However, despite accumulating evidence, the precise mechanisms underlying thyroid toxicity associated to interferon, especially in cancer patients, remain to be elucidated.

Levothyroxine (LT4) therapy is indicated as treatment of interferon-induced hypothyroidism and withdrawal of interferon is not generally needed. When destructive thyroiditis is present, treatment with corticosteroids is needed and β-blockers are often useful to control the signs and symptoms of thyrotoxicosis. When interferon causes hyperthyroidism, antithyroid agents such as methimazole or propylthiouracil may be administered, if clinically indicated. In patients with relapsing flares of thyroiditis during prolonged courses of interferon-α, ablation with ^{131}I during remission may be offered to prevent further episodes of the condition [46].

Despite specific recommendations for patients treated with interferon-α for oncological diseases are lacking, it appears rational to apply the recommendations available for patients with hepatitis C [47]. In particular, the same serological screening is suggested, including pretreatment TSH and anti-TPO antibodies evaluation, followed by TSH serum measurement every 2 months and then every six months in the case of negative anti-thyroid peroxidase (anti-TPO) antibodies [1].

3.1.2. Interleukin-2

Interleukin-2 is a cytokine involved in several mechanisms of immune response, including activation of natural killer cells and antigen-specific T-cells. These properties are used to stimulate tumor cell killing, also in combination with interferon or lymphokine-activated killer cells. Interleukin-2 is approved for the treatment of metastatic melanoma and RCC, although its use has been recently reduced in concomitance with the availability of more effective and better tolerated agents.

Several autoimmune side-effects have been associated to interleukin-2 therapy, including thyroid disease with an incidence of 10%–50% [48-54]. Hypothyroidism usually occurs 4–17 weeks after initiation of treatment [48,49]. It may be reversible following discontinuation of the drug [49,55]. Most patients who developed hypothyroidism showed positive anti-TG or anti-TPO antibodies. In addition to hypothyroidism, thyroiditis and thyrotoxicosis have also been reported at a lesser frequency [55,56]. An early phase of presumably destructive thyrotoxicosis is common, with variable degrees of hyperthyroidism [57].

Evidence suggests that thyroid disease associated to interleukin-2 may be induced by stimulating autoreactive lymphocytes, leading to autoimmune thyroiditis. Patients under treatment with interleukin-2 showed high levels of interferon-γ and tumor necrosis factor-α, which may trigger autoimmunity by enhancing the presentation of human leukocyte antigen class II and associated autoantigens by thyrocytes. Also, interleukin-2 may have direct effects on thyrocyte functioning [58,59]. Increase in serum thyroid autoantibodies levels [48,53] and lymphocyte infiltration of the thyroid gland [57] were found in patients treated with interleukin-2, suggesting a cell-mediated autoimmune mechanism. Similarly to interferon, preexisting positivity of thyroid autoantibodies seems to predict an increased risk of developing hypothyroidism during interleukin-2 treatment [49].

Occurrence of hypothyroidism was associated with a favorable response to treatment [48,60], but other studies did not confirm these results [61]. It has been suggested that thyroid dysfunction may develop more often in the responders because they receive longer courses of the treatment [46,62]. Patients with interleukin-2-induced hypothyroidism may be treated with LT4, while thyrotoxicosis only requires symptom control with β-blockers and corticosteroids. Measuring TSH before treatment and then every 2–3 months during treatment with interleukin-2 is advisable [1].

3.2. Thalidomide and lenalidomide

Thalidomide and lenalidomide are immunomodulatory drugs with antineoplastic activity [63,64]. These agents enhance T-cell stimulation and proliferation, induce endogenous cytokine release, and increase number and function of natural killer cells, thus enhancing immune-mediated destruction of tumor cells. They also inhibit proliferation and induce apoptosis of tumor cells and exert antiangiogenic activity [63,64].

Thalidomide and lenalidomide are approved for the treatment of multiple myeloma. Lenalidomide has also been approved for 5q myelodysplastic syndrome. Both agents are under evaluation for the treatment of several solid tumors, including thyroid cancer [65-67] and for a range of autoimmune diseases [68].

Hypothyroidism has been associated to treatment with these drugs with varying grades and frequency [68-71]. In a recent study on patients affected by multiple myeloma and treated with thalidomide [69], subclinical hypothyroidism was reported in 20% of participants, and 7% showed overt hypothyroidism, mostly occurring 1–6 months after initiating treatment [69].

Lenalidomide is more potent and showed a more favorable toxicity profile compared to thalidomide [72,73]. Hypothyroidism due to lenalidomide has been reported in 5%–10% of patients [74,75]. Thyroid abnormalities were found in 10 out of 170 patients who received lenalidomide for various hematological cancers. After a median of 5 months of therapy the patients reported both hypothyroidism and thyrotoxicosis. However, many of them had been exposed to prior radiation or thalidomide [76].

Many mechanisms have been suggested for the hypothyroidism induced by these drugs [69], including inhibition of thyroid hormone secretion [77] or a reduction of iodine uptake into follicular cells [78]. Most probably, since thalidomide and lenalidomide exert an antiangiogenic activity, compromise the blood flow to the thyroid may explain thyroid toxicity [69]. In some patients, TSH suppression has been documented before the development of hypothyroidism, suggesting ischemic thyroiditis [69]. Alternatively, a thyrotoxicosis triggered by an immune-mediated destructive thyroiditis may be hypothesized. This condition may be induced by deregulation of cytokine levels or through direct effects on T-lymphocytes [69]. A direct toxic effect on thyroid cells is also possible, but this has not been evaluated. TSH measurement before treatment and then every 2–3 months during treatment is recommended [1,79].

3.3. Anti-CTLA4 monoclonal antibodies

Ipilimumab and tremelimumab are monoclonal antibodies directed against cytotoxic T-lymphocyte-associated antigen 4 (CTLA-4) (anti–CTLA-4 mAbs), a receptor expressed on T-cells that exerts a suppressive effect on the immune response after T-cell/antigen-presenting cell interaction [80]. Blocking the receptor, an increased T-cell activation and antitumor effects are obtained. Ipilimumab is approved for the treatment of unresectable or metastatic melanoma.

These agents have been associated with several immune-related adverse events (IRAEs), most frequently enterocolitis, hepatitis, cutaneous reactions [81-83]. The spectrum of autoimmune endocrine adverse events experienced by patients treated with anti–CTLA-4 mAbs includes hypopituitarism, primary thyroid disease, and sporadically primary adrenal insufficiency [84]. The prevalence of autoimmune hypophysitis varies among different studies (0%–17%) [85], being 3-5% in larger studies. Similarly to classical autoimmune hypophysitis, secondary hypothyroidism has been reported in patients who develop hypophysitis induced by anti-CTLA-4 monoclonal antibodies.

Direct damage to the thyroid induced by these agents presents two clinical common forms: hyperthyroidism in Graves' disease and thyroid destruction with hypothyroidism in Hashimoto's thyroiditis. Since these conditions are classically included in autoimmune thyroid diseases phenotype and previous studies suggested that *CTLA-4* is a candidate gene conferring susceptibility to thyroid autoimmunity [86], an autoimmune pathogenesis has also been suggested for thyropathies induced by anti-CTLA4-mAbs (anti-CTLA4-IT). The incidence of these conditions varies from 0 to 4% among the different trials. In two studies [87,88], tremelimumab (15 mg/Kg body weight) was associated with thyreopathy (hyper-/hypothyroidism, autoimmune-thyroiditis, or Graves' disease) in 4% of cases. In studies on ipilimumab, the reported incidence of anti-CTLA4-IT was apparently lower, namely 0-2%, being mild hypothyroidism the most frequent thyroid side-effect. Recently, Hodi et al. in a large phase III trial, reported for the first time an improvement in overall survival obtained by ipilimumab in pretreated patients affected by metastatic melanoma [89]. The treatment was associated with thyroid disorders or abnormal thyroid function tests in approximately 2% of patients. In a randomized phase II study on a cohort of 115 patients affected by metastatic melanoma, evaluating the potential protective effect of budesonide on IRAEs induced by ipilimumab, hypothyroidism was diagnosed in 5.3% of patients who received ipilimumab with placebo (3 out of 57 patients; with severe hypothyroidism in one of them, 1.8%), compared with no cases in the group of patients treated with budesonide as well. These data suggest a potential protective effect of budesonide in terms of reduced incidence of ipilimimab-related thyroiditis, but this hypothesis needs to be confirmed in specifically designed clinical trials [90].

In a phase I study [91] evaluating the combination of ipilimumab (10 mg/Kg every 3 weeks for 4 cycles, than every 3 months) with bevacizumab (7.5 mg/kg - Cohort 1; 15 mg/kg - cohort 2 every 3 weeks) in a group of 21 patients affected by unresectable stage III or stage IV melanoma, thyroiditis was diagnosed in 4 (19%) patients. No cases of endocrine-IRAEs were reported in a trial on 36 patients who received both ipilimumab (0.1-3 mg/kg; 24 patients received the higher dose) and interleukin-2 (720,000 IU/kg every 8 hours) which is not infrequently associated with autoimmune thyroiditis [92].

The onset of anti-CTLA4-IT appears rather earlier than other IRAEs, occurring after 2-4 infusions. In most cases the anti-CTLA4-ITs have a subclinical course or may be transient. Alternatively, this condition may be characterized either by hypothyroidism with increased serum TSH concentrations, normal free-T4, and presence of anti-TPO antibodies, less frequently anti-TG antibodies or evolve in permanent hypothyroidism, requiring thyroid hormone supplementation [93].

Sporadic cases of Graves' ophthalmopathy associated with ipilimumab therapy in euthyroid patients have been reported [82,94]. In these cases the effective treatment was to administer a high dose of glucocorticoids in the acute phase, rapidly tapered down and continue with hydrocortisone, if required. None of the patients affected by anti-CTLA4-IT showed concomitant hypophysitis or other IRAEs.

Patients who need to receive anti–CTLA-4 mAbs should be carefully informed on the importance of observing and early reporting signs or symptoms potentially related to IRAEs, and that these symptoms may occur weeks to months after starting treatment. In these patients, TSH, free-T4, serum electrolytes, serum glucose, and blood cell counts should be assessed before initiating treatment and before each cycle.

3.4. Tyrosine kinase inhibitors

Tyrosine kinase inhibitors (TKIs) have emerged as a new class of molecular targeted anti-cancer agents with proven efficacy in several types of carcinoma and in some hematologic cancers. At the moment, about 150 kinase-targeted drugs are in clinical development and many more are in various stages of preclinical development [95].

The registered kinase inhibitors are small molecules, that, with sporadic exceptions, exert their pharmacological action at the ATP-site of a wide variety of tyrosine kinases critical for tumor cell survival and proliferation and angiogenesis. TKIs compete with ATP for binding to the catalytic domain that act by preventing ATP binding to these targets with different selectivity, potency and pharmacokinetic properties. However, despite their inherent selectivity, the available TKIs showed a variable grade of affinity for the different tyrosine kinases, but none specific for a single kinase. In addition, interference is frequently extended to off-target intracellular processes of normal cells. As a direct consequence, TKIs may cause a number of infrequent or even new toxicities. TKI-induced endocrine side effects mainly include thyroid dysfunction and disease, but also may be responsible for gonadal and adrenal dyfunction, bone and glucose altered metabolism, impairment in linear growth and fetal development [96].

Two types of thyroid dysfunctions have been observed with TKIs [97]. The first is worsening of hypothyroidism in patients under satisfactory treatment with thyroid hormone replacement. This effect was initially noted in patients under treatment with imatinib, but also other TKIs were found responsible for increase in LT4 supplementation in hypothyroid patients [98-102]. The second type of thyroid disturbance is primary hypothyroidism in patients with previously normal thyroid function. Almost all TKIs are responsible, at a variable extent, of primary hypothyroidism, with the exception of gefitinb and erlotinib.

The mechanisms of TKI-induced thyroid dysfunction are unclear. An increase in the requirement of replacement therapy with LT4 during certain TKIs has been suggested to be dependent on possible interference of the drug at nondeiodination clearance of LT4 [98]. Several drugs (e.g. phenobarbital, phenytoin, carbamazepine, rifampicin, and nicardipine) can increase thyroid hormone clearance through the induction of hepatic microsomal enzymes, including mixed function oxygenases and uridine diphosphate–glucuronosyltransferases [103]. These drugs can cause hypothyroidism in patients who undergo LT4 [11,104-106]. For example, imatinib is a potent competitive inhibitor of several mixed function oxygenases (CYP2C9, CYP2D6, and CYP3A4/5), and the induction of uridine diphosphate–glucuronosyl transferases has been hypothesized to be a possible mechanism of interference of imatinib on levothyroxine metabolism [98]. Alternatively, an interference of sunitinib with thyroid hormone action at the pituitary level has been suggested [122].

TKI-induced hypothyroidism (*de novo* primary hypothyroidism) may have several explanations. In some cases thyrotoxicosis may precede the development of hypothyroidism, suggesting a thyroiditis-induced thyrotoxicosis [107,108,123]. Other possible mechanisms include direct toxic effects on thyrocytes, namely the reduced synthesis of thyroid hormones related to inhibition of thyroid peroxidase activity [109], impaired iodine uptake [110], the drug induced regression of the gland vascular bed with significant capillary alteration and reduction in density [111]. However, a role for iodine uptake in TKI-hypothyroidism was not confirmed by *in vitro* studies [112] and anti-peroxidase effect seems unable to provide an explanation for cases with initial destructive thyrotoxicosis, or with thyroid atrophy.

Induction of Hashimoto thyroiditis has also been proposed [113], although Hashimoto thyroiditis is unlikely to be the main mechanism because of the low prevalence of anti-TPO antibodies.

The most likely explanation is that the thyroid dysfunction may be related to the effects of these agents on tyrosine kinase receptors involved in vascular function, such as vascular endothelial growth factor (VEGF) receptor (VEGFR). This could cause a reduction in thyroid blood flow to this extremely vascular gland. If the blood flow decreases rapidly, an ischemic thyroiditis could result, leading to a transient period of thyrotoxicosis. If the decreased blood flow develops more slowly, gradual thyroid destruction may occur with resulting hypothyroidism [114]. Supporting evidence for this theory include findings that thyroid cells express VEGF and VEGFR mRNA, and preclinical studies in mouse models have shown glandular capillary regression with TKI exposure [115]. In humans, case reports demonstrated reduced thyroid volume and reduced vascularity by Doppler ultrasound [116,117], with rapid increase in the size of the thyroid with cessation of sunitinib. This reduced thyroid volume secondary to reduced blood flow, may also explain the impaired radioactive iodine uptake *in vivo*, but not *in vitro* [118]. However, the role of VEGF in thyroid signaling is uncertain. Unlike treatment with antiangiogenic TKIs, bevacizumab is not associated with altered thyroid homeostasis [119]. In addition, *in vitro* experiments showed that VEGF reduces TSH induced iodine uptake by thyroid cells, and inhibition of VEGF restores iodine uptake [120]. Other factors, such as platelet derived growth factor α and c-KIT, contribute to maintaining thyroid homeostasis, but so far no data on their role in this toxicity have been published.

3.4.1. *Imatinib*

Imatinib inhibits the kinase activity of the tyrosine kinases of breakpoint cluster region proto-oncogene ABL1 (BCR-ABL fusion protein), c-Kit and platelet derived growth factor receptor (PDGFR) α/β. It is currently approved for the treatment of chronic myeloid leukemia, gastrointestinal stromal tumors (GIST) and dermatofibrosarcoma protuberans. The influence of daily 400–800 mg imatinib on LT4 was reported in a cohort of 11 patients (10 with medullary thyroid carcinoma and 1 with GIST) [98]. Among the patients with medullary thyroid carcinoma, eight underwent thyroidectomy and received LT4 and three had thyroid carcinoma *in situ*. Thyroid function was evaluated before, during and 2 weeks after therapy with imatinib or LT4. Symptoms of hypothyroidism occurred in all patients who had undergone thyroidectomy, but not in those with intact thyroid. Patients who had undergone thyroidectomy had markedly elevated TSH levels, and required an increase of LT4 during imatinib dosing. The effect was reversible after discontinuation of treatment, suggesting that imatinib might be the causative agent.

In another study on 68 patients with intact thyroid gland who received imatinib for chronic myeloid leukemia, no case of drug-induced alterations in thyroid laboratory parameters was observed. These data sustain the hypothesis that imatinib-induced thyroid dysfunction is limited to athyreotic patients and are not the consequence of a direct action of the drug on thyroid gland [121], but more probably of an interference of the drug in the nondeiodination clearance of LT4 through the induction of hepatic microsomal enzymes [98].

3.4.2. *Sunitinib*

Sunitinib is an oral, multitarget inhibitor of VEGF receptor 1 (VEGFR1), VEGFR2, Fms-like tyrosine kinase 3 (Flt3), colony stimulating factor 1 receptor (CSF1R), RET, c-Kit, and PDGFR. This agent has been found to influence the thyroid function of patients with GIST or RCC.

In total, 2 out of 56 patients with RCC and a history of well controlled hypothyroidism, and 7 out of 21 patients with imatinib-resistant GIST, had a worsening hypothyroidism during sunitinib treatment [109,111,122], reported the case of a woman with GIST who was resistant to imatinib and received LT4 after thyroidectomy and ^{131}I-ablation for follicular thyroid carcinoma. The patient's dose of LT4 needed to be increased after sunitinib treatment. In this report, the marked increase in TSH levels has been attributed to a potential interference of sunitinib with thyroid hormone action at the pituitary level [122].

Desai *et al.* [123] prospectively evaluated the thyroid function tests (TFTs) in a phase I/II study of sunitinib therapy in 42 patients with imatinib-resistant GIST. Most patients received 50 mg sunitinib daily every 4–6 weeks, each consisting of 2–4 weeks of sunitinib followed by 2 weeks of wash-out. Initially, TFT were performed only if clinically indicated. Thereafter, serum TSH was evaluated before each sunitinib cycle. In total, 42 patients with normal baseline TFT who received at least 3 sunitinib treatment cycles for a median of 37 weeks were evaluated. Abnormal serum TSH concentrations were documented in 26 patients (62%). Sunitinib caused persistent primary hypothyroidism in 15 patients (36%), after an average of 50 weeks of therapy (range 12–94 weeks). Seven additional patients (17%) experienced transient, mild serum TSH elevation (5.0–7.0 mU/L). In 4 patients TSH was suppressed, but they discontinued treatment before the TFTs could be repeated. Out of

15 patients with hypothyroidism, 6 (40%) had at least one TSH value below 0.5 mU/L before developing the condition, which suggests a thyroiditis-induced thyrotoxicosis. The risk of hypothyroidism increased with the duration of sunitinib therapy. Subclinical or overt hypothyroidism was observed in 4 out of 22 patients [18%] who received sunitinib for 9 months, and in 5 of 17 patients (29%) who received sunitinib for longer than 12 months. In patients treated for longer than 96 weeks, 90% developed increased levels of TSH. The mean time to onset of hypothyroidism was 50 weeks. Among the patients with TSH concentrations greater than 10 mU/L, none had spontaneous biochemical resolution. During the titration of LT4, serum TSH values remained elevated for a median of 17 weeks (range 4–117 weeks). The TSH concentrations returned to normal in all patients who received conventional doses of LT4. Interestingly, in 2 patients with hypothyroidism and normal baseline TFTs, ultrasonography revealed atrophic thyroid tissue, which suggests destructive thyroiditis. This clinical trial was the first to report the prevalence of sunitinib related hypothyroidism [123].

Rini *et al.* [111] described thyroid abnormalities in a retrospective study of 66 patients with metastatic RCC treated with sunitinib. In all, 30 patients were pretreated with cytokine-based therapy (6 of them were treated with bevacizumab), and 30 patients were treatment-naive. All patients received the standard sunitinib dose of 50 mg daily for 4 weeks, followed by 2 weeks off therapy. TFT assessment, including free thyroxine index, was initiated in 29 patients (and subsequently in another 37 patients) as a routine laboratory assessment at baseline and on day 28 of every even numbered cycle. Out of the 66 patients, 56 (85%) had one or more TFT abnormality. These abnormalities were consistent with hypothyroidism in all patients and primarily included the elevation of TSH, decreased levels of T3 and, less commonly, decreases in T4 and/or of the free thyroxine index. TFT abnormalities were detected early (the median time of detection was at cycle 2). Among patients with abnormal TFTs, signs and symptoms related to hypothyroidism were found in 47 patients (84%). These symptoms included fatigue, cold intolerance, anorexia, periorbital edema, fluid retention, and alterations in skin or hair. LT4 therapy was given at the discretion of the physician, on the basis of the degree of biochemical abnormality and/or clinical symptoms. A resolution of biochemical abnormalities occurred in all 17 patients treated with LT4, and an improvement of symptoms was recorded in 9 patients. Anti-TG antibodies were measured in 44 patients and were abnormal in 13 (30%). No association was observed between the presence of anti-TG antibodies and the incidence or severity of TFT abnormalities [111].

Feldman *et al.* [124] reported that hypothyroidism was found in 14 (18%) out of the 80 patients enrolled in a prospective clinical trial that investigated the efficacy of sunitinib in metastatic RCC. Serum TSH levels were obtained only from symptomatic patients and ranged from 6.0 to 146.4 mU/L (normal range 0.35–5.5 mU/L). Hypothyroidism was detected after a median time of 10 months of therapy (range 1–26 months), being fatigue the predominant symptom. The Authors highlighted that the lower incidence of hypothyroidism reported might depend on the fact that TFT assessment was performed on symptomatic patients only [124].

Wong *et al.* [109] explored the potential effects of sunitinib on thyroid function in a cohort of 40 patients affected by different tumor histotypes, the majority of whom were affected by imatinib-resistant GIST. In this study a new onset or worsening condition of hypothyroidism occurred in 21 out of 40 patients (53%) patients who underwent TFTs. Patients developed elevated TSH levels after a median of 5 months of treatment (range, 1–36 months). The median TSH level was 21.4 mU/L (range, 4.6–174 mU/L). The influence of sunitinib on peroxidase activity was assessed by testing its effects on guaiacol oxidation and protein iodination caused by lactoperoxidase. The potency of sunitinib antiperoxidase activity was about 25% of that noted with propylthiouracil. The Authors proposed that the antithyroid effect of sunitinib is mediated by the inhibition of peroxidase activity, which is involved in the synthesis of the thyroid hormone [109].

Wolter *et al.* [125] prospectively evaluated the incidence of hypothyroidism in patients with GIST or metastatic RCC treated with sunitinib at the standard dose [125]. TFTs included assessment of serum TSH, T3, free thyroxine index and thyroid antibodies (anti-TG, anti-TPO antibodies, and TSH receptor antibodies) and was measured on days 1 and 28 of each treatment cycle. The analysis revealed that 16 patients (27%) developed sub- or clinical hypothyroidism requiring thyroid hormone replacement and 20 patients (34%) showed at least one thyroid test abnormality. The median time to develop thyroid dysfunction was 4 weeks and patients who did not develop hypothyroidism within the first cycles did not develop hypothyroidism later during therapy.

In another prospective phase I-II study, Mannavola *et al.* [110] evaluated TFT (serum TSH, free T3 and T4, thyroglobulin, anti-TG and anti-TPO antibodies) in 24 patients with GIST who were treated with sunitinib (4 weeks of 50 mg daily and 2 weeks of withdrawal). Urinary iodine was measured in 18 patients and urinary fluorine was assessed in 10 patients. Thyroid ultrasonography and echocolor-Doppler were performed, both at enrollment and after a variable number of treatment cycles. To study thyroid function, ^{123}I thyroidal uptake and scintigraphy were performed in 6 unselected patients at the end of the treatment and withdrawal periods. Hypothyroidism was documented in 46% of patients, and a transient elevation of TSH levels in 25% of cases. The overall prevalence of elevated TSH levels after sunitinib was 71%. At onset, hypothyroidism was subclinical in all but one patient with Hashimoto thyroiditis, the only one with detectable antithyroid autoantibodies. TSH levels were found to fluctuate according to whether treatment was given or withdrawn, and progressively increased during treatment. In most cases, progressive worsening of hypothyroidism was shown, but in a few cases a sudden development of severe hypothyroidism was observed. The normal echographic and echocolor-Doppler patterns, obtained both at baseline and during treatment, indicate that hypothyroidism is unlikely to be the consequence of a direct toxic effect on thyroid cells or secondary to an autoimmune process. Inhibition of iodine uptake seems to be a more likely explanation for hypothyroidism. Indeed, radioiodine uptake impairment has been demonstrated by a reduced uptake at the end of treatment periods, with a partial or total recovery during the withdrawal phase. Of particular interest was the observation of a blunted early ^{123}I uptake curve, which suggests an alteration in the uptake phase rather than in the organification process. The Authors noted that after sunitinib withdrawal, TSH levels returned to the normal range in a maximum of 60 days.

Interestingly, the association between TKI-induced thyroid dysfunction and clinical efficacy has been demonstrated in two larger studies. Schmidinger *et al.* [126] in a prospective analysis of 87 patients with metastatic RCC who were to receive treatment with sunitinib or sorafenib, thyroid function was monitored every 4 weeks during the first 2 months of treatment and every 2 to 4 weeks thereafter. Subclinical hypothyroidism was present in five patients at baseline and was diagnosed in 30 patients (36.1%) within the first 2 months of therapy. Patients with subclinical hypothyroidism had a statistically significant objective remission rate of 28.3% *versus* 3.3% in euthyroid patients ($p<0.001$) and median duration of survival (not reached *versus* 13.9 months in euthyroid patients; $p=0.016$). In addition, in a multivariate analysis, the development of subclinical hypothyroidism within 2 months of treatment was found to be an independent predictor of survival ($p=0.014$). In another study on patients with metastatic RCC who received sunitinib or sorafenib, Riesenbeck *et al.* [127] found that 21 (38.1%) out of the 66 evaluable patients developed hypothyroidism. Hypothyroidism was associated with a longer PFS (16.0 ± 0.8 months *versus* 6.0 ± 0.8 months, $p=0.032$). In agreement with the study by Schmidinger *et al.* [126], hypothyroidism was found to be an independent predictor of survival ($p=0.01$) in a multivariate analysis.

3.4.3. Sorafenib

Sorafenib is an oral multikinase inhibitor that inhibits the kinase activity of RAF/MEK/ERK, VEGFR2 and VEGFR3, Flt3, fibroblast growth factor receptor 1, RET, cMET, PDGFR β, Kit and other receptors involved in tumor progression and angiogenesis. It is approved for the treatment of advanced RCC and unresectable hepatocellular carcinoma. In addition, it is under clinical evaluation in a number of tumor types, including lung, pancreatic, prostate, melanoma and differentiated thyroid cancer. Tamaskar *et al.* [114] retrospectively investigated the incidence of TFT abnormalities in 39 patients with metastatic RCC treated with 400 mg sorafenib twice daily. Most patients had received at least one prior treatment. Out of the 39 patients, 16 (41%) had one or more serum TFT values outside the laboratory normal reference range during treatment with sorafenib. The median timing of the abnormal test was 1.8 months (range 0.6–7.3 months). Biochemical hypothyroidism occurred in 7 out of 39 patients (18%) during treatment, which was first observed 2–4 months after sorafenib initiation. Six of these patients had mild TSH level elevations (5.5–10.0 mU/L). Another patient showed a rapid onset of hypothyroidism with TSH level rising from 5.74 to 160.64 mU/L, and T3 level decreasing from 72 to 49 ng/dl over 1.5 months. One patient had normal TSH concentration (2.42 mU/L) but low T3 and T4 at 4 months after starting sorafenib treatment, these abnormalities worsened over the next 4 months with further reductions of T3 and T4 levels, and abnormal TSH (9.930 mU/L). Both these patients received LT4. In two of the seven hypothyroid patients anti-TG antibody titers increased; two patients had persistent serum TSH elevation and in one case a normalization of the TSH values was observed.

Clement *et al.* [128] prospectively monitored thyroid function in 38 patients with metastatic RCC who were treated with sorafenib 400 mg twice daily. Thyroid function was assessed at baseline and on day 1 of each treatment cycle. Out of 23 patients with normal baseline thyroid function, seven patients (30%) developed at least one elevated serum TSH and 1 patient (5%) developed low TSH levels. For these abnormalities no therapy was required. In addition, out of 15 patients with either thyroid dysfunction at baseline or previous treatment potentially interfering with thyroid function, two patients with baseline subclinical hypothyroidism (defined as an increase in serum TSH above normal and ≤ 10 mU/L, with normal T3 and T4 values) developed clinical hypothyroidism (TSH ≥ 10 mU/L or T3 and T4 values below the normal range) requiring thyroid hormone replacement therapy.

In another prospective observational study [129] on 69 Japanese patients affected by metastatic RCC refractory to cytokine therapy and subsequently treated with sorafenib for at least 12 weeks, thyroid function was assessed before and every 4 weeks after the initiation of sorafenib treatment. Forty-six (67.7%) patients developed hypothyroidism. Interestingly, 11 (23.9%) of these patients first showed a suppressed TSH value accompanying the increase in free T3 and/or free T4, before developing hypothyroidism. This pattern clearly suggests that sorafenib may have induced thyroiditis. LT4 was needed by 4 patients (5.8%) who presented severe clinical symptoms caused by hypothyroidism. Among several factors examined, only age was significantly associated with the risk of developing hypothyroidism.

Sorafenib-associated thyroid dysfunction was not reported in two registration trials in patients affected by advanced hepatocellular carcinoma (HCC). More recently, in a series of 38 consecutive patients with HCC treated with sorafenib, 5 (13%) of them developed subclinical hypothyroidism (TSH levels, 7,41 μIU/mL; range, 6,38-8,94 μIU/mL (unpublished data) [130]. Other case reports of patients affected by HCC showed progressive destructive thyroiditis after taking sorafenib. These data highlight the possibility that also hypothyroidism induced by sorafenib may be the result of an initial thyrotoxicosis [131].

Abdulrahman *et al.* [132] in a small prospective study on 21 patients with progressive nonmedullary thyroid carcinoma treated with sorafenib, measured serum total T4, free T4, total T3, free T3, reverse T3, and TSH concentrations at baseline and after 26 weeks of treatment with sorafenib. Results from this study suggested that sorafenib enhances T4 and T3 metabolism, which may be probably caused by an increased type 3 deiodination.

3.4.4. *Motesanib*

Motesanib diphosphate is a highly selective, oral inhibitor of VEGFR-1, -2, and -3; PDGFRs and c-KIT. The association between motesanib and thyroid function was recognized in a phase II study of 93 patients with progressive radioiodine-resistant differentiated thyroid cancer who daily received motesanib diphosphate [102]. All the patients had previously undergone thyroidectomies and were on thyroid hormone replacement therapy. Increased serum TSH concentrations, hypothyroidism or both were observed in 20 patients (22%). The Authors suggested that alterations in the absorption or metabolism of LT4 may explain changes in thyroid hormone levels while on motesanib.

In a phase II study [101] on 91 patients affected by locally advanced or metastatic medullary thyroid cancer (MTC), motesanib was taken orally at the standard dose for up to 48 weeks or until unacceptable toxicity or disease progression. Thirty-seven patients (41%) had elevated serum TSH levels compared with baseline and/or hypothyroidism.

In another phase II study assessing the tolerability and activity of motesanib in 138 patients with imatinib-resistant GIST, only 3 patients (2%) developed hypothyroidism, but only in one case related to treatment [133].

3.4.5. *Vandetanib*

Vandetanib is an oral inhibitor of VEGFR-2 and -3, RET kinases, and at higher concentrations, the epidermal growth factor receptor kinases. This drug has been approved in the United States for unresectable locally advanced or metastatic MTC and is under evaluation in phase III trials on patients affected by several cancer types [134].

In a phase II study of vandetanib, 19 patients with advanced hereditary MTC received vandetanib 100 mg daily [135]. All patients had undergone prior total thyroidectomy and were receiving LT4 therapy. In all 17 patients who had available baseline TFTs, an increase in serum TSH levels was observed. TSH elevation reached a maximum by day 84 after the start of vandetanib treatment with a median 7.3-fold increases over baseline. No patients were reported to have symptomatic hypothyroidism, but LT4 was increased in two patients.

Interestingly, in a study on 39 patients with progressive medullary or differentiated thyroid cancer included in two randomized placebo-controlled trials using vandetanib 300 mg/day [136] LT4 had to be increased by 50 µg/d to maintain serum TSH within the normal range, probably by increased type 3 deiodinase activity as described using sorafenib [132].

3.4.6. *Axitinib*

Axitinib is an oral TKI that acts selectively inhibiting all VEGFR kinases [137]. The drug is approved by the FDA for the treatment of advanced RCC after the failure of one prior systemic therapy. In a Japanese study on 18 patients affected by various solid tumors receiving axitinib at different dosage, 16 (89%) patients experienced elevation in serum TSH above the upper limit of normal range [138].

In a phase II study on 60 patients with thyroid cancers resistant or not appropriate for ^{131}I, who received axitinib (starting dose, 5 mg orally twice daily), no thyroid tests abnormalities were registered, except for the initial decreases in thyroglobulin seen in most patients, regardless of their clinical response to therapy. In another phase II study on 62 patients with metastatic RCC refractory to prior therapies, including sorafenib, G1-2 hypothyroidism was registered in 29% of patients [139]. In preclinical studies with axitinib inhibition of VEGFR-2 and VEGFR-3 induced by axitinib lead to thyroid capillary regression [115,140]. Again, destructive thyroiditis mediated by the destruction of thyroid capillary appears a plausible mechanism of action explaining axitinib-associated hypothyroidism.

3.4.7. *Nilotinib*

Nilotinib is a second-generation TKI with greater potency and specificity for BCR-ABL inhibition compared with imatinib [141,142]. It is approved for the treatment of Philadelphia-positive chronic myeloid leukemia (Ph-positive CML). Kim et al. [143] retrospectively assessed the effect of nilotinib on TFT in 55 patients with Ph-positive CML. In 12 patients (22%), TFTs were consistent with hypothyroidism (6 subclinical, 6 clinical) and in 18 (33%) patients with hyperthyroidism (10 subclinical, 8 clinical) at some point during their therapy. Six (11%) of these patients were on thyroid medication prior to starting the nilotinib and in most patients an increase in LT4 dose was not required. In 4 patients evidence of thyroiditis was found (3 had positive anti-thyroid antibodies) with an episode of hyperthyroidism preceding the development of hypothyroidism.

Recently, a case of overt hypothyroidism following initiation of treatment with nilotinib has been described in a 76-year-old euthyroid male with CML [144]. Serum TSH was 30.23 μU/mL with low free T4 and free T3, and negative anti-thyroid antibodies. The ultrasound examination showed a normal size gland, markedly decreased inhomogeneous echo signals and slightly reduced vascularity, all compatible with thyroiditis. In this case symptoms dramatically regressed following the initiation of LT4 and nilotinib was not withdrawn.

3.4.8. *Dasatinib*

Dasatinib is another second-generation TKI with activity against BCR-ABL and Src family kinases that is approved for the treatment of imatinib-resistant Ph-positive CML and Ph-positive acute lymphoblastic leukemia [145]. In a retrospective survey on patients with Ph-positive CML who received dasatinib, 5 (50%) patients had TFT abnormalities consistent with hypothyroidism (4 subclinical, 1 clinical) and 2 patients (20%) had thyroid values consistent with subclinical hyperthyroidism. No patient required LT4, except one patient who developed hypothyroidism and was also taking amiodarone, a medication known to cause thyroid dysfunction. Two patients were on LT4 prior to starting dasatinib and modification of LT4 was not required [143].

3.4.9. *Pazopanib*

Pazopanib is an oral angiogenesis inhibitor targeting VEGFR-1, PDGFR, and c-Kit. Pazopanib is under clinical development for the treatment of multiple tumor types and has been recently approved for the treatment of advanced RCC. Preliminary data on the incidence and severity of thyroid dysfunction in patients who received pazopanib as treatment for RCC in 3 prospective trials have been recently reported [146]. TFTs were systematically assessed in 578 patients with serum TSH values collected at baseline and every 12 weeks and serum free T3 and T4 at baseline and if TSH was abnormal during the treatment. Elevated TSH (>5 μUI/mL) before initiating pazopanib was found in 37 (6%) patients. TSH value >5 μUI/mL during the treatment was found in 167 (29%) patients. Overt hypothyroidism was diagnosed in 34 (6%) patients. Hyperthyroidism was seen in 8 (1%)

patients. Only 20 (3%) patients with a TSH elevation received LT4. Hypothyroidism was registered as a Grade 1/2 adverse event in 26 (4%) patients. Thyroid dysfunction was never reported as a severe adverse event in any patient.

3.4.10. Cediranib

Hypothyroidism was also reported with cediranib, another blocker of VEGFR 1-3 and c-Kit kinases in 45% of patients affected by advanced non-small-cell lung cancer enrolled in a randomized, double-blind trial of carboplatin and paclitaxel taking either oral cediranib or placebo daily [147]. Similarly, in a randomized phase II study on 46 patients affected by recurrent epithelial ovarian or fallopian tube cancer and treated with cediranib as single agent, Grade 2 hypothyroidism occurred in 56% of patients [148]. Details regarding the rate of patients requiring LT4 or effects of this treatment on hypothyroidism-related symptoms was not reported.

3.5. Bexarotene

Bexarotene is a selective agonist of the retinoid X receptor (RXR), a nuclear hormone receptor. It is approved for the treatment of cutaneous T cell lymphoma and has been found to induce secondary hypothyroidism [102]. Bexarotene appears to interfere with the normal feedback of thyroid hormone on the pituitary gland [102,149]. T3 binding to its receptor in the pituitary leads to heterodimerization of the receptor with RXR, which suppresses transcription of the β-subunit of TSH, which is required for thyroid stimulation. Bexarotene also has TSH-independent effects on thyroid hormone metabolism. Thyroidectomized thyroid cancer patients receiving thyroid hormone replacement who started bexarotene had a dramatic decrease in total T3 and T4, and free T4 levels with TSH levels that failed to rise appropriately [150].This may be probably due to an effect on peripheral thyroid hormone metabolism via non-deiodinase mechanisms.

4. Why is it important to assess thyroid function in cancer patients?

Abnormalities of thyroid function induced by anticancer drugs are variably common, accordingly to the agent used. Identifying thyroid dysfunction and disease in cancer patients may have important consequences for diagnostic, therapeutic and prognostic purpose.

Diagnostic challenges are tendered by symptoms of thyroid dysfunction. For example, fatigue and constipation are present in the majority of patients with hypothyroidism, but they may be caused also by underlying malignancy, antineoplastic treatment(s) received, or medications used for control of other symptoms (i.e. nausea or pain) [1]. Similarly, many symptoms of thyrotoxicosis are similar to those attributable to other complications, such as sepsis. Inability to diagnose the presence of thyroid dysfunction or disease as treatment-related toxic effects may lead to misguided treatment strategies, unjustified dose reduction or even to treatment withdrawal [1]. In addition, unrecognized hypothyroidism or thyrotoxicosis may affect the metabolism of other medications [151]. Finally, it should be considered that thyroid dysfunction, although rarely, can lead to life-threatening consequences in cancer patients, as warned by case reports of patients who experienced myxedematous coma [152] or impaired cardiac function [153,154] as a complication of TKI-induced hypothyroidism (i.e. sunitinib).

Therefore, clinicians should maintain an adequate level of surveillance for thyroid abnormalities when patients receive certain anticancer treatments, such as TKI or certain immunomodulatory drugs, present with symptoms consistent with hypothyroidism (i.e. constipation, bradycardia, hypothermia, unexpected weight gain, dry skin or dry hair and brittle nails) or thyrotoxicosis (i.e. palpitations, weight loss, heat intolerance, frequent bowel movements, tremor, proximal muscle weakness, tachycardia, lid retraction or lid lag, insomnia, irritability, fever). Of note, hypophysitis has recently emerged as an unusual, peculiar side effect of ipilimumab/tremelimumab. Symptoms like headache, visual impairment, nausea, vomiting, loss of appetite, fatigue, weakness, asthenia, fever, lethargy, hypotension, hypoglycemia and hyponatremia in patients recently treated with ipilimumab should lead physicians to suspect hypophysitis. The early diagnosis of this side-effect allows to prevent primarily a life-threatening complication such as adrenal insufficiency, but also central hypothyroidism and other endocrine consequences of hypopituitarism [84]. Monitoring thyroid function even in asymptomatic patients has emerged as a prognostic tool as well. A lower cancer risk and a more indolent disease has been noted in patients with primary hypothyroidism and breast cancer [155]. The association between the appearance of treatment-induced hypothyroidism has been related to an increased likelihood of response to therapy and even of better outcomes. The development of hypothyroidism following radiotherapy for head and neck cancer was associated with better survival [156]. Propylthiouracil-induced hypothyroidism was associated with improved survival in patients with glioma [157]. Thyroid autoimmunity may predict an improved tumor response to interleukin 2 therapy for melanoma [62] and RCC [48,49,60]. When patients with RCC are treated with sorafenib or sunitinib, a higher rate of remission and better overall survival are seen in those who developed hypothyroidism compared to those who did not [126,158]. Studies of anti-CTLA4 monoclonal antibodies suggest that the presence of immune-related adverse events, including hypophysitis and thyroiditis, is associated with better clinical outcomes [159].

In patients who are going to start drugs potentially associated with thyroid side-effects, an accurate screening for thyroid function should be carried out at baseline and monitored throughout the period of treatment and follow-up. Despite specific guidelines generated by high level evidence are lacking, rational approaches have been proposed [1,160].

Successful treatment of thyroid dysfunction such as hypo- and hyperthyroidism, is likely to improve patient quality of life and may prevent erroneous withdrawal from effective anticancer therapies. Patients with TSH greater than 10 mIU/L or with low free T4 levels, should receive thyroid hormone replacement with LT4 at an average dose of 1.6 μg/kg per day. In the case of coronary artery disease, a lower initial dose (e.g. 50 μg/d) should be used for the first few weeks [1]. Monitoring thyroid hormone replacement is usually carried out by serum TSH measurements, aimed at maintaining TSH within the normal range. On the contrary, in patients who develop central hypothyroidism (i.e. secondary to bexarotene and anti-CTLA4 monoclonal antibodies), TSH concentrations cannot be used, and free T4 levels should be monitored, with a goal of about 1–1.5 ng/dL [1].

The treatment of subclinical hypothyroidism (TSH 5–10 mIU/L with a normal free T4) is questionable in cancer patients. In general, treatment of this condition is discouraged in a healthy population because there is insufficient evidence of benefit [161,162]. However, it may be offered to patients with subclinical hypothyroidism and antiTPO/anti-TG antibodies, hypercolesterolemia, thyroid nodules, or symptoms (i.e. fatigue) that may greatly worsen quality of life of patients [5]. In one study [111], at least half of patients who started LT4 for sunitinib-associated hypothyroidism had improvement of their symptoms of fatigue [111]. Conversely, Garfield et al. [163] warned that some preclinical, epidemiological and clinical evidence suggests that LT4 is permissive for tumor growth. Possible actions of thyroid hormones on cancer cells include the amplification of *EGFR*, phosphorylation of insulin-like growth factor 1 receptor, stimulation of migration, a direct trophic effect on tumor cells, cell specific anti apoptotic activity and angiogenesis [164].

Practical suggestions for the treatment of individual cancer patients showing TKI-induced subclinical hypothyroidism are available [5]. However, the best approach seems to to start low-dose LT4 in individual patients as a therapeutic trial [1]. This prudent method may be extended to patients who develop this condition as a side effect of other anticancer agents. However, specific prospective studies evaluating the influence of thyroid replacement therapy in cancer patients, not only in term of quality of life, but also in term of survival, are urgently needed [165]. Thyrotoxicosis induced by anticancer drugs may result from an Hashi-toxocosis or Graves' disease. Thyrotoxicosis from thyroiditis is generally self-limiting and specific treatment is not required. Corticosteroid and β-blockers, usually propranolol, can be efficacious in symptom control. However, patients with this side effect should be monitored for subsequent hypothyroidism. Patients presenting with Graves disease, are usually treated with antithyroid drugs (i.e. methimazole), followed by ^{131}I ablation if indicated. However, due to its complexity, anticancer drug-induced thyrotoxicosis is advisable to be managed under close consultation with an endocrinologist [1].

5. Conclusions

Thyroid dysfunctions are emerging as a variably common endocrine toxicity of several highly selective anticancer drugs. Routine testing for thyroid abnormalities in patients receiving these agents are recommended at baseline, during the treatment and follow up. Furthermore, thyroid function tests should be included in routine toxicity assessment of TKIs and possibly in other classes of targeted drugs under clinical evaluation. Hypothyroidism *per se* is not an indication for dose reduction or discontinuation of these agents. The clinical relevance of overt and subclinical hypothyroidism, the value of thyroid hormone replacement in individuals with abnormal serum TSH levels following anticancer systemic therapy, and the correct timing of thyroid replacement therapy need to be more accurately defined. Additional prospective clinical trials are necessary to investigate these important aspects. In parallel, these trials could offer the unique opportunity to clarify the molecular mechanisms underlying thyroid toxicities induced by an increasing number of anticancer agents.

Author details

Francesco Torino
Department of Internal Medicine, Chair of Medical Oncology, University of Rome "Tor Vergata", Rome, Italy

Agnese Barnabei, Roberto Baldelli and Marialuisa Appetecchia*
Endocrinology Unit, National Institute of Cancer "Regina Elena", Rome, Italy

6. References

[1] Hamnvik OP, Larsen PR, Marqusee E. Thyroid dysfunction from antineoplastic agents. J Natl Cancer Inst 2011;103(21):1572-87.
[2] Yeung SC, Chiu AC, Vassilopoulou-Sellin R, Gagel RF. The endocrine effects of nonhormonal antineoplastic therapy. Endocr Rev 1998;19(2):144–172.
[3] Stava CJ, Jimenez C, Vassilopoulou-Sellin R. Endocrine sequelae of cancer and cancer treatments. J Cancer Surviv 2007;1(4):261-274.
[4] Torino F, Barnabei A, De Vecchis L, Appetecchia M, Strigari L, Corsello SM. Recognizing menopause in women with amenorrhea induced by cytotoxic chemotherapy for endocrine-responsive early breast cancer. Endocr Relat Cancer 2012;19(2):R21-33.
[5] Torino F, Corsello SM, Longo R, Barnabei A, Gasparini G. Hypothyroidism related to tyrosine kinase inhibitors: an emerging toxic effect of targeted therapy. Nat Rev Clin Oncol 2009;6(4):219-228.
[6] van der Molen AJ, Thomsen HS, Morcos SK. Effect of iodinated contrast media on thyroid function in adults. Eur Radiol 2004;14(5):902–907.
[7] Markou K, Georgopoulos N, Kyriazopoulou V, Vagenakis AG. Iodine-induced hypothyroidism. Thyroid 2001;11(5):501–510.
[8] Schneider AB, Sarne DH. Long-term risks for thyroid cancer and other neoplasms after exposure to radiation. Nat Clin Pract Endocrinol Metab 2005;1(2):82–91.
[9] Hancock SL, Cox RS, McDougall IR. Thyroid diseases after treatment of Hodgkin's disease. N Engl J Med 1991;325(9):599–605.
[10] Beex L, Ross A, Smals A, Kloppenborg P. 5-fluorouracil-induced increase of total serum thyroxine and triiodothyronine. Cancer Treat Rep 1977;61(7):1291–1295.
[11] Surks MI, Sievert R. Drugs and thyroid function. N Engl J Med 1995;333(25):1688–1694.

* Corresponding Author

[12] Dong BJ. How medications affect thyroid function. West J Med 2000;172(2):102–106.
[13] Mamby CC, Love RR, Lee KE. Thyroid function test changes with adjuvant tamoxifen therapy in postmenopausal women with breast cancer. J Clin Oncol 1995;13(4):854–857.
[14] Garnick MB, Larsen PR. Acute deficiency of thyroxine-binding globulin during L-asparaginase therapy. N Engl J Med 1979;301(5):252–253.
[15] Ferster A, Glinoer D, Van Vliet G, Otten J. Thyroid function during L-asparaginase therapy in children with acute lymphoblastic leukemia: difference between induction and late intensification. Am J Pediatr Hematol Oncol 1992;14(39:192–196.
[16] Heidemann PH, Stubbe P, Beck W. Transient secondary hypothyroidism and thyroxine binding globulin deficiency in leukemic children during polychemotherapy: an effect of L-asparaginase. Eur J Pediatr 1981;136(3):291–295.
[17] Massart C, Le Tellier C, Lucas C, Gibassier J, Leclech G, Nicol M. Effects of cisplatin on human thyrocytes in monolayer or follicle culture. J Mol Endocrinol 1992;8(3):243–248.
[18] Daffara F, De Francia S, Reimondo G, Zaggia B, Aroasio E, Porpiglia F, Volante M, Termine A, Di Carlo F, Dogliotti L, Angeli A, Berruti A, Terzolo M. Prospective evaluation of mitotane toxicity in adrenocortical cancer patients treated adjuvantly. Endocr Relat Cancer. 2008;15(4):1043-1053.
[19] Zatelli MC, Gentilin E, Daffara F, Tagliati F, Reimondo G, Carandina G, Ambrosio MR, Terzolo M, Degli Uberti EC. Therapeutic concentrations of mitotane [o,p'-DDD] inhibit thyrotroph cell viability and TSH expression and secretion in a mouse cell line model. Endocrinology 2010;151(6):2453-2461.
[20] Allolio B, Fassnacht M. Adrenocortical carcinoma: clinical update. Journal of Clinical Endocrinology and Metabolism 2006; 91(6):2027-37.
[21] Stuart NS, Woodroffe CM, Grundy R, Cullen MH. Long-term toxicity of chemotherapy for testicular cancer—the cost of cure. Br. J. Cancer 1990;61(3):479–484.
[22] Sutcliffe SB, Chapman R, Wrigley PF. Cyclical combination chemotherapy and thyroid function in patients with advanced Hodgkin's disease. Med. Pediatr Oncol 1981;9(5):439–448.
[23] Ogilvy-Stuart AL, Shalet SM, Gattamaneni HR. Thyroid function after treatment of brain tumors in children. J Pediatr 1991;119(5):733–737.
[24] Paulino AC. Hypothyroidism in children with medulloblastoma: a comparison of 3600 and 2340 cGy craniospinal radiotherapy. Int J Radiat Oncol Biol Phys 2002;53(3):543–547.
[25] Jonasch E, Haluska FG. Interferon in oncological practice: review of interferon biology, clinical applications, and toxicities. Oncologist 2001;6(1):34–55.
[26] Fried MW, Shiffman ML, Reddy KR, Smith C, Marinos G, Goncales FL Jr., Haussinger D, Diago M, Carosi G, Dhumeaux D, Craxi A, Lin A, Hoffman J, Yu J. Peginterferon alfa-2a plus ribavirin for chronic hepatitis C virus infection. N Engl J Med 2002;347(13):975–982.
[27] Sroczynski G, Esteban E, Conrads-Frank A, Schwarzer R, Muhlberger N, Wright D, Zeuzem S, Siebert U. Long term effectiveness and cost-effectiveness of antiviral treatment in hepatitis C. J Viral Hepat 2010;17(1):34–50.

[28] Tomer Y, Blackard JT, Akeno N. Interferon alpha treatment and thyroid dysfunction. Endocrinol Metab Clin North Am 2007;36(4):1051–1066.

[29] Tran HA, Malcolm Reeves GE, Gibson R, Attia JR. Development of thyroid diseases in the treatment of chronic hepatitis C with alpha-interferon may be a good prognosticator in achieving a sustained virological response: a metaanalysis. J Gastroenterol Hepatol 2009;24(7):1163–1168.

[30] Kakizaki S, Takagi H, Murakami M, Takayama H, Mori M. HLA antigens in patients with interferon-alpha-induced autoimmune thyroid disorders in chronic hepatitis C. J Hepatol 1999;30(5):794–800.

[31] Dumoulin FL, Leifeld L, Sauerbruch T, Spengler U. Autoimmunity induced by interferon-alpha therapy for chronic viral hepatitis. Biomed Pharmacother 1999;53(5–6):242–254.

[32] Marcellin P, Pouteau M, Benhamou JP. Hepatitis C virus infection, alpha interferon therapy and thyroid dysfunction. J Hepatol 1995;22(3):364–369.

[33] Koh LK, Greenspan FS, Yeo PP. Interferon-alpha induced thyroid dysfunction: three clinical presentations and a review of the literature. Thyroid 1997;7(6):891–896.

[34] Okanoue T, Sakamoto S, Itoh Y, Minami M, Yasui K, Sakamoto M, Nishioji K, Katagishi T, Nakagawa Y, Tada H, Sawa Y, Mizuno M, Kagawa K, Kashima K.et al. Side effects of high-dose interferon therapy for chronic hepatitis C. J Hepatol 1996;25(3):283–291.

[35] Wong V, Fu AX, George J, Cheung NW. Thyrotoxicosis induced by alpha-interferon therapy in chronic viral hepatitis. Clin Endocrinol [Oxf]. 2002;56(6):793–798.

[36] Gisslinger H, Gilly B, Woloszczuk W, Mayr WR, Havelec L, Linkesch W, Weissel M. Thyroid autoimmunity and hypothyroidism during long-term treatment with recombinant interferon-alpha. Clin Exp Immunol 1992;90(3):363–367.

[37] Scalzo S, Gengaro A, Boccoli G, Masciulli R, Giannella G, Salvo G, Marolla P, Carlini P, Massimini G, Holdener EE, et al. Primary hypothyroidism associated with interleukin-2 and interferon alpha-2 therapy of melanoma and renal carcinoma. Eur J Cancer 1990;26(11–12):1152–1156.

[38] Fattovich G, Giustina G, Favarato S, Ruol A. A survey of adverse events in 11,241 patients with chronic viral hepatitis treated with alfa interferon. J Hepatol 1996;24(1):38–47.

[39] Tran HA, Jones TL, Ianna EA, Reeves GE. The natural history of interferon-alpha induced thyroiditis in chronic hepatitis C patients: a long term study. Thyroid Res 2011;4(1):2. doi:10.1186/1756-6614-4-2

[40] Marazuela M, Garcia-Buey L, Gonzalez-Fernandez B, García-Monzón C, Arranz A, Borque MJ, Moreno-Otero R. Thyroid autoimmune disorders in patients with chronic hepatitis C before and during interferon-alpha therapy. Clin Endocrinol [Oxf] 1996;44(6):635–642.

[41] Deutsch M, Dourakis S, Manesis EK, Gioustozi A, Hess G, Horsch A, Hadziyannis S. Thyroid abnormalities in chronic viral hepatitis and their relationship to interferon alfa therapy. Hepatology 1997;26(1):206–210.

[42] Roti E, Minelli R, Giuberti T, Marchelli S, Schianchi C, Gardini E, Salvi M, Fiaccadori F, Ugolotti G, Neri TM, Braverman LE. Multiple changes in thyroid function in patients with chronic active HCV hepatitis treated with recombinant interferon-alpha. Am J Med 1996;101(5):482–487.

[43] Corssmit EP, de Metz J, Sauerwein HP, Romijn JA. Biologic responses to IFN-alpha administration in humans. J Interferon Cytokine Res 2000;20(12):1039–1047.

[44] Yue SJ, Enomoto T, Matsumoto Y, Kawai K, Volpe R. Thyrocyte class I and class II upregulation is a secondary phenomenon and does not contribute to the pathogenesis of autoimmune thyroid disease. Thyroid 1998;8(9):755–763.

[45] Caraccio N, Giannini R, Cuccato S, Faviana P, Berti P, Galleri D, Dardano A, Basolo F, Ferrannini E, Monzani F. Type I interferons modulate the expression of thyroid peroxidase, sodium/iodide symporter, and thyroglobulin genes in primary human thyrocyte cultures. J Clin Endocrinol Metab. 2005;90(2):1156–1162.

[46] Barbesino G. Drugs affecting thyroid function. Thyroid 2010;20(7):763-70.

[47] Ward DL, Bing-You RG. Autoimmune thyroid dysfunction induced by interferon-alpha treatment for chronic hepatitis C: screening and monitoring recommendations. Endocr Pract 2001;7(1):52–58.

[48] Weijl NI, Van der Harst D, Brand A, Kooy Y, Van Luxemburg S, Schroder J, Lentjes E, Van Rood JJ, Cleton FJ, Osanto S. Hypothyroidism during immunotherapy with interleukin-2 is associated with antithyroid antibodies and response to treatment. J Clin Oncol 1993;11(7):1376–1383.

[49] Atkins MB, Mier JW, Parkinson DR, Gould JA, Berkman EM, Kaplan MM. Hypothyroidism after treatment with interleukin-2 and lymphokine-activated killer cells. N Engl J Med 1988;318(24):1557–1563.

[50] Fraenkel PG, Rutkove SB, Matheson JK, Fowkes M, Cannon ME, Patti ME, Atkins MB, Gollob JA. Induction of myasthenia gravis, myositis, and insulin-dependent diabetes mellitus by high-dose interleukin-2 in a patient with renal cell cancer. J Immunother 2002;25(4):373–378.

[51] Krouse RS, Royal RE, Heywood G, Weintraub BD, White DE, Steinberg SM, Rosenberg SA, Schwartzentruber DJ. Thyroid dysfunction in 281 patients with metastatic melanoma or renal carcinoma treated with interleukin-2 alone. J Immunother Emphasis Tumor Immunol 1995;18(4):272–278.

[52] Vialettes B, Guillerand MA, Viens P, Stoppa AM, Baume D, Sauvan R, Pasquier J, San Marco M, Olive D, Maraninchi D. Incidence rate and risk factors for thyroid dysfunction during recombinant interleukin-2 therapy in advanced malignancies. Acta Endocrinol [Copenh] 1993;129(1):31–38.

[53] Schwartzentruber DJ, White DE, Zweig MH, Weintraub BD, Rosenberg SA. Thyroid dysfunction associated with immunotherapy for patients with cancer. Cancer 1991;68(11):2384–2390.

[54] Jacobs EL, Clare-Salzler MJ, Chopra IJ, Figlin RA. Thyroid function abnormalities associated with the chronic outpatient administration of recombinant interleukin-2 and recombinant interferon-alpha. J Immunother 1991;10(6):448–455.

[55] Vassilopoulou-Sellin R, Sella A, Dexeus FH, Theriault RL, Pololoff DA. Acute thyroid dysfunction [thyroiditis] after therapy with interleukin-2. Horm Metab Res 1992;24(9):434–438.
[56] Kragel AH, Travis WD, Feinberg L, Pittaluga S, Striker LM, Roberts WC, Lotze MT, Yang JJ, Rosenberg SA. Pathologic findings associated with interleukin-2-based immunotherapy for cancer: a postmortem study of 19 patients. Hum Pathol 1990;21(5):493–502.
[57] Pichert G, Jost LM, Zobeli L, Odermatt B, Pedia G, Stahel RA. Thyroiditis after treatment with interleukin-2 and interferon alpha-2a. Br J Cancer. 1990;62[1]:100–104.
[58] Gemlo BT, Palladino MA Jr., Jaffe HS, Espevik TP, Rayner AA. Circulating cytokines in patients with metastatic cancer treated with recombinant interleukin 2 and lymphokine-activated killer cells. Cancer Res 1988;48(20):5864–5867.
[59] Pang XP, Hershman JM, Chung M, Pekary AE. Characterization of tumor necrosis factor-alpha receptors in human and rat thyroid cells and regulation of the receptors by thyrotropin. Endocrinology 1989;125(4):1783–1788.
[60] Franzke A, Peest D, Probst-Kepper M, Buer J, Kirchner GI, Brabant G, Kirchner H, Ganser A, Atzpodien J. Autoimmunity resulting from cytokine treatment predicts long-term survival in patients with metastatic renal cell cancer. J Clin Oncol 1999;17(2):529–533.
[61] Krouse RS, Royal RE, Heywood G, Weintraub BD, White DE, Steinberg SM, Rosenberg SA, Schwartzentruber DJ. Thyroid dysfunction in 281 patients with metastatic melanoma or renal carcinoma treated with interleukin-2 alone. J Immunother Emphasis Tumor Immunol 1995;18(4):272–278.
[62] Phan GQ, Attia P, Steinberg SM, White DE, Rosenberg SA. Factors associated with response to high-dose interleukin-2 in patients with metastatic melanoma. J Clin Oncol 2001;19(15):3477–3482.
[63] Anderson KC. Lenalidomide and thalidomide: mechanisms of action—similarities and differences. Semin Hematol 2005;42(4;suppl 4):S3–S8.
[64] Kotla V, Goel S, Nischal S, Heuck C, Vivek K, Das B, Verma A. Mechanism of action of lenalidomide in hematological malignancies. J Hematol Oncol 2009;;2(8):36. doi:10.1186/1756-8722-2-36
[65] Choueiri TK, Dreicer R, Rini BI, Elson P, Garcia JA, Thakkar SG, Baz RC, Mekhail TM, Jinks HA, Bukowski RM Phase II study of lenalidomide in patients with metastatic renal cell carcinoma. Cancer 2006;107(11):2609–2616.
[66] Bartlett JB, Tozer A, Stirling D, Zeldis JB. Recent clinical studies of the immunomodulatory drug [IMiD] lenalidomide. Br J Cancer 2005;93(6):613–619.
[67] Ain KB, Lee C, Williams KD. Phase II trial of thalidomide for therapy of radioiodine-unresponsive and rapidly progressive thyroid carcinomas. Thyroid 2007;17(7):663–670.
[68] de Savary N, Lee R, Vaidya B. Severe hypothyroidism after thalidomide treatment. J R Soc Med 2004;97(9):443. doi: 10.1258/jrsm.97.9.443

[69] Badros AZ, Siegel E, Bodenner D, Zangari M, Zeldis J, Barlogie B, Tricot G. Hypothyroidism in patients with multiple myeloma following treatment with thalidomide. Am. J. Med 2002;112(5):412–413.

[70] Erdem F, Gundogdu M, Kiki I, Capoglu I. Autoimmune thyroiditis during thalidomide treatment. Am J Hematol 2006;81(2):152. DOI: 10.1002/ajh.20480

[71] Chowta MN, Chowta NK. Hypothyroidism caused by thalidomide. Indian J Med Sci 2006;60(10):424–426.

[72] Mateos MV. Management of treatment-related adverse events in patients with multiple myeloma. Cancer Treat Rev 2010;36(suppl 2):S24–S32.

[73] Gay F, Hayman SR, Lacy MQ, Buadi F, Gertz MA, Kumar S, Dispenzieri A, Mikhael JR, Bergsagel PL, Dingli D, Reeder CB, Lust JA, Russell SJ, Roy V, Zeldenrust SR, Witzig TE, Fonseca R, Kyle RA, Greipp PR, Stewart AK, Rajkumar SV. Lenalidomide plus dexamethasone versus thalidomide plus dexamethasone in newly diagnosed multiple myeloma: a comparative analysis of 411 patients. Blood 2010;115(7):1343–1350.

[74] List A, Dewald G, Bennett J, Giagounidis A, Raza A, Feldman E, Powell B, Greenberg P, Thomas D, Stone R, Reeder C, Wride K, Patin J, Schmidt M, Zeldis J, Knight R Lenalidomide in the myelodysplastic syndrome with chromosome 5q deletion. N Engl J Med 2006;355(14):1456–1465.

[75] Dispenzieri A, Lacy MQ, Zeldenrust SR, Hayman SR, Kumar SK, Geyer SM, Lust JA, Allred JB, Witzig TE, Rajkumar SV, Greipp PR, Russell SJ, Kabat B, Gertz MA. The activity of lenalidomide with or without dexamethasone in patients with primary systemic amyloidosis. Blood 2007;109(2):465–470.

[76] Figaro MK, Clayton W Jr, Usoh C, Brown K, Kassim A, Lakhani VT, Jagasia S. al. Thyroid abnormalities in patients treated with lenalidomide for hematological malignancies: results of a retrospective case review. Am J Hematol 2011;86(6):467–470.

[77] Somers GF. Pharmacological properties of thalidomide [alpha-phthalimido glutarimide], a new sedative hypnotic drug. Br J Pharmacol Chemother 1960;15(1):111–116.

[78] Murdoch JM, Campbell GD. Antithyroid activity of N-phthalyl glutamic acid imide [K17]. Br Med J 1958;1(5062):84–85.

[79] Giagounidis A, Fenaux P, Mufti GJ, Muus P, Platzbecker U, Sanz G, Cripe L, Von Lilienfeld-Toal M, Wells RA. Practical recommendations on the use of lenalidomide in the management of myelodysplastic syndromes. Ann Hematol 2008;87(5):345–352.

[80] Ledford H. Melanoma drug wins US approval. Nature 2011;471(7340):561. doi:10.1038/471561a

[81] Ribas A, Camacho LH, Lopez-Berestein G, et al. Antitumor activity in melanoma and anti-self responses in a phase I trial with the anti-cytotoxic T lymphocyte-associated antigen 4 monoclonal antibody CP-675,206. J Clin Oncol 2005;23(35):8968–8977.

[82] Min L, Vaidya A, Becker C. Thyroid autoimmunity and ophthalmopathy related to melanoma biological therapy. Eur J Endocrinol 2011;164(2):303–307.

[83] Bashey A, Medina B, Corringham S, Pasek M, Carrier E, Vrooman L, Lowy I, Solomon SR, Morris LE, Holland HK, Mason JR, Alyea EP, Soiffer RJ, Ball ED. CTLA4 blockade

with ipilimumab to treat relapse of malignancy after allogeneic hematopoietic cell transplantation. Blood 2009;113(7):1581–1588.
[84] Torino F, Barnabei A, De Vecchis L, Salvatori R, Corsello SM. Hypophysitis induced by monoclonal antibodies to cytotoxic T lymphocyte antigen 4: challenges from a new cause of a rare disease. Oncologist 2012;17(4):525-35.
[85] Dillard T, Yedinak CG, Alumkal J, Fleseriu M. Anti-CTLA-4 antibody therapy associated autoimmune hypophysitis: Serious immune related adverse events across a spectrum of cancer subtypes. Pituitary 2010;13(1):29 –38.
[86] Chistiakov DA, Turakulov RI. CTLA-4 and its role in autoimmune thyroid disease. J Mol Endocrinol. 2003;31(1): 21–36. doi: 10.1677/jme.0.0310021
[87] Ribas A, Hauschild A, Kefford R, Punt CJ, Haanen JB, Marmol M, et al. Phase III, open-label, randomized, comparative study of tremelimumab [CP-675,206] and chemotherapy [temozolomide [TMZ] or dacarbazine [DTIC]] in patients with advanced melanoma. J Clin Oncol 2008;26:9011. http://meeting.ascopubs.org/cgi/content/abstract/26/15_suppl/LBA9011.
[88] Kirkwood JM, Lorigan P, Hersey P, Hauschild A, Robert C, McDermott D, Marshall MA, Gomez-Navarro J, Liang JQ, Bulanhagui CA. Phase II trial of tremelimumab [CP-675,206] in patients with advanced refractory or relapsed melanoma. Clin Cancer Res 2010;16(3):1042-1048.
[89] Hodi FS, O'Day SJ, McDermott DF, Weber RW, Sosman JA, Haanen JB, Gonzalez R, Robert C, Schadendorf D, Hassel JC, Akerley W, van den Eertwegh AJ, Lutzky J, Lorigan P, Vaubel JM, Linette GP, Hogg D, Ottensmeier CH, Lebbe C, Peschel C, Quirt I, Clark JI, Wolchok JD, Weber JS, Tian J, Yellin MJ, Nichol GM, Hoos A & Urba WJ. Improved survival with ipilimumab in patients with metastatic melanoma. N Engl J Med 2010;363(8):711–723. doi:10.1056/NEJMoa1003466
[90] Weber J, Thompson JA, Hamid O, Minor D, Amin A, Ron I, Ridolfi R, Assi H, Maraveyas A, Berman D, Siegel J, O'Day SJ. A randomized, double-blind, placebo-controlled, phase II study comparing the tolerability and efficacy of ipilimumab administered with or without prophylactic budesonide in patients with unresectable stage III or IV melanoma. Clin Cancer Res 2009;15(17):5591–5598.
[91] Hodi FS, Friedlander PA, Atkins MB et al. A phase I trial of ipilimumab plus bevacizumab in patients with unresectable stage III or stage IV melanoma. J Clin Oncol 2011;29(15 suppl):8511.
[92] Maker AV, Phan GQ, Attia P, Yang JC, Sherry RM, Topalian SL, Kammula US, Royal RE, Haworth LR, Levy C, Kleiner D, Mavroukakis SA, Yellin M, Rosenberg SA. Tumor regression and autoimmunity in patients treated with cytotoxic T lymphocyte-associated antigen 4 blockade and interleukin 2: a phase I/II study. Ann Surg Oncol. 2005;12(12):1005-1016.
[93] Di Giacomo AM, Biagioli M, Maio M. The emerging toxicity profiles of anti-CTLA-4 antibodies across clinical indications. Semin Oncol 2010;37(5):499-507.
[94] Borodic G, Hinkle DM, Cia Y. Drug-induced graves disease from ctla-4 receptor suppression. Ophthal Plast Reconstr Surg. 2011; 27(4):e87-88.

[95] Fabbro D, Cowan-Jacob SW, Möbitz H, Martiny-Baron G. Targeting cancer with small-molecular-weight kinase inhibitors. Methods Mol Biol 2012;795:1-34.

[96] Lodish MB, Stratakis CA. Endocrine side effects of broad-acting kinase inhibitors. Endocr Relat Cancer. 2010;17(3):R233-44. doi: 10.1677/ERC-10-0082

[97] Brown RL. Tyrosine kinase inhibitor-induced hypothyroidism: incidence, etiology, and management. Targ Oncol (2011) 6:217–226 DOI 10.1007/s11523-011-0197-2

[98] de Groot JW, Zonnenberg BA, Plukker JT, van Der Graaf WT, Links TP. Imatinib induces hypothyroidism in patients receiving levothyroxine. Clin Pharmacol Ther 2005;78(4):433–438.

[99] Kundra P, Burman KD. The effect of medications on thyroid function tests. Med Clin North Am 2012;96(2):283-95.

[100] Gupta-Abramson V, Troxel AB, Nellore A, Puttaswamy K, Redlinger M, Ransone K, Mandel SJ, Flaherty KT, Loevner LA, O'Dwyer PJ, Brose MS. Phase II trial of sorafenib in advanced thyroid cancer. J Clin Oncol 2008;26(29):4714–4719.

[101] Schlumberger MJ, Elisei R, Bastholt L, Wirth LJ, Martins RG, Locati LD, Jarzab B, Pacini F, Daumerie C, Droz JP, Eschenberg MJ, Sun YN, Juan T, Stepan DE, Sherman SI. Phase II study of safety and efficacy of motesanib in patients with progressive or symptomatic, advanced or metastatic medullary thyroid cancer. J Clin Oncol 2009;27(23):3794–3801.

[102] Sherman SI, Wirth LJ, Droz JP, Hofmann M, Bastholt L, Martins RG, Licitra L, Eschenberg MJ, Sun YN, Juan T, Stepan DE, Schlumberger MJ. Motesanib diphosphate in progressive differentiated thyroid cancer. N Engl J Med 2008;359(1):31–42.

[103] Curran PG, DeGroot LJ. The effect of hepatic enzyme-inducing drugs on thyroid hormones and the thyroid gland. Endocr Rev 1991;12(2):135–150.

[104] Schröder-van der Elst JP, van der Heide D, DiStefano JJ 3rd, van der Bent C, Kaptein E, Visser TJ. Effects of 5, 5'-diphenylhydantoin on the metabolic pathway of thyroid hormone in rats. Eur. J. Endocrinol 1997;136(3):324–329.

[105] De Luca F, Arrigo T, Pandullo E, Siracusano MF, Benvenga S, Trimarchi F. Changes in thyroid function tests induced by 2 month carbamazepine treatment in L-thyroxine-substituted hypothyroid children. Eur J Pediatr 1986;145(1-2):77–79.

[106] Takasu N, Takara M, Komiya I. Rifampin induced hypothyroidism in patients with Hashimoto's thyroiditis. N Engl J Med 2005;352(5):518–519.

[107] Grossmann M, Premaratne E, Desai J, Davis ID. Thyrotoxicosis during sunitinib treatment for renal cell carcinoma. Clin Endocrinol [Oxf] 2008;69(4):669–672.

[108] Faris JE, Moore AF, Daniels GH. Sunitinib [sutent]- induced thyrotoxicosis due to destructive thyroiditis: a case report. Thyroid 2007;17(11):1147–1149.

[109] Wong E, Rosen LS, Mulay M, Vanvugt A, Dinolfo M, Tomoda C, Sugawara M, Hershman JM. Sunitinib induces hypothyroidism in advanced cancer patients and may inhibit thyroid peroxidase activity. Thyroid 2007;17(4):351–355.

[110] Mannavola D, Coco P, Vannucchi G, Coco P, Vannucchi G, Bertuelli R, Carletto M, Casali PG, Beck-Peccoz P, Fugazzola L. A novel tyrosine-kinase selective inhibitor,

sunitinib, induces transient hypothyroidism by blocking iodine uptake. J Clin Endocrinol Metab 2007;92(9):3531–3534.

[111] Rini BI, Tamaskar I, Shaheen P, Salas R, Garcia J, Wood L, Reddy S, Dreicer R, Bukowski RM. Hypothyroidism in patients with metastatic renal cell carcinoma treated with sunitinib. J Natl Cancer Inst 2007;99(1):81–83.

[112] Salem AK, Fenton MS, Marion KM, Hershman JM. Effect of sunitinib on growth and function of FRTL-5 thyroid cells. Thyroid 2008;18(6):631–635.

[113] Alexandrescu DT, Popoveniuc G, Farzanmehr H, Dasanu CA, Dawson N, Wartofsky L. et al. Sunitinib-associated lymphocytic thyroiditis without circulating antithyroid antibodies. Thyroid 2008;18(7):809–812.

[114] Tamaskar I, Bukowski R, Elson P, Ioachimescu AG, Wood L, Dreicer R, Mekhail T, Garcia J, Rini BI. Thyroid function test abnormalities in patients with metastatic renal cell carcinoma treated with sorafenib. Ann Oncol 2008;19(2):265–268.

[115] Kamba T, Tam BY, Hashizume H, Haskell A, Sennino B, Mancuso MR, Norberg SM, O'Brien SM, Davis RB, Gowen LC, Anderson KD, Thurston G, Joho S, Springer ML, Kuo CJ, McDonald DM. VEGF-dependent plasticity of fenestrated capillaries in the normal adult microvasculature. Am J Physiol Heart Circ Physiol 2006;290(2):H560–H576.

[116] Makita N, Miyakawa M, Fujita T, Iiri T. Sunitinib induces hypothyroidism with a markedly reduced vascularity. Thyroid 2010;20(3):323–326.

[117] Rogiers A, Wolter P, Op de Beeck K, Thijs M, Decallonne B, Schöffski P. Shrinkage of thyroid volume in sunitinib-treated patients with renal-cell carcinoma: a potential marker of irreversible thyroid dysfunction? Thyroid 2010;20(3):317–322.

[118] Hershman JM, Liwanpo L. How does sunitinib cause hypothyroidism? Thyroid 2010;20(3):243–244.

[119] Willett CG, Boucher Y, di Tomaso E, Duda DG, Munn LL, Tong RT, Chung DC, Sahani DV, Kalva SP, Kozin SV, Mino M, Cohen KS, Scadden DT, Hartford AC, Fischman AJ, Clark JW, Ryan DP, Zhu AX, Blaszkowsky LS, Chen HX, Shellito PC, Lauwers GY, Jain RK. Direct evidence that the VEGF specific antibody bevacizumab has antivascular effects in human rectal cancer. Nat Med 2004;10(2):145–147.

[120] Willett CG, Boucher Y, Duda DG, di Tomaso E, Munn LL, Tong RT, Kozin SV, Petit L, Jain RK, Chung DC, Sahani DV, Kalva SP, Cohen KS, Scadden DT, Fischman AJ, Clark JW, Ryan DP, Zhu AX, Blaszkowsky LS, Shellito PC, Mino-Kenudson M, Lauwers GY. Surrogate markers for antiangiogenic therapy and dose-limiting toxicities for bevacizumab with radiation and chemotherapy: continued experience of a phase i trial in rectal cancer patients. J Clin Oncol 2005;23(31):8136–8139.

[121] Dora JM, Leie MA, Netto B, Fogliatto LM, Silla L, Torres F, Maia AL. Lack of imatinib-induced thyroid dysfunction in a cohort of non-thyroidectomized patients. Eur J Endocrinol 2008;158(5):771–772.

[122] de Groot JW, Links TP, van der Graaf WT. Tyrosine kinase inhibitors causing hypothyroidism in a patient on levothyroxine. Ann Oncol 2006;17(11):1719–1720. doi: 10.1093/annonc/mdl112.

[123] Desai J, Yassa L, Marqusee E, George S, Frates MC, Chen MH, Morgan JA, Dychter SS, Larsen PR, Demetri GD, Alexander EK. Hypothyroidism after sunitinib treatment for patients with gastrointestinal stromal tumors. Ann Intern Med 2006;145(9):660–664.

[124] Feldman DR, Martorella AJ, Robbins RJ, Motzer RJ. Re: hypothyroidism in patients with metastatic renal cell carcinoma treated with sunitinib. J Natl Cancer Inst 2007;99(12):974–975.

[125] Wolter P, Stefan C, Decallonne B, Dumez H, Bex M, Carmeliet P, Schoffski P. The clinical implications of sunitinib-induced hypothyroidism: a prospective evaluation. Br J Cancer 2008;99(3):448–454. doi:10.1038/sj.bjc.6604497

[126] Schmidinger M, Vogl UM, Bojic M, Lamm W, Heinzl H, Haitel A, Clodi M, Kramer G, Zielinski CC. Hypothyroidism in patients with renal cell carcinoma: blessing or curse? Cancer 2011;117(3)::534–544. doi: 10.1002/cncr.25422.

[127] Riesenbeck LM, Bierer S, HoVmeister I, Köpke T, Papavassilis P, Hertle L, Thielen B, Herrmann E. Hypothyroidism correlates with a better prognosis in metastatic renal cancer patients treated with sorafenib or sunitinib. World J Urol 2011;29(6):807–813. DOI 10.1007/s00345-010-0627-2

[128] Clement P WP, Stefan C, Decallonne B, Dumez H, Wildiers H, Schöffski P. J Clin Oncol 2008;26(20 suppl): abstr 16145.

[129] Miyake H, Kurahashi T, Yamanaka K, Kondo Y, Muramaki M, Takenaka A, Inoue TA, Fujisawa M. Abnormalities of thyroid function in Japanese patients with metastatic renal cell carcinoma treated with sorafenib: a prospective evaluation. Urol Oncol 2010;28(5):515–519.

[130] Iavarone M, Perrino M, Viganò M, Beck-Peccoz P, Fugazzola L. Sorafenib-induced destructive thyroiditis. Thyroid 2010;20(9):1043-1044.

[131] van Doorn L, Eskens FA, Visser TJ, van der Lugt A, Mathijssen RH, Peeters RP. Sorafenib induced thyroiditis in two patients with hepatocellular carcinoma. Thyroid 2011;21(2):197-202.

[132] Abdulrahman RM, Verloop H, Hoftijzer H, Verburg E, Hovens GC, Corssmit EP, Reiners C, Gelderblom H, Pereira AM, Kapiteijn E, Romijn JA, Visser TJ, Smit JW. Sorafenib-induced hypothyroidism is associated with increased type 3 deiodination. J Clin Endocrinol Metab 2010;95(8):3758-62.

[133] Benjamin RS, Schöffski P, Hartmann JT, Van Oosterom A, Bui BN, Duyster J, Schuetze S, Blay JY, Reichardt P, Rosen LS, Skubitz K, McCoy S, Sun YN, Stepan DE, Baker L. Efficacy and safety of motesanib, an oral inhibitor of VEGF, PDGF, and Kit receptors, in patients with imatinib-resistant gastrointestinal stromal tumors. Cancer Chemother Pharmacol 2011;68(1):69-77.

[134] Brassard M, Rondeau G. Role of vandetanib in the management of medullary thyroid cancer. Biologics 2012;6:59-66. doi: 10.2147/BTT.S24220

[135] Robinson BG, Paz-Ares L, Krebs A, Vasselli J, Haddad R. Vandetanib [100 mg] in patients with locally advanced or metastatic hereditary medullary thyroid cancer. J Clin Endocrinol Metab 2010;95(6):2664–2671. doi: 10.1210/jc.2009-2461

[136] Brassard M, Neraud B, Trabado S, Salenave S, Brailly-Tabard S, Borget I, Baudin E, Leboulleux S, Chanson P, Schlumberger M, Young J. Endocrine effects of the tyrosine kinase inhibitor vandetanib in patients treated for thyroid cancer. J Clin Endocrinol Metab 2011;96(9):2741–2749.

[137] Kelly RJ, Rixe O. Axitinib [AG-013736]. Recent Results Cancer Res 2010;184:33–44

[138] Fujiwara Y, Kiyota N, Chayahara N, Suzuki A, Umeyama Y, Mukohara T, Minami H. Management of axitinib [AG-013736]-induced fatigue and thyroid dysfunction, and predictive biomarkers of axitinib exposure: results from phase I studies in Japanese patients. Investig New Drugs. 2012;30(3):1055-64. doi:10.1007/ s10637-011-9637-1

[139] Rini BI, Wilding G, Hudes G, Stadler WM, Kim S, Tarazi J, Rosbrook B, Trask PC, Wood L, Dutcher JP. Phase II study of axitinib in sorafenib-refractory metastatic renal cell carcinoma. J Clin Oncol 2009;20(27):4462-4468.

[140] Baffert F, Le T, Sennino B, Thurston G, Kuo CJ, Hu-Lowe D, McDonald DM. Cellular changes in normal blood capillaries undergoing regression after inhibition of VEGF signaling. Am J Physiol Heart Circ Physiol 2006;290(2):H547–H559. doi: 10.1152/ ajpheart.00616.2005

[141] Weisberg E, Catley L, Wright RD, Moreno D, Banerji L, Ray A, Manley PW, Mestan J, Fabbro D, Jiang J, Hall-Meyers E, Callahan L, DellaGatta JL, Kung AL, Griffin JD. Beneficial effects of combining nilotinib and imatinib in preclinical models of BCR-ABL+ leukemias. Blood 2007;109(5):2112–2120. doi: 10.1182/blood-2006-06-026377

[142] Manley PW, Drueckes P, Fendrich G, Furet P, Liebetanz J, Martiny-Baron G, Mestan J, Trappe J, Wartmann M, Fabbro D. Extended kinase profile and properties of the protein kinase inhibitor nilotinib. Biochim Biophys Acta 2010;1804(3):445–453.

[143] Kim TD, Schwarz M, Nogai H, Grille P, Westermann J, Plockinger U, Braun D, Schweizer U, Arnold R, Dorken B, le Coutre P. Thyroid dysfunction caused by second-generation tyrosine kinase inhibitors in Philadelphia chromosomepositive chronic myeloid leukemia. Thyroid 2011; 20(11):1209–1214.

[144] Yoshizato T, Nannya Y, Yoshiki Y, Nakamura F, Imai Y, Ichikawa M, Kurokawa M. Nilotinib-induced hypothyroidism in a patient with chronic myeloid leukemia. Int J Hematol 2011;93(3):400–402.

[145] Ohanian M, Cortes J, Kantarjian H, Jabbour E. Tyrosine kinase inhibitors in acute and chronic leukemias. Expert Opin Pharmacother 2012;13(7):927-938.

[146] Wolter P, McCann L, Sternberg CN, Hutson TE, Mehmud F, Pandite LN, Schoffski P. Incidence of thyroid dysfunction in renal cell carcinoma [RCC] patients treated with pazopanib in prospective clinical trials. J Clin Oncol 2011; (29 suppl); abstr 4633.

[147] Goss GD, Arnold A, Shepherd FA, Dediu M, Ciuleanu TE, Fenton D, Zukin M, Walde D, Laberge F, Vincent MD, Ellis PM, Laurie SA, Ding K, Frymire E, Gauthier I, Leighl NB, Ho C, Noble J, Lee CW, Seymour L. Randomized, double-blind trial of carboplatin and paclitaxel with either daily oral cediranib or placebo in advanced non-small-cell lung cancer: NCIC clinical trials group BR24 study. J Clin Oncol 2010;28(1):49–55.

[148] Matulonis UA, Berlin S, Ivy P, Tyburski K, Krasner C, Zarwan C, Berkenblit A, Campos S, Horowitz N, Cannistra SA, Lee H, Lee J, Roche M, Hill M, Whalen C,

Sullivan L, Tran C, Humphreys BD, Penson RT. Cediranib, an oral inhibitor of vascular endothelial growth factor receptor kinases, is an active drug in recurrent epithelial ovarian, fallopian tube, and peritoneal cancer. J Clin Oncol 2009;20(33):5601-5606.
[149] Sharma V, Hays WR, Wood WM, et al. Effects of rexinoids on thyrotrope function and the hypothalamic-pituitary-thyroid axis. Endocrinology 2006;147(3):1438–1451.
[150] Smith JW, Stokkel MP, Pereira AM, Romijn JA, Visser TJ. Bexarotene-induced hypothyroidism: bexarotene stimulates the peripheral metabolism of thyroid hormones. J Clin Endocrinol Metab 2007;92(7):2496–2499.
[151] O'Connor P, Feely J. Clinical pharmacokinetics and endocrine disorders. Therapeutic implications. Clin Pharmacokinet 1987;13(6):345–364.
[152] Chen SY, Kao PC, Lin ZZ, Chiang WC, Fang CC. Sunitinib-induced myxedema coma. Am J Emerg Med 2009;27(3):370.e1–370.e3.
[153] Collinson F, Vasudev N, Berkin L, Khan MM, Selby PJ, Brown JE. Sunitinib-induced severe hypothyroidism with cardiac compromise Med Oncol 2010;28(Suppl 1):S699-701. doi:10.1007/s12032-010-9757-z.
[154] Di Lorenzo G, Autorino R, Bruni G, Cartenì G, Ricevuto E, Tudini M, Ficorella C, Romano C, Aieta M, Giordano A, Giuliano M, Gonnella A, De Nunzio C, Rizzo M, Montesarchio V, Ewer M, De Placido S. Cardiovascular toxicity following sunitinib therapy in metastatic renal cell carcinoma: a multicenter analysis. Ann Oncol 2009;20(9):1535–1542.
[155] Cristofanilli M, Yamamura Y, Kau SW, Bevers T, Strom S, Patangan M, Hsu L, Krishnamurthy S, Theriault RL, Hortobagyi GN. Thyroid hormone and breast carcinoma. Primary hypothyroidism is associated with a reduced incidence of primary breast carcinoma. Cancer 2005;103(6):1122–1128.
[156] Nelson M, Hercbergs A, Rybicki L, Strome M. Association between development of hypothyroidism and improved survival in patients with head and neck cancer. Arch Otolaryngol Head Neck Surg 2006;132(10):1041–1046.
[157] Hercbergs AA, Goyal LK, Suh JH, Lee S, Reddy CA, Cohen BH, Stevens GH, Reddy SK, Peereboom DM, Elson PJ, Gupta MK, Barnett GH. Propylthiouracil-induced chemical hypothyroidism with high-dose tamoxifen prolongs survival in recurrent high grade glioma: a phase I/II study. Anticancer Res 2003;23(1B):617–626.
[158] Wolter P, Stefan C, Decallonne B, et al. Evaluation of thyroid dysfunction as a candidate surrogate marker for efficacy of sunitinib in patients [pts] with advanced renal cell carcinoma [RCC]. J Clin Oncol 2008;26(15S): abstract 5126.
[159] Yang JC, Hughes M, Kammula U, Royal R, Sherry RM, Topalian SL, Suri KB, Levy C, Allen T, Mavroukakis S, Lowy I, White DE, Rosenberg SA. Ipilimumab [anti-CTLA4 antibody] causes regression of metastatic renal cell cancer associated with enteritis and hypophysitis. J Immunother 2007;30(8):825–830.
[160] Eisen T, Sternberg CN, Robert C, Mulders P, Pyle L, Zbinden S, Izzedine H, Escudier B. Targeted therapies for renal cell carcinoma: review of adverse event management strategies. J Natl Cancer Inst 2012;104(2):93-113.

[161] Baskin HJ, Cobin RH, Duick DS, Gharib H, Guttler RB, Kaplan MM, Segal RL. American Association of Clinical Endocrinologists medical guidelines for clinical practice for the evaluation and treatment of hyperthyroidism and hypothyroidism. Endocr Pract 2002;8(6):457–469.
[162] Surks MI, Ortiz E, Daniels GH, Sawin CT, Col NF, Cobin RH, Franklyn JA, Hershman JM, Burman KD, Denke MA, Gorman C, Cooper RS, Weissman NJ. Subclinical thyroid disease: scientific review and guidelines for diagnosis and management. JAMA 2004;291(2):228–238. doi: 10.1001/jama.291.2.228
[163] Garfield DH, Hercbergs A, Davis PJ. Re: Hypothyroidism in patients with metastatic renal cell carcinoma treated with sunitinib. J Natl Cancer Inst 2007;99(12):975–976.
[164] Davis PJ, Davis FB, Lin HY, Bergh JJ, Mousa S, Hercbergs A, Fenstermaker RA, Ciesielski MJ. Cell surface receptor for thyroid hormone and tumor cell proliferation. Exp Rev Endocrinol Metabol 2007;1(6):753-761. DOI 10.1586/17446651.1.6.753
[165] Torino F, Corsello SM, Longo R, Barnabei A, Gasparini G. Is hypothyroidism a clinically relevant toxicity of tyrosine kinase inhibitors? Thyroid 2009;19(5):539-40.

Section 6

Experimental Advances

Chapter 13

Thyroid Culture from Monolayer to Closed Follicles

Clara Spinel, Magnolia Herrera and Jhon Rivera

Additional information is available at the end of the chapter

1. Introduction

1.1. Morphology

The thyroid is an endocrine gland formed by two lobes (Figure 1A L) located on each side of the trachea and the larynx; they are joined by an isthmus (ultimo-branchial origin) (Figure 1A clear arrow) located between the trachea's second and third cartilage rings (Figure 1A black arrow).

1.1.1. Histology

A fibrous connective tissue capsule covers each lobe from where the septa go inside, partially dividing the glandular parenchyma containing a very developed network of capillaries surrounding the follicles and irrigating the glandular parenchyma. The gland also contains adipocytes, nerve fibres, mastocytes and occasionally lymphocytes and macrophages [2].

The thyroid parenchyma mainly consists of follicles which are the thyroid's functional unit (Figure 1B). It has an oval or spherical structure whose wall consists of a layer of cubic epithelial cells (thyrocytes) (Figure 1B black arrow) surrounding a viscous solution of proteins called colloid (Figure 1B Co) [2,3] containing 80% thyroglobulin (Tg) or thyroid hormone [4,5]. Follicle size varies according to an individual's age, its localisation in the gland and animal species; for example, diameter varies from 50 to 150 μm in rats and mice where peripheral follicles are larger than the central ones (Figure 1A L), whilst diameter varies from 150 to 500 μm in humans and pigs, the largest ones occurring towards the inside of the gland, even though their location could vary [6,2]. As well as follicle cells or thyrocytes, it has been found that 1% to 2% of neural crest cells in different mammals' thyroids are parafollicular or clear cells, appearing clearer in different types of histological staining. These are located at the base of follicles but do not come into contact with the colloid and secrete calcitonin [7].

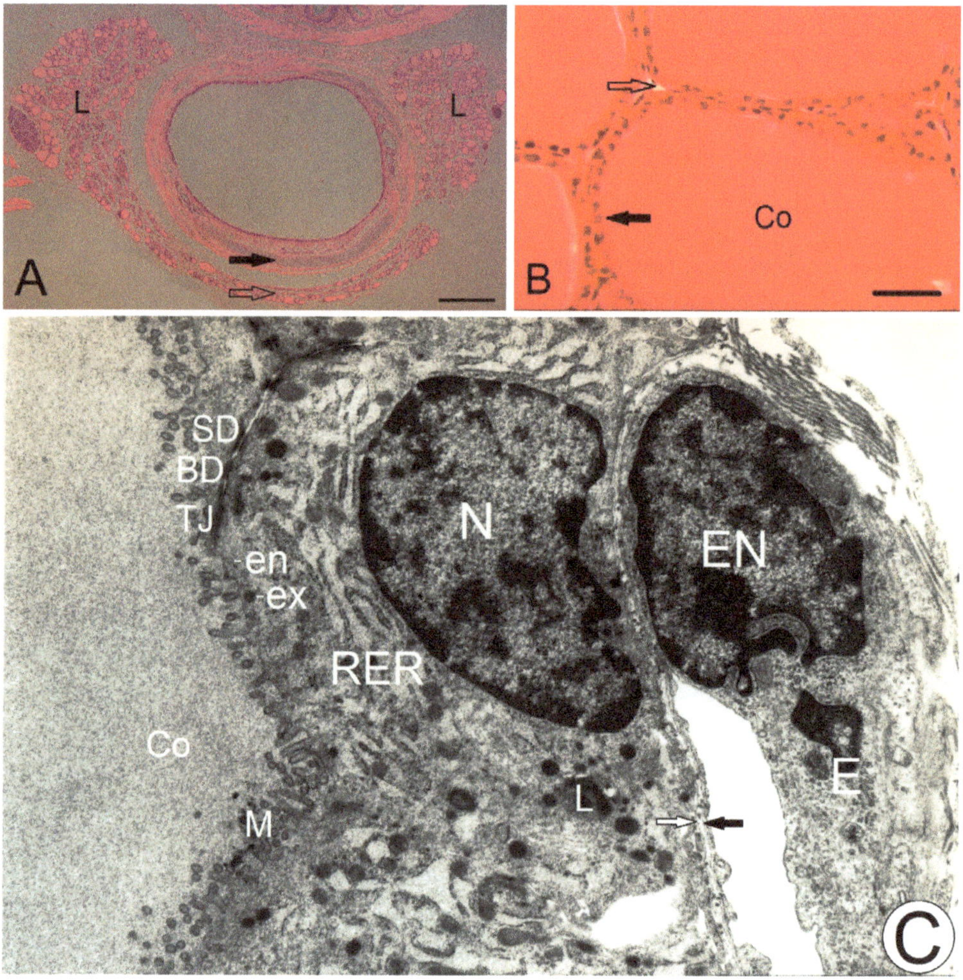

Figure 1. A. Histological cross-section of mouse trachea, showing cartilage (black arrow) and mouse thyroid lobes (L) and isthmus (clear arrow) adhering to connective tissue between cartilage and thyroid. The thyroid parenchyma consists of follicles which look like spherical or oval structures. **B.** The appearance of pig follicles in the lobe's central region. Each follicle consists of simple cubic epithelium (black arrow) limits the follicle centre full of colloid (Co) which follicular cells or thyrocytes secrete. The capillaries surrounding the follicles can be seen (clear arrow). **C.** Rat thyrocyte ultra-structure or cytology. The rugose endoplasmic reticulum (RER) can be seen around the nucleus (N) and Golgi complex in supranuclear position; these organelles and lysosomes (L) occupy the cells' base region. Different vesicles can be seen at apical level, from exocytosis (ex) being denser than electrons and endocytosis (en) and having the same density as electrons and colloid (Co), and the apical membrane forming microvellosities (M) in contact with colloid in the centre of the follicles. The binding complex can be observed in the lateral membrane at apical level: tight junctions (TJ) followed by belt desomosome (BD) and spot desmosome (SD). The thyrocytes' basement membrane or basal lamina (white arrow) is in close contact with the endothelium's (E) fenestrated capillaries' basement membrane (black arrow); the endothelium cell nucleus (EN) can be seen (A and B H-E, MO. Scale bar A 1mm, B 40 μm. C TEM. 7300X).

1.1.2. Ultra-structure

Endocrine gland cells are usually not polarised with their central nucleus and organelles; however, thyrocytes are exceptionally polarised endocrine cells and the nucleus and organelles are located in the cell's basal region like exocrine epithelium cells. This is due to the larynx's embryonic development by polarised cells involuting inside it. Such morphological and exocrine functional characteristics are conserved within follicles for thyroid hormone synthesis, storing and secretion (Figure 1C). The thyrocytes' basal membrane is directly related to the follicles' basement membrane or basal lamina (Figure 1C white arrow), in turn, being in direct contact with the fenestrated capillaries' endothelial (Figure 1C E) basement membrane (Figure 1C black arrow). The thyrocytes' apical membrane is in direct contact with colloid forming microvellosities (Figure 1C M) whose length and amount vary according to a gland's functional state [8]. Exocytotic vesicles (Figure 1C ex) can be seen in the apical region, some of them being more electron dense than less electron dense endocytic vesicles (Figure 1C en) and some coated at the base of microvellosities [5].

The thyrocytes' lateral membranes have binding complexes in the apical region formed by tight junction, belt desmosome and spot desmosome (Figure 1C TJ, BD, SD) isolating and separating colloid from the intercellular spaces and basolateral apical membranes [9].

The thyrocytes' nucleus is surrounded by abundant RER in the cells' basal region (Figure 1C RER) and the GC is in the supra-nuclear region in normal physiological conditions (Figure 1C N). The lysosomes are located in the thyrocytes' basal media region (Figure 1C L). The mitochondria are distributed throughout the whole cell.

The thyrocytes form depends on their functional state; they are cubic in normal conditions (euthyroid morphology) and have the aforementioned ultra-structure (Figure 1C). Without thyrotrophic or thyrotropin-stimulating hormone (TSH), endocytic vesicles disappear at the beginning and exocytosis increases and microvellosities become reduced. The lysosomes increase in size and have very heterogeneous content following several days without TSH; the follicular cavity increases after a few days and cells become thin and atrophied because the RER and GC become reduced. Such cells disappear following 20 or 30 days' suppression of TSH (hypothyroid morphology). A rapid increase in exocytic vesicles (micropendocytosis) occurs when the gland is stimulated by TSH and the apical membrane forms cytoplasmic expansions or pseudopods forming large macroendocytic vesicles called colloid droplets; such vesicles merge with lysosomes which migrate to the cells' apical region [10]. When TSH stimulation is sustained for more than 5 days, microvellosities' length and amount increase, follicular cavities become reduced and the thyrocytes become cylindrical and hypertrophied because the RER and GC increase, occupying almost the whole of a cell (hyperthyroid morphology) [2,8,10,11].

1.2. Function

T_3 (3,5,3′-triiodine-thyronine) and T_4 thyroid hormone (3,5,3′,5′- tetraiodine-thyronine) synthesis reflects thyrocytes' follicular morphology and ultra-structure which can be divided into 3 stages (Figure 2 circles): stage 1, Tg synthesis and colloid secretion at

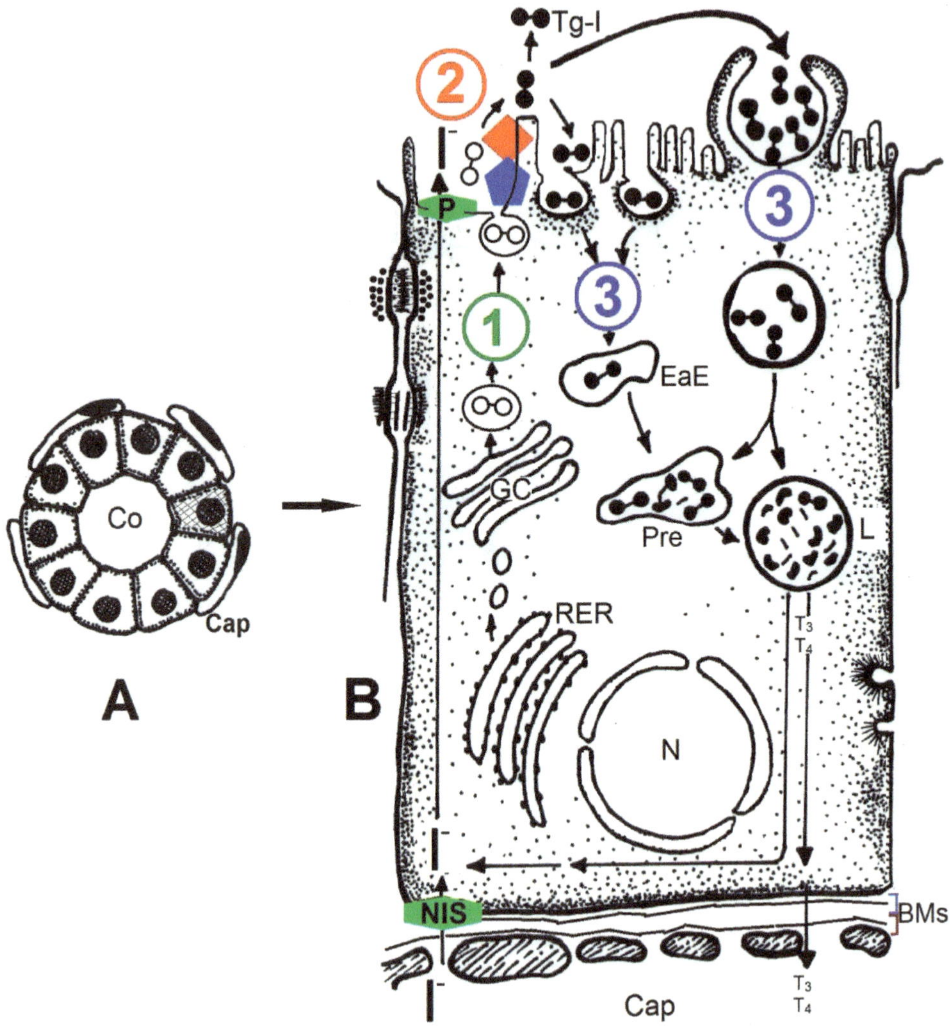

Figure 2. **A.** A diagram of a thyroid follicle surrounded by capillaries (Cap); Co: colloid. **B.** A diagram of a thyrocyte showing the physiology of thyroid hormone synthesis. Iodide is captured in the basement membrane by the *sodium/*iodide symporter or Na^+/I^- symporter (NIS) and rapidly transported to colloid, mainly via pendrin (P); it is used there for thyroid hormone synthesis. Tg is synthsised in the RER and *N*-osidic glycosylation culminates in the GC; Tg is secreted to colloid by exocytic vesicles (green circle 1). Once in colloid, thyroperoxidase (blue) with thyroid oxidase 1 or 2 (red) fixes iodide to Tg (red circle 2) forming iodine-thyronine on Tg (Tg-I). When thyroid hormones are required, Tg-I is endocyted by microvesicles or macrovesicles (blue circle 3) when TSH stimulates the thyroid. Tg-I becomes degraded by lysosomal enzymes (L) releasing T_3 and T_4 into the blood stream. N: nucleus; RER: rugose endoplasmic reticle; GC: Golgi complex; I^-: ion iodide; NIS: Na^+/I^- symporter; EeE: early endosome; Pre: prelysosome or late endosome; L: lysosome; BMs: basements membranes or basals laminas; T_3 and T_4: thyroid hormones. Diagram modified from Spinel (2003) [12].

intracellular level; stage 2, iodide accumulation and its organification regarding Tg in colloid at thyrocyte extracellular level; and stage 3, endocytosis and intracellular hormone secretion [5,12].

The first stage occurs at intracellular level, Tg is synthesised and glycosylated (*N*-osidic glycosylation) in RER and then glycosylation in culminates in the GC. Tg is transported in exocytic vesicles which emerge from the GC (Figure 2 green circle 1) and is released to the colloid [5]. Iodide accumulation takes place in the basal membrane via the sodium/iodide symporter (NIS) or Na^+/I^- symporter (Figure 2 NIS) [13]. It then passes through colloid via pendrin (I^-/Cl^- apical exchanger) [14] (Figure 2 P), regulated by the apical region's ClC-5 channel [15].

The second stage happens at extracellular level. Thyroperoxidase (TPO) is found in the base of microvellosities anchored to the apical membrane which oxides iodide (Figure 2 blue) and thyroid oxidases 1 or 2 (Duox1 and 2) forming H_2O_2 (Figure 2 red). TPO fixes one or two iodines on specific Tg thyrosins in colloid (iodide organification), thereby forming mono- and di-iodinethyrosins (Figure 2 circle 2). TPO couples the iodinethyrosins, producing iodine-thyronine or T_3 and T_4 hormones on Tg19S or thyroid prohormone (Figure 2 Tg-I); in both processes TPO reduces H_2O_2 [16,17].

The third stage is intracellular. Tg19S is endocyted [10] (Figure 2 blue circle 3) and degraded in prelysosomes [18] and in lysosomes (Figure2 Pre, L), releasing the hormones which become diffused through the basal membrane to the blood stream [19] where they are transported by three families of blood proteins to an organism's cells [20,21].

Due to the thyroid's morphological characteristics and its function, "it is an exquisitely regulated gland", [22]. Its function is essentially controlled by the hypothalamus-hypophysis and also by the nervous system and other thyroid systems [22]. Thyroid gland function and growth is controlled by TSH secreted by adenohypophysis thyreotropic cells. TSH secretion is stimulated by thyrotropin releasing hormones (TRH) secreted by the hypothalamus. TSH and TRH concentration in circulation are regulated by T_3 and T_4 concentration; thyroid and TSH concentrations are regulated by iodide concentration in the blood stream obtained during daily intake [2,3,22,23,24,25].

TSH mainly activates the AMPc route which stimulates transcription factors (CREB, TTF-1 and -2, PAX8) and culminates by activating the transcription and expression of molecules implicated in T_3 and T_4 hormone synthesis (i.e. NIS in basal membrane, Tg in RER and its exocytosis, TPO and Douxs in the apical membrane and H_2O_2 formation). TSH's effect can be shown by increased T_3 and T_4 in the blood stream [26,27].

Normal iodide in circulation ranges from 10E-9 to 10E-7 M. Concentrations of this ion greater than 10E-5 inhibit T_3 and T_4 organification and synthesis during the first 48 h (called the Wolff-Chaikoff effect) [1], regardless of TSH concentration. Iodide organification inhibition directly depends on iodide intrathyroid accumulation [28]. This thyroid auto-regulatory effect happens when inorganic iodine concentration in blood exceeds a set threshold (overload) and the gland blocks iodine's organic binding for 48 h [1]. The gland adapts once such 48 h have elapsed and organified iodide escapes, producing new hormones [29]; NIS expression becomes reduced at this time, as does iodide capture [30]. It has been suggested that there is a reduction in the function of the molecules implicated in organification and hormone formation: TPO, Duox 1 and 2, pendrin and Tg [30,31]. Thyrocytes in culture in the presence of 10-E3 M iodide reduce NIS expression and inhibit TPO and Tg synthesis [32]. Such reduction of NIS does not happen in hypothyroid mice, nor is Duox 1 and 2, TPO, pendrin and Tg gene expression modified [33]. An excess of iodide leads to iodide organification inhibition depending on TPO and not on NIS. TSH effects become reduced in the presence of strong concentrations of iodide, resulting in them adopting antagonic roles [34].

2. Thyroid culture

2.1. Introduction

Thyroid tissue fragments were kept on glass in saline solution, or *in vitro* (as this involved a glass vessel). Established the neuron cell theory, it has since been established that the unit of life is a cell (i.e. cell theory 1910) and cell culture or *in vitro* study began [35]. Cell cultures were then developed, thereby leading to studying cell functions in controlled conditions and different descriptions of culture mediums, supports and conditions have been developed from 1910. Fibroblasts in culture leave a matrix on culture surface on which endothelium cells from blood capillaries can be cultured; this has been called an extracellular matrix (ECM) [36]. Extracellular supports close to the ECM surrounding cells *in vivo* (such as collagen, laminin, fibronectin or matrigel) are currently being used [37].

New culture techniques were developed in 1975 in view of the close structure-function relationship, recognising the importance of organs' functional units, such as isolating and culturing isles of Langerhans from the pancreas [38] or "acini" regions from the lactant mammary gland or epithelial structures which needed to be conserved in polarised cell culture [39]. Thyroid follicle incubations and cultures could also be mentioned here.

A brief description of the most pertinent techniques for culturing the thyroid, isolated thyrocytes and/or thyroid follicles is given below.

2.2. Organotypical culture or organ culture

Organ culture or organotypical culture consists of culturing an organ's fragments or explants. Regarding the thyroid, this began with 2 to 3 h incubations (the term usually used to refer to cultures lasting less than 24h) of sheep thyroid fragments in the presence of radioactive iodide thereby demonstrating *in vitro* the ion's incorpoproportion into diiodinethyronine (DIT) and T_4 [40]. When the transmission electron microscope was developed in the 1970s, this led to an ultra-structural description of thyrocytes *in vitro*; the first descriptions of thyrocytes' morphological changes in different culture conditions were made. It was shown that organ culture thyrocytes had reduced RER and GC in the absence of TSH [41,42]. Thyrocyte follicular architecture and ultra-structure were rapidly lost in some of the models which were described. Approaching the 1990s attempts were made to use very small fragments (less than 1mm^3) in organ cultures (called mini organ cultures) which lasted 2 to 3 days without necrosis, exhibited iodide, sulphate and phosphate transport, synthesised a 19S Tg (normally glycosylated and iodised) [43] and were maintained for up to 7 days without cell death when coated with collagen [44]

2.3. Isolation and monolayer culture or cell culture

Monolayer culture (better known as cell culture) mainly deals with a single cell type. This implies tissue dissociation by enzymatic digestion or mechanical action and the isolation of cellular types by different sepaproportion methods. Isolated cells are placed on different types of supports where they adhere and proliferate in a single layer until reaching confluence (called primary culture). Secondary culture consists of sowing cells removed from the primary culture in fresh recipients and so on. The term passage is used to indicate the number of successive secondary culture sowings, thus the 1st secondary culture is the 1st cell passage. Thyrocytes were first cultured in 1911 [45]. Using this dissociation technique and continuous shaking during culture has shown that sheep thyrocytes concentrate radioactive iodide and incorporate it in iodine-thyronine: MIT, DIT and T_4 [46]. Isolated and small cells, aggregates of 10 to 15 thyrocytes, are obtained after dissociation with trypsin [47,48]. One of the greatest drawbacks is the loss of cultured thyrocytes' cellular polarity when one wishes to study thyroid physiology since such polarity is fundamental in conserving thyrocyte membrane domains, and thus the expression of domain-specific molecules guaranteeing hormone synthesis [49].

Thyrocyte cultures were developed in dual chambers during the 1990s on cubic monolayers as *in vivo* with binding complexes in the lateral membranes' apical region, separating in thyrocytes' the apical membrane domains from the basolateral membrane domains, TSH favouring such cellular polarisation [50]. This model has demonstrated that ion flow is determined by thyrocytes' polarity, thereby corroborating the fact that ion channels are different in both thyrocytes membrane domains when thyrocytes' cubic form is conserved. A new channel has been described for the thyrocytes' apical membrane [51]; this new channel is CLC5 which is located in the apical region *in vivo* and it has been proposed that thyrocytes have a position in the apical membrane for controlling pendrin, the I^-/Cl^- transporter [15].

The foregoing has shown the importance of conserving cell polarity and cubic form in thyrocyte culture for studying the gland's physiology and biochemistry.

Cell lines are continually growing and indefinitely proliferating cell cultures because they have lost control over their own cell division, contrary to primary and secondary cell cultures which die after a finite number of passes or subcultures, as is genetically determined in normal cells. Thethyrocyte cell line was described [52,53]; Fischer rat thyroid cell line or FRTL is most used around the world as it has a more similar ultra-structure to thyrocytes and synthesised Tg. These have been very useful in studying gene expression, cytoskeleton modification with different factors, iodide flow and that of other ions.

Such studies have led to advances being made in knowledge regarding some precise processes but there are limitations for extrapolating this to the gland *in vivo* because they are cells which lost certain control over their tissue of origin.

2.4. Pseudofollicles

Some of the main problems involved in thyroid physiology *in vitro* studies are the loss of follicle architecture, thyrocyte polarity and T3 and T4 hormone synthesis [54]. As mentioned above, the follicle lumen disappears in the monolayer with its colloid and the thyrocyte membrane domain polarity necessary for carrying out hormone synthesis [55,56]. However, tridimensional structures can be induced by covering monolayers with ECM elements, they become re-organised into two- to four-cell structures around the intercellular cavity in the presence of TSH, called pseudofollicles by some authors and "follicles" by others [54,56,57,58,59,60,61,62]. These pseudofollicles are unstable, short-duration structures and do not reproduced *in vitro* the function of iodide incorporation in Tg or synthesis of T_3 or T_4, and shown that follicle structures' thyrocyte polarity is necessary for studying thyroid physiology and the molecular processes implicated in such function [63].

3. Follicles

A new culture technique was developed from 1965 to 1980 where the functional unit of different epithelial organs, isles of Langerhans in the pancreas [64,65] or the acinar region of the mammary gland [39] are isolated and cultivated, conserving *in vivo* morphology.

It is clear that conserving multicellular structures *in vitro* forming exocrine glands' functional units depends on preserving apical-basal polarity for imitating *in vivo* functions; this is why attempts at characterising the factors generating polarity and which molecules allow maintaining 3D structures *in vitro* in mammary gland acini [66], the endocrine pancreas [67] or kidneys [68] are continued.

The 1980s saw the beginning of 24-h thyroid follicle cultures [23,69,70,71,72,73,74] on agarose, to avoid cell adhesion and monolayer formation [75]. Such incubations showed that iodide organification and H_2O_2 production took place in colloid [23,72] and that rat thyrocitos of open and closed follicles incubated for 12 h on agarose conserved their apical-basal polarity and *in vivo* ultra-structure, in basal region nucleus surrounded by RER, supranuclear GC, in apical region vesicles' and microvellosities. As well as responding to TSH-forming pseudopods [16,23,75], synthetic TSH peptides bound in the basolateral membrane [76]. Closed follicles were maintained for up to 3 days [69] and responded to thyrocytes' TSH, increasing RER [23]. TSH has stimulated pig and human open follicle thyrocyte function in culture during the first two days [49,74]. Pig open follicles cultured for 48 h with forskolin have been used for determining the function of H_2O_2 formation which is important in hormone synthesis [77]. The presence of TSH- or forskolin-induced cyclic adenosine monophosphate (AMPc) route stimulants has been seen to be indispensable in these cultures and has reiterated the importance of conserving follicle structure in culture for promoting hormone formation, as happens with thyroid gland apical membrane *in vivo*. It is so important that specific genes have been described which govern follicle formation and maintain follicle architecture, the gene transcribing the thyroid-specific enhancer-binding protein (T/ebp or Nkx2.1) regulating the transcription of genes implicated in hormone synthesis: NIS, TPO, TSH receptor and Tg and re-organised transfecteds thyrocites in follicles [78]. Human goitre follicle structure has been covered with collagen to preserve it longer and cavities in human [79,80] and mouse thyrocyte [78] thin cell bilayers have persisted 2 days more. Collagen's importance in preserving epithelial cells' apical-basal polarity has been described for obtaining MDKC (Madin-Darby canine kidney epithelial cell line) cell 3D cultures, but hepatic growth factor (HGF) was added to cultures [81].

The methodology developed by our group for reproducibly obtaining closed follicles, conserving their architecture and function in culture analogously to that of the gland *in vivo* is described below.

4. Method used

Most of the first work on rat follicle culture was open and became disorganised during the first days of culture [16,23,72]. We based our approach on these rat thyroid dissociation techniques. We describe the importance of isolating closed follicles, their culture and long-term response to TSH and iodide (9 and 12 days) and to increasing doses of iodide. Details are given of the isolation methodology, the morphological study of these isolated follicles and in culture at morphological level by inverted (IM) optical (OM), electron (TEM) and (CM) confocal microscope and their functional study: iodide accumulation and organification, Tg, T_3, T_4 synthesis and NIS localisation.

4.1. Isolation and closed follicle culture

Wistar rat (200g) and ICR mouse (30g) thyroid was used; the animals were obtained from the Universidad Nacional de Colombia's Bioterium. Pig Cialta and strain 769 thyroid was provided by two slaughterhouses in Bogotá. Some having sub-clinical hyperthyroidism due to β- energetic injection, having T_3 (1.34 ng/dL) and T_4 (107.0 ng/dL) within the normal range and excessively low TSH (<0.005 mUI/mL), were called hypothyroidic, as morphologically and functionally described in mice [33], whilst the others were called euthyroidic. The animals were handled according to Colombian considerations for animals being used in research and care of animals for domestic consumption.

The methodology mainly involved rat thyroid and was corroborated in mouse thyroid. Obtaining human thyroid fragments is difficult; pig was thus used due to its similarity with human metabolism [82,83,84,85,86], even though it is hoped to begin cultures with human thyroid in the near future. The differences between rodents and pig had to be considered. General metabolism regulated by the thyroid gland in rodents is 10 times greater than that in pigs and humans. Follicle diameter ranges from 50 to 150 μm in rodents, whilst this is 150 to 500 μm in pigs and humans. Rodent lobes range from 3 to 5 mm^3 at their widest whilst this is 3 to 5 cm^3 in pigs and humans, meaning that many rodents must be sacrificed for each experiment; 30% to 40% of a pig's lobe is used. Rodents' capsule is thin and the parenchyma does not have large amounts of connective tissue; this capsule is thick in pigs and connective tissue septa are very abundant and extensive. Shaving razors are used for stereoscopic micro-dissection. The capsule of rat and mice lobes is eliminated; each is cut in two along its major axis whilst pig lobes are opened in two with a scalpel and cut into 7 to 10 mm^3 fragments. Connective tissue is then eliminated as far as possible using stereoscopic microdissection with razors without affecting the parenchyma. Around 3 mm^3 fragments are obtained (similar to rodent fragments) without connective tissue visible by stereoscope.

The thyroid fragments are put together and washed 3 times with COON medium [55], enzymatically dissociated with collagenase II which digests collagen (250 U/mL rodents; 400 U/mL pig) and 2 µg/mL DNase 1 (nb, the original article [82] read "2 mg/ml DNase I" when it should have been 2 µg/ml). Dead cells form aggregates which are avoided with DNase which only dead cells' DNA digest and become fragmented; live follicle cells or fragments become attached to these aggregates if DNase is not added [23].

Thyroid fragments become dissociated in enzyme solution in COON medium at 37ºC and being shaken at 140 oscillations per minute; without delay, they are mechanically dissociated in this solution, aspirating and expelling enzyme solution containing thyroid fragments with 20 mL pipettes (3 to 5mm distal diameter; extreme for liquid entry and exit from pipettes), 10 times. The technique with rodent fragments continues with 10mL pipettes (1.5 mm distal diameter), 10 times. Such pipette dissociation is done at 10 min intervals during enzyme dissociation (i.e. the supernatant containing isolated follicles is collected every 10 min after pipette dissociation and fresh enzyme solution added for the following 10 min). This is done three times x 10 min with rodent thyroid and 6 x 10 min with pig thyroid; this is a modification of already described dissociation [16,23,72] and is most important for avoiding follicle opening. Most follicles are isolated during a second dissociation for rats and mice and in a third and fourth for pigs.

The follicles isolated during each 10 min interval are washed 3 times with COON + 2% foetal calf serum (FCS) spun at 50*g* for rodent follicles and 30*g* for pig follicles. This must be done in a free rotor centrifuge using low centrifugal force, otherwise centrifugal pressure opens up many follicles. All the follicles are placed together and filtered through 100 µm pore diameter mesh for rodents; those for pigs are left to decant at 1*g* for 10 min. Dissociation pre-incubation or recuperation time is continued for 4 h for rats and mice and 12 h for pigs in COON medium + 0.5% FCS in a 95% air - 5% CO_2 atmosphere and 100% humidity on 1% agarose type I (less grouping than with agarose type II) to avoid cells adhering to the support [44,75]. Culture medium (the same as pre-incubation) is changed for aspiration with follicles; it is spun at 50*g* for rodents and 30*g* for pigs. The supernatant is skimmed off and fresh medium added to begin culture in the same ambient conditions and on agarose type I; the same is done for changing medium when making the culture.

Undissociated fragments (around 0.8 mm^3) remaining after enzyme dissociation are washed 3 times with COON + 2 % FCS and cultured in the same conditions as for follicles but with 2% FCS. This has been called mini organ culture, according to Bauer and Herzog [43].

Different supports have been tried for maintaining follicular architecture, such as glass, plastic, collagen or collagen coated (1mg/mL), and 1%, 5% and 10% FCS concentration. Closed follicles are conserved in culture; however, thyrocyte monolayers grow proportionally to serum concentration in the medium. Monolayer growth should be avoided because this increases iodide accumulation values and interferes with analysis of iodide organification function; fresh enzyme dissociation must be carried out to recover the follicles [82,86]. When follicular cell fragments are cultured in collagen they do not reform follicles as has been described for human [79,80] and mouse thyrocytes [78]; some MDKC epithelial cells are organised in follicle-like structures requiring HGF [81]. The foregoing meant that the use of glass, plastic and collagen for follicle culture was rejected and agarose type I used instead.

Follicles' functional and morphological state was controlled before beginning the cultures by 5% Trypan blue exclusion exam [87], cell viability was determined by IM which also allowed visualising open or closed follicle architecture. Thyrocyte viability is usually around 100% immediately after isolation and before beginning pre-incubation. Cells which do not exclude Trypan blue are usually endothelium cells bound to follicle periphery (Figure 3B solid black arrows) or follicular fragment aggregate thyrocytes (Figure 3B circle).

Iodide accumulation and organification is determined (5 μCi/mL $Na^{125}I$, 4 h) for ensuring a high percentage of closed follicles; the importance of this control before beginning culture is described and discussed ^{125}I in 6.1. Importance of obtaining closed follicles.

Follicles are culture for 0, 1, 3, 6, 9 and 12 days with TSH and without TSH (1 and 0.1 mU/mL rat; 1 mU/mL pig) in the same conditions as for pre-incubation. Culture medium is changed during these days aspirating it with the follicles and spinning at 50*g* for rat and 30 *g* pig, discarding the supernatant which usually contains cell and follicle fragments. The follicles are examined by IM during each stage. 5 μCi/mL $Na^{125}I$ is added each culture day 4 h before collecting the follicles for morphological and functional studies.

The follicles are cultured for 1 day with and without TSH (0.1 mU/mL rats; 1 mU/mL pigs) for studying the effect of different iodide concentrations. The medium is changed and the follicles cultured for 0.5, 3, 8, 12, 24 and 48 h with 10E-10, 10E-7, 10E-5, 10E-3 M $Na^{127}I$ and $Na^{125}I$ 5 μCi/mL (kindly donated by Manuel E Patarroyo) with and without TSH. The follicles are collected after such treatment for morphological and functional analysis.

4.2. Morphological studies

Morphological study involves impregnating follicles in Epon resin; follicles are spun at 300*g* for dehydratation before being impregnated in the resin [23,82,83]. Semi-fine, autoradiographed slices are observed by OM and ultra-fine slices by TEM.

Protein synthesis and NIS expression reduce excess iodide [30,31,32] and (bearing in mind that NIS has not been described in closed follicle cultures) the presence of NIS is determined in culture in the presence of different iodide and TSH concentrations, with anti-NIS/GS antibodies (1:500, kindly donated by Thierry Pourcher) and Alexa 488 anti-rabbit secondary antibodies (1:1,000). The nuclei are visualised using DAPI/PBS (1:9,000). Follicles are compressed on commercial laminas as their diameter is greater than that of cells; a 1 mm high chamber was constructed to enable observing by CM without follicular compression.

4.3. Functional studies

Iodide organification (which is essential in thyroid hormone synthesis) becomes lost during the first days in the thyroid culture models described to date. Functional analysis of follicles in culture for determining whether follicular architecture is conserved has advantages over other cultures regarding hormone synthesis.

Follicles' accumulated and organified ^{125}I-radiactivity is determined by γ well counter. Rat follicles are washed 3 times for 5 min at 50*g* and at 30*g* for pig follicles with COON + Na^{127}I (cold) 100 times the concentration of radioactive iodide used in culture and the radioactivity arising from accumulated (A) is determined. 10% trichloroacetic acid + Na^{127}I 100 times the radioactive iodide concentration used in culture is then added and the radioactivity present in protein precipitate corresponding to protein binding iodide (PBI) or iodide organification (O) is determined.

The precipitate is used for determining the amount of DNA by diphenylamine method [88], Tg19S by HPLC and iodine-thyronine (MIT, DIT, T_3, rT_3 and T_4) in Tg by inverse-phase HPLC [89]. The results are expressed in % iodide dose in µg DNA. Follicle structure does not allow the number of cells to be counted and statistical analysis requires having a parameter letting the results be homogenised; based on 1 pg DNA/mL equals 2E5 cells, the number of cells present in cultures can be determined and the results statistically correlated [82].

4.4. Statistical analysis

Data given in the text are expressed as mean standard deviation for N values. Significant differences are established between some times for A and O variables by Student's t-test.

5. Results

Closed follicular architecture is indispensable in agarose culture since open follicles become dissociated and cells die; it is thus essential to begin with maximum closed follicles possible to avoid this. The following item gives the criteria determined important for beginning culture. Then, the long-term culture results in which closed and isolated follicle morphology and function were compared. Last, the morphological and functional results in the presence of different doses of iodide and TSH.

5.1. The importance of obtaining closed follicles for culturing them

Many isolated cells and follicular fragments were obtained when thyrocytes became detached after 30 contiguous min, instead of 10 minute enzyme dissociation time (Figure

3A); these thyrocytes were eliminated 24 h later when culture medium was changed. If some fragments persisted after 1 or 2 days' culture they became dissociated and thyrocytes died because they could not adhere to the agarose covered culture support [75] since normal cells require support for growing in culture. Trypan blue allowed an approximation of follicles'

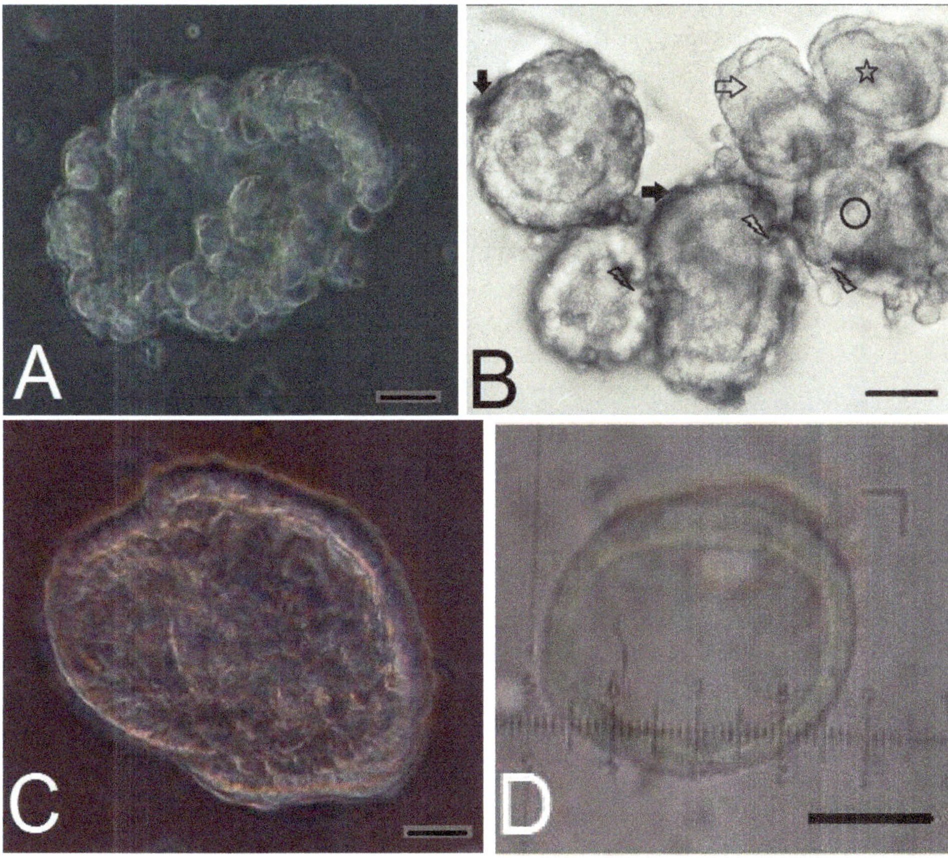

Figure 3. **A.** A follicle fragment from euthyroidic pig thyroid dissociated for 30 min without interruption pre-incubated for 12 h. Note the contour of thyrocytes which became detached from the follicular fragment and cell waste in culture support. **B.** Trypan blue for recently isolated rat thyroid follicles by strong dissociation (Strong dissociation, Table 1). Follicles which did not open (star) conserved colloid birefrigence and a clear and continuous boundary between colloid and cells, whilst those which became resealed (clear arrow) lost colloid birefrigence and the boundary between cavity and cells was not clear. Openings could be seen in those which did not reseal (triangles beam). Cells which did not exclude stain were mainly endothelium cells found in follicle periphery (solid arrows). Follicle fragments presented non-viable thyrocyte aggregates (circle). **C.** Pig euthyroid resealed follicles 12 h pre-incubation. Note that the thyrocytes' apical boundaries could be distinguished due to a lack of colloid. **D.** Trypan blue of closed follicle with colloid birefrigence of pig hypothyroids pre-incubated for 12 h; colloid was birefrigent and the boundary between colloid and thyrocytes was clear and continuous (IM. Scale bar: A 20 μm, B 50 μm, C 15 μm, D 70 μm).

closed or open state (Figure 3B); those conserving colloid showed up due to birefringence in IM and there was a clear boundary between colloid and cells (Figures 3B star and 3D) whilst those which became resealed lost their colloid birefringence and the boundary between cavity and cells was not clear (Figures 3B clear arrow and 3C). Openings in follicles which did not become resealed appeared (Figure 3B triangles beam) as did colloid loss. Cells which did not exclude the stain were mainly endothelium cells which were found on follicle periphery (Figure 3B black arrows). Follicle fragments could be seen because they lost follicular structure and organisation continued from thyrocytes' epithelial layer (Figure 3B circle).

Follicle morphology and function were analysed after 4 hours' labelling with radioactive iodide, varying according to the dissociation procedure used with and without pre-incubation. If pipette dissociation after each 10 min enzyme digestion was done in such a way that hydrodynamic forces were produced with turbulence, this was called **strong dissociation,** but when this was done slowly without turbulence in the liquid and avoiding air-bubble formation it was called **mild dissociation.**

Iodide which did not bind to molecules was eliminated in fixation liquid until being impregnated in resin; labelling in autoradiographs (following pre-incubation, added for 2 h in the presence of $Na^{125}I$ 5 µCi/mL) was that which bound to proteins and was equivalent to organified iodide. The number of closed follicles could thus be counted and distinguished from open ones by autoradiographs. Open follicles were numerous in strong dissociation; they could be seen because no organified iodide was concentrated within follicle interior (Figure 4A star) even though histological cross-sections seemed to suggest that the cubic epithelial layer continued (Figure 4A circle). There were much fewer open follicles if dissociation was mild (Figure 4B). Follicles which resealed could be distinguished because, even though the labelling was homogeneous, it was less intense in colloid than in those which remained closed (Figure 4B arrow).

Pre-incubation time was another key aspect for obtaining a maximum of closed follicles at the beginning of culture (4 h for rat follicles and 12 h for pig follicles when this was divided into 4 initial hours in which medium was changed by aspirating the medium with follicles and spinning at 30*g* x 5 min followed by pre-incubation for 8 h). The pre-incubation period was essential since this time allowed cells to recover from the aggression of the enzyme used for dissociation.

Pre-incubation time following dissociation promoted an increase in closed follicles with two dissociations (strong or mild, 33% and 46%, respectively, Table 1). Open follicles which did become resealed or follicular fragments (Figure 4A) became disorganised and were discarded in the supernatant when changing the medium and spinning to wash them.

Morphological modifications included modification of the amount of iodide accumulated and organified by follicles (Table 1); if dissociation was mild, iodide accumulation (A) and organification (O) values and O/A percentage increased following pre-incubation time, whereas if dissociation was strong then these values were lower.

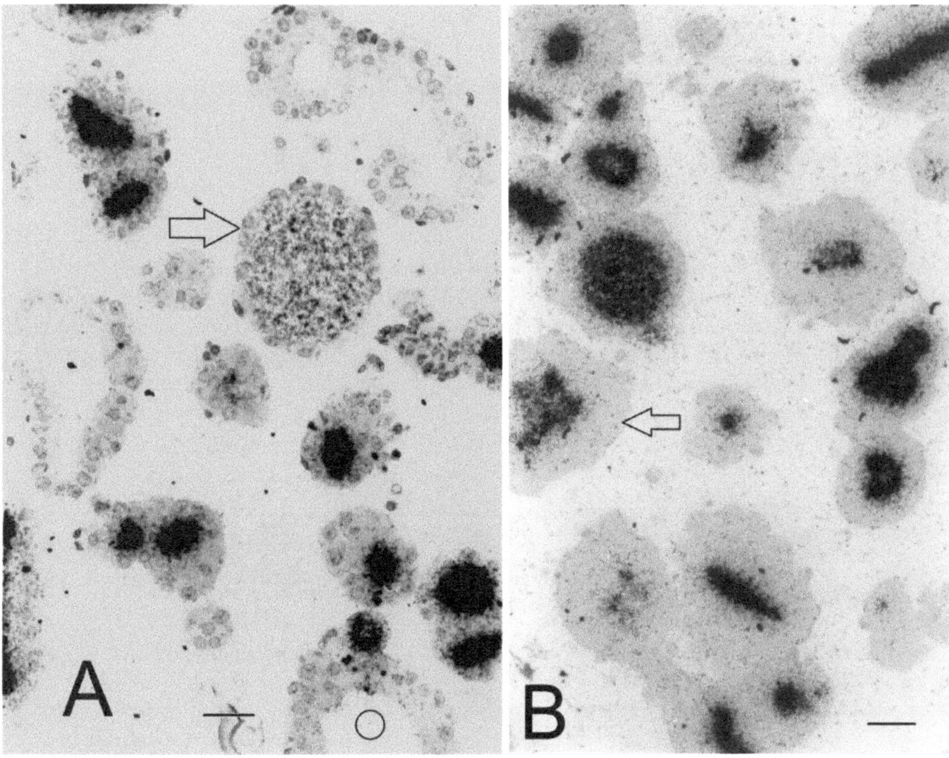

Figure 4. Autoradiograph of dissociated follicles (following pre-incubation, they were added for 2 h in the presence of 5 μCi/mL $Na^{125}I$). Iodide ions which did not bind to proteins were eliminated while washing the histotechnic preparation until being impregnated in resin. Closed follicles were labelled in the follicle centre even though they became resealed (arrow). **A.** Follicles isolated by strong dissociation (aliquot of follicles from Table 1, strong dissociation with pre-incubation). Follicles seeming to be closed by histological cross-section but which did not accumulate organified iodide in colloid were open follicles (circle). **B.** Most follicles isolated by mild dissociation (aliquot of follicles from Table 1, mild dissociation with pre-incubation) were closed because of intense labelling within follicular cavities (OM. Toluidine bleu. Scale bar: 25 μm).

Closed follicles counted on autoradiographies corresponded to O/A proportion percentage; thus mild dissociation gave 83% closed follicles and 85% O/A proportion whilst strong dissociation gave 45% closed and 58% O/A proportion (Table 1).

Follicles isolated by mild dissociation, following 2 h with radioactive iodide, accumulated iodide 4.8 times and 7.8 times more with 0.1 and 1 mU/mL TSH, respectively, regarding without TSH. TSH did not modify morphology regarding follicular architecture or O/A proportion (Table 2).

This follicle isolation method can be applied to other thyroid tissues from other species, such as rabbits or humans. The percentage of open follicles was greater in pig or human thyroid follicles and more tissue was obtained per experiment; 12 h was thus allowed for pre-incubation (Figures 4C and 4D).

Digestion conditions	% follicles closes	A	O	% O/A
Without pre-incubation				
Mild dissociation	57 ± 1,4	1.14 ± 0,01	0.89 ± 0,01	78
Strong dissociation	45 ± 5,7	1.84 ± 0,37	1.08 ± 0,14	58
With pre-incubation 4 hours				
Mild dissociation	83 ± 1,4	1.93 ± 0,24	1.64 ± 0,17	85
Strong dissociation	60 ± 7,1	1.32 ± 0,17	0.91 ± 0,01	68

Table 1. Influence of dissociation conditions and pre-incubation time on the percentage of rat thyroid isolated and closed follicles and their function. It can be seen that the percentage of organified iodide on accumulated iodide (O/A) was equivalent to the percentage of closed follicles concentrating radioactive ion determined by follicle count using accumulated grains in follicular colloid in autoradiography of semi-fine cross-sections (Figure 4). Average values for two culture dishes ± SD. Following pre-incubation, $^{125}I^-$ accumulation (A) and incorporation in proteins (O) were determined following 2 h in the presence of $Na^{125}I$ 5 μCi/mL and expressed in μg/dose/μg DNA.

TSH	A	O	% O/A
None	0.73 ± 0,18	0.58 ± 0,11	79
0,1mU/mL	3.48 ± 0,17	2.78 ± 0,04	80
1mU/mL	5.71 ± 0,72	4.98 ± 0,67	87

Table 2. Influence of TSH on iodide accumulation and organification in isolated rat follicles expressed in μg/dose/μg DNA. Follicles were cultured for 2 h in the presence of $Na^{125}I$ 5 μCi/mL immediately following pre-incubation. TSH was stimulated by $Na^{125}I$ but O/A proportion was around 80% with or without TSH. The value without TSH represented the percentage of closed follicles obtained following correct mechanical dissociation and pre-incubation of follicles. Average values for culture dishes ± SD (these values were representative of 3 experiments).

A good approximation of the percentage of closed follicles following pre-incubation must thus be born in mind (this corresponded to day 0 in our cultures). It can thus be generalised that O/A proportion values should be greater than 80% before beginning culture (day 0, Table 2) and that there should be a potentially high number of closed follicles, even though follicle diameter may vary in each species or come from different thyroid functional states [85,86,90]. Open follicles' ability to reveal themselves during the course of pre-incubation probably depended on the degree of initial opening. Even though groupings of rat thyroid cells became organised in the presence of TSH and on agarose, they became reorganised into 6- to 10-cell follicles which could be cultured for 3 days [69,73]. In our results, rat or pig follicles which became resealed did not require TSH for conserving their follicular architecture.

5.2. Long-term closed follicle culture

5.2.1. Functional study

On **day zero** (4 h pre-incubation in the presence of radioactive iodide) follicles accumulated 3.5 ± 2.1% of the dose in the medium **without TSH** (9 experiments in rats). Organified iodide percentage varied according to closed follicle percentage at the start of each experiment.

O/Aprioportion was 57% in experiment 1 and 91% in experiment 2 (Table 3); more than two thirds of organified iodide bound to stable Tg19S (Table 4), the rest of the molecules having lower molecular weight. Capture increased in the presence of **TSH** regarding without TSH 250 ± 210% (9 experiments in rats), but O/A percentage remained constant. The effect of TSH was evident on A and O, and higher than values without TSH (Tables 2, 3 and 4). Iodide accumulation on Tg19S slightly increased with TSH, but not significantly so (Table 4).

	Exp. 1			Exp. 2		
TSH	0.0	0.1	1.0	0.0	0.1	1.0
Culture, day						
0	57	46	69	91	93	94
1	69	75	71	78	94	93
3	64	85	85	84	86	87
6	0	58	83	60	51	84
9	2	51	71	59	78	91
12	0	54	82	50	73	90

Table 3. Evolution of $^{125}I^-$ organification/accumulation in rat follicle culture. Comparing two experiments where rat closed follicle percentage varied during the course of two experiments (Exp. 1 and Exp. 2). 80% of follicles were closed at the start of culture counted in autoradiographs of culture aliquots in experiment 2 (*cf* 65% in experiment 1). $Na^{125}I$ 5 μCi/mL was added 4 h before collecting follicles during each day of the experiment, expressed in %/dose/μg DNA. Each value was the average of two samples or culture dishes. Experiment 2 was representative of 7 independent experiments. TSH: mU/mL.

Following **one day**'s culture without TSH, accumulation was low at the start of culture; it did not become modified, but if it was high it became reduced, whilst incorpoproportion of iodide in Tg became reduced (Table 4). T_3 and T_4 proportion in regarding Tg was not modified. Iodide accumulation increased in the presence of TSH, O/A percentage remained high and in starting values (Table 3). Iodide incorpoproportion in Tg19S was better (Table 4) and Tg19S content in follicles did not vary.

Accumulation fell abruptly on the **third day** without TSH when starting with a low percentage of closed follicles, just like O/A percentage, whilst it became reduced with a high percentage of closed follicles, but O/A was maintained. O/A values were high in the presence of TSH and remained higher than 80% (Table 3).

Accumulation and organification values and their O/A percentage differed on the **sixth day** regarding closed follicle percentage; A and O could not be determined in experiment 1 which began with 57% (Table 3. Exp. 1) whilst experiment 2 began with 94% and became reduced to 60% (Table 3. Exp. 2). There was a reduction in all O/A percentages in rat or pig cultures by the sixth day which also differed with the percentage of closed follicles (Table 5), animal species and functional state at the start of culture. The percentage of iodide on Tg19S also became reduced (Table 4).

	A			$^{125}I^-$ in Tg19S*		
TSH	0.0	0.1	1.0	0.0	0.1	1.0
Culture. Day						
Without NaI						
0	5.8	5.5	7.2	59	63	67
1	1.4	2.7	3.1	43	66	65
3	1.3	4.5	8.7	46	50	52
6	0.7	1.2	4.0	25	13	42
9	0.2	0.6	4.0	16	17	55
12	0.2	0.7	8.0	15	25	52
With NaI						
0	5.8	7.8	9.3	60	61	66
1	1.1	1.8	3.1	31	58	64
3	0.7	4.2	7.6	49	49	52
6	0.1	1.4	3.4	10	22	39
9	0.2	1.6	2.6	14	32	38
12	0.1	1.9	2.9	11	33	58

Table 4. Evolution of iodide accumulation (A) and its incorporation in stable Tg19S in rat follicle culture. Effect of adding a small dose of cold iodide (10E-10 M $Na^{127}I$). A was expressed in %/dose/μg DNA. Radioactivity determined in stable Tg19S was expressed in % $^{125}I^-$ accumulation/dose/μg DNA. The results without NaI were those expressed in experiment 2, Table 3. $Na^{125}I$ 5 μCi/mL 4 h was added before collecting follicles during each day of the experiment. Each value was the average of two samples or culture dishes.

O/A retained the same values on **day 9 and 12** as those for day 6 in both experiments without TSH, whilst with TSH this increased in experiment 1 regressed to day 1 values and then maintained similar values to those of the two first days. The percentage of iodide on Tg19S with and without TSH was conserved (Table 4).

The presence of a small dose of iodide (10E-10 M NaI) did not modify iodide accumulation values at the start of culture (Table 4), but responded better to TSH. Tg19S had more T_3 and T_4 and TSH increased the percentage of T_3. O/A percentage increased with 0.1mU/mL TSH on days 6, 9 and 12 whilst it fell with 1 mU/mL (not significantly). Iodide had no effect on stable Tg19S content in follicles; more than two thirds of accumulated iodide was incorporated in Tg19S (Table 4) even in the absence of TSH where iodide accumulation was very low on day 12.

Preserving the function of pig follicle thyrocytes during culture also depended on the percentage of closed follicles since the beginning. However, this differed from those for rats in the absence of TSH, because this began with 43% O/A equivalent to the percentage of closed follicles presenting iodide organification on days 6 and 9 (Table 5, euthyroidic follicles) contrary to rat follicles which was zero (Table 3. Exp. 1). As 7 times more material was obtained from pig thyroids than rat follicles, a greater number of recovered follicles were conserved in changes of medium by centrifuging, or different species having variations in response to the same medium conditions.

		Euthyroid		Hipothyroid	
Culture, day	TSH	% O/A	N	% O/A	N
	0	43.4. ±.5.9	4	82.4. ±.7.2	4
0	1mU/mL	61.5. ±.4.6	4	80.5. ±.3.7	4
	0	56.94. ±.4.7	3	77.0. ±.3.8	4
1	1mU/mL	71.4. ±.7.1	2	76.44. ±.3.9	4
	0	37.4. ±.6.6	2	82.24. ±.4.1	3
3	1mU/mL	43.2. ±.5.9	2	76.44. ±.5.3	2
	0	9.16. ±.2.2	2	23.3. ±.9.4	2
6	1mU/mL	15.0. ±.3.7	2	52.32. ±.4.2	2
	0	52.66. ±.2.2	2	16.62. ±.1.5	3
9	1mU/mL	64.8. ±.4.3	2	53.6. ±.5.0	3

Table 5. Evolution of $^{125}I^-$ organification/accumulation (O/A proportion) percentage for pig follicles. Hypothyroid follicles had high O/A percentage at the start regarding euthyroids (representative results from 4 experiments). This experiment began with less than 50% O/A in euthyroids for comparing with Table 3, experiment 1; however, when 3 experiments began with euthyroid follicles having 80% or more O/A they behaved like those for rat follicles in experiment 2, Table 3. 5 µCi/mL $Na^{125}I$ were added 4 h before collecting follicles on each day of the experiment expressed in %/dose/µg DNA. Average values for the number (N) of culture dishes ± SD.

The difference between euthyroidic rat or pig follicles regarding hypothyroid ones was that hypothyroids responded to TSH on the sixth and ninth culture days, perhaps due to adapting to normal culture conditions, like hypothyroid glands' response *in vivo* when the effect induced by hypothyroidism stimulated with TSH was eliminated [24].

We compared isolated follicles' iodide accumulation and organification with their respective pig mini organ cultures lasting up to 9 days. Euthyroidic tissue became disorganised after the sixth day and functionality could not be determined after this day. Some follicles were conserved in the hypothyroids on the outside of the cultured fragment and presented this function on days 6 and 9 (Table 6). Mini organ culture functional values were higher than those of follicles isolated on the first day, but these were not significant; they were higher from the first day onwards in isolated follicles, maintaining higher values up to day 9 (euthyroidic and hypothyroid) (Table 6).

TSH	A	O	% A/O	N	TSH	A	O	% A/O	N
		Euthyroid, follicles				**Euthyroid, mini organ culture**			
0	0.049	0.025	51.6 ± 0.052	4	0	CND	CND		3
1mU/mL	0.074	0.048	65.3 ± 0.043	4	1mU/mL	CND	CND		3
		Hypothyroid, follicles				**Hypothyroid, mini organ culture**			
0	0.122	0.0633	36.75 ± 0.67	4	0	0,115	0.025	22.7 ± 1.5	3
1mU/mL	0.122	0.0655	53.6± 0.050	4	1mU/mL	0.723	0.278	38.5 ± 0.067	2

Table 6. Determining iodide accumulation (A) and organification (O) for isolated follicles and mini organ cultures from the same pig thyroids after 9 days' culture. 5 µCi/mL $Na^{125}I$ was added 4 h before collecting follicles and mini organ cultures on each day of the experiment expressed in %/dose/µg DNA. Average µg of follicle DNA was 4.5 and 14.7 for mini organ cultures. Values represent the average number (N) of culture dishes ± SD. CND: could not be determined.

It has been described that pig thyroid mini organ cultures enables studying "thyroid tissue structural and functional integrity *in vitro* [54]"; however, we have considered that studying thyroids *in vitro* is better done with isolated follicles than using mini organ cultures. Since closed follicles maintain their architecture throughout culture time, thyrocytes are viable and their basement membrane is in direct contact with the medium and not with capillaries whose endothelial cells die rapidly in culture during the first 24 h (Figure CB).

DNA content per culture dish did not show a significant change during 12 days' rat follicle culture (1.55 ± 0.52 µg/dish, N = 16) or 9 days' pig follicle culture (5.35 ± 0.36 µg/dish, N = 25).

Even though closed and isolated follicles in culture had differences regarding stable Tg19S, the amount of T_3 and T_4 and iodide accumulation between different treatments with and without TSH and with or without 10E-10 M NaI, the follicles did have more iodide organification, iodised Tg19S and T_3 and T_4 at 12 days' culture, even without TSH [83,86], than in all other culture models published to date except of the group [83,84,85,86]. Such variations were homologous to glands *in vivo* in the same study conditions.

Our culture system has different characteristics distinguishing it from other models described up to now. Monolayers lose their function on the first day [48], become reorganised in pseudofollicles on the third day and only 2% to 4 % become incorporated or organified in iodine accumulated in poorly iodised Tg (Tg16S) [91], even though higher than 90% O/A with TSH has been reported for a matrigel-covered monolayer culture forming a double cell layer having cavities [61]. Different models mentioning culturing "follicles" [92,93,94,95] have not shown these functions in their results; others culturing pig "follicles" for 2 days, based on Björkman and Ekholm [16] as we, require 5% FCS, 1 mU/mL TSH and non-physiological molecules such as forskolin or 8-(4-chlorophenylthio)-cAMP for maintaining thyrocyte functions [77]. Using closed follicles enables functional parameters to be conserved and measured: iodide accumulation, iodide organification and, particularly, Tg19S equivalent to that *in vivo* and T_3 and T_4 formation throughout culture with or without TSH. We have also shown that maintaining closed follicular architecture is an indispensable condition for conserving such thyroid functions in culture *in vitro*. If follicular architecture is to be conserved, it is not enough to maintain functions at the same values as those at the start of culture as TSH is required and culture becomes improved by adding iodide, as thyroid function *in vivo* is governed by TSH and iodide.

5.2.2. *Morphological study*

Pig hypothyroid follicles cultured 1 and 3 days without TSH have a very thin epithelial layer (Figure 5A) like original tissue's follicle epithelium. The epithelium became cubic after day 6 and was preserved up to day 9 (Figure 5C). It was seen that follicles conserving colloid had a birefrigent aspect when observed by IM, thereby showing that this was conserved during culture. Epithelium thickness increased in the presence of TSH, becoming cubic on the first day of culture (Figure 5B) and being maintained so until day 9.

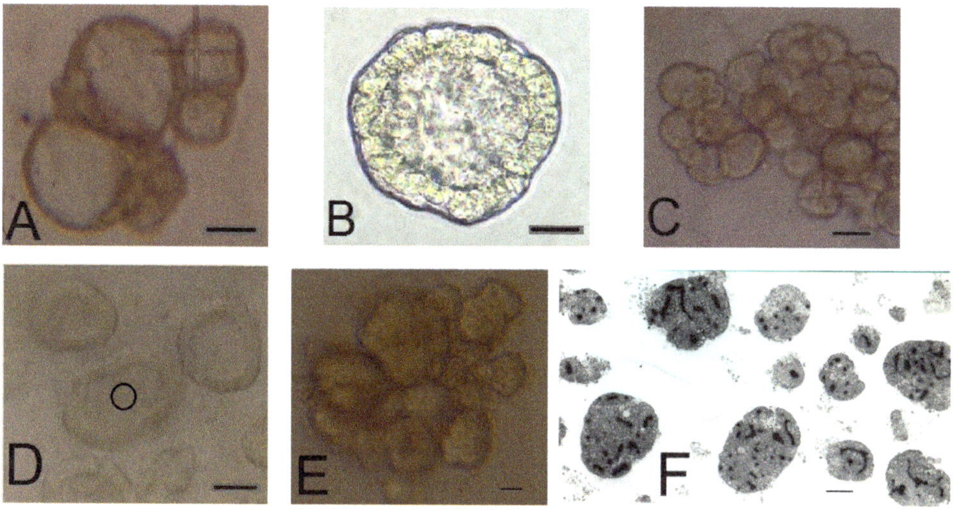

Figure 5. Morphological aspect of follicles in culture. A. Hypothyroid follicle 1 day's culture without TSH; birefringent colloid and thin follicle epithelium can be seen. **B.** Hypothyroid follicle 1 day's culture with 1mU/mL TSH; cubic epithelium and thyrocytes' apical poles typical of a resealed follicle can be seen. **C.** Hypothyroid follicles in 9 days' culture without TSH; the epithelium is cubic and colloid birefringence can be seen in all follicles. **D.** Euthyroid follicle 1 day culture without TSH. A resealed follicle (circle) having irregular contour between thyrocytes and cavity can be seen in the centre. Closed follicles preserve colloid birefringence and regular boundary between thyrocytes and colloid since the start of culture. **E** Pig euthyroid follicles in the presence of 1 mU/mL TSH; follicular cavities are difficult to distinguish. **F.** Autoradiography of rat follicles cultured 12 days in the presence of TSH (1 mU/mL) corresponding to experiment 2, Table 3. Follicle cavities are evident due to the organified iodide found only in very narrow follicular cavities (Scale bar: A and D 50 μm, B 25 μm, C 130 μm, E 100 μm, IM. F 150 μm, OM. Toluidina bleu).

Rat or pig euthyroid follicles without TSH kept the same follicular architecture throughout the whole culture time (Figure 5D). Colloidal cavities became reduced from the third day in the presence of TSH and were difficult to distinguish on day 9 and 12 by IM (Figure 5E); however, they could be seen by autoradiography where only iodide bound to molecules could be identified and they were only located in follicles' very narrow colloidal cavities (Figure 5F). Colloidal cavities' boundaries could also be seen by labelling thyrocytes' apical membrane protein SLC5A8 (short-chain fatty acids transporter) [84].

Rat thyrocyte and pig euthyroid follicle ultra-structure in **one day** culture without TSH (Figure 6A) and with TSH (Figure 6B) was comparable to that for cells *in vivo* (Figure 1C). They conserved their polarity and organelles, but exocytic vesicles were difficult to distinguish from those from endocytosis. RER was more abundant in the presence of TSH and microvellosities were more evident than without TSH.

Thyrocytes had vacuolated and reduced RER and GC following **3 days'** culture without TSH; the GC could be seen in supra-nuclear position (Figure 6C G) as could numerous autophagic vacuoles (Figure 6C arrow) and secondary lysosomes. This became modified in

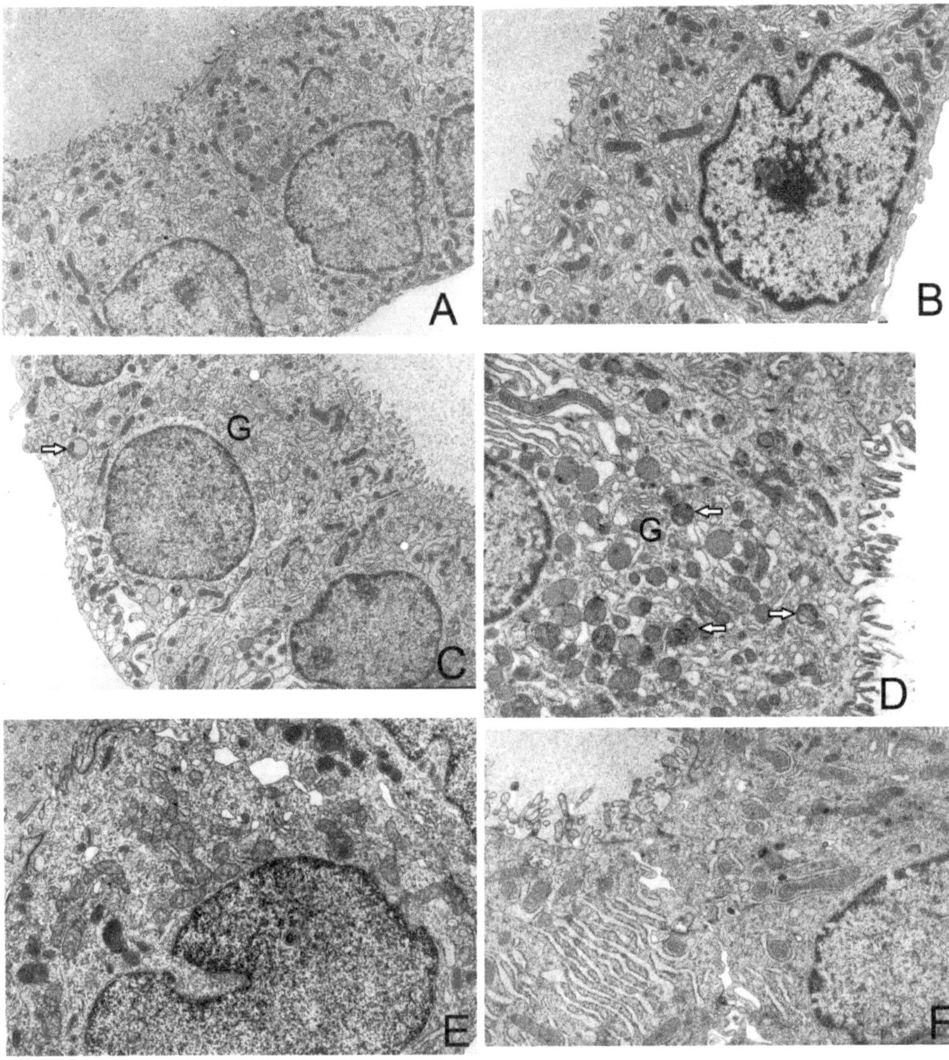

Figure 6. Ultra-structure of thyrocytes from follicles cultured without TSH A 1 day, C 3 days, D 12 days and with 1 mU/mL TSH B 1 day, D 3 days and F 12 days. Binding complexes were preserved in thyrocytes' lateral membrane apical region during all the times with and without TSH. **A.** Thyrocytes conserved their polarisation; microvellosities in contact with electron-dense colloid. Binding complexes were located in lateral membrane's apical region between cells. The rugose endoplasmic reticulum (RER) was found to be slightly vesiculated. **B.** Thyrocyte ultra-structure was comparable to without TSH, even though RER was more abundant. **C. and D.** Ultra-structure was conserved in thyrocytes; the supranuclear Golgi complex (G) and more abundant RER in thyrocytes in the presence of TSH can be seen. Autophagic vacuoles (C. arrow) and secondary lysosomes (D, arrows) with or without TSH can be seen. **E.** Thyrocyte polarity was conserved. Colloid was electron-dense and separated from follicle exterior. Thyrocytes had exiguous RER and G. **F.** Organelles were well conserved. RER was well developed and occupied thyrocytes' apical region (TEM. A and C 7,300 X, B 7,500 X, D 7,438 X, E 9,810 X, F 8,260 X).

the presence of TSH, presenting abundant RER and GC (Figure 6D G) and containing more autophagic vacuoles and secondary lysosomes in thyrocytes' apical region (Figure 6D arrows) than without TSH. RER and GC became more reduced by the **sixth day** without TSH and thyrocytes became thin. Whilst autophagic vacuoles and secondary lysosomes became reduced with TSH, RER and GC also did so by day 3.

Thyrocytes were thin by **day 9** and **12** without TSH and had exiguous RER and GC and reduced microvellosities. The nuclei contained very little heterochromatin (Figure 6E). Follicular centres were very narrow in the presence of TSH, thyrocytes had abundant GC and RER reaching the cells' apical regions (Figure 6F) and the other organelles had the same distribution as on the first days of culture.

Adding 10E-10 M NaI did not modify thyrocytes' follicular architecture or ultra-structure; however, RER and GC were preserved up to day 12 without TSH.

Pig thyrocyte and hypothyroid follicle ultra-structure had exiguous RER and GC when culture began (Figure 7A), like original gland hypothyroids *in vivo*, and culture (even without TSH) developed these organelles from the third day of culture [86]. These hypothyroid follicles' thyrocytes became cubic in the presence of TSH (Figure 5B) from the first day of culture and it was seen that the RER and GC developed and became more evident on the **sixth** and **ninth day** of culture (Figure 7B), similar to rat or pig euthyroid follicle response with TSH, but follicular cavity did not become reduced.

Thyrocytes had normal mitochondria in rat follicle and pig euthyroidic and hypothyroid cultures for all culture times.

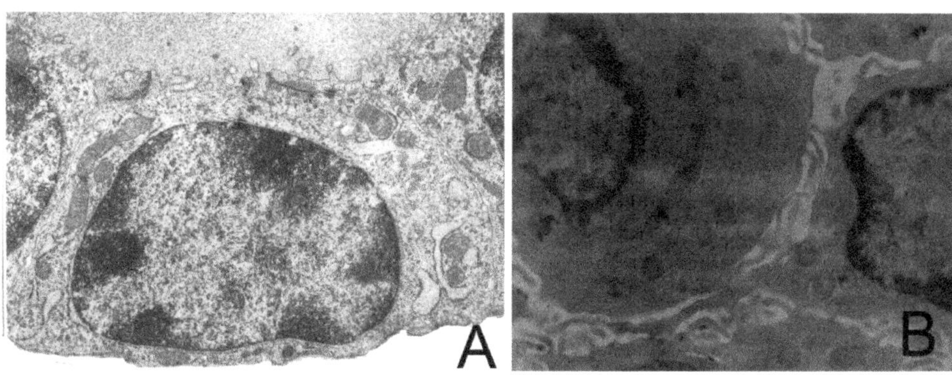

Figure 7. Pig hypothyroid follicle culture. **A.** RER and GC were exiguous and cells were thin 1 day in the absence of TSH. **B.** 9 days in the presence of 1 mU/mL TSH. Cross-section of thyrocyte follicle basal pole. Abundant RER can be seen around the nucleus (TEM. A 7,800 X, B 9,000 X).

Similar culture models to these have been described. Pig follicle culture has highlighted the importance of thyrocyte polarity, but OM morphological study was limited on day 1 [74,94]. Another, dealing with "normal" human follicle culture of thyroidectomy for goitre requiring

TSH [93] had a TEM image showing thyrocytes having the ultra-structure for cells in the process of cell death with lysed mitochondria, without RER or GC. Using this human follicle culture model enabled analyzing the effect of TSH [95] or cytokines [95,96] without presenting culture morphology.

Our results showed that if culture was begun with closed follicles then extracellular matrix support elements were not required [56,57,79,80] nor was TSH for maintaining follicular cavity, as has been described in most pseudofollicle or follicle cultures reconstructed from monolayers, or similar structures called "follicles" [57,50,60,61,62,79,96], thereby demonstrating that if closed follicles are used from the start of culture they conserve their morphology, having the correct polarity as that of their thyrocytes in culture and have a binding complex (tight junction, belt desmosome and spot desmosome) in lateral membranes' apical part as well as *in vivo* [9]. Such closed follicles in culture responded to TSH, like other *in vitro* models [42] or like gland follicles in normal *in vivo* to TSH stimulus [3,25], epithelium thickness, RER and GC becoming increased, and follicular cavities becoming notably reduced [11,83,90]. Follicle response to the absence of TSH both *in vivo* [24] and *in vitro* [42] was also comparable as these organelles became reduced. This effect became reverted *in vivo* when TSH was added, reactivating thyroid functions [11,33,97].

Pig closed and isolated hypothyroid follicles behaved like the gland *in vivo* when the hypothyroid effect was deleted [24], RER and GC increased, follicular epithelium became thin to cubic and culture time became faster in the presence of TSH, but follicular cavity did not become reduced during the 9 days of culture.

Our results thus showed that long-term thyroid follicle function and morphology can be maintained *in vitro*, being equivalent to the gland *in vivo*.

The next section describes the effect of increasing doses of iodide on closed follicles in culture.

5.3. Closed follicle cultures reproduce the Wolff-Chaikoff effect described *in vivo*

5.3.1. Functional study

Follicles were cultured for 1 day before starting to analyse the effect of different iodide concentrations.

Follicles accumulated iodide linearly for 6 h in the presence of 10E-10 and 10E-7 M NaI; accumulation was at its maximum after the first 30 min with 10E-5 M and 10E-3 M NaI (Table 7); they became accumulated 100 times more than with 10E-10 M NaI in the presence of 10E-7 M NaI. Whilst high O/A percentages in follicles were maintained in the presence of 10E-10 and 10E-7 M NaI, organification began after 2 h with 10E-5 M, accounting for only 5% of accumulated iodide, these values being maintained for 6 h, whilst O/A proportion was zero for all times with 10E-3 M NaI (Table 7), even though accumulation could have been 100 times greater to that presented by follicles in the presence of 10E-7 M NaI [98].

	% O/A			
M, NaI	10E-10	10E-7	10E-5	10E-3
Culture, hours				
0.5	82	64	0	0
1	84	42	0	0
2	88	90	5	0
3	92	88	3	0
4	95	87	6	0
5	88	89	6	0
6	84	93	4	0

Table 7. Response of organification percentage regarding iodide accumulation (O/A proportion) by rat follicles cultured in the presence of increasing doses of iodide (NaI, M) and $Na^{125}I$ 5 μCi/mL. The follicles were cultured on agarose with 0.5% FCS for 1 day, medium was changed and culture began with NaI and TSH experimental points. Each value was the average of two samples or culture dishes expressed in %/dose/μg DNA.

Iodide accumulation and organification in rat follicles could be assimilated to biochemical reactions after 30 min with and without TSH and thus define a constant (Km) and maximum speed (Vmax). Accumulation apparent Km without TSH was 5x10E-6 M and 10E-7 M de NaI with TSH; iodide organification apparent Km was 5x10E-7 M and was not modified by the presence of TSH (Figure 8). Iodide accumulation by isolated follicles corresponded well with saturable iodide transport characteristics [15,99] and stimulated TSH thereby reducing Km but not Vmax (Figure 8). It should be stated that organification had to be inhibited and

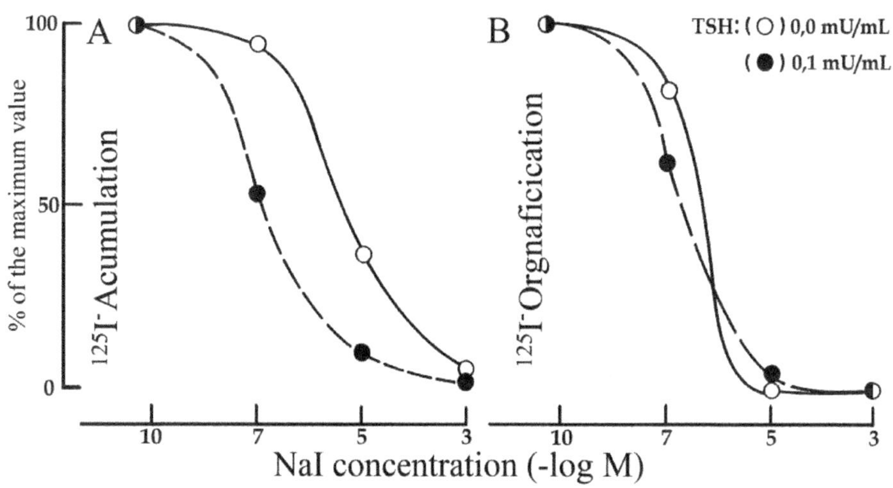

Figure 8. Initial $^{125}I^{-}$iodide accumulation (**A**) and organification (**B**) for follicles in culture measured following half an hour in the presence of increasing doses of ^{127}-I Na and 5 μCi/mL ^{125}-I Na expressed in -log M with and without TSH. The follicles were cultured on agarose with 0.5% FCS for 1 day, the medium was changed and culture began with NaI and TSH experimental points. The results were the average of two samples and were expressed as percentage of maximum value.

the time between the end of the culture and the moment when accumulation was determined had to be reduced for measuring exact iodide transport parameters. The washing times meant that part of $^{125}I^-$ concentrated in follicles would be released before radioactivity was determined and this would induce under-stimulation of accumulation and perhaps overstimulation of O/A percentage.

The presence of TSH for 30 min suppressed the inhibiting effect on iodide organification at 10E-5 M, but did not suppress such iodide effect on organification in the presence of 10E-3 M TSH (Table 8).

	M, NaI	10E-10			10E-7		
Culture	TSH	A	O	% O/A	A	O	% O/A
0.5	-	2.58	1.29	50 ± 5*	360.9	156.34	43 ± 6*
	+	8,06	4,52	56 ± 2*	676,69	406,02	60 ± 14*
3	-	10.88	8.16	75 ± 10*	902.26	525.24	58 ± 7
	+	14,84	11,81	79 ± 1*	1308,27	1079,24	82 ± 1
8	-	35.97	29.84	83 ± 11	2255.64	1602.81	71 ± 4*
	+	32,26	28,06	87 ± 23	1736,84	1371,98	79 ± 10*
12	-	ND			1849.62	1191.13	64 ± 9
	+	ND			1353,38	853,23	63 ± 13
24	-	ND			1714.29	1421.05	83 ± 10
	+	ND			1759,4	1254,17	71 ± 8
48	-	ND			1917.29	1361.98	71 ± 10*
	+	ND			3969,92	3194,23	80 ± 6*
	M, NaI	10E-5			10E-3		
Culture	TSH	A	O	% O/A	A	O	% O/A
0.5	-	14749.09	0	0 *	233469.39	0	0
	+	12480,01	2,63	21 ± 16*	244244,9	0	0
3	-	15272.73	1553.64	10 ± 6	520816.33	0	0
	+	17541,82	2987,27	17 ± 2	466938,78	0	0
8	-	16495.45	2397.15	14 ± 5	574693.88	0	0
	+	20770,91	4450,91	21 ± 2	790204,08	0	0
12	-	ND			* 718367.35	0	0
	+	ND			* 1957551,02	0	0
24	-	ND			* 3071020.41	0	0
	+	ND			* 682448,98	0	0
48	-	ND			664489.8	0	0
	+	ND			484897,96	0	0

Table 8. The effect of I^- dose on the accumulation (A) and organificación (O) of the rat follicles. Follicles cultured on agarose with 0.5% FCS for 1 day; the medium was changed and culture began with different experimental points. The follicles were keep in culture along the time (culture in hours) with 5 μCi/mL $Na^{125}I$, with (+) or without 0.1 mU/mL TSH (-) and doses of $Na^{127}I$ (NaI). Each value was the average of two samples expressed in μg/dose/μg DNA. This result was representative of 5 independent experiments. O/A: percentage of the proportion O/A ± SD. *$p< 0.05$. ND: not determinated.

Follicle culture in the presence of the same iodide dose with 0.1 mU/mL and without TSH led up to 8 h with 10E-10 M and 10E-5 M NaI and up to 48 h with 10E-7 M and 10E-3 M NaI. An iodide accumulation function directly proportional to NaI concentration was reproduced as in table 7.

Accumulation in follicles became saturated after 8 h in the presence of **10E-7 M** NaI with and without TSH, becoming slightly reduced at 12 and 24 h and increasing at 48 h; iodide accumulation with TSH was lower at 8, 12 and 24 h than without TSH (significant only at 12 h, $p< 0.05$). Percentage of the proportion O/A was maintained high values with and without TSH, difference with and without TSH at 30 min and 48 h being significant (Table 8).

Iodide accumulation satuproportion was reproduced in follicles in the presence of **10E-5 M** NaI, whether with or without TSH. TSH significantly stimulated organification inhibited by 10E-5 M NaI ($p< 0.05$) at 30 min, even though O/A percentage was slightly higher than at other times (but was not significant) (Table 8).

Iodide accumulation in follicles in the presence of **10E-3 M** NaI with and without TSH reached a *plateau* at 3 h (Table 8) and was greater in follicles without TSH than with TSH at 12, 24 and 48 h; however, this difference was only significant at 12 and 48 h ($p< 0.05$). Iodide accumulation became reduced with and without TSH at 48 h to 3 h values, even though without TSH this was greater but not significantly so. Iodide organification was zero with such strong dose of iodide with and without TSH at all times examined (Table 8).

Pig euthyroidic follicles had the same response as rat follicles when culturing for 48 h in the presence of increasing doses of iodide with or without TSH. Organification was zero at all times in the presence of 10-E3 M NaI with and without TSH (Table 9).

	M, NaI	10E-10		10E-7		10E-3	
Culture	TSH	% O/A	N	% O/A	N	% O/A	N
0.5	-	30.4 ± 0.56	2	30.4 ± 0.63	2	0	3
	+	34.7 ± 9.21	2	72.7 ± 2.84	2	0	3
3	-	67.0 ± 1.54	2	63.2 ± 9.14	2	0	3
	+	79.5 ± 6.79	2	73.6	1	0	3
12	-	71.8 ± 2.35	2	52.4 ± 2.63	1	0	3
	+	78.9 ± 2.63	2	77.6 ± 3.15	2	0	3
24	-	59.7 ± 2.09	2	87.6 ± 1.97	2	0	4
	+	68.8 ± 7.13	2	85.7 ± 0.99	2	0	3

Table 9. The effect of I^- dose on the proportion accumulation/organificación pourcentage (% A/O) in euthyroidic pig follicles cultured. Follicles cultured on agarose with 0.5% FCS for 1 day; the medium was changed and culture began with different experimental points. The follicles were keep in culture along the time (culture in hours) with 5 µCi/mL $Na^{125}I$, with (+) or without 1 mU/mL TSH (-) and doses of $Na^{127}I$ (NaI). Each value was the average of accumulated or organified (O/A) iodide expressed in %/dose/µg DNA per number (N) of culture dishes ± SD.

Pig hypothyroid follicles had a different response to the presence of increasing doses of iodide than rat and pig euthyroidic follicles (Table 10). They accumulated 40 to 100 times more in the three doses than euthyroidic follicles, presenting organification in the presence of 10E-3 M NaI with or without TSH. Iodide accumulation in these follicles in the presence of perchlorate (30 μM) was only inhibited at 12 h in the presence of 10E-3 M NaI and at 3 h in the presence of 10E-7 M NaI (euthyroidic follicles in the presence of 30 μM perchlorate inhibited iodide capture at all concentrations) and O/A percentages in follicles in the presence of 10E-7 M NaI were greater in the absence of TSH than in their presence (Table 10), such value becoming reduced with culture time.

	NaI	10E-10 M		10E-7 M		10E-3 M	
Culture	TSH	% O/A	N	% O/A	N	% O/A	N
0.5	-	77.9 ± 0.61	4	74.9 ± 0.63	4	6.3 ± 0.63	3
	+	57.3 ± 0.78	4	71.6 ± 2.84	4	15.1 ± 0.63	3
3	-	75.8 ± 0.49	4	68.7 ± 9.14	4	5.4 ± 0.63	3
	+	60.6 ± 0.68	4	57.2 ± 9.14	4	3.0 ± 0.63	3
12	-	ND		87.3 ± 2.63	4	10.4 ± 0.63	3
	+	ND		72.8 ± 3.15	4	3.8 ± 0.63	3
24	-	ND		44.3 ± 1.97	4	11.6 ± 0.63	4
	+	ND		28.7 ± 0.99	4	9.7 ± 0.63	3

Table 10. The effect of I^- dose on the proportion accumulation/organificación pourcentage (% A/O) in pig hypothyroid follicles cultured. Follicles cultured on agarose with 0.5% FCS for 1 day; the medium was changed and culture began with different experimental points. The follicles were keep in culture along the time (culture in hours) with 5 μCi/mL $Na^{125}I$, with (+) or without 1 mU/mL TSH (-) and doses of $Na^{127}I$ (NaI). Each value was the average of iodide accumulated or organified (O/A) iodide expressed in %/dose/μg DNA per number (N) of culture dishes ± SD. ND: not determinated.

Iodide accumulation values in the presence of 10E-3 M NaI in hypothyroid follicles were 2 times greater in follicles in the presence of TSH than without TSH, had organification in similar proportions to euthyroidic follicles in the presence of 10E-5 M NaI. Percentage of the proporction O/A was higher at 30 min without TSH than with TSH; it was lower at the other times. Without TSH increased with culture time whilst values became reduced regarding time with TSH (Table 10). Organification in this case was not nil, but the organified iodine did not exceed 11% for accumulated iodide.

Mouse follicles cultured 3 days in the presence of 10E-7 M NaI was more intense in the presence of reactive species at the boundary between apical membrane microvellosities and colloid and the oxide reduction system became completely closed down with an excess of iodide (10E-4 M NaI) [100]. This proved that an excess of iodide inhibited the enzymes responsible for organification in closed follicles as we have thought should be in the gland *in vivo.*

Euthyroidic follicles accumulated iodide regarding medium constant proportion concentration. Accumulated iodide was organified in the presence of 10E-10 M and 10E-7 M NaI; organification was extremely reduced in the presence of 10E-5 M and zero with 10E-3 M NaI as described *in vivo* [1]. Accumulation was greater in follicles without TSH than with TSH in the presence of 10E-3 M NaI at 12, 24 and 48 h; this reduction was similar to that of the gland *in vivo* [101,102].

Hypothyroid follicles in the presence of 10-3 M NaI accumulated more iodide without TSH than with TSH at the beginning (30 min), even though proportion of O/A percentage was greater at 30 min than at other times; this effect (different to euthyroidic ones) was similar to that described *in vivo* in hypothyroid glands [28]. They also responded by reproducing the effect observed in animals suffering experimental goitre as, when excess iodide was added to food, they did not respond to TSH [24]. 50% of human endemic goitre has responded to an iodine-rich diet and some of these to TSH [25] as hypothyroid follicles in the presence of TSH and 10E-3 M NaI have responded by becoming less organified than in the absence of TSH. It should be stated that there is no consensus regarding what should be the correct dose for defining low, medium or high iodide concentration in human alimentation [25].

Closed and isolated follicles thus responded to 10E-5 M and 10E-3 M NaI inhibiting iodide organification in a similar way to that described for the gland *in vivo* in 1948 [1] (i.e. reproducing the Wolff-Chaikoff effect).

5.3.2. Morphological study

Hypothyroid follicles conserved follicular architecture during 48 h of culture in the presence of different doses of iodide with and without TSH (Figures 9A, 9B and 9C). Rat follicles and pig euthyroidic follicles at all iodide doses in the presence or absence of TSH conserved follicular architecture for 48 h (Figure 9D).

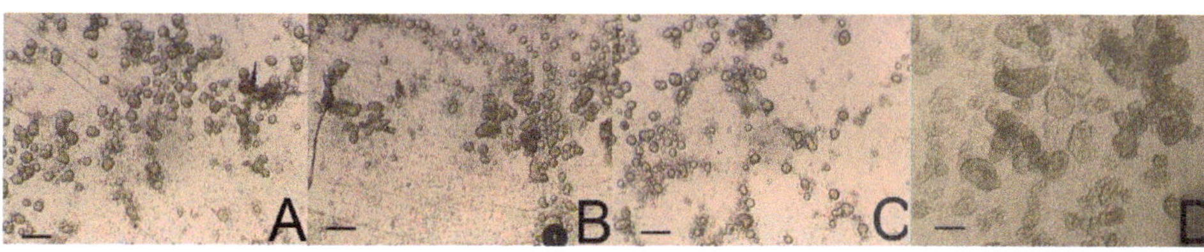

Figure 9. Appearance of pig follicles cultured on agarose with 0.5% FCS for 1 day; the medium was changed and culture lasted 48 h. A. Hypothyroid s follicles in the presence of 10E-10M NaI. **B.** Hypothyroid follicles in the presence of 10E-7M NaI. **C.** Hypothyroid follicles in the presence of 10E-3M NaI. **D.** Euthyroidic follicles in the presence of 10E-3M NaI. The follicular architecture of the gland *in vivo* was conserved in all cultures; hypothyroids (A, B and C) had thin epithelium and euthyroidic (D) ones cubic epithelium (IM. Scale bar: A, B, C 800 μm, D 200 μm).

The Trypan blue exclusion exam of thyrocytes from follicles cultured with 10E-3 M NaI did not have an alteration to their membranes and excluded the stain, whether being pig euthyroidic follicles cultured 48 h (Figure 10A) or rat ones cultured for 6 days (Figure 10B). The cells of cell aggregates which did not have follicular structure became stained (Figure 1C), the same as isolated cells (Figure 10B) or those found in follicles.

The ultra-structure of thyrocytes in all treatments and times preserved cell polarisation and organelle distribution (Figure 11), like the gland *in vivo* (Figure 1C); endocytic vesicles can be seen in thyrocytes' apical region (Figure 11) like follicles after 3 days of culture (Figures 6C and 6D).

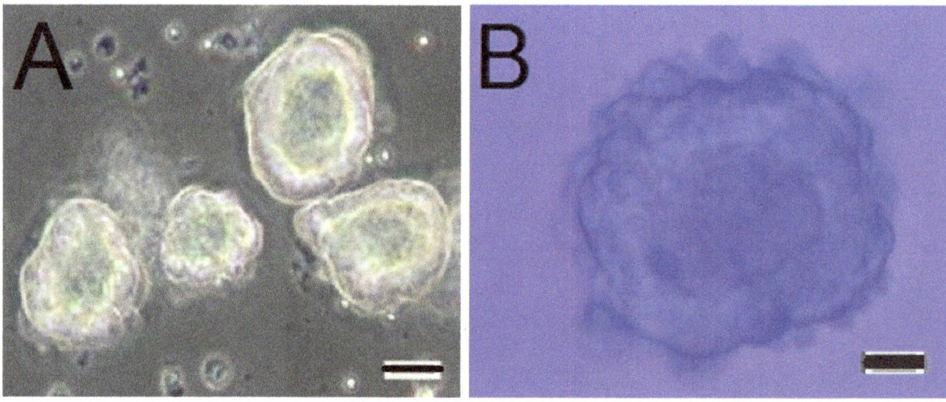

Figure 10. Trypan blue exclusion exam of culture aliquots for follicles cultured on agarose with 0.5% FCS 1 day; the medium was changed and culturing involved 10E-3 M NaI. **A.** 2 day rat follicle culture. **B.** 6 day pig euthyroid follicle culture. The thyrocytes from the follicles excluded the stain whilst isolated cells did not exclude it, whether separated from the follicle (A) or on the follicle (B) (IM, Scale bar A 60 μm, B 15 μm).

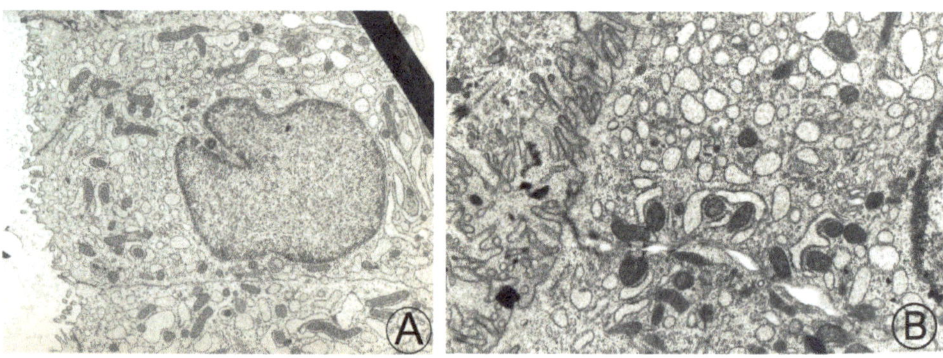

Figure 11. The ultra-structure of rat follicle rat thyrocytes cultured on agarose with 0.5% FCS for 1 day; the medium was changed and 48-h culture involved different experimental points: **A.** 10E-7 M NaI. **B.** 10E-3 M NaI + 0.1 mU/mL TSH. Thyrocytes kept their polarisation; microvellosities were in contact with electron-dense colloid. The binding complexes were located in the lateral membrane's apical region between cells. The RER was slightly vesiculated. Thyrocytes did not have cytological differences regarding iodide dose; follicular centres only became narrowed in the presence of TSH (B) (TEM. A 8,720 X, B 10,720 X)

Follicles in the presence of TSH narrowed their follicle centres at all iodide doses used (Figures 12B and 12D), but did not undergo any ultra-structural modification in strong iodide concentrations: 10E-5M or 10E-3 M NaI. Organelle distribution was comparable to normal gland *in vivo* (Figure 1C) or follicles in long-term culture (Figures 6C and 6D).

Lysosome fusion occurred in follicles in the presence of 10E-10 M NaI and 0.1 mU/mL TSH for 8 h (Figure 12B) while this did not happen in thyrocytes' apical region (Figure 12B insert) in the absence of TSH (Figures 12A and 12C). This was also observed en thyrocytes from follicles cultured for 8 h with 10E-3 M NaI and TSH, but colloid droplets were only located in the apical region in this dose (Figure 12D). Thyrocytes also had endocytic vesicles in this dose without TSH but also located in cells' apical region (Figure 12C). Thyrocytes ultra-structure in the presence of strong concentrations of iodide did not have morphological modifications, or distribution of organelles regarding normal or non-stimulated cells *in vivo* (Figure 1C) or *in vitro* (Figures 6C and 6D).

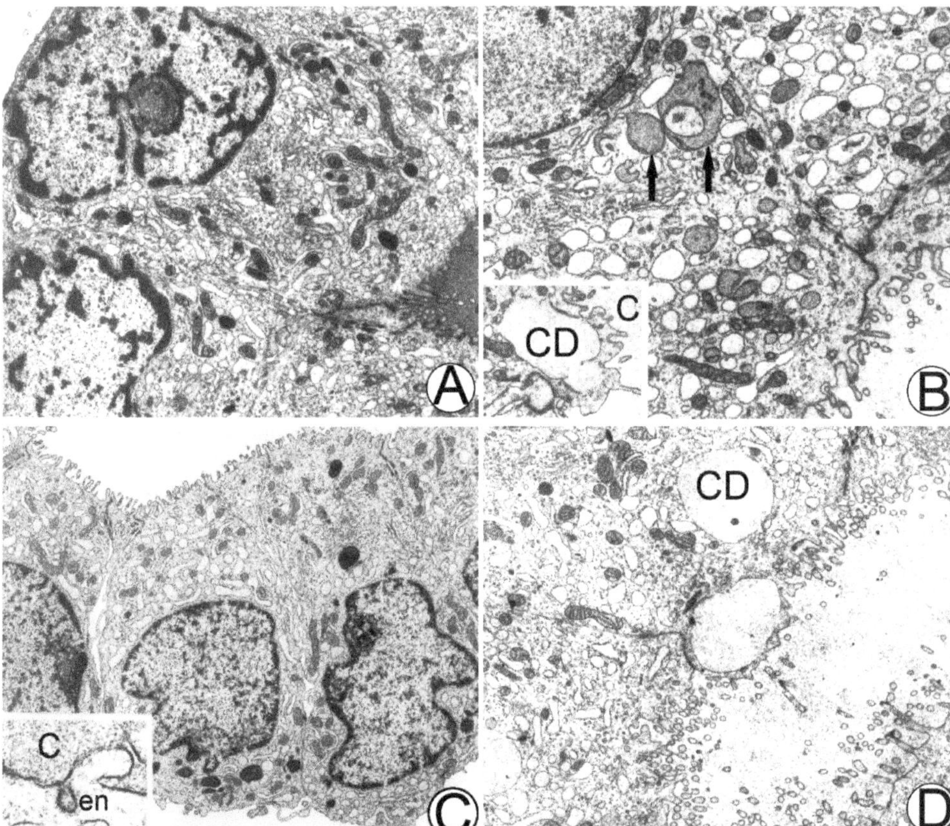

Figure 12. The ultra-structure of rat follicle thyrocytes cultured on agarose with 0.5% FCS for 1 day; the medium was changed and 8 h of culture involved different experimental points: A. 10-E10 M NaI. B. 10-E10 M NaI + 0.1 mU/mL TSH. C. 10-E3 M NaI. D. 10-E3 M NaI + 0.1 mU/mL TSH. A. The ultra-structure of thyrocytes in the absence of TSH was identical to that of thyrocytes from follicles cultured for 1 day. B. Lysosomes close to the nucleus and few *colloid droplets* located in the apical pole (insert) were observed in the presence of TSH. C. They were well conserved in the presence of TSH, even in this strong dose of NaI. Endocytic vesicles were present in such strong dose of iodide. D. Colloid droplets were also observed in the presence of TSH, having the same density as colloid and were located in the thyrocytes' apical pole. Follicle centre was narrow and had abundant microvellosities (TEM. A 8,720 X, B 12,510 X, box 10,720 X, C 7,430 X, box 70,950 X, D 13,450 X).

The thyrocytes from follicles cultured from 30 min up to 6 days in the presence of 10E-3 M NaI did not have cytotoxic signs and all follicular cells were viable, like normal animals' thyroid glands' *in vivo* when fed with excess iodide for 3 weeks [103].

Open human follicle culture in the presence of 10E-3 M NaI with and without TSH for 24 h had ultra-structural alterations related to cytotoxicity [92] involving free radical attack and lipid peroxidation. Excess iodide in pig follicles led to thyrocyte apoptosis because iodine production in lactone became reduced, but did not present morphology. Our results showed that conserving closed follicles did not lead to signs of cell death with 10E-5 M or 10E-3 M NaI or disorganisation or alteration of thyrocyte ultra-structure. The difference with [92] and [94] was that they were open follicle cultures and thyrocytes died simply because they were cultured on a support which inhibited cellular adhesion, like our cell aggregates.

Closed follicles were present (Figure 12), as described for the gland. There was apical membrane turnover between microvellosities which is important for maintaining Tg synthesis and its secretion to colloid [8]. Coated endocytic vesicles (Figure 12C insert) were also present in the base of microvellosities, like micro-endocytosis *in vivo* [5], and those stimulated by TSH formed pseudopods and colloid droplets (Figures 12B insert and 12C letter DC), called *in vivo* macro-endocytosis [10]. Thyrocyte fusion with prelysosomes or late endosomes from the lysosome route was also observed (Figure 12B arrows) for Tg degradation and thyroid hormones were formed *in vivo* [19] and *in vitro* [18].

Closed rat and pig euthyroidic follicles responded to increasing doses of iodide, as *in vivo*, thereby producing the Wolff-Chaikoff effect [1], and presented no modifications in thyrocytes' follicular architecture or ultra-structure, being comparable to a gland *in vivo*.

5.3.2.1. Na^{+}/I^{-} symporter determination

Many thyrocyte culture studies have described reduced RNAm and NIS protein expression when maintained in the presence of strong iodide concentrations (10E-6 to 10E-4 M of iodide). We wanted to determine NIS in rat follicles cultured with strong iodide concentrations with and without TSH 0.1 mU/mL.

Follicles cultured at **12 h** in the presence of 10E-7 M NaI and without TSH had NIS in basolateral membranes (Figure 13A) and labelling was more intense in lateral membranes in the presence of TSH (Figure 13B). In the presence of 10E-3 M NaI NIS was mainly located in vesicles between nucleus and basolateral membranes (Figure 13C), and in the presence of TSH; as well as being presented in vesicles they were observed in basolateral membranes (Figure 13D). It could have been that inhibiting vesicular movement in the presence of 10E-3 M NaI in the apical region (Figures 11C and 11D), as well as inhibiting the movement of the vesicles forming in the basement region with NIS symporter for avoiding excessive iodide entry to thyrocytes.

The NIS symporter was located in the basolateral members in the presence of 10E-10 M NaI at 48 h (E and F), labelling being more intense in the presence of TSH. The NIS symporter was found in the cytoplasmatic vesicles with TSH (F). NIS symporter expression in the presence of 10E-3 M NaI for 48 h (G and H) was so low that confocal microscope parameters

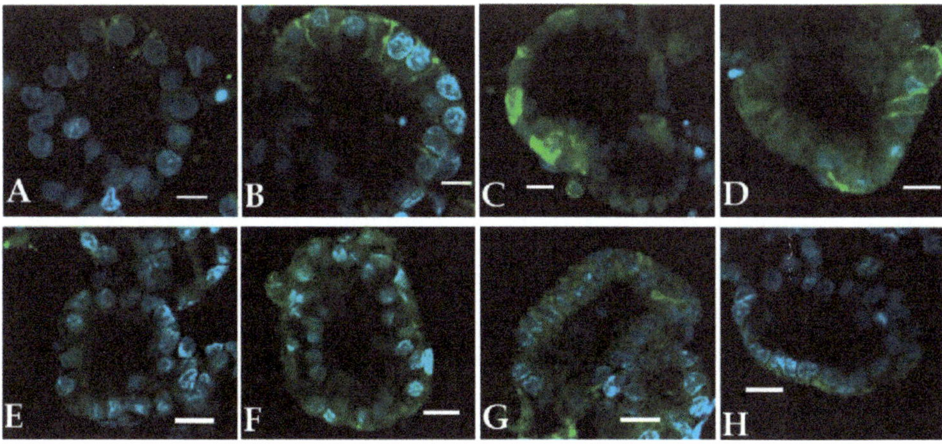

Figure 13. Indirect immunofluorescence of NIS symporter (green) expression and localisation and DAPI-labelled nuclei (blue) in follicles isolated from rats cultured for 1 day on agarose with 0.5% FCS for 1 day; the medium was changed and were cultured for 12 h (A, B, C and D) and for 48 h (E, F, G and H), with different experimental points: NaI with and without 0.1 mU/mL TSH. **A.** 10E-7 M NaI, **B.** 10E-7 M NaI + TSH. **C.** 10E-3 M NaI. **D.** 10E-3 M NaI + TSH. **E.** 10E-7 M NaI. **F.** 10E-7 M NaI + TSH. **G.** 10E-3 M NaI. **H.** 10E-3 M NaI + TSH. NIS symporter was located in the basolateral membranes in the presence of 10E-10 M NaI at 12 h (A and B). TSH intensified labelling (B). NIS symporter was located in cytoplasmatic vesicles near thyrocytes' basolateral membranes in the presence of 10E-3 M NaI at 12 h (C and D). There was more intense labelling in some thyrocytes' basolateral membranes in the presence of TSH (D). [104]

(laser intensity, detector gain, scanning time) had to be adjusted again to increase labelling intensity. NIS protein was mainly observed in cytoplasmatic vesicles in these follicles, being more intense than labelling without TSH (G). Basement membranes had exiguous NIS labelling (CM. Scale bar: 10 μm).

The NIS symporter in follicles cultured for **48 h** in the presence of 10E-7 M NaI were located in vesicles and basolateral membranes (Figure 13E); TSH intensified such labelling (Figure 13F). NIS expression was very reduced regarding the other treatments in the presence of 10E-3 M NaI with and without TSH and microscope parameters had to be readjusted for observing fluorescence. NIS was located in cytoplasmatic vesicles in this strong dose of NaI and without TSH (Figure 13G). TSH was located in vesicles in the base region but labelling was less intense (Figure 13H) than with TSH.

NIS has normally been located in thyrocytes' basolateral members *in vivo* [13], and a reduction in its normal expression has been associated with escape from the Wolff-Chaikoff effect [30] following 48 h in the presence of strong iodide concentrations [29]. Being found in vesicles has reduced NIS in its normal position for thyrocytes from follicles in the presence of a strong dose of NaI [104] and has thus suppressed I^-transport for thyroid hormone production.

These results were similar in the FRTL5 cell line where the same dose did not alter NIS RNAm percentage, but protein became reduced by 50% and 78 % at 24 and 48 h, respectively [32]. NIS RNAm became reduced in dogs with goitre at 48 h with a comparable iodide dose [105]. This was perhaps presented by reduced AM2Pc levels at 48 h, as excess I^- inhibited an increase in AMPc stimulated by TSH in hypophysectomised rats [106] and mice [34], which could have explained the low NIS level during Wolff-Chaikoff effect and in follicles at 48 h in the presence of excess iodide (Figure s13G and 13H). Excess I^- inhibited IP_3 production and increased Ca^{2+} flow induced by TSH, which could have led to reduced peroxide production during Wolff-Chaikoff effect [107,108]. The organification observed in the presence of 10E-5 M (Table 8) did not completely inhibit TPO and had no effect on NIS in the presence of 10E-3 M NaI (Figures 13E and 13H), thereby demonstrating that organification depends on TPO and not on NIS as in cells transfected with the TPO gene [34]. TSH did not stimulate the organification of iodide captured in 10E-3 M but did so in 10E-5 M NaI (Tables 8 and 10), as it has been described that the effect of TSH on thyroid physiology becomes reduced in the presence of excess I^-, meaning that antagonic roles are assumed *in vivo* [102].

TSH modulated relative NIS expression and its subcellular localisation in the thyrocytes of isolated and closed follicles *in vitro*. These results were similar to those found in FRTL5cells, where it has been demonstrated that *de novo* synthesis [32], half-life time, NIS targeting and/or retention regarding cytoplasmatic membrane requires TSH to be located throughout cell membrane, due to loss of polarity [109].

Thyrocyte disposition in follicles has not been necessary for iodide accumulation, since it has been present in foetal thyroids before follicular lumen formation [110] and also in primary cultures from normal thyrocytes [111] or goitre patients [112] and in the FRTL cell line [113]; however, these cultures have required TSH, hormones and other molecules for maintaining them. Nevertheless, isolating the colloidal cavity from the exterior must be ensured for iodide accumulation and incorporation in Tg, T_3 and T_4 hormone synthesis, as demonstrated with rat or pig isolated and closed follicle cultures.

Rat and pig follicles thus inhibited iodide organification in the presence of strong concentrations of iodide, i.e. performed the Wolff-Chaikoff effect. Neither thyrocytes' follicular architecture nor ultra-structure was modified and no sign of cell death was presented. The TSH and iodide effects observed *in vivo* during the Wolff-Chaikoff effect were reproduced.

6. Conclusion

Loss of follicular structure during the first 24 h of culture has been the main drawback of *in vitro* thyroid studies and, therefore, hormone synthesis. It is not enough to conserve thyrocytes' apical-basal polarity in culture in this specific tissue for maintaining colloid's extracellular functions for the enzymes implicated in iodide fixation on Tg and hormone synthesis.

We have shown that follicular architecture must be conserved in culture, especially the follicular cavity isolated from extracellular medium as this is indispensable for maintaining ultra-structure and the polarity of thyrocytes around the follicular cavity; such premise conserving the idea of Tg19S synthesis usually being glycosylated and iodised, as also T_3 and T_4 hormone synthesis. Follicular morphological conservation is necessary for reproducing the Wolff-Chaikoff effect *in vitro*, as has been described *in vivo*. NIS symporter localisation in thyrocytes depends on I and TSH concentration.

This culture may be used for obtaining follicles from pathologies of human tissue whose epithelium may be thin plate-like cells for *in vitro* studies in controlled and homologous conditions regarding the pathology *in vivo*. It will also enable studying normal or pathological thyroid's physiological, cellular and molecular mechanisms (for example CLC-5 channel) in a homologous model of the gland *in vivo*.

Author details

Clara Spinel[1,3], Magnolia Herrera[3] and and Jhon Rivera[2,3]
Membrane Biophysics and Biology Group,
[1]Biology Department, Science Faculty, Universidad Nacional de Colombia, Colombia
[2]Chemistry Department, Science Faculty, Universidad Nacional de Colombia, Colombia
[3]International Physics Center, Bogotá, Colombia

Acknowledgement

This work was supported by grants from the Colombian Science, Technology and Innovation Department (COLCIENCIAS) programmes Ecos-Nord and Jóvenes Investigadores P 2009-0745, by the Universidad Nacional de Colombia's Research Department and Fundacion Instituto de Inmunología de Colombia (FIDIC). We would like to extend our most sincere thanks to Marcela Camacho, Marie France van den Hove, Thierry Pourcher, Jean-François Denef, Hernando Curtidor and Manuel E Patarroyo for their support and encouragement for carrying out basic research in Colombia.

We would also like to thank the students who carried out and who are carrying out BSc, MSc and PhD thesis experiments: Sandra Perdomo, Gabriela Delgado, Cristina Zapata, Ricardo Cabezas, Alejandro Ondo, Leslie Leal, Oscar Vivas, Claudia Moreno, Eleonora Bernal, Anyela González, Mauren Ortíz, Carolina Ochoa and Luz Marina Porras; this work could not have been completed without their input.

7. References

[1] Wolff J, Chaikoff IL (1948). Plasma inorganic iodide as a homeostatic regulator of thyroid function. J Biol Chem. 174:555-64.
[2] Wollman S (1980) Structure of the thyroid gland. In: Vissher M, editor. The thyroid gland. New York: Raven Press. pp. 1-19.
[3] Werner C, Ingbar H (1971) The thyroid. A fundamental and clinical text, pp.5-40. London: Harper & Row. 914p.

[4] Smeds S (1972) A microgel electrophoretic analysis of the colloid proteins in single rat thyroid follicles. I. The quantitative protein composition of the colloid in normal thyroid. Endocrinology 91:1288-99.
[5] Ekholm R, Björkman U (1972) Thyroid structure and synthesis of thyroglobulin. Ann Clin Res 4:64-9.
[6] Nadler NJ (1974) Anatomical features. In: Greep RO, Aswhood EB, editors. Handbook of physiology. Washington DC: Am Physiol Soc. pp.39-54.
[7] Ekholm R, Ericson LE (1968) The ultrastructure of the parafollicular cells of the thyroid gland in the rat. J. Ultrastruct Res 23:378-402
[8] Wollman SH, Loewenstein JE (1973) Rates of colloid droplet and apical vesicle production and membrane turnover during thyroglobulin secretion and resorption. Endocrinology 93(1):248-52.
[9] Engström G, Ericson LE (1981) Effect of graded doses of thyrotropin on exocytosis and early phase of endocytosis in the rat thyroid. Endocrinology 108(2):399-405.
[10] Tice LW, Carter RC, Wollman SH (1976) Gap junctions in thyroid epithelium of the rat. Endocrinology 98(3):800-1.
[11] Denef J-F, Cordie AC, Mesquita M, Haumont S (1979) The influence of fixation procedure, embedding medium and section thickness on morphometric data in thyroid gland. Histochemistry 63:163-71.
[12] Spinel C (2003) Biología molecular de la cellula eucariótica animal, pp. 201-214. Medellín: Biogénesis Fondo Editorial. 420p.
[13] Carrasco N (1993) Iodide transport in the thyroid gland. Biochim Biophys Acta 1154:65-82.
[14] Kopp P (1999) Pendred's syndrome: identification of the genetic defect a century after its recognition. Thyroid 9(1): 65-9.
[15] van den Hove MF, Croizet-Berger K, Jouret F, Guggino SE, Guggino WB, Devuyst O, *et al.* (2006) The loss of the chloride channel, ClC-5, delays apical iodide efflux and induces a euthyroid goiter in the mouse thyroid gland. Endocrinology. 147(3):1287-96.
[16] Björkman U, Ekholm R (1984) Generation of H_2O_2 in isolated porcine thyroid follicles. Endocrinology 115:392-8.
[17] Medeiros-Neto G, Targovnik H, Vassart G (1993) Defective thyroglobulin synthesis and secretion causing goiter and hypothyroidism. Endocr Rev. 14(2):165-83.
[18] Dubois B, Couvreur M, Spinel C, Denef J-F, van den Hove M-F (1991) Thyroglobulin (Tg) hydrolysis starts in prelisosomes. Netherlands: Proceeding of the 10th International Thyroid Conferences. pp.111.
[19] van den Hove-Vandenbroucke (1980) Secretion of thyroid hormones. In: De Visscher M, editors. The thyroid gland. New York: Raven Press. pp. 61-79.
[20] Gershengorn MC, Cheng S-Y, Lippoldt RE, Lord RS, Robbins J (1977). Characterizaction of human thyroxine-binding globulin. Evidence for a single polypeptide chain. J Biol Chem. 252: 8713-8.
[21] Richardson SJ (2007) Cell and molecular biology of transthyretin and thyroid hormones. Int Rev Cyt. 258:137-93.

[22] Yen P (2001) Physiological and molecular basis of thyroid hormone action. Physiol Rev. 81:1097- 42.
[23] Denef J-F, Björkman U, Ekholm R (1980) Structural and functional characteristics of isolated thyroid follicles. J Ultrastruct Res. 71:185-202.
[24] Many MC (1982) L'involution de la hyperplasie thyroïdienne chez la souris C3H. [PhD thesis]. Brussels: Univ Catholique de Louvain.
[25] Gaitán E, Nelson N, Poole G (1991) Endemic goiter and endemic thyroid disorders, World J Surg.15(2):205-15.
[26] Cardoso LC, Martins DC, Campos DV, Santos LM, Correa da Costa VM, Rosenthal D, *et al.* (2002) Effect of iodine or iopanoic acid on thyroid Ca2+/NADPH-dependent H2O2-generating activity and thyroperoxidase in toxic diffuse goiters. EurJ Endocrinol. 147 293-8.
[27] Dumont J, Optiz R, Christophe D, Vassart G, Roger P, Maenhaut C (2011) Ontogeny, anatomy metabolism and physiology of the thyroid. In: Thyroid Disease Manager. Available at: http://www.thyroidmanager.org/chapter/ontogeny-anatomy-metabolism-and-physiology-of-the-thyroid/
[28] Raben MS (1949) The paradoxical effects of thiocyanate and of thyrotropin on the organic binding of iodine by the thyroid in the presence of large amounts of iodide. Endocrinology 45:296-304.
[29] Wolff J, Chaikoff IL, Goldberg R, Meier J (1949) The temporary nature of the inhibitory action of excess iodine on organic iodine synthesis in the normal thyroid. Endocrinology 45:504-13.
[30] Eng PH, Cardona GR, Fang SL, Previti M, Alex S, Carrasco N, Chin WW, Braverman LE (1999) Escape from the acute Wolff-Chaikoff effect is associated with a decrease in thyroid sodium/iodide symporter messenger ribonucleic acid and protein. Endocrinology 140:3404-10.
[31] Ferreira AC, Lima LP, Araujo Rl, Muller G, Rocha RP, Rosenthal D *et al.* (2005) Rapid regulation of thyroid sodium-iodide symporter activity by thyrotrophin and iodine. J Endocrinol 184:69-76.
[32] Eng PH, Cardona GR, Previti MC, Chin WW, Braverman LE (2001) Regulation of the sodium iodide symporter by iodide in FRTL-5 cells. Eur J Endocrinol 144:139-44.
[33] Li HS, Carayanniotis G (2007) Induction of goitrous hypothyroidism by dietary iodide in SJL mice. Endocrinology 148(6):2747-52.
[34] Wenzel A, Upadhyay G, Schmitt TL, Loos U (2003) Iodination of proteins in TPO transfected thyroid cancer cells is independent of NIS. Mol Cell Endocrinol 213:99–108.
[35] Harrison RG (1910). The outgrowth of the nerve fiber as a mode of protoplasmic movement. J Exp Zool. 9(4):787–846.
[36] Gospodarowicz D, Ill C (1980) Extracellular matrix and control of proliferation of vascular endothelial cells. J Clin Invest. 65(6):1351-64.
[37] Kleinman HK, Martin GR (2005) Matrigel: basement membrane matrix with biological activity. Semin Cancer Biol 15(5):378-86.
[38] Lacy PE, Kostianovsky M (1967) Method for the isolation of intact islets of Langerhans from the rat pancreas. Diabetes 16(1):35-9.

[39] Bissell MJ (1981) The differentiated state of normal and malignant cells or how to define a "normal" cell in culture. Int Rev Cytol. 70:27-100.
[40] Morton, ME, Chaikoff IL (1943) The formation *in vitro* of thyroxine and diiodotyrosine by thyroid tissue with radioactive iodine as indicator. Journal of Biological Chemistry 147(1):1-9.
[41] Pantic V, Pavlovic-Hnac M, Rappaport L (1970) Relation entre l'ultrastructure de cultures et des greffes de glandes thyroïdes de rats et leur pouvoir de synthèse de la thyroglobuline. J Ultrastruct Res. 31:37–45.
[42] Baker TG, Young BA (1973) Organ culture of the rat thyroid gland. Experiantia 29(12):1548-50.
[43] Bauer MF, Herzog V (1988) Mini organ culture of thyroid tissue: a new technique for maintaining the structural and functional integrity of thyroid tissue *in vitro*. Lab Invest. 59(2):281-91.
[44] Toda S, Watanabe K, Yokoi F, Matsumura S, Suzuki K, Ootani A, et al. (2002) A new organotypic culture of thyroid tissue three-dimensional follicles with C cells for a long term. Biochem Biophys Res Comun. 294: maintains 906-11.
[45] Carrel A, Burrows MT (1911) Cultivation *in vitro* of the thyroid gland. J Exp Med. 13(4):416-21.
[46] Tong W, Kerkof PR, Chaikoff IL (1962) Iodine metabolism of dispersed thyroid cells obtained by trypsinization of sheep thyroid glands. Biochim Biophys Acta. 60:1-19
[47] Rodesh F, Dumont JE (1967) Metabolic properties of isolated sheep thyroid cells. Exp Cell Res. 47(1):386-96
[48] Tong W (1962) The isolation and culture of the thyroid cells. Methods Enzymol. 32(Part B):745-58.
[49] Kuliawat R, Lisanti Mp, Arvan P (1995) Polarized distribution and delivery of plasma membrane proteins in the thyroidal follicular epithelial cells. J Biol Chem. 270(6):2478-82.
[50] Nilsson M, Björkmann U, Ekholm R, Ericson LE (1990) Iodide transport in primary cultured thyroid follicle cells: evidence of a TSH-regulated channel mediating iodide efflux selectively across the apical domain of the plasma. Eur J Cell Biol. 52:270-281.
[51] Nilsson M (1991) Integrity of the occluding barrier in high-resistant thyroid follicular epithelium in culture. I. Dependence of extracellular Ca2+ is polarized. Eur J Cell Biol. 56(2):295-307.
[52] Ambesi-Impiombato FS, Coon HG (1979) Thyroid cells in culture. *Int Rev Cytol Suppl.* (10):163-72
[53] Avvedimento EE, Monticelli A, Tramontano D, Polistina C, Nitsch L, Di Lauro R (1985) Differential expression of thyroglobulin gene in normal and transformed thyroid cells. Eur J Biochem. 149(3):467-72.
[54] Lissitzky S, Fayet G, Giraud A, Verrier B, Torresani J (1971) Thyrotropine-induced aggregation and reorganization into follicles of isolated porcine-thyroid cells. 1. Mechanism of action of thyrotrophin and metabolic properties. Eur J Biochem. 24(1):88-99.

[55] Ambesi-Impiombato FS, Parks LA, Coon HG (1980) Culture of hormone-dependent functional epithelial cells from rat thyroids. Proc Natl Acad Sci USA 77(6):3455-9.
[56] Eggo MC, Quiney M, Campbell VS (2003) Local factors regulating growth and and function of human thyroid cells *in vitro* and *in vivo*. Mol Cell Endocrinol. 213:47-58.
[57] Fayet G, Michel-Béchet M, Lissitizke S (1971) Induced aggregation and reorganization into follicles of isolated porcine-thyroid cells in culture. 2. Ultrastructural studies. Eur J Biochem. 24(1):100-11.
[58] Chambard M, Gabrion J, Mauchamp J (1981) Influence of collagen gel on the orientation of epithelial cell polarity: Follicle formation from isolated thyroid cells and from preformed monolayers. J Cell Biol. 91:157-166
[59] Toda S, Yonemitsu N, Minami Y, Sugihara H (1993) Plural cells organize thyroid follicles through aggregation and linkage in collagen gel culture of porcine follicle cells. Endocrinology. 1993;133(2):914-20.
[60] Mauchamp J, Mirrione A, Alquier C André F (1998) Follicle-like structure and polarized monolayer: role of the extracellular matrix on thyroid cell organization in primary culture. Biol Cell. 90:369-80.
[61] Pellerin S, Croizet K, Rabilloud R, Feige J, Rousset B (1999) Regulation of the three-dimensional organization of thyroid epithelial cells into follicle structures by the matricellular protein, thrombospondin-1. Endocrinology 140(3):1094-103.
[62] Kogai T, Curcio F, Hyman S, Cornford E, Brent G, Hershman J (2000) Induction of follicle formation in long-term cultured normal human thyroid cells treated with thyrotropin stimulates iodide uptake but not sodium/iodide symporter messenger RNA and protein expression. J Endocrinol 167:125-35.
[63] Bernier-Valentin F, Trouttet-Masson S, Rabilloud R, Selmiodideruby S, et al. (2006) Three-dimensional organization of thyroid cells into follicle structures is a pivotal factor in the control of sodium/iodide symporter expression. Endocrinology 147:2035-42
[64] Moskalewski S (1965) Isolation and culture of the islets of Langerhans of the guinea pig. Gen Comp Endocrinol. 5(3):342-53.
[65] Andersson A, Borg H, Groth CG, Gunnarsson R, Hellerström C, Lundgren G *et al.* (1976) Survival of isolated human islets of Langerhans maintained in tissue culture. J Clin Inves. 57(5):1295-301.
[66] Inman JL, Bissell MJ (2010) Apical polarity in three-dimensional culture systems: where to now? J Biol 9:1-5.
[67] Teramura Y, Iwata H (2009) Islet encapsulation with living cells for improvement of biocompatibility. Biomaterials 30:2270-5
[68] Schwarz RP, Goodwin TJ, Wolf DA (1992) Cell culture for three-dimensional modeling in rotating-wall vessels: An application of simulated microgravity. Methods Cell Sci. 14(2):51-7.
[69] Nitsch L, Wollman SH (1980) Suspension culture of separated follicles consisting of differentiated thyroid epithelial cells. Proc Natl Acad Sci USA 77(1): 472-6.
[70] Nitsch L, Wollman SH (1980) Thyrotropin preparations are mitogenic for thyroid epithelial cells in follicles in suspension culture. Proc Natl Acad Sci USA 77(5):2743-7.

[71] Herzog V, Miller F (1981) Structural and functional polarity of insade-out follicles prepared from pig thryoid gland. Eur J Cell Biol. 24:74-84.
[72] Björkman U, Ekholm R, Denef J-F (1981) Cytochemical localization of hydrogen peroxide in isolated thyroid follicles. J Ultrastruct Res. 74:105-15
[73] Karlsson F, Westermark K, Westermark B (1982) Functional properties of porcine-thyroid follicles in suspension. Mol Cell Endocrinol. 28: 99-112.
[74] Gärtner R, Greil W, Stübner D, Permanetter W, Horm K, Pickardt CR (1985) Preparation of porcine thyroid follicles with preserved polarity: functional and morphological properties in comparison to inside-out-follicles. Mol Cell Endocrinol.40:9-16.
[75] Westermark K, Karlsson Fe, Westermark B (1985) Thyrotropin modulates EGF receptor function in porcine thyroid follicles cells. Mol Cell Endocrinol 40:17-23.
[76] Orozco J, Guzmán F, Orozco O, Spinel C (1997) Deteccion en tirocitos humanos de peptidos sintéticos derivados de la hormone tireotrópica. Rev Boliva. Endocrinol. 6 (1):14-20.
[77] Morand S, Chaaraoui M, Kaniewski J, Deme D, Ohayon R, Noel-Hudson MS, et al. (2003) Effect of iodide on nicotinamide adenine dinucleotide phosphate oxidase activity and duox2 protein expression in isolated porcine thyroid follicles. Endocrinology 144(4):1241-8.
[78] Kusakabe T, Kawaguchi A, Hoshi N, Kawaguchi R, Hoshi S, Kimura S (2006) Thyroid-specific enhancer-binding protein/NKX2.1 is required for the maintenance of ordered architecture and function of the differentiated thyroid. Mol Endocrinol. 20:1796-809.
[79] Takasu N, Ohno S, Komiya I, Yamada T (1992) Synthesis; cytoskeletons and iodine metabolism in polarized monolayer cells on collagen gel and in double layered, follicle-forming cells. Endocrinology 131(3):1143-8.
[80] Massart C, Gibassier J, Raoul Ml, Le Gall F, Lancien G, Genetet N, *et al*. (1997) Action of peripheral or intrathyroidal lymphocytes on autologous thyrocytes cultured in follicles in collagen gel. J Mol Endocrinol. 18:137-45.
[81] Elia N, Lippincott-Schwartz J (2009) Culturing three dimensional MDCK cells for analyzing intracellular dynamics. Curr Protoc Cell Biol. Available: http://www.ncbi.nlm.nih.gov/pmc/articles/PMC2786266/
[82] Spinel C (1987) Aspects morphologiques et fonctionnels des follicules thyroïdiens en culture. [PhD thesis]. Brussels: Univ Catholique de Louvain. Brussels.
[83] Spinel C, Colin I, van den hove M-F, Denef J-F (1990) Correlated morphological and functional study of isolated rat thyroid follicles in culture. Mol Cell Endocrinol. 213:47-58.
[84] Herrera M, Ondo A, Spinel C (2007) Culture of follicles isolated and closed in the long term of pig thyroid and its morphologic study. Acta Microsc. 16(1-2) Supp 2: 315-6.
[85] Cabezas R, Ondo A, Arias J, Spinel C (2005) Isolation and culture of closed thyroid follicles in mouse, pig and man. Thyroid 15 (Suppl. 15):84-5.
[86] Herrera M, Ondo A, Spinel C (2008) Estudio morfolǿgico del cultivo a largo plazo de foloculos aislados y cerrados de tiroides de cerdo. Acta biol Colom. 13(3):49-60.
[87] Phillips HS (1973) Dye exclusion tests for cell viability. In: Kruse PF, Patterson MK, editors. Tissue culture methods and applications. New York: Academic Press. pp.406-8.

[88] Schneider WC (1957) Determination of nucleic acids in tissues by pentose analysis. Meth Enz. 3:680-4.

[89] van den Hove MF, Paternoster S, Couvreur M (1986) Hormonogenic peptides of thyroglobulin aer released during the coupling of iodotyrosines. Ann Endocrinol. 47: 62A.

[90] Herrera M, Rivera J, Spinel C (2010) Swine follicles in three-dimensional morph-functional culture are homologous to the thyroid *in vivo* and by morphometric analyze can determinate the functional status. Paris: Abstract Book 14th International Thyroid Congress. OC-125.

[91] Tachetti C, Zurzolo C, Monticelli A, Nitsch L 1986) Funtional properties of normal and inverted rat thyroid follicles in suspension culture. J Cell Physiol. 126(1):93-8.

[92] Many MC, Mestdagh C, van den Hove M-F, Denef J-F (1992) *In vitro* study of acute toxic effects of high iodide doses in human thyroid follicles. Endocrinology 131:621-30.

[93] Sato K, T. Satoh T, K, Shizume K, M, Ozawa M, D. Han D, H. Imamura H, *et al.* (1990) Inhibition of ^{125}I-organification and thyroid hormone release by interleukin-l, tumor necrosis factor-α, and interferon-γ in human thyrocytes in suspension culture. J Clin Endocrinol Metab. 70: 1735-43.

[94] Langer R, Burzler C, Bechtner G, Gärtner R (2003) Influence of iodide and iodolactones on thyiroid apoptosis. Exp Clin Endocrinol Diabetes 111, 325-9.

[95] Yamasaki K, Suzuki K, Yamada E, Yamada T, Takeshita F, Matsumoto, *et al.* (2007) Suppression of iodide uptake and thyroid hormone synthesis with stimulation of the type I interferon system by double-stranded ribonucleic acid in cultured human thyroid follicles. Endocrinology 148(7):3226-35.

[96] Yamazaki K, Yamada E, Kanaji Y, Shizume K, Wang DS, Maruo N, *et al.* (1996) Interleukin-6 (IL-6) inhibits thyroid function in the presence of soluble IL-6 receptor in cultured human thyroid follicles. Endocrinology 137:4857-63.

[97] Hilfer SR, Searls RL (1980) Differentiation of the thyroid in the hypophysectomized chick embryo. Dev Biol. 79(1):107-18.

[98] Spinel C, Yildiz I (1991) High doses of iodide are not toxic for rat thyroid follicles in culture. Netherlands: Proceeding of the 10th International Thyroid Conference. pp.259.

[99] Bastomsky CH (1974) Thyroid iodide transport. In: Greer MA, Solomon DH, editors. Handbook of Physiology Sec. 7, Vol. 3. Washington DC: American Physiological Society, 1974, pp 81-99.

[100] Bernal E, Spinel C, Ondo A. (2010) Amiodarone and NIS in the mice thyroid. Paris: Book of Abstracts from the 14th International Thyroid Congress. P-0294.

[101] Follis RH, Jr. (1964) Further observations on thyroiditis and colloid accumulation in hyperplastic thyroid glands of hamsters receiving excess iodine. Lab Invest 13:1590-99.

[102] Hashizume K, Akasu F, Takazawa K, Endo W, Onaya T (1976) The inhibitory effect of acute administproportion n of excess iodide on the formation of adenosine 3', 5'-monophosphate induced by thyrotropin in mouse thyroid lobes. Endocrinology 99:1463-8.

[103] Mahmoud I, Colin I, Many MC, Denef JF (1986) Direct toxic effect of iodide in excess on iodine-deficient thyroid glands: epithelial necrosis and inflammation associated with lipofuscin accumulation. Exp Mol Pathol. 44:259-71.

[104] Rivera J, Herrera M, Ochoa C, Spinel C (2010) Swine and mice closed follicular thyroid in a three-dimensional culture reproduce the Wolff-Chaikoff effect. Paris: Book of Abstracts from the 14th International Thyroid Congress. P-0053.

[105] Uyttersprot N, Pelgrims N, Carrasco N, Gervy C, Maenhaut C, Dumont JE, *et al.* (1997) Moderate doses of iodide *in vivo* inhibit cell proliferation and the expression of thyroperoxidase and NaI/I- symporter mRNAs in dog thyroid. Mol Cell Endocrinol. 131:195–203.

[106] Rapoport B, West MN, Ingbar SH (1975) Inhibitory effect of dietary iodine on the thyroid adenylate cyclase response to thyrotropin in the hypophysectomized rat. J Clin Invest 56:516-519.

[107] Corvilain B, Laurent E, Lecomte M, Vansande J, Dumont JE (1994) Role of the cyclic adenosine 3',5'-monophosphate and the phosphatidylinositol-$Ca2^{+}$ cascades in mediating the effects of thyrotropin and iodide on hormone synthesis and secretion in human thyroid slices. J Clin Endocrinol Metab. 79:152-9.

[108] Hashizume K, Ichikawa K, Komiya I, Onaya T (1984) Thyrotropin-induced acceleration of calcium efflux from mouse thyroid: evidence for inhibition by excess iodide. Endocrinology 114:1672-7.

[109] Riedel C, Levy O, Carrasco N (2001) Post-transcriptional regulation of the sodium/iodide symporter by thyrotropin. J Biol Chem. 276:21458-63.

[110] Hodges R, Evans T, Bradbury J, Keettel W (1955) The Accumulation of radioactive iodine by human fetal thyroids. J Clin Endocrinol Metab. 15(6): 661-7.

[111] Sherwin JR, Tong W (1974) The actions of iodide and TSH on thyroid cells showing a dual control system for the iodide pump. Endocrinology 94:1465-1474.

[112] Saito T, Endo T, Kawaguchi A, Ikeda M, Nakazato M, Kogai T, Onaya T (1997) Increased expression of the Na+/I- symporter in cultured human thyroid cells exposed to thyrotropin and in Grave's thyroid tissue. J Clin Endocrinol Metab. 82:3331-6.

[113] Weiss SJ, Philp NJ, Ambesi-Impiombato FS, Grollman EF (1984) Thyrotropin-stimulated iodide transport mediated by adenosine 3' 5'-monophosphate and dependent on protein synthesis. Endocrinology 114:1099-107.

Permissions

The contributors of this book come from diverse backgrounds, making this book a truly international effort. This book will bring forth new frontiers with its revolutionizing research information and detailed analysis of the nascent developments around the world.

We would like to thank Dr. Neeraj Kumar Agrawal, for lending his expertise to make the book truly unique. He has played a crucial role in the development of this book. Without his invaluable contribution this book wouldn't have been possible. He has made vital efforts to compile up to date information on the varied aspects of this subject to make this book a valuable addition to the collection of many professionals and students.

This book was conceptualized with the vision of imparting up-to-date information and advanced data in this field. To ensure the same, a matchless editorial board was set up. Every individual on the board went through rigorous rounds of assessment to prove their worth. After which they invested a large part of their time researching and compiling the most relevant data for our readers. Conferences and sessions were held from time to time between the editorial board and the contributing authors to present the data in the most comprehensible form. The editorial team has worked tirelessly to provide valuable and valid information to help people across the globe.

Every chapter published in this book has been scrutinized by our experts. Their significance has been extensively debated. The topics covered herein carry significant findings which will fuel the growth of the discipline. They may even be implemented as practical applications or may be referred to as a beginning point for another development. Chapters in this book were first published by InTech; hereby published with permission under the Creative Commons Attribution License or equivalent.

The editorial board has been involved in producing this book since its inception. They have spent rigorous hours researching and exploring the diverse topics which have resulted in the successful publishing of this book. They have passed on their knowledge of decades through this book. To expedite this challenging task, the publisher supported the team at every step. A small team of assistant editors was also appointed to further simplify the editing procedure and attain best results for the readers.

Our editorial team has been hand-picked from every corner of the world. Their multi-ethnicity adds dynamic inputs to the discussions which result in innovative outcomes. These outcomes are then further discussed with the researchers and contributors who give their valuable feedback and opinion regarding the same. The feedback is then collaborated with the researches and they are edited in a comprehensive manner to aid the understanding of the subject.

Apart from the editorial board, the designing team has also invested a significant amount of their time in understanding the subject and creating the most relevant covers. They scrutinized every image to scout for the most suitable representation of the subject and create an appropriate cover for the book.

The publishing team has been involved in this book since its early stages. They were actively engaged in every process, be it collecting the data, connecting with the contributors or procuring relevant information. The team has been an ardent support to the editorial, designing and production team. Their endless efforts to recruit the best for this project, has resulted in the accomplishment of this book. They are a veteran in the field of academics and their pool of knowledge is as vast as their experience in printing. Their expertise and guidance has proved useful at every step. Their uncompromising quality standards have made this book an exceptional effort. Their encouragement from time to time has been an inspiration for everyone.

The publisher and the editorial board hope that this book will prove to be a valuable piece of knowledge for researchers, students, practitioners and scholars across the globe.

List of Contributors

José María Fernández-Santos, Jesús Morillo-Bernal, Rocío García-Marín, José Carmelo Utrilla and Inés Martín-Lacave
Department of Cytology and Histology, School of Medicine, University of Seville, Spain

Irmgard D. Dietzel
Department of Molecular Neurobiochemistry, Ruhr-University Bochum, Bochum, Germany

Sivaraj Mohanasundaram
Department of Molecular Neurobiochemistry, Ruhr-University Bochum, Bochum, Germany
International Graduate School of Neuroscience (IGSN), Ruhr-University Bochum, Germany

Vanessa Niederkinkhaus
Department of Molecular Neurobiochemistry, Ruhr-University Bochum, Bochum, Germany
International Graduate School of Neuroscience (IGSN), Ruhr-University Bochum, Germany

Gerd Hoffmann
Department of Molecular Neurobiochemistry, Ruhr-University Bochum, Bochum, Germany
PFM Medical AG, Köln, Germany

The late Jens W. Meyer
JM Technische Entwicklungen, Bochum, Germany

Christoph Reiners
Department of Nuclear Medicine, University Hospital, Würzburg, Germany

Christiana Blasl
Department of Nuclear Medicine, University Hospital, Würzburg, Germany
Diagnostische Gemainschaftspraxis Karlstrasse, Karlsruhe, Germany

Katharina Bohr
Neuro Reha Zentrum Plau, Plau am See, Germany

Pradip K. Sarkar
Department of Basic Sciences, Parker University, Dallas, Texas, USA

Asano Ishikawa and Jun Kitano
Ecological Genetics Laboratory and JST PRESTO, National Institute of Genetics, Mishima, Japan

R.G. Ahmed
Division of Anatomy and Embryology, Zoology Department, Faculty of Science, Beni-Suef University, Egypt

N.K. Agrawal and Ved Prakash
Department of Endocrinology and Metabolism, Institute of Medical Sciences, Banaras Hindu University, Varanasi, India

Manuj Sharma
Department of Medicine, Gandhi Medical College, Bhopal

Giuseppe Pasqualetti, Angela Dardano, Sara Tognini, Antonio Polini and Fabio Monzani
Geriatrics Unit, Department of Internal Medicine, University of Pisa, Italy

Renata de Azevedo Melo Luvizotto, Sandro José Conde, Miriane de Oliveira, Maria Teresa De Sibio, Keize Nagamati Jr and Célia Regina Nogueira
Department of Internal Medicine, Botucatu School of Medicine, University of São Paulo State, Botucatu, SP, Brazil

Einav Yehuda-Shnaidman, Bella Kalderon and Jacob Bar-Tana
Human Nutrition and Metabolism, Hebrew University Medical School, Jerusalem, Israel

Eva Feigerlova, Marc Klein, Anna Angelousi, Lelia Groza and Georges Weryha
Department of Endocrinology, CHU Nancy, Vandoeuvre, France

Bruno Leheup
Department of Pediatric Endocrinology, CHU Nancy, Vandoeuvre, France

Emina Kasumagic-Halilovic
Department of Dermatovenerology, Sarajevo University Clinical Center, Sarajevo, Bosnia and Herzegovina

Begler Begovic
Department of Clinical Pharmacology, Sarajevo University Clinical Center, Sarajevo, Bosnia and Herzegovina

Francesco Torino
Department of Internal Medicine, Chair of Medical Oncology, University of Rome "Tor Vergata", Rome, Italy

Agnese Barnabei, Roberto Baldelli and Marialuisa Appetecchia
Endocrinology Unit, National Institute of Cancer "Regina Elena", Rome, Italy

Clara Spinel
Membrane Biophysics and Biology Group, Biology Department, Science Faculty, Universidad Nacional de Colombia, Colombia

Jhon Rivera
Chemistry Department, Science Faculty, Universidad Nacional de Colombia, Colombia

Clara Spinel, Magnolia Herrera and Jhon Rivera
International Physics Center, Bogotá, Colombia